D0764262

Essentials of Nuclear Medicine Imaging

Essentials of Nuclear Medicine Imaging

6th Edition

FRED A. METTLER, JR., MD, MPH
Imaging Service
New Mexico Veteran's Affairs Heath Care System
Clinical and Emeritus Professor
University of New Mexico School of Medicine
Albuquerque, New Mexico

MILTON J. GUIBERTEAU, MD
Professor of Clinical Radiology and Nuclear Medicine
University of Texas Medical School at Houston
Academic Chief, Department of Medical Imaging
Director of Nuclear Medicine
St. Joseph Medical Center
Houston, Texas

ELSEVIER
SAUNDERS

ELSEVIER
SAUNDERS

1600 John F. Kennedy Blvd.
Ste 1800
Philadelphia, PA 19103-2899

ESSENTIALS OF NUCLEAR MEDICINE IMAGING, 6th Edition   ISBN: 978-1-4557-0104-9
Copyright © 2012, 2006, 1998, 1991, 1985, 1983 by Saunders, an imprint of Elsevier Inc.

No part of this publication may be reproduced or transmitted in any form or by any means, electronic or mechanical, including photocopying, recording, or any information storage and retrieval system, without permission in writing from the publisher. Details on how to seek permission, further information about the Publisher's permissions policies and our arrangements with organizations such as the Copyright Clearance Center and the Copyright Licensing Agency, can be found at our website: www.elsevier.com/permissions.

This book and the individual contributions contained in it are protected under copyright by the Publisher (other than as may be noted herein).

Notice

Knowledge and best practice in this field are constantly changing. As new research and experience broaden our knowledge, changes in practice, treatment, and drug therapy may become necessary or appropriate. Readers are advised to check the most current information provided (i) on procedures featured or (ii) by the manufacturer of each product to be administered, to verify the recommended dose or formula, the method and duration of administration, and contraindications. It is the responsibility of practitioners, relying on their own experience and knowledge of the patient, to make diagnoses, to determine dosages and the best treatment for each individual patient, and to take all appropriate safety precautions. To the fullest extent of the law, neither the publisher nor the editors assume any liability for any injury and/or damage to persons or property arising out of or related to any use of the material contained in this book.

Library of Congress Cataloging-in-Publication Data

Mettler, Fred A., 1945-
  Essentials of nuclear medicine imaging / Fred A. Mettler Jr., Milton
J. Guiberteau. -- 6th ed.
    p. ; cm.
Includes bibliographical references and index.
ISBN 978-1-4557-0104-9 (pbk. : alk. paper)
I. Guiberteau, Milton J. II. Title.
[DNLM: 1. Nuclear Medicine--methods. 2. Radionuclide Imaging. 3.
Radiopharmaceuticals. 4. Radiotherapy. WN 445]

616.07575--dc23

                                                    2011040394

Acquisitions Editor: Don Scholz
Developmental Editor: Lora Sickora
Publishing Services Manager: Anne Altepeter
Project Managers: Kiruthiga Kasthuri/Louise King
Marketing Manager: Tracie Pasker

Working together to grow
libraries in developing countries

www.elsevier.com | www.bookaid.org | www.sabre.org

ELSEVIER   BOOK AID International   Sabre Foundation

Printed in China

Last digit is the print number: 9 8 7 6 5 4 3 2

*To our parents, our families,
and those who spend their time teaching residents*

Preface

Six years have elapsed since publication of the fifth edition of *Nuclear Medicine Imaging,* and it has been 34 years since the first edition. In this sixth edition, we have made revisions that reflect changes in the current practice of nuclear medicine and molecular imaging, while maintaining our focus on the essential elements. We have also endeavored to retain the book's prior extent and affordability. Since the previous edition, there has been continued change, not only in the patterns of use of existing nuclear medicine studies but also notably in the evolution of radiopharmaceuticals and instrumentation, such as the widespread use of hybrid imaging (especially PET/CT and SPECT/CT).

The progressive integration of traditional nuclear medicine techniques with those of diagnostic radiology, providing both anatomic and functional information on a single set of coregistered images, has added powerful tools to the diagnosis of disease and the assessment of treatment effectiveness. At the same time, it has increased the need for imagers to broaden their imaging skills. These considerations are addressed in this edition. Further, enhanced equipment automation has allowed information about quality control to be condensed and included in Chapters 1 and 2.

We have updated all chapters to include recent developments in instrumentation and radiopharmaceuticals. We have also limited content on less common and outmoded procedures, and removed outdated content. We have added new material on procedure guidelines (such as GI emptying studies and Na-^{18}F bone scanning). The expanded use of PET has permitted material on PET and PET/CT imaging for CNS and cardiac applications to be relocated to those organ-specific chapters, and we have organized separate chapters on non-PET and PET neoplasm imaging. Information relative to the duties and expectations of an authorized user (AU) has been updated and clarified.

We have noted that residents supplement their clinical case experience with atlases and casebooks. There are more than 400 figures in this edition, and about 40% of the illustrations are entirely new. We have also included in the text, where appropriate, information on how to use radiation (dosing) wisely. At the end of the text, we have updated and revised the Unknown Case Sets in a more familiar and, hopefully, instructive format. Review of the sets will allow readers to assess their knowledge in a commonly employed format and to gain familiarity with commonly encountered nuclear imaging entities.

Fred A. Mettler, Jr.
Milton J. Guiberteau

Acknowledgments

We would like to recognize the many residents, technologists, and others who provided suggestions, as well as a number of our colleagues who provided images, background material, and suggestions. We also would like to thank RuthAnne Bump for her help with the illustrations.

Contents

1 Radioactivity, Radionuclides, and Radiopharmaceuticals

BASIC ISOTOPE NOTATION

The atom may be thought of as a collection of protons, neutrons, and electrons. The protons and neutrons are found in the nucleus, and shells of electrons orbit the nucleus with discrete energy levels. The number of neutrons is usually designated by N. The number of protons is represented by Z (also called the *atomic number*). The atomic mass number, or the total number of nuclear particles, is represented by A and is simply the sum of N and Z. The symbolism used to designate atoms of a certain element having the chemical symbol X is given by $^A_Z X_N$. For example, the notation $^{131}_{53}I_{78}$ refers to a certain isotope of iodine. In this instance, 131 refers to the total number of protons and neutrons in the nucleus. By definition, all isotopes of a given element have the same number of protons and differ only in the number of neutrons. For example, all isotopes of iodine have 53 protons.

Nuclear Stability and Decay

A given element may have many isotopes, and some of these isotopes have unstable nuclear configurations of protons and neutrons. These isotopes often seek greater stability by decay or disintegration of the nucleus to a more stable form. Of the known stable nuclides, most have even numbers of neutrons and protons. Nuclides with odd numbers of neutrons and protons are usually unstable. Nuclear instability may result from either neutron or proton excess. Nuclear decay may involve a simple release of energy from the nucleus or may actually cause a change in the number of protons or neutrons within the nucleus. When decay involves a change in the number of protons, there is a change of element. This is termed a *transmutation*. Isotopes attempting to reach stability by emitting radiation are *radionuclides*.

Several mechanisms of decay achieve stability. One of these is *alpha-particle emission*. In this case, an alpha (α) particle, consisting of two protons and two neutrons, is released from the nucleus, with a resulting decrease in the atomic mass number (A) by four and reduction of both Z and N by two. The mass of the released alpha particles is so great that they travel only a few centimeters in air and are unable to penetrate even thin paper. These properties cause alpha-particle emitters to be essentially useless for imaging purposes.

Beta-particle emission is another process for achieving stability and is found primarily in nuclides with a neutron excess. In this case, a beta (β^-) particle (electron) is emitted from the nucleus accompanied by an antineutrino; as a result, one of the neutrons may be thought of as

1

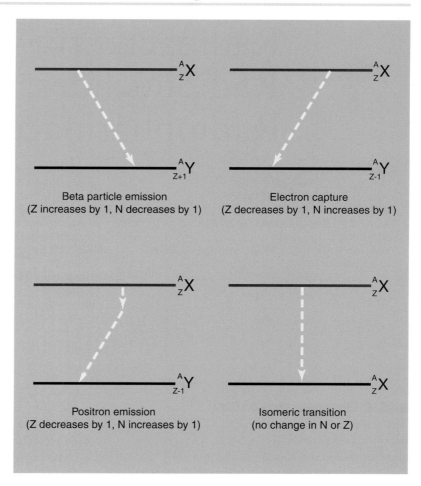

Figure 1-1. Decay schemes of radionuclides from unstable states (*top line* of each diagram) to more stable states (*bottom line*).

being transformed into a proton, which remains in the nucleus. Thus, beta-particle emission decreases the number of neutrons (N) by one and increases the number of protons (Z) by one, so that A remains unchanged (Fig. 1-1). When Z is increased, the arrow in the decay scheme shown in Figure 1-1 points toward the right, and the downward direction indicates a more stable state. The energy spectrum of beta-particle emission ranges from a certain maximum down to zero; the mean energy of the spectrum is about one third of the maximum. A 2-MeV beta particle has a range of about 1 cm in soft tissue and is therefore not useful for imaging purposes.

Electron capture occurs in a neutron-deficient nuclide when one of the inner orbital electrons is captured by a proton in the nucleus, forming a neutron and a neutrino. This can occur when not enough energy is available for positron emission, and electron capture is therefore an alternative to positron decay. Because a nuclear proton is essentially changed to a neutron, N increases by one, and Z decreases by one; therefore, A remains

unchanged (see Fig. 1-1). Electron capture may be accompanied by gamma emission and is always accompanied by characteristic radiation, either of which may be used in imaging.

If, in any of these attempts at stabilization, the nucleus still has excess energy, it may be emitted as nonparticulate radiation, with Z and N remaining the same. Any process in which energy is given off as gamma rays and in which the numbers of protons and neutrons are not changed is called *isomeric transition* (see Fig. 1-1). An alternative to isomeric transition is *internal conversion*. In internal conversion, the excess energy of the nucleus is transmitted to one of the orbital electrons; this electron may be ejected from the atom, which is followed by characteristic radiation when the electron is replaced. This process usually competes with gamma-ray emission and can occur only if the amount of energy given to the orbital electron exceeds the binding energy of that electron in its orbit.

The ratio of internal conversion electrons to gamma-ray emissions for a particular radioisotope

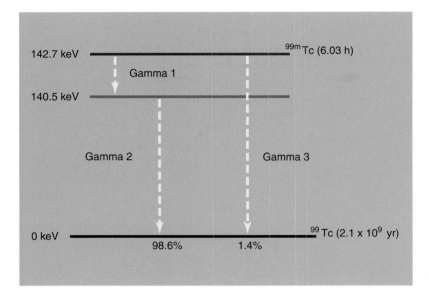

Figure 1-2. Decay scheme of technetium-99m.

is designated by the symbol α. (This should not be confused with the symbol for an alpha particle.) For an isotope such as technetium-99m (^{99m}Tc), α is low, indicating that most emissions occur as gamma rays with little internal conversion. A low conversion ratio is preferable for in-vivo usage because it implies a greater number of gamma emissions for imaging and a reduced number of conversion electrons, which are absorbed by the body and thus add to the patient's radiation dose.

In many instances, a gamma-ray photon is emitted almost instantaneously after particulate decay. If there is a measurable delay in the emission of the gamma-ray photon and the resulting decay process is an isomeric transition, this intermediate excited state of the isotope is referred to as *metastable*. The most well-known metastable isotope is ^{99m}Tc (the *m* refers to metastable). This isotope decays by isomeric transition to a more stable state, as indicated in Figure 1-2. In the decay scheme, the arrows point straight down, showing that there is no change in Z. Also, ^{99m}Tc may decay by one of several routes of gamma-ray emission.

In cases in which there are too many protons in the nucleus (a neutron-deficient nuclide), decay may proceed in such a manner that a proton may be thought of as being converted into a neutron. This results in *positron* (β⁺) *emission*, which is always accompanied by a neutrino. This obviously increases N by one and decreases Z by one, again leaving A unchanged (see Fig. 1-1). The downward arrow in the

decay scheme again indicates a more stable state, and its leftward direction indicates that Z is decreased. Positron emission cannot occur unless at least 1.02 MeV of energy is available to the nucleus.

When a positron is emitted, it travels for a short distance from its site of origin, gradually losing energy to the tissue through which it moves. When most of its kinetic energy has been lost, the positron reacts with a resident electron in an annihilation reaction. This reaction generates two 511-keV gamma photons, which are emitted in opposite directions at about (but not exactly) 180 degrees from each other (Fig. 1-3).

RADIONUCLIDE PRODUCTION

Most radioactive material that does not occur naturally can be produced by particulate bombardment or fission. Both methods alter the neutron-to-proton ratio in the nucleus to produce an unstable isotope. Bombardment essentially consists of the irradiation of the nuclei of selected target elements with neutrons in a nuclear reactor or with charged particles (alpha particles, protons, or deuterons) from a cyclotron. Bombardment reactions may be summarized by equations in which the target element and bombarding particle are listed on the left side of the equation and the product and any accompanying particulate or gamma emissions are indicated on the right. For example,

$$^{A}_{Z}X + n \text{ (neutron)} \rightarrow ^{A+1}_{Z}X + \gamma \text{ or more specifically}$$
$$^{98}_{42}Mo + n \text{ (neutron)} \rightarrow ^{99}_{42}Mo + \gamma$$

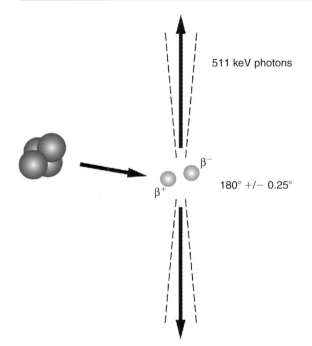

511 keV photons

β⁻

β⁺

180° +/− 0.25°

Figure 1-3. **Positron decay.** After the positron (β⁺) is emitted from the radionuclide, it travels some distance before interacting with an electron (β⁻) and undergoing annihilation, resulting in emission of two 511-keV photons at 180-degrees from each other.

These equations may be further abbreviated using parenthetical notation. The molybdenum reaction presented previously is thus represented as ^{98}Mo (n, γ) ^{99}Mo. The target and product are noted on the outside of the parentheses, which contain the bombarding particle on the left and any subsequent emissions on the right.

Once bombardment is completed, the daughter isotope must be physically separated from any remaining and unchanged target nuclei, as well as from any target contaminants. Thus, it is obvious that the completeness of this final separation process and the initial elemental purity of the target are vital factors in obtaining a product of high specific activity. Because cyclotron isotope production almost always involves a transmutation (change of Z) from one element to another, this process aids greatly in the separation of the radionuclides to obtain *carrier-free* isotopes (i.e., isotopes that have none of the stable element accompanying them). Radionuclides made by neutron bombardment, which does not result in a change of elemental species (e.g., ^{98}Mo [n, γ] ^{99}Mo), are not carrier free because the chemical properties of the products are identical, and thus radionuclides are not as easily separated.

Fission isotopes are simply the daughter products of nuclear fission of uranium-235 (^{235}U) or plutonium-239 (^{239}Pu) in a reactor and represent a multitude of radioactive materials, with atomic numbers in the range of roughly half that of ^{235}U. These include iodine-131 (^{131}I), xenon-133 (^{133}Xe), strontium-90 (^{90}Sr), molybdenum-99 (^{99}Mo), and cesium-137 (^{137}Cs), among others. Because many of these isotopes are present together in the fission products, the desired isotope must be carefully isolated to exclude as many contaminants as possible. Although this is sometimes difficult, many carrier-free isotopes are produced in this manner.

Neutron bombardment and nuclear fission almost always produce isotopes with neutron excess, which decay by beta emission. Some isotopes, such as ^{99}Mo, may be produced by either method. Cyclotron-produced isotopes are usually neutron deficient and decay by electron capture or positron emission. Some common examples of cyclotron-produced isotopes include iodine-123 (^{123}I), fluorine-18 (^{18}F), gallium-67 (^{67}Ga), indium-111 (^{111}In), and thallium-201 (^{201}Tl). In general, cyclotron-generated radionuclides are more expensive than are those produced by neutron bombardment or fission.

Positron-emitting radionuclides are most commonly produced in cyclotrons by bombarding a stable element with protons, deuterons, or helium nuclei. The produced radionuclides have an excess of protons and decay by the emission of positrons.

RADIOACTIVE DECAY

The amount of radioactivity present (the number of disintegrations per second) is referred to as *activity*. In the past, the unit of radioactivity has been the curie (Ci), which is 3.7×10^{10} disintegrations per second. Because the curie is an inconvenient unit, it has been largely replaced by an international unit called a becquerel (Bq), which is one disintegration per second. Conversion tables are found in Appendixes B-1 and B-2. *Specific activity* refers to the activity per unit mass of material (mCi/g or Bq/g). For a carrier-free isotope, the longer the half-life of the isotope, the lower is its specific activity.

Radionuclides decay in an exponential fashion, and the term *half-life* is often used casually to characterize decay. Half-life usually refers to the *physical half-life,* which is the amount of time necessary for a radionuclide to be reduced to half of its existing activity. The physical half-life (T_p) is equal to $0.693/\lambda$, where λ is the decay constant. Thus, λ and the physical half-life have characteristic values for each radioactive nuclide. Decay tables for various radionuclides are presented in Appendix C.

A formula that the nuclear medicine physician should be familiar with is the following:

$$A = A_0 e^{-0.693 / T_p \,(t)}$$

This formula can be used to find the activity (A) of a particular radioisotope present at a given time (t) and having started with activity (A_0) at time 0. For instance, if you had 5 mCi (185 MBq) of ^{99m}Tc at 9 AM today, how much would remain at 9 AM tomorrow? In this case, T_p of ^{99m}Tc is 6 hours, t is 24 hours, and e is a mathematical constant. Thus,

$$A = A_0 e^{\frac{-0.693}{T_p}\,(t)}$$

$$A = A_0 e^{\frac{-0.693}{6\,\text{hours}}\,(24\,\text{hours})}$$

$$A = 5\,\text{mCi}\; e^{\frac{-0.693}{6\,\text{hours}}\,(24\,\text{hours})}$$

$$A = 5\,\text{mCi}\; e^{-0.1155\,(24\,\text{hours})}$$

$$A = 5\,\text{mCi}\; e^{-2.772}$$

$$A = 5\,\text{mCi}\; e^{\frac{1}{2.772}}$$

$$A = 5\,\text{mCi}\; e^{\left(\frac{1}{15.99}\right)}$$

$$A = 0.31\,\text{mCi}$$

Thus, after 24 hours, the amount of ^{99m}Tc remaining is 0.31 mCi (11 MBq).

In addition to the physical half-life or physical decay of a radionuclide, two other half-life terms are commonly used. *Biologic half-life* refers to the time it takes an organism to eliminate half of an administered compound or chemical on a strictly biologic basis. Thus, if a stable chemical compound were given to a person, and half of it were eliminated by the body (perhaps in the urine) within 3 hours, the biologic half-life would be 3 hours. The *effective half-life* incorporates both the physical and biologic half-lives. Therefore, when speaking of the effective half-life of a particular radiopharmaceutical in humans, one needs to know the physical half-life of the radioisotope used as a tag or label as well as the biologic half-life of the tagged compound. If these are known, the following formula can be used to calculate the effective half-life:

$$T_e = (T_p \times T_b) / (T_p + T_b)$$

where

T_e = effective half-life
T_p = physical half-life
T_b = biologic half-life

If the biologic half-life is 3 hours and the physical half-life is 6 hours, then the effective half-life is 2 hours. Note that the effective half-life is *always shorter* than either the physical or biologic half-life.

RADIONUCLIDE GENERATOR SYSTEMS

A number of radionuclides of interest in nuclear medicine are short-lived isotopes that emit only gamma rays and decay by isomeric transition. Because it is often impractical for an imaging laboratory to be located near a reactor or a cyclotron, generator systems that permit on-site availability of these isotopes have achieved wide use. Some isotopes available from generators include technetium-99m, indium-113m (^{113m}In), krypton-81m (^{81m}Kr), rubidium-82 (^{82}Rb), strontium-87m (^{87m}Sr), and gallium-68 (^{68}Ga).

Inside the most common generator (^{99}Mo-^{99m}Tc), a radionuclide "parent" with a relatively long half-life is firmly affixed to an ion exchange column. A ^{99}Mo-^{99m}Tc generator consists of an alumina column on which ^{99}Mo is bound. The parent isotope (67-hour half-life) decays to its radioactive daughter, ^{99m}Tc, which is a different element with a shorter half-life (6 hours). Because the daughter is only loosely bound on the column, it may be removed, or washed off, with an elution liquid such as normal (0.9%) saline. Wet and dry ^{99}Mo-^{99m}Tc generator systems are available and differ only slightly. A *wet system* has a saline reservoir and a vacuum vial that draws saline across the column. With a *dry system*, a specific amount of saline in a vial is placed on the generator entry port and drawn across by a vacuum vial (Fig. 1-4).

After the daughter is separated from the column, the buildup process is begun again by the residual parent isotope. Uncommonly, some of the parent isotope (^{99}Mo) or alumina is removed from the column during elution and appears in the eluate containing the daughter isotope. This is termed *breakthrough*.

To make efficient use of a generator, elution times should be spaced appropriately to allow for reaccumulation of the daughter isotope on the column. The short-lived daughter reaches maximum activity when the rate of decay of the daughter equals its rate of production. At this equilibrium point, for instance, the amount of daughter ^{99m}Tc is slightly greater than the activity of the parent ^{99}Mo (Fig. 1-5). When the parent isotope has a half-life somewhat greater than that of the daughter, the equilibrium attained is said to be a *transient equilibrium*. This is the case in a ^{99}Mo-^{99m}Tc generator.

Most generators used in hospitals have ^{99}Mo activity levels of about 1 to 6 Ci (3.7 to 22.0 GBq). The amount of ^{99m}Tc in the generator reaches about half the theoretical maximum in one half-life (6 hours). It reaches about three fourths of the theoretical maximum in about two half-lives, and so on (see Appendix C-1). This indicates that if one elutes all of the ^{99m}Tc daughter from an ^{99}Mo generator, 24 hours later (four half-lives), the amount of ^{99m}Tc present in the generator will have returned to about 95% of the theoretical maximum.

Other, much less common photon-emitting radionuclide generator systems include rubidium-81 (^{81}Rb) (4.5 hours)/^{81m}Kr (13 seconds), tin-13 (^{113}Sn) (115 days)/^{113m}In (1.7 hours), yttrium-87 (^{87}Y) (3.3 days)/^{87m}Sr (2.8 hours), and tellurium-132 (^{132}Te) (3.2 days)/^{132}I (2.3 hours). Although generator systems are most often used to produce photon-emitting radionuclides, certain generators can produce positron emitters. These include strontium-82 (^{82}Sr) (25 days)/^{82}Rb (1.3 minutes). ^{82}Rb is a potassium analog and can be used for myocardial perfusion

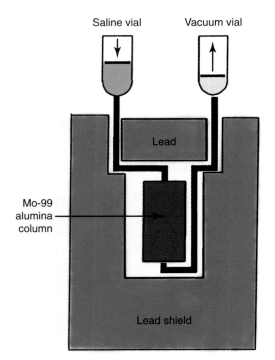

Figure 1-4. Generator. Schematic of dry molybdenum-99/technetium-99m generator system.

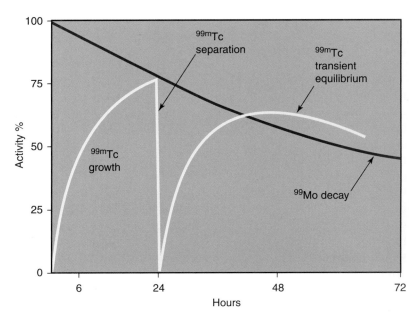

Figure 1-5. Radionuclide buildup and decay in a generator. Molybdenum-99 (^{99}Mo) decay and technetium-99m (^{99m}Tc) buildup in a generator eluted at 0 hours and again at 24 hours.

imaging using position emission tomography. Gallium-68 (6.5 hours) is another positron emitter that can be produced from a germanium-69 (^{69}Ge) (271 days) generator.

RADIONUCLIDES AND RADIOPHARMACEUTICALS FOR IMAGING

In evaluating the choice of a radionuclide to be used in the nuclear medicine laboratory, the following characteristics are desirable:

■ Minimum of particulate emission
■ Primary photon energy between 50 and 500 keV
■ Physical half-life greater than the time required to prepare material for injection
■ Effective half-life longer than the examination time
■ Suitable chemical form and reactivity
■ Low toxicity
■ Stability or near-stability of the product

The radionuclides most commonly used for imaging are shown in Tables 1-1 and 1-2. A radionuclide that has desirable imaging properties can usually be used to make a variety of radiopharmaceuticals. This is done by coupling the radionuclide with various stable compounds that are localized by organs or disease states. Many of radionuclides are radiopharmaceuticals in their own right and can be administered without alteration to obtain useful images. Commonly used radiopharmaceuticals are shown in Table 1-3. The biologic behavior of most of these radionuclides can be markedly altered by a combination with additional substances to form other radiopharmaceuticals.

Mechanisms of localization for some of these radiopharmaceuticals are listed in Table 1-4. The various radiopharmaceuticals used in imaging procedures are additionally discussed in the appropriate chapters. Dosimetry and protocols for the various radionuclides are presented in Appendix E-1. Issues related to pediatric dose and pregnancy and breastfeeding are in Appendixes D and G.

Although the localizing properties of radiopharmaceuticals are generally sufficient to obtain adequate diagnostic images, the localizing mechanisms may be altered by various conditions in an individual patient, including the administration of other medications. A list of these agents and their effects on the distribution of particular radiopharmaceuticals is given in Appendix E-2.

Technetium-99m

Technetium-99m fulfills many of the criteria of an ideal radionuclide and is used in more than 80% of nuclear imaging procedures in the United States. It has no particulate emission, a 6-hour half-life, and a predominant (98%) 140-keV photon with only a small amount (10%) of internal conversion.

Technetium-99m is obtained by separating it from the parent ^{99}Mo (67-hour half-life) in a generator system. Molybdenum-99 for generators is generally produced by neutron irradiation of ^{98}Mo or by chemical separation of ^{235}U fission products. In the latter case, ^{99}Mo is nearly carrier free and has a high specific activity. In the alumina generator system, the molybdenum activity is absorbed on an alumina column. By passing physiologic saline over the column, ^{99m}Tc is eluted or washed off as *sodium pertechnetate* (Na ^{99m}TcO$_4^-$).

Technetium can exist in a variety of valence states, ranging from –1 to +7. When eluted from an alumina column generator, ^{99m}Tc is present primarily as heptavalent (+7) pertechnetate (TcO$_4^-$). In the preparation of radiopharmaceuticals, ^{99m}Tc pertechnetate can be reduced from +7 to a lower valence state, usually +4, to permit the labeling of various chelates. This is generally accomplished with stannous (tin) ions.

As pertechnetate, the technetium ion is a singly charged anion and is similar in size to the iodide ion. After intravenous injection, ^{99m}Tc pertechnetate is loosely bound to protein and rapidly leaves the plasma compartment. More than half leaves the plasma within several minutes and is distributed in the extracellular fluid. It rapidly concentrates in the salivary glands, choroid plexus, thyroid gland, gastric mucosa, and functioning breast tissue; during pregnancy, it crosses the placenta.

Excretion is by the gastrointestinal and renal routes. Although ^{99m}Tc pertechnetate is excreted by glomerular filtration, it is partially reabsorbed by the renal tubules; as a result, only 30% is eliminated in the urine during the first day. The ion is also secreted directly into the stomach and colon, with a much smaller amount coming from the small bowel. The colon is the critical organ and receives about 1 to 2 rad/10 mCi (0.04 mGy/ MBq) of ^{99m}Tc pertechnetate administered. The biodistribution of ^{99m}Tc pertechnetate is shown in Figure 1-6. The principal emission (140-keV photon) of ^{99m}Tc has a half-value layer (HVL) of

TABLE 1–1	Characteristics of Commonly Used Radionuclides		
	SYMBOL	**PHYSICAL HALF-LIFE**	**APPROXIMATE ENERGY**
Photon-Emitting Radionuclides for Imaging			**Gamma (keV)**
Technetium-99m	$^{99m}_{43}Tc$	6 hr	140
Molybdenum-99	$^{99}_{42}Mo$	67 hr	181, 740, 780
Iodine-123	$^{123}_{53}I$	13.2 hr	159
Iodine-131	$^{131}_{53}I$	8.0 day	364
Xenon-133	$^{133}_{54}Xe$	5.3 day	81
Gallium-67	$^{67}_{31}Ga$	78.3 hr	93, 184, 296, 388
Indium-111	$^{111}_{49}In$	67 hr	173, 247
Indium-113m	$^{113m}_{49}In$	1.7 hr	392
Thallium-201	$^{201}_{81}Tl$	73.1 hr	69, 81 (x-rays from mercury daughter)
Krypton-81m	$^{81m}_{36}Kr$	13 sec	191
Positron-Emitting Radionuclides for Imaging			**Positron (MeV)**
Carbon-11	$^{11}_{6}C$	20.3 min	0.960
Nitrogen-13	$^{13}_{7}N$	10 min	1.198
Oxygen-15	$^{15}_{8}O$	124 sec	1.730
Fluorine-18	$^{18}_{9}F$	110 min	0.634
Rubidium-82	$^{82}_{32}Rb$	1.27 min	3.150
Unsealed Radionuclides Used for Therapy			**Emissions**
Phosphorus-32	$^{32}_{15}P$	14.3 day	1.71 MeV max; 0.7 MeV mean beta
Strontium-89	$^{89}_{38}Sr$	50.5 day	1.46 MeV max; 0.58 MeV mean beta; 910 keV gamma (0.01%)
Yttrium-90	$^{90}_{39}Y$	64 hr	2.2 MeV max; 0.93 MeV mean beta
Iodine-131	$^{131}_{53}I$	8.0 day	0.19 MeV mean beta; 364 keV gamma (82%)
Samarium-153	$^{153}_{62}Sm$	46 hr	0.81 MeV max; 0.23 MeV mean beta; 103 keV gamma (28%)
Rhenium-186	$^{186}_{75}Re$	90 hr	0.34 MeV mean beta; 186 keV gamma (9%)
Gold-198	$^{198}_{79}Au$	2.7 day	0.96 MeV max; 0.31 MeV mean beta; 412 keV gamma (96%)

Note: The approximate range (cm) of beta particle in tissue is the energy (MeV) divided by two.

0.028 cm in lead and 4.5 cm in water. Because tissue is close to water in terms of attenuation characteristics, it is clear that about 2 inches of tissue between the radionuclide and the detector removes about half of the photons of interest, and 4 inches removes about three fourths.

Iodine-123 and -131

Two isotopes of iodine (^{123}I and ^{131}I) are clinically useful for imaging and may be administered as iodide. Iodine-123 has a 13.2-hour half-life and decays by electron capture to tellurium-123 (^{123}Te). The photons emitted are 28-keV (92%)

TABLE 1–2	Characteristics of Common PET Radionuclides					
NUCLIDE (DECAY PRODUCT)	**PHYSICAL HALF-LIFE**	**DECAY MODE**	**MAXIMAL AND AVERAGE POSITRON ENERGY (KeV)**	**MAXIMUM AND MEAN RANGE IN WATER (mm)**	**PRODUCTION REACTION**
Carbon-11 (Boron-11)	20.3 min	99.8% positron 0.2% electron capture	960, 385	4.1, 1.1	$^{14}N(p,alpha)^{11}C*$
Nitrogen-13 (Carbon-13)	10 min	100% positron	1198, 491	5.1, 14	$^{16}O(p,alpha)^{13}N$ $^{13}C(p,n)^{13}N$
Oxygen-15 (Nitrogen-15)	124 sec	99.9% positron	1730, 735	7.3, 1.5	$^{15}N(p,n)^{15}O$ $^{14}N(d,n)^{15}O$
Fluorine-18 (Oxygen-18)	110 min	97% positron 3% electron capture	634, 250	2.4, 1.0	$^{18}O(p,n)^{18}F$ $^{20}Ne(d, alpha)^{18}F$ $^{16}O(^{3}He, alpha)^{18}F$
Rubidium-82	75 sec	96% positron 4% electron capture	3150, 1385	14.1, 5.9	^{82}Sr generator (T1/2 25.3 days)

*This symbolism means that a proton is accelerated into an atom of nitrogen-14, causing the ejection of an alpha particle from the nucleus to produce an atom of carbon-11.

and 159-keV (84%) gamma rays. Iodine-123 is usually produced in a cyclotron by bombardment of antimony-121 (^{121}Sb) or tellurium-122 or -124 (^{122}Te or ^{124}Te). Another method is to bombard iodine-127 (^{127}I) to produce ^{123}Xe and let this decay to ^{123}I. Contamination with ^{124}I may increase the radiation dose; because ^{124}I is long lived, its proportion in an ^{123}I preparation increases with time.

Iodine-131 is a much less satisfactory isotope from an imaging viewpoint because of the high radiation dose to the thyroid and its relatively high photon energy. However, it is widely available, is relatively inexpensive, and has a relatively long shelf life. Iodine-131 has a half-life of 8.06 days and decays by beta-particle emission to a stable ^{131}Xe. The principal mean beta energy (90%) is 192 keV. Several gamma rays are also emitted, and the predominant photon is 364 keV (82% abundance) (HVL in water of 6.4 cm).

When iodine is orally administered as the iodide ion, it is readily absorbed from the gastrointestinal tract and distributed in the extracellular fluid. It is concentrated in a manner similar to that for ^{99m}Tc pertechnetate in the salivary glands, thyroid, and gastric mucosa. As with pertechnetate, there is renal filtration with significant tubular reabsorption. Urinary excretion is the predominant route (35% to 75% in 24 hours), although there is some fecal excretion as well. Iodide trapped and organified by the normal thyroid has an effective half-life of

about 7 days. Iodine is a useful radionuclide because it is chemically reactive and is used to produce a variety of radiopharmaceuticals, which are discussed in later clinical chapters.

Xenon-133

Xenon is a relatively insoluble inert gas and is most commonly used for pulmonary ventilation studies. Xenon is commercially available in unit-dose vials or in 1 Ci (37 GBq) glass ampules. Xenon is highly soluble in oil and fat, and there is some adsorption of xenon onto plastic syringes.

Xenon-133 has a physical half-life of 5.3 days. The principal gamma photon has an energy of 81 keV and emits a 374-keV beta particle. With normal pulmonary function, its biologic half-life is about 30 seconds. Some disadvantages of ^{133}Xe include its relatively low photon energy, beta-particle emission, and some solubility in both blood and fat.

Gallium-67

Gallium-67 has a physical half-life of 78.3 hours and decays by electron capture, emitting gamma radiation. It can be produced by a variety of reactions in a cyclotron. The principal gamma photons from ^{67}Ga are 93 keV (40%), 184 keV (24%), 296 keV (22%), and 388 keV (7%). An easy way to remember these energies is to round off the figures (i.e., 90, 190, 290, and 390 keV).

TABLE 1–3 Imaging Radiopharmaceuticals

RADIONUCLIDE	RADIOPHARMACEUTICAL	USES
Carbon-11	Acetate	Prostate
Nitrogen-13	Ammonia	Cardiac perfusion
Oxygen-15	Gas	Brain perfusion
Fluorine-18	FDG (fluorodeoxyglucose)	Tumor, cardiac viability, brain metabolism, infection
	Sodium	Bone
Gallium-67	Citrate	Infection, tumor
Krypton-81m	Gas	Pulmonary ventilation
Rubidium-82	Chloride	Myocardial perfusion
Technetium-99m	Diphosphonate	Bone
	DISIDA (diisopropyl iminodiacetic acid)	Biliary
	DMSA (dimercaptosuccinic acid)	Renal cortical
	DTPA (diethylenetriamine pentaacetic acid)	Renal dynamic, brain, lung ventilation
	ECD (ethyl cysteinate dimmer)	Brain perfusion
	Glucoheptonate	Brain, renal dynamic
	HMPAO (hexamethylpropyleneamine oxine)	Brain perfusion
	HMPAO labeled white cells	Infection
	Labeled red cells	GI blood loss, cardiac function, hepatic hemangioma
	MAA (macroaggregated albumin)	Lung perfusion, leVeen shunt patency, intraarterial liver.
	MAG3 (mercaptoacetyltriglycine)	Renal
	Mebrofenin	Biliary
	Pertechnetate	Thyroid, salivary glands, Meckel diverticulum, testicular.
	Sestamibi	Myocardial perfusion, parathyroid, breast
	Sulfur colloid	Liver/spleen, red bone marrow, esophageal transit, gastric emptying
	Sulfur colloid (filtered)	Lymphoscintigraphy
	Teboroxime	Myocardial perfusion
	Tetrofosmin	Myocardial perfusion
Indium-111	DTPA	CSF flow, gastric liquid emptying
	Oxine labeled white cells	Infection
	Pentetreotide	Somatostatin receptor tumors
Iodine-123	Sodium	Thyroid
	MIBI (metaiodobenzylguanidine)	Pheochromocytoma, adrenal medullary, neural crest tumors
Iodine-131	Sodium	Thyroid cancer
Xenon-127 or 133	Gas	Lung ventilation
Thallium-201	Chloride	Myocardial perfusion

CSF, Cerebrospinal fluid; *GI*, gastrointestinal.

TABLE 1–4	**Mechanisms of Localization and Examples**
Capillary blockade	Macroaggregated albumin in lung
Diffusion	Filtration of DTPA by kidney
Sequestration	Leukocytes for abscess scanning
	Labeled platelets (damaged endothelium)
	Heat-damaged red blood cells for splenic scanning
Phagocytosis	Colloid scanning for liver and spleen, bone marrow, and lymph nodes
Receptor binding	Neuroreceptor imaging
Active transport	Iodocholesterol in adrenal scanning
	Iodine or pertechnetate (accumulation by choroid plexus, Meckel diverticulum, salivary gland, stomach, and thyroid)
	Technetium-99m IDA analogs in liver/biliary tract
	Orthoiodohippurate in renal tubules
	Thallous ions in myocardium
Metabolism	Fluorodeoxyglucose imaging of brain, tumor, and myocardium
Compartmental containment	Labeled red blood cells for gated blood pool studies
Compartmental leakage	Labeled red blood cells for detection of gastrointestinal bleeding
Physicochemical adsorption	Phosphate bone-scanning agents
Antibody–antigen reactions	Tumor imaging, monoclonal antibodies

DTPA, Diethylenetriaminepentaacetic acid; IDA, iminodiacetic acid.

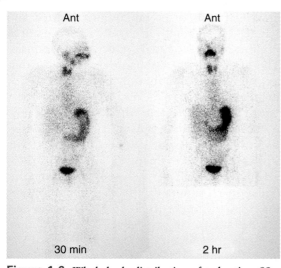

Figure 1-6. Whole-body distribution of technetium-99m sodium pertechnetate. Activity is seen in the salivary glands, thyroid gland, saliva, stomach, and bladder.

When injected intravenously, most ^{67}Ga is immediately bound to plasma proteins, primarily transferrin. During the first 12 to 24 hours, excretion from the body is primarily through the kidneys, with 20% to 25% of the administered dose being excreted by 24 hours. After that time, the intestinal mucosa becomes the major route of elimination. Overall, these modes of excretion account for the elimination of about one third of the administered dose. The remaining two thirds is retained in the body for a prolonged period. Typically on images, activity is seen in the liver and to a lesser extent the spleen. In addition to activity within the axial skeleton, liver, spleen, and bowel, concentration is also seen in the salivary and lacrimal glands as well as in the breasts and external genitalia. If imaging is performed in the first 24 hours, kidney and bladder activity may also be noted.

A common problem encountered in the interpretation of abdominal images is the physiologic presence of gallium in the bowel, which may mimic lesions or mask disease. Bowel activity is particularly notable in the colon and may be diffuse or focal. Frequently, activity is seen in the region of the cecum, hepatic and splenic flexures, and rectosigmoid. These accumulations may appear as early as a few hours after injection. Various bowel preparations have been investigated as possible means of eliminating such interfering activity in the colon, but none has proved consistently successful. The progress of excreted gallium through the colon on sequential images may provide the best evidence of physiologic activity. Persistence of gallium in a given area of the abdomen should be viewed as abnormal. Activity is seen in the osseous pelvis, particularly in the sacrum and sacroiliac joints on posterior views. On early images, bladder activity may be noted, and later, concentrations may be seen in the region of male or female genitalia. As in the abdomen, cecal or rectosigmoid accumulation may present a problem in interpretation. As a weak bone agent, gallium is noted throughout the normal skeleton and in areas of benign skeletal remodeling.

Indium-111

Indium is a metal that can be used as an iron analog; it is similar to gallium. Isotopes of interest are ^{111}In and ^{113m}In. Indium-111 has a physical half-life of 67 hours and is produced by a cyclotron. The principal photons are 173 keV (89%) and 247 keV (94%). Indium-113m can be conveniently produced by using a ^{113}Sn generator system. It has a physical half-life of 1.7 hours and a photon of about 392 keV. Indium-111 can be prepared as a chelate with diethylenetriaminepentaacetic acid (DTPA). Because of its long half-life, the ^{111}In chelate can be used for intracranial cisternography. Indium-111 is also used to label platelets, white cells, monoclonal antibodies, and peptides. Indium-111 oxine labeled white cells are commonly used to scan for infections. On these images, activity is seen mostly in the spleen and to a lesser extent in the liver and bone marrow (see Chapter 12).

Thallium-201

When a thallium metal target is bombarded with protons in a cyclotron, lead 201 (^{201}Pb) is produced, which can be separated from the thallium target and allowed to decay to ^{201}Tl. Thallium-201 has a physical half-life of 73.1 hours and decays by electron capture to mercury-201 (^{201}Hg). Mercury-201 emits characteristic x-rays with energies from 68 to 80 keV (94.5%) and much smaller amounts of gamma rays with higher energies. The relatively low energy of the major emissions can cause significant attenuation by tissue between the radionuclide and the gamma camera. The HVL in water is about 4 cm. For these reasons, attenuation correction methodologies have been developed (see Chapter 2). Because ^{201}Tl is produced by a cyclotron, it is expensive. Thallium-201 is normally administered as a chloride and rapidly clears from the blood with a half-life between 30 seconds and 3 minutes. Because it is roughly a potassium analog, it is rapidly distributed throughout the body, particularly in skeletal and cardiac muscle. Thallium-202 (95% photon at 439 keV) contamination should be less than 0.5% and, if present in greater quantities, can significantly degrade images.

Fluorine-18 and Other Positron Emitters

The most commonly used positron-emitting radiopharmaceutical in clinical imaging is the glucose analog fluorine-18 fluorodeoxyglucose (^{18}F-FDG). Many tumor cells use large amounts of glucose as an energy source and possess increased expression of glucose transporters (especially GLUT1) and increased hexokinase activity (especially HK2). Glucose transporters transfer glucose and fluorodeoxyglucose into the cells, where they are phosphorylated by hexokinases (Fig. 1-7). The rate-limiting step in this process is at the hexokinase level and not at glucose transport. Although phosphorylated glucose can be further metabolized, phosphorylated FDG cannot be rapidly metabolized and ^{18}F-FDG is essentially trapped within the cell in proportion to the rate of glucose metabolism. This allows sufficient time to image its distribution in normal and abnormal bodily tissues. A notable exception to the trapping of phosphorylated FDG is the liver, in which an abundance of phosphatases causes enhanced dephosphorylation of FDG-6-phosphate, which accelerates its washout from that organ.

Although ^{18}F-FDG reaches a plateau of accumulation in tumors at about 45 minutes after injection, the tumor-to-background ratio is best at 2 to 3 hours. Highest activity levels at 2 hours are seen in the brain, heart (if not fasting), and urinary system.

The effective dose to the patient for most ^{18}F-FDG PET scans is about 0.1 rem (1 mSv) or about 0.093 rem/mCi (0.025 mSv/MBq). Pregnancy and breastfeeding are common concerns when administering radionuclides to women. Fetal dose estimates after administration of 13.5 mCi (500 MBq) of ^{18}F-FDG to the mother are about 1400 mrem (14 mSv) in early pregnancy and about 400 mrem (4 mSv) at term. Although ^{18}F-FDG can accumulate in breast

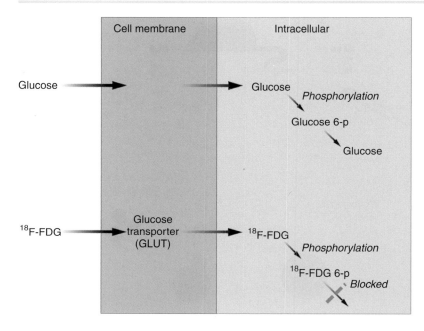

Figure 1-7. ^{18}F-FDG metabolism. Although ^{18}F-FDG is transported into the cell in the same manner as glucose, it cannot be dephosphorylated and remains in the cell. *FDG,* Fluorodeoxyglucose.

tissue, it is not secreted to any significant degree in the milk. It is usually recommended that the mother not cuddle or breastfeed the infant for about 8 hours after injection.

Fluorine-18 is also used in a sodium form as skeletal imaging agent. Excretion is predominantly via the kidneys. Images are similar to those obtained with technetium phosphate compounds. This is discussed in further detail in Chapter 8.

The positron emitters carbon-11, nitrogen-13, and oxygen-15 are not used commonly in clinical practice primarily because of the need for an on-site cyclotron. Carbon-11 acetate and palmitate are metabolic agents, carbon monoxide can be used for blood volume determinations, and there are a few carbon-11 labeled receptor binding agents. Nitrogen-13 ammonia is a perfusion agent and nitrogen glutamate is a metabolic agent. Oxygen-15 carbon dioxide and water are perfusion agents and oxygen as a gas is a metabolic agent.

Rubidium-82 chloride is obtained from a generator and used for myocardial perfusion studies; however, widespread clinical use has been limited by cost issues.

Monoclonal Antibodies

During the past several years, much interest has been generated in the development of labeled antibodies for the immunodetection and immunotherapy of a variety of diseases, particularly those of an oncologic nature. However, it was not until the development of methods of producing and labeling monoclonal antibodies that the clinical potential of such agents could be seriously explored. Growing interest in antibody therapies developed to antigens on subgroups of tumors and even tumors from individual patients has given rise to prospects for realizing the potential for development of patient-specific oncologic therapies.

Monoclonal antibodies are so named because when developed against a given antigen, they are absolutely identical to one another. The technique for producing monoclonal antibodies first involves the immunization of an animal, generally a mouse, with a specific antigen (Fig. 1-8). This antigen can be virtually anything capable of inducing the B lymphocytes to begin producing antibodies against the injected substance. Once this is done, the B lymphocytes are harvested from the mouse and placed in a tube containing mouse myeloma cells. Fusion of these myeloma cells with the B lymphocytes then takes place, forming what is known as *hybridoma.* This hybridoma has the ability to continue producing antigen-specific antibodies based on the B-lymphocyte parent and, at the same time, to perpetuate itself based on the characteristic of continual mitosis conferred on it by the myeloma cells.

Hybridomas can then be grown in clones and separated out until a clone is developed that

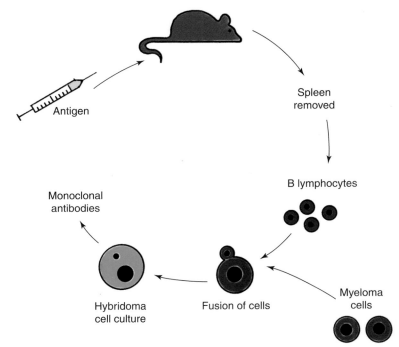

Figure 1-8. Schematic for production of monoclonal antibodies.

produces an antibody of particular interest. When such clones are developed, they are grown in the peritoneal cavities of mice, and the antibody produced is secreted into the ascitic fluid. This ascitic fluid is harvested and processed to provide a purified form of the antibody. Large quantities of monoclonal antibodies can be obtained in this way. Bulk production of monoclonal antibodies is also possible by using a synthetic approach in vitro.

Once produced, monoclonal antibodies, or fragments thereof, may be labeled with radionuclides and used to map the distribution of specific antigens in vivo. Although the concept initially appears simple, substantial problems exist that limit the clinical application of monoclonal antibodies for tumor imaging. Not the least of these problems is the selection of an appropriate specific antigen, the successful labeling of the antibody, significant cross-reactivity with other antigens, and poor target-to-nontarget ratios in vivo. Immune responses to the foreign antibody protein in humans have provided a further barrier to successful widespread use. When the antibodies are produced in a murine system, human antimouse antibody (HAMA) develops in up to 40% of patients receiving a single dose of the whole antibody. HAMA limits the success of future administrations by complexing with the antibody radiopharmaceutical, thereby

reducing the amount of antibody available for imaging. Monoclonal antibody fragments or antibodies of human or chimeric origin (human–mouse) appear to reduce HAMA production. As solutions to these drawbacks are devised, monoclonal antibodies are gradually becoming part of the radiopharmaceutical armamentarium of diagnostic and therapeutic nuclear medicine. Radiolabels currently include radioiodines, ^{111}In, ^{99m}Tc, and ^{90}Y.

Adverse Reactions

As drugs, radiopharmaceuticals are extremely safe: mild reactions are uncommon, and severe reactions are very rare. There are less than 200 serious reactions reported in the worldwide literature even though tens of millions of doses are administered annually. An *adverse reaction* may be defined as an unanticipated patient response to the nonradioactive component of a radiopharmaceutical; this reaction is not caused by the radiation itself. Overdoses of radioactivity represent reportable events (see Chapter 13) and are not adverse reactions. The only adverse effect of a radiopharmaceutical that is required to be reported is one associated with an investigational drug.

The incidence of reactions to radiopharmaceuticals in the United States is about 2.3 per 100,000 administrations. Most reported adverse reactions are allergic in nature, although some vasovagal reactions have occurred. The clinical manifestations of most reactions are rash, itching, dizziness, nausea, chills, flushing, hives, and vomiting. These reactions may occur within 5 minutes or up to 48 hours after injection. Late-onset rash or itching, dizziness, and/or headache have most commonly been reported with ^{99m}Tc bone agents. Severe reactions involving anaphylactic shock or cardiac arrest are reported in less than 3% of adverse reactions. In addition to allergic or vasomotor reactions, adverse effects with albumin particulates have been reported owing to pulmonary capillary vascular blockage in patients with diminished pulmonary vascular capacity. Positron emission tomography (PET) radiopharmaceuticals are also extremely safe, with no reported adverse reactions in more than 80,000 administered doses. An isolated case report of anaphylaxis after MIBG (metaiodobenzylguanidine) has been reported.

Reactions related to pyrogens or additives have become exceedingly rare because of the extensive quality control used in the manufacture and preparation of radiopharmaceuticals. Pyrogen reactions may be suspected if more than one patient receiving a dose from a single vial of a radiopharmaceutical has experienced an adverse effect.

Common nonradioactive pharmaceuticals used in nuclear medicine are dipyridamole and glucagon. Adverse reactions (usually headache) have been reported to occur in up to 45% of patients. Severe reactions to these occur in about 6 per 100,000 administrations and include prolonged chest pain, syncope (dipyridamole), and anaphylaxis (glucagon). Anaphylactic reactions have also been reported in up to 1% of patients receiving isosulfan blue dye during sentinel lymph node procedures.

Investigational Radiopharmaceuticals

Any new radiopharmaceutical must be treated as an investigational new drug (IND) and must go through the process outlined in the *Guidelines for the Clinical Evaluation of Radiopharmaceutical Drugs* of the Food and Drug Administration (FDA). Either manufacturers or health practitioners can file an IND application. Initially, the application must include complete composition of the drug, source, manufacturing data, and preclinical investigations, including animal studies.

Clinical investigation of INDs occurs in three phases. Phase one is early testing in humans to determine toxicity, pharmacokinetics, and effectiveness. These studies usually involve a small number of people and are conducted under carefully controlled circumstances. Phase two trials are controlled trials to test both for effectiveness in treatment of a specific disease and for evaluation of risk. Phase three, clinical investigation, involves extensive clinical trials, provided that information obtained in phases one and two demonstrates reasonable assurance of safety and effectiveness. Phase-three studies acquire necessary information for complete drug labeling, including the most desirable dose and the safety and effectiveness of the drug. Most reimbursement organizations and third-party payers will not pay for a drug unless it is fully approved by the FDA.

RADIOPHARMACY QUALITY CONTROL

Most nuclear medicine departments now get "unit doses" from commercial radiopharmacies. Such doses are prepared in an off-site commercial radiopharmacy, placed in a syringe, labeled (radiopharmaceutical, activity, and patient name), and calibrated for a certain amount of activity to be injected at a specific time. The only quality controls that may be performed in the department are dose calibration and photopeak analysis at the time of imaging. Additional quality control should be requested from the radiopharmacy if the images demonstrate an unexpected distribution of activity (Fig. 1-9).

Because most departments no longer use ^{99}Mo/^{99m}Tc generators to elute technetium or compound radiopharmaceuticals from kits, the burden of most radiopharmaceutical quality assurance issues has been shifted to others. However, it is still important to understand the quality control processes and principles in case there is an adverse reaction or the radiopharmaceutical does not localize in the patient's tissues as expected.

For those who continue to prepare radiopharmaceuticals in the nuclear medicine department, there are new, complex, and potentially very expensive requirements (U.S. Pharmacopeia Chapter 797) concerning the compounding of sterile preparations. This USP chapter provides strict requirements for inspection standards, licensing, and accreditation. Preparation

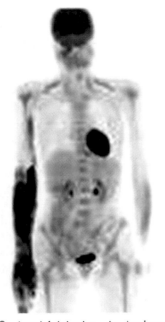

Figure 1-9. Arterial injection. An inadvertent arterial injection during administration of ^{18}F-FDG caused intense activity distal to the injection site. This is known as the "glove phenomenon." (Case courtesy Harry Agress, MD.)

of kits is considered "low-risk level" but still requires ISO Class 5 laminar airflow hood in an ISO Class 8 clean room with an ante area. These areas must also be routinely monitored for cleanliness and there must be a specific quality assurance program, written proof of staff training, equipment maintenance, and calibration. Regardless of whether radiopharmaceuticals are commercially obtained or prepared in-house, there are strict NRC requirements for receipt, management, and disposal. These are outlined in Chapter 13.

Generator and Radionuclide Purity

The first step in quality control is to ensure that the radionuclide is pure (Table 1-5). This is expressed as the percentage of activity present that is due to the radionuclide of interest. Because ^{99m}Tc normally is obtained by eluting or "milking" a molybdenum generator, there must be assurance that only ^{99m}Tc is eluted. Most ^{99}Mo-^{99m}Tc generators are fission produced, and radionuclide impurities such as ^{99}Mo, iodine-131 (^{131}I), and ruthenium-103 (^{103}Ru) may be present. The amount of ^{99}Mo contamination, or

TABLE 1-5	**Radiopharmaceutical Quality Control**			
TESTS	**PROBLEM**	**LIMITS**	**COMMENT**	
Radionuclide purity Mo-99/Tc-99m generator	Mo-99 breakthrough	0.15μCi Mo-99 /mCi Tc-99m (0.15 kBq Mo-99/MBq Tc-99m)	Test every generator elution for Mo-99. Note: Because of the longer half-life of Mo-99, a dose that was just compliant at the time of preparation may not be compliant at the time of administration.	
Sr-82/Rb-82 generator	Sr-82 breakthrough	0.02 μCi Sr-82/ mCi Rb-82 (0.02 kBq Sr-82/MBq Rb-82)	Test every generator elution. Limits are at time of patient administration.	
	Sr-85 contamination	0.2 μCi Sr-85/mCi Rb-82 (0.2kBq Sr-85/MBq Rb-82)		
Radiochemical purity	Tc-99m not in +7 valence state Free Tc-99m pertechnetate, hydrolyzed, or reduced moieties	95% or more must be in +7	Most radiopharmaceuticals must be at least 90% pure (i.e., 90% of the radioisotope bound in the desired chemical form). The +4, +5 and +6 valence states are impurities. Detect with thin layer chromatography (TLC). Detect with instant thin layer chromatography (TLC).	
Chemical purity Mo-99/Tc-99m generator	Alumina breakthrough	<10 μg/mL	Detected visually by paper colorimetric test. Done for every generator elution.	

breakthrough, during elution is normally determined by placing the eluate from the generator in a lead shield and measuring the penetration of any ^{99}Mo (740- and 780-keV) photons. The presence of other radionuclides may be determined by multichannel analysis or by counting of the eluate at different times to allow for decay. The latter method indicates whether the half-life of the contaminant is or is not consistent with that of ^{99}Mo.

The NRC and USP regulations allow no more than 0.15 μCi (0.005 MBq) of ^{99}Mo per 1 mCi (37 MBq) of ^{99m}Tc at the time of administration. Because ^{99m}Tc decays much faster than ^{99}Mo, the relative amount of any molybdenum contaminant rises with time. Thus, if the ^{99}Mo in an eluate from a generator was barely acceptable at 8 AM, it will likely become unacceptable later the same day.

The elution column inside the generator is made of alumina (Al$_2$O$_3$). If, during elution, sufficient alumina breaks through, the eluate may become cloudy. The presence of aluminum ion (Al^{3+}) should be ascertained at the time of eluting ^{99m}Tc from the generator. Small amounts of aluminum ion may be detected with an indicator paper similar to the pH paper used in chemistry. If aluminum ion is present, a red color develops. The maximum permissible amount of aluminum ion is 10 μg/mL of ^{99m}Tc eluate with a fission generator. If too much aluminum is present, technetium–aluminum particles form, which are manifested clinically by hepatic uptake. Excessive aluminum ion may also cause aggregation of sulfur colloid preparations, resulting in lung uptake (Fig. 1-10). The purpose of ethylenediaminetetra-acetic acid (EDTA) in sulfur colloid kits is to bind excess Al3+ and thus to prevent such problems. Agglutination of red blood cells may also occur when inordinate amounts of aluminum ion are contained in ^{99m}Tc pertechnetate solutions.

Product standards and quality control requirements for PET radiopharmaceuticals are provided by both the U.S. Pharmacopeia and guidance from the FDA (which, in some instances, is more restrictive). For ^{18}F-FDG injection, the FDA indicates that (1) the solution must be colorless and free from particulate matter when observed visually (appearance), (2) the half-life must be measured to be between 105 and 115 minutes (radionuclide identity), (3) no more than 4% of free ^{18}F- must be present in an

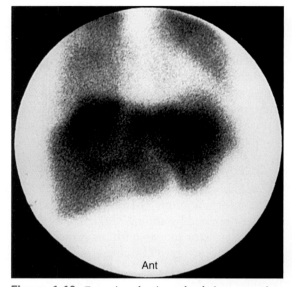

Figure 1-10. Excessive aluminum levels in preparation. A liver and spleen scan demonstrates activity above the liver in both lungs owing to aggregation of the sulfur colloid causing larger particles.

injection (radiochemical impurity), (4) no less than 90% of the radioactivity must locate at a specific spot on chromatography (radiochemical purity), and (5) additional tests for chemical purity must assure that various reagents, unwanted products, or residual organic solvents are not present in excess.

Radiochemical Labeling

Once radionuclide purity is ensured, a prepackaged kit containing an unlabeled pharmaceutical may be used to produce a radiochemical compound. The biodistribution of that radiochemical in a patient can then easily be visualized with a gamma camera system. Assessment of chemical purity of ^{99m}Tc radiopharmaceuticals is performed by determining the degree of successful tagging of the agent contained in the kit and the amount of residual (unbound ^{99m}Tc) in the preparation. The degree of purity may reflect the proficiency of those who prepare the kits or simply any lot-to-lot or manufacturer-to-manufacturer variability in the kits.

Instant thin-layer chromatography is usually performed to assess radiochemical purity, using silica gel impregnated in glass fiber sheets or strips. By using various solvents, impurities can be identified by their different migrations in the particular solvent used.

A drop of the radiochemical compound to be analyzed is placed on the strip, and the solvent is applied. As the solvent approaches the end of the sheet, an assessment is made of the radioactivity present at the point of origin and at the advancing solvent front. Although this may be performed by various scanning methods, the simplest way is to cut the fiber strip into segments and count them individually in a well counter. If this is done, the technician must be extremely careful to put only a very small amount of activity at the spot of origin because well counters are efficient, and it is easy to exceed their count rate capability.

The most common ^{99m}Tc radiopharmaceuticals are prepared by adding ^{99m}Tc freshly eluted from a generator to a cold kit, as prescribed by the kit manufacturer. The eluate of the generator should be ^{99m}TcO$_4^-$ (+7) (i.e., pertechnetate). Because pertechnetate in this valence state is relatively stable, it cannot tag a cold kit preparation and must be reduced to a lower valence state (+3, +4, +5). This is done by using a reducing agent such as stannous chloride, which is generally present in the reaction vial.

Most radiochemical impurities obtained in a kit preparation are the result of interaction of either oxygen or water with the contents of the kit or vial. If air reaches the vial contents, stannous chloride may be oxidized to stannic chloride even before introduction of ^{99m}Tc into the vial. If this happens, the production of reactive technetium is no longer possible, and free pertechnetate becomes an impurity. If moisture reaches the vial contents, stannous chloride becomes hydrolyzed, and the formation of stannous hydroxide, a colloid, results.

Reactive reduced technetium may also become hydrolyzed, forming technetium dioxide. This hydrolyzed, reduced form of technetium is insoluble and is another impurity that must be tested. Technetium that has been tagged to a compound can reoxidize and revert to pertechnetate.

To minimize oxidation problems, most cold kits are purged with nitrogen, and additional antioxidants, such as ascorbic acid, may also have been added. It is still extremely important not to inject air into the reaction vial when preparing a radiopharmaceutical. An often overlooked source of problems is the sterile saline used in preparation of the kits. This saline should be free of preservatives because bacteriostatic agents often interfere with the tagging process.

To check for the presence of free pertechnetate, the radiopharmaceutical is placed on the chromatographic strip, and acetone is used as the solvent. Most tagged radiopharmaceuticals remain at the origin, whereas the free pertechnetate advances with the solvent front (Fig. 1-11). To assess the presence of hydrolyzed technetium or technetium dioxide, saline is used as the solvent. In this case, technetium dioxide remains at the origin, whereas those radiopharmaceuticals that are soluble in saline, such as diethylenetriaminepentaacetic acid (DTPA) and pertechnetate, advance with the solvent front. For some compounds that are insoluble in saline, such as macroaggregated albumin, it is not possible to assess the presence of technetium dioxide by using instant thin-layer chromatography.

USP regulations define the lower limits of acceptability for radiochemical purity as 95% for pertechnetate, 92% for ^{99m}Tc sulfur colloid, and 90% for all other ^{99m}Tc radiopharmaceuticals. Once the chromatographic procedures are established, they take little time to perform and ideally should be done before patient injection.

One reason for performing thin-layer chromatography before patient injection is that simple errors can cause the radiolabeling to be completely ineffective. For example, in the production of sulfur colloid, one kit normally calls for injection of syringe A first and then for injection of syringe B into the reaction vial. If these two injections are reversed, no sulfur colloid is produced, and there is a large amount of free ^{99m}Tc pertechnetate. Thus, a liver scan is not possible with the agent. Free ^{99m}Tc pertechnetate is seen as unexpected activity in both the thyroid and stomach (Fig. 1-12).

The ^{99m}Tc radiopharmaceuticals that are produced with stannous chloride reduction or stannous chelates include macroaggregated albumin, phosphate compounds, and glucoheptonate. The only one in common use that is produced without reduction or chelation by tin is sulfur colloid. The compounds in which the presence of hydrolyzed technetium (Tc dioxide) may need to be checked are DTPA, phosphate compounds, glucoheptonate, and iminodiacetic acid (IDA) derivatives.

Excessive stannous agents can cause quality control problems during radiopharmaceutical preparation that become evident in the actual clinical images. Excess stannous ions (tin) may cause liver uptake on bone scans by formation of a tin colloid (Fig. 1-13). Residual stannous ions in the blood may also cause red blood cell labeling.

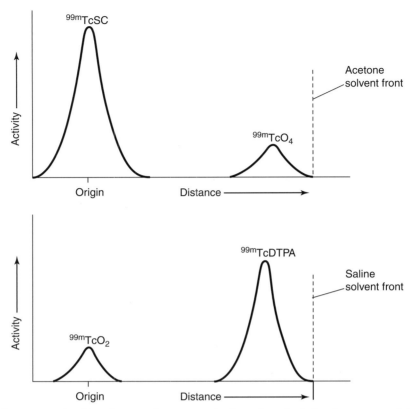

Figure 1-11. Chromatography. *Top*, Acetone chromatography is used to check for the presence of free pertechnetate, which migrates with the acetone solvent front. *Bottom*, To check for technetium dioxide ($^{99m}TcO_2$), saline is used; those radiopharmaceuticals that are soluble in saline advance with the solvent.

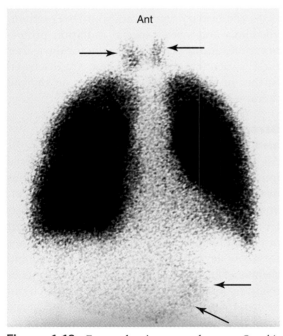

Figure 1-12. Free technetium pertechnetate. On this ^{99m}Tc-MAA lung scan, unexpected activity in the thyroid (*top arrows*) and stomach (*bottom arrows*) indicates the presence of unlabeled free technetium pertechnetate. *MAA,* Macroaggregated albumin.

Stannous ions may remain in the blood after a bone scan, so that a ^{99m}Tc pertechnetate thyroid or Meckel diverticulum scan attempted within 1 week may result in red blood cell labeling.

Particle size of certain compounds may be checked by a hemocytometer as part of the quality control procedure. The USP maximum diameter recommendation for macroaggregated albumin is 150 μm, with 90% of particles between 10 and 90 μm. Most physicians prefer particles less than 100 μm in size for pulmonary perfusion imaging. Slightly large particle size in preparations of ^{99m}Tc sulfur colloid results in relatively more uptake in the spleen and may give a false impression of hepatocellular dysfunction.

UNSEALED RADIONUCLIDES USED FOR THERAPY

Radionuclides can be administered to patients for therapeutic purposes in sealed or unsealed forms. Unsealed radionuclides may be given orally, administered intravenously, or placed directly into a body cavity (such as a knee joint or peritoneum). Most unsealed radionuclides

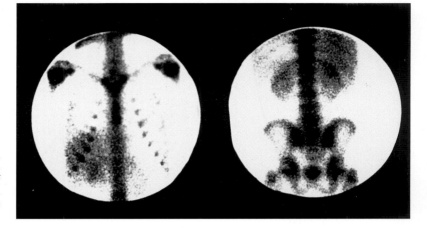

Figure 1-13. **Excess tin.** Images from a bone scan show unexpected hepatic activity because of poor quality control and excess tin causing formation of colloid-size particles.

are predominantly beta emitters. As such, they usually present little hazard to the public or family members. A few radionuclides also emit gamma photons, which can be helpful in imaging the localization of the material; however, a large amount of gamma emissions will present a radiation hazard and give a significant radiation dose to nontarget tissues. Issues related to the release of patients in accordance with U.S. Nuclear Regulatory Commission regulation are included in Appendix G. Sealed radionuclides are administered to patients in an encapsulated form for regional radiotherapy. Because they are generally used in the practice of radiation oncology, sealed radionuclides will not be discussed in this text.

Phosphorus-32, Yttrium-90 and Gold-198

All three of these radionuclides have been used for radioisotopic therapy. Currently, they are rarely used in colloidal form for intracavitary administration for abdominopelvic serosal metastases or knee joint synovectomy. Intravenous phosphorus-32, as an ionic phosphate, has been used in the past to treat polycythemia vera, but has largely been replaced by nonradioisotopic drugs. Yttrium-90 (^{90}Y) can be coupled with a localization agent to deliver antineoplastic therapy. Yttrium-90 labeled microspheres, injected through a transfemoral catheter into the hepatic artery, lodge in the small blood vessels of liver neoplasms to deliver a therapeutic dose. ^{90}Y-labeled monoclonal antibodies can

be injected intravenously to treat some non-Hodgkin lymphomas.

Iodine-131

Iodine-131 is discussed earlier in the section on imaging radionuclides; however, large administered activities of sodium ^{131}I are commonly used for treatment of hyperthyroidism and thyroid cancer. Although ^{131}I is a beta emitter, there is a predominant energetic gamma emission (364 keV), which can be used to image the biodistribution. This gamma photon also can result in measurable absorbed radiation doses to persons near the patient. Because excretion is via the urinary tract, and, to a lesser extent, via saliva and sweat, special radiation protection precautions need to be taken for days after these patients are treated. These are discussed further in Chapter 4 in the section on thyroid therapy and in Appendix G.

Strontium-89, Samarium-153, and Rhenium-186

All three of these radionuclides are administered intravenously and used to treat painful osseous metastases from prostate and breast cancer. Strontium-89 (^{89}Sr) is essentially a pure beta emitter and poses virtually no hazard to medical staff or patient families, except for urinary precautions for a few days. Both samarium-153 (^{153}Sm) and rhenium-186 (^{186}Re) also emit small amounts of relatively low-energy gamma photons, which can be used to image distribution. These are discussed in more detail at the end of Chapter 8.

PEARLS & PITFALLS

- The superscript before a radionuclide symbol or the number following in regular text is the mass number (A) which is the sum of the number of neutrons (N) and protons (Z). Thus, ^{131}I (iodine-131) has 53 protons and 78 neutrons to equal 131.

- All isotopes of a given element have the same number of protons and only differ in the number of neutrons.

- Effective half-life of a radionuclide is always less than either the physical or biologic half-life.

- A becquerel is 1 disintegration per second. A curie is 3.7×10^{10} disintegrations per second.

- Cyclotron-produced isotopes are often carrier free (do not contain any of the stable element) because the process involves transmutation. Isotopes produced by neutron bombardment are not usually carrier free because they involve bombardment of the same element. Radionuclides produced by fission in a reactor can be carrier free because they are produced by splitting other elements.

- A generator system for producing radionuclides uses a long-lived parent that decays into another shorter lived element that can be chemically separated.

- In most generators used, there comes a time when the ratio of the daughter to the parent becomes constant (transient equilibrium) and for ^{99}Mo-^{99m}Tc generators, the ^{99m}Tc activity slightly exceeds the ^{99}Mo activity. This takes several days. Once eluted, a ^{99}Mo-^{99m}Tc generator will reach 95% of maximal ^{99m}Tc activity in about 24 hours.

- Once produced, most excited states of an atom decay almost instantaneously to a more stable configuration. The "m" in technetium-99m refers to metastable, meaning that there is an excited state of the isotope that persists for some time before there is emission of a gamma ray.

- Severe adverse reactions of radiopharmaceuticals are extremely rare (about 2 per 100,000). Adverse reactions to non-radioactive pharmaceuticals used in nuclear medicine are much more common.

- Technetium-99m as eluted is in a +7 valence state. Tin is used as a reducing agent to allow labeling of other compounds.

- Molybdenum breakthrough in a generator eluate is detected by the penetration of 740- and 780-keV photons through a lead shield that attenuates the 140-keV photons of technetium.

- Aluminum ion breakthrough in the eluate from a ^{99}Mo-^{99m}Tc generator is detected by using a special test paper that changes color. Excessive aluminum indicates the lack of stability of the generator column.

- Radionuclide purity of a sample is performed by examining the energy of the photons emitted and comparing it to those expected for a given radionuclide.

- Radiochemical purity related to radiopharmaceutical labeling is tested by using thin-layer chromatography with either acetone or saline as the solvent. Usually, 95% tagging is required.

- Free ^{99m}Tc pertechnetate is usually seen as unexpected activity in the stomach, thyroid, and salivary glands.

SUGGESTED READINGS

Bushberg JT, Seibert JA, Leidholdt EM, Boone JM. The Essential Physics of Medical Imaging. 2nd ed. Baltimore: Williams & Wilkins; 2002, chapters 18-20. (3rd ed. In press).

Hendee WR, Ritenour ER. Medical Imaging Physics. 4th ed. New York: Wiley-Liss; 2002, chapters 2-4.

Silberstein EB. Positron-emitting radiopharmaceuticals: how safe are they? Cancer Biother Radiopharm 2001; 16:13-5.

Silberstein EB, Ryan J. Pharmacopeia Committee of the Society of Nuclear Medicine: Prevalence of adverse reactions in nuclear medicine. J Nucl Med 1996;37:185-92.

Simpkin DJ. The AAPM/RSNA Physics Tutorial for Residents: Radiation interactions and internal dosimetry in nuclear medicine. RadioGraphics 1999;19:155-67.

2 Instrumentation and Quality Control

GEIGER-MUELLER COUNTER

Geiger-Mueller (GM) counters are handheld, very sensitive, inexpensive survey instruments used primarily to detect small amounts of radioactive contamination. The detector is usually pancake shaped, although it may also be cylindrical (Fig. 2-1). The detector is gas-filled and has a high applied voltage from the anode to the cathode. This causes one ionization to result in an "avalanche" of other electrons, allowing high efficiency for detection of even a single gamma ray. The avalanche of electrons takes some time to dissipate; as a result, "dead time" must occur before the next ionization can be detected. This precludes use of GM counters in high radiation fields. They are usually limited to exposure rates of up to about 100 mR (2.5×10^{-5} C/kg)/hour. Most GM counters are equipped with a thin window that also allows detection of most beta rays. Very weak beta rays (such as those from tritium) cannot be detected.

IONIZATION CHAMBER

Ionization chambers are handheld survey instruments used to measure low or high exposure rates (Fig. 2-2). They have an air or gas-filled chamber but a low efficiency for detection of gamma rays. These instruments have a relatively low applied voltage from anode to cathode; as a result, there is no avalanche effect and no dead time problem. Ionization chambers typically are useful at exposure rates ranging from 0.1 mR (2.5×10^{-8} C/kg)/hour to 100 R (2.5×10^{-2} C/kg)/hour. A dose calibrator is a special form of an ionization chamber.

SODIUM IODIDE WELL COUNTER

Well counters are common in nuclear medicine laboratories for performing in vitro studies as well as quality control and assurance procedures. Many sodium iodide well counters are designed for counting radioactive samples in standard test tubes. Generally, there is a solid

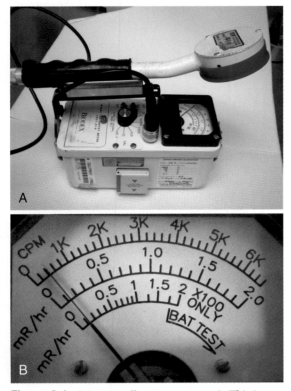

Figure 2-1. Geiger-Mueller survey meter. A, This instrument is used for low levels of radiation or activity. On the instrument, the pancake detector is located at the end of the handle and the face is covered with a red plastic cap. The selector knob has various multipliers to use with the displayed reading. Note the radiation check source affixed to the side, which is used to make sure the instrument is functional. Also there is a calibration sticker. **B,** The dial reads in either counts per minute (CPM) or milliroentgens per hour (mR/hr). There is also a battery test range that is used when the battery check button is pushed or the selector knob is switched to battery check.

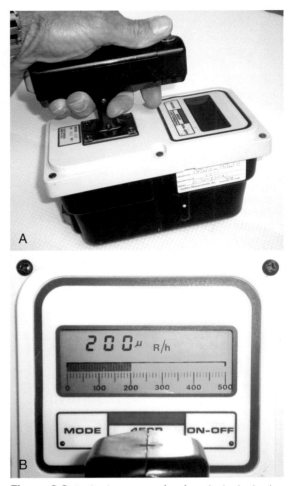

Figure 2-2. Ionization survey chamber. A, An ionization chamber must be used if there are high levels of activity or radiation. For this handheld model, the detector is inside the body of the instrument. **B,** The scale reads in units of radiation exposure.

cylindrical sodium iodide crystal with a cylindrical well cut into the crystal, into which the test tube is placed (Fig. 2-3). A photomultiplier tube (PMT) is optically coupled to the crystal base. Radiation from the sample interacts with the crystal and is detected by the PMT, which feeds into a scalar. The scalar readout directly reflects the amount of radioactivity in the sample and is usually recorded in counts for the time period during which the sample is measured.

Reflected light and scattering inside the well surface and the thickness of the crystal limit the energy resolution of the standard well counter. Because the sample is essentially surrounded by the crystal, the geometric efficiency for detection of gamma rays is high. *Geometric efficiency*

is defined as the fraction of emitted radioactivity that is incident on the detection portion of the counter, in this case, the crystal. Because the crystal is relatively thick, most low energy photons undergo interaction, and few pass through undetected. As a result, in the energy ranges below 200 keV, the overall crystal detection efficiency is usually better than 95%.

Because the top of the well in the crystal is open, it is important to keep the sample volume in the test tube small. If varying sample volumes are placed in the well counter, different amounts of radiation escape near the top of the crystal, resulting in unequal geometric efficiencies. Absorption of gamma rays within the wall of the test tube is a factor when lower energy sources, such as iodine-125 (^{125}I), are counted;

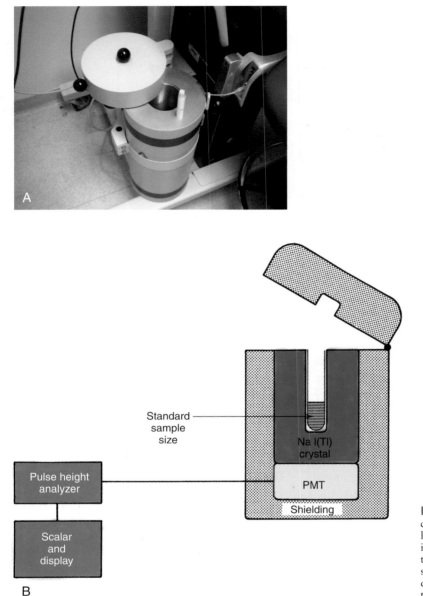

Figure 2-3. **Well counter. A,** Well counters are heavily shielded scintillation crystals used to measure and identify small amounts of radioactivity contained in small volumes such as a test tube. **B,** Schematic diagram. *PMT,* Photomultiplier tube.

therefore the sample tubes should also be identical.

Because sodium iodide well counters have such a high detection efficiency, there is a serious problem with electronic dead time. If high levels of activity are used, much of the radiation is not detected. In general, well counters can typically count activity only up to about 1 μCi (37 kBq). Attempts to measure amounts of activity greater than this in a well counter can lead to serious underestimates attributable to dead-time counting errors.

SINGLE PROBE COUNTING SYSTEMS

Single probe counting systems using only one crystalline detector are primarily used for measuring thyroid uptake of radioactive iodine. The probe used for thyroid counting is actually similar to the standard well counter in concept (Fig. 2-4), although it does not have the central hole in the sodium iodide crystal. The typical crystal is 5 cm in diameter and 5 cm in thickness, with a cone shaped (flat field) collimator. As with the well counter, a PMT is situated at the crystal

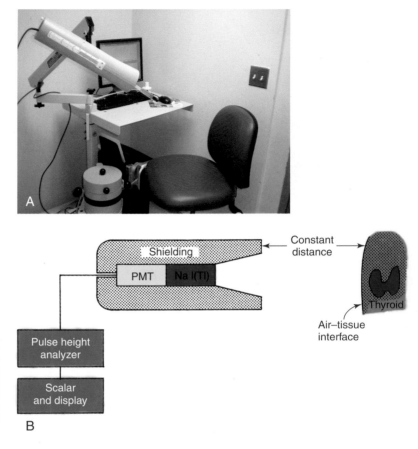

Figure 2-4. Single probe counting system. **A,** Single crystal thyroid probe used for measuring radioiodine uptake. The end of the barrel is placed a fixed distance from the sitting patient's neck. **B,** Schematic diagram. *PMT,* Photomultiplier tube.

base. When these probes are used, it is important for quantitative consistency to maintain a fixed distance from the object being measured to the face of the crystal and to eliminate all extraneous sources of background radiation.

In addition to the larger type probes there are also handheld intraoperative probes most commonly used to identify and localize sentinel lymph nodes and parathyroid adenomas. These need to have excellent spatial resolution and are highly collimated counting devices with solid state scintillation or semiconductor detectors. Scintillation based detectors have an NaI(Tl), CsI(Tl), or bismuth germanate crystal connected to a photomultiplier tube and are best for medium to high energy photons. Semiconductor (CdZn, CdZnTe, or HgI$_2$) detectors are less sensitive but have higher energy resolution. Some of the devices have interchangeable probes and can detect gamma, beta, or positron emissions and thus can be used for a variety of radionuclides, including ^{99m}Tc, ^{111}In, and ^{18}F.

DOSE CALIBRATOR

Because it is extremely important to calibrate a dose of isotope before injection, the dose calibrator is an essential piece of equipment in any nuclear medicine laboratory. A standard sodium iodide well counter is not useful because the upper limit of sample activity that can be measured accurately is in the microcurie (37 kBq) range. A dose calibrator is essentially a well-type ionization chamber capable of measuring quantities in the millicurie (37 MBq) range. It does not contain a sodium iodide crystal. The chamber is cylindrical and holds a defined volume of pressurized inert gas (usually argon). Within the chamber is a collecting electrode (Fig. 2-5). As radiation emanates from the radiopharmaceutical in the syringe, it enters the chamber and interacts with the gas, causing ionization. An electrical differential applied between the chamber and the collecting electrode causes the ions to be captured and measured. This measurement is used to calculate the dose contained in the

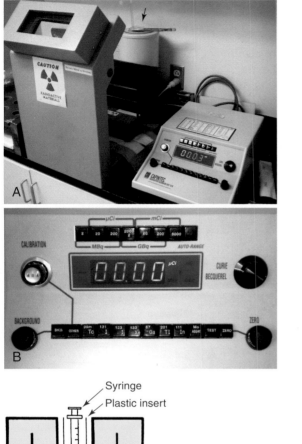

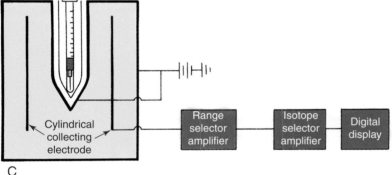

Syringe
Plastic insert

Cylindrical collecting electrode

Range selector amplifier

Isotope selector amplifier

Digital display

C

Figure 2-5. Dose calibrator. **A,** The sample is placed in the shielded ionization chamber (*arrow*) which is behind the technologist's protective shielding. **B,** The selector buttons on the control panel and display require the user to select the appropriate radionuclide in order to display the correct activity. **C,** Schematic diagram.

syringe. Limits for maximum activity to be measured by dose calibrators are usually specified for ^{99m}Tc.

As with other radiopharmaceuticals, the activity of positron emitters may be measured in a typical dose calibrator before administration to the patient. Although a dose calibrator (ionization chamber) cannot determine the energy of emitted photons, the amount of electrical current in the chamber produced by the photons varies directly with photon energy. Because the 511 keV annihilation photons are substantially more energetic than are ^{99m}Tc photons, the current produced is about three times greater. Therefore the maximum activity limit for ^{18}F is about one third that specified for ^{99m}Tc. Consequently, a dose calibrator with relatively high specified maximum activity is preferred. In addition, more lead shielding around the dose calibrator is required for measurement of ^{18}F. It should be at least 5 cm or greater compared with the 4- to 6-mm thickness usually supplied with a standard dose calibrator.

GAMMA SCINTILLATION CAMERA

The most widely used imaging devices in nuclear medicine are the simple gamma scintillation (Anger) camera and the single-photon emission computed tomography (SPECT) capable gamma camera. A gamma camera converts photons emitted by the radionuclide in the patient into a light pulse and subsequently into a voltage signal. This signal is used to form an image of the distribution of the radionuclide. The basic components of a gamma camera system (Fig. 2-6) are the collimator, the scintillation crystal, an array of photomultiplier tubes (PMTs), preamplifiers, a pulse height analyzer (PHA), digital correction circuitry, a cathode ray tube (CRT), and the control

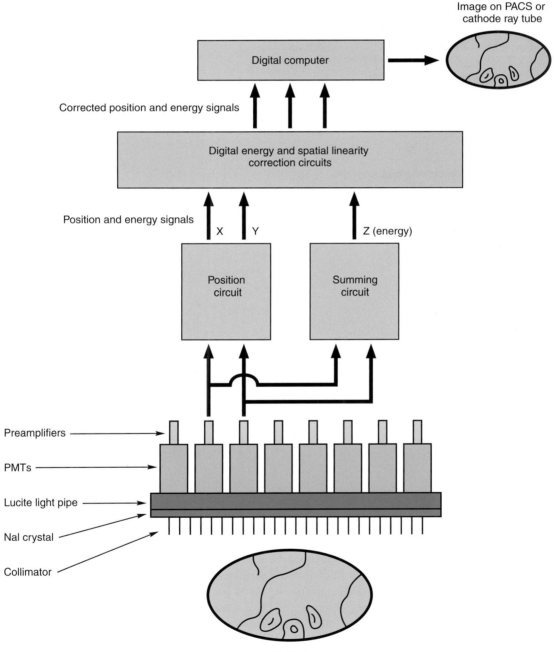

Figure 2-6. Gamma camera schematic. A cross-sectional image of the patient is shown at the *bottom*, with a final image seen on the computer console at the *top*.

console. A computer and picture archiving systems (PACs) are also integral parts of the system. Most of the newer cameras incorporate digital features. Even the most advanced digital cameras, however, start with the analog signal in the scintillation crystal and return to an analog signal for CRT or PACs display of the image. Typical performance parameters are shown in Table 2-1.

Collimator

The collimator is made of perforated or folded lead and is interposed between the patient and the scintillation crystal. It allows the gamma camera to localize accurately the radionuclide in the patient's body. Collimators perform this function by absorbing and stopping most radiation except that arriving almost perpendicular

TABLE 2–1 Properties of Typical Nuclear Medicine Imaging Equipment

CHARACTERISTIC	SPECT GAMMA CAMERA
Radionuclides imaged	Any with gamma or x-ray in the energy range 40-520 keV
Collimators	Low energy all-purpose and high resolution, medium and high energy, pinhole
Detector	Rotating dual head with various configurations, including non circular orbits
Crystal material	Sodium iodide crystal (thallium doped) usually single
Crystal size	60 × 50 cm
Crystal thickness	9.5 mm (3/8 inches) or 15.9 mm (5/8 inches)
Photomultiplier tubes	40-90
Spatial resolution (intrinsic)	3-10 mm (varies with type of reconstruction)
Energy window	40-520 keV (capable of six energy windows simultaneously)
Field uniformity	2%-5%
Maximum count rate	300-350 kcps
Axial resolution (FWHM)	8-9 mm FWHM (low energy all-purpose collimator)
Energy resolution (FWHM)	≤10%
Attenuation correction	Optional, either gadolinium-153 source or CT on SPECT/CT camera
PET/CT Scanner	
Radionuclides imaged	Positron emitters
Detector array	Rings (usually 18-64)
Detector (crystal material)	NaI curved, BGO, LSO, GSO, LYSO, semiconductor
Crystal number and size	Variable but in state-of-the-art ring systems with block detectors about 10,000-20,000 small crystals (about 4 × 4 × 30 mm) with 36-170 crystals per block
Counting rates	High
Algorithm for location	Specific detector
Acquisition	2 or 3 dimensional and time-of-flight
Spatial resolution	High (5-6 mm)
Coincidence window	4-12 nsec
Energy window	≈350-650 keV
System sensitivity (cps/kBq)	5-10
Axial resolution (FWHM)	≈4.5-7 mm
Energy resolution (FWHM)	≈10%-25%
Attenuation correction	CT

BGO, Bismuth germanate; *FWHM*, full width at half-maximum; *GSO*, gadolinium oxyorthosilicate; *LSO*, lutetium oxyorthosilicate; *LYSO*, lutetium yttrium oxyorthosilicate; *NaI*, sodium iodide; *PET*, positron emission tomography; *SPECT*, single-photon emission computed tomography; *Tl*, thallium.

to the detector face. Most radiation striking the collimator at oblique angles is not included in the final image. Of all the photons emitted by an administered radiopharmaceutical, more than 99% are "wasted" and not recorded by the gamma camera; less than 1% are used to generate the desired image. Thus the collimator is the "rate limiting" step in the imaging chain of gamma camera technology.

The two basic types of collimators are *pinhole* and *multihole*. A *pinhole collimator* operates in a manner similar to that of a box camera (Fig. 2-7). Radiation must pass through the pinhole aperture to be imaged, and the image is always inverted on the scintillation crystal. Because little of the radiation coming from the object of interest is allowed to pass through the pinhole over a given time period, the pinhole collimator has very poor sensitivity. Collimator sensitivity refers to the percentage of incident photons that pass through the collimator. The poor sensitivity of a pinhole collimator makes placement near the organ of interest critical, and bringing the object of interest close to the pinhole magnifies the image. Because magnification is a function of distance, if the object of interest is not relatively flat or thin, the image may be distorted. Pinhole collimators are routinely used for very high resolution images of small organs, such as the thyroid, and for certain skeletal regions, such as hips or wrists, especially in pediatric patients.

The holes in a *multihole collimator* may be aligned in a parallel, diverging, or converging manner. The *parallel hole collimator* is the most widely used multihole collimator in nuclear medicine laboratories. It consists of parallel holes with a long axis perpendicular to the plane of the scintillation crystal. The lead walls between the holes are referred to as *septa*. The septa absorb most gamma rays that do not emanate from the direction of interest; therefore a collimator for high energy gamma rays has much thicker septa than does a collimator for low energy rays. The septa are generally designed so that septal penetration by unwanted gamma rays does not exceed 10% to 25%.

A parallel hole collimator should be chosen to correspond to the energy of the isotope being imaged. Low energy collimators generally refer to a maximum energy of 150 keV, whereas

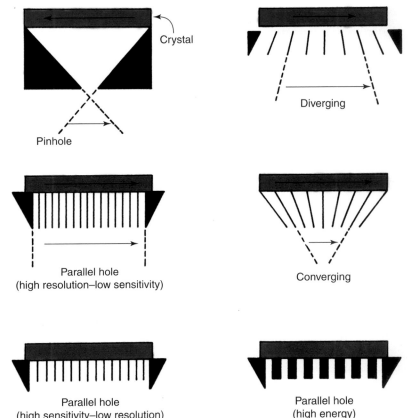

Figure 2-7. Types of gamma camera collimators. As the energy of the radionuclide increases, the best collimator usually has thicker and longer septa. For a given septal thickness, spatial resolution of a collimator increases with septal length but sensitivity decreases.

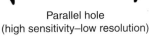

medium energy collimators have a maximum suggested energy of about 400 keV. Collimators are available with different lengths and different widths of septa. In general, the longer the septa, the better the resolution but the lower the count rate (sensitivity) for a given amount of radionuclide. The count rate is inversely proportional to the square of the collimator hole length. If the length of the septa is decreased, the detected count rate increases, and resolution decreases (Fig. 2-8).

The difference between typical low energy, general-purpose collimators and low-energy, high-sensitivity collimators is that high-sensitivity collimators may allow about twice as many counts to be imaged, although the spatial resolution is usually degraded by about 50%. A high resolution, low energy collimator has about three times the resolving ability of a high sensitivity, low energy collimator.

With a parallel hole collimator, neither the size of the image nor the count rate changes significantly with the distance of the object of interest from the collimator. This is because as the object is moved small distances away from the crystal, the inverse square law reduces the number of counts. However, this is compensated for by the increased viewing area of the collimator. On the other hand, resolution is best when the object of interest is as close to the collimator face as possible (Figs. 2-9 and 2-10), and scans with multihole collimators are usually obtained with the collimator in contact with or as close as possible to the patient. With a

parallel hole collimator, scattered photons emitted from the patient perpendicular to the crystal face may be imaged (Fig. 2-11). These photons and those that penetrate the septa degrade spatial resolution.

Crystal and Other Photon Detector Devices

Radiation emerging from the patient and passing through the collimator typically interacts with a thallium activated sodium iodide crystal. Crystals also can be made with thallium or sodium activated cesium iodide or even lanthanum bromide, but these are uncommon. Interaction of the gamma ray with the crystal may result in ejection of an orbital electron (photoelectric absorption), producing a pulse of fluorescent light (scintillation event) proportional in intensity to the energy of the gamma ray. PMTs situated along the posterior crystal face detect this light and amplify it. About 30% of the light from each event reaches the PMTs. The crystal is fragile and must have an aluminum housing that protects it from moisture, extraneous light, and minor physical damage.

The crystal may be circular and up to about 22 inches in diameter, but most newer ones are square or rectangular. For most cameras, a 6- to 10-mm thick crystal is used. A larger diameter crystal has a larger field of view and is more expensive but has the same inherent resolution as does a smaller diameter crystal. The thicker the crystal becomes, the worse the spatial resolution but the more efficient the detection of gamma

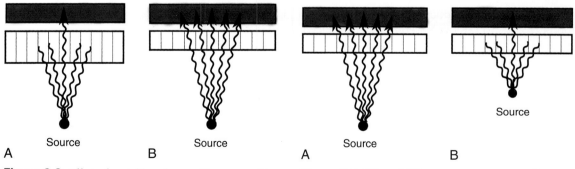

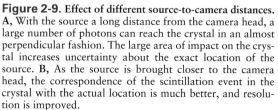

Figure 2-8. Effect of septal length on collimator sensitivity and resolution. **A,** Longer septa in the collimator attenuate most photons, except those exactly perpendicular to the crystal face. This increase in selectivity increases the resolution and decreases the count rate detected. **B,** Shortening the length of the septa allows more photons to reach the crystal; thus the count rate is higher. The spatial resolution, however, is decreased because the photons coming through a hole in the collimator are from a larger area.

Figure 2-9. Effect of different source-to-camera distances. **A,** With the source a long distance from the camera head, a large number of photons can reach the crystal in an almost perpendicular fashion. The large area of impact on the crystal increases uncertainty about the exact location of the source. **B,** As the source is brought closer to the camera head, the correspondence of the scintillation event in the crystal with the actual location is much better, and resolution is improved.

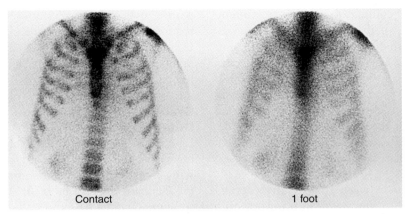

Contact   1 foot

Figure 2-10. **Effect of increasing the patient-to-detector face distance on clinical images.** When the camera is in contact with this patient, who is having a bone scan, the osseous structures are well defined. Increasing the distance to 1 foot has a major adverse effect on resolution.

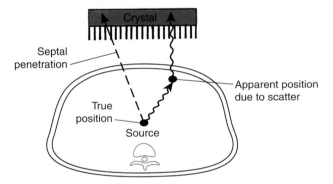

Figure 2-11. **Scintillation events that degrade images.** Both septal penetration and photon scattering within the patient's body cause events to be recorded in locations other than their true positions.

rays. In general, with a 12-mm thick crystal, the efficiency for detection of gamma rays from xenon-133 (^{133}Xe) (81 keV) and technetium-99m (^{99m}Tc) (140 keV) is almost 100%; that is, few of the photons pass through the crystal without causing a light pulse. As the gamma energy of the isotope is increased, the efficiency of the crystal is markedly reduced. For example, with iodine-131 (^{131}I) (364 keV), efficiency is reduced to about 20% to 30%. With a thinner crystal, the overall sensitivity (count rate) decreases by about 10% because more photons pass through, but there is about a 30% increase in spatial resolution because the PMTs are closer to the event and thus can localize it more accurately, and because there is an increase in light collection. Some newer cameras have pixilated detectors in which the field of view is covered by an array of detectors with a face size of 2 to 3 mm instead of a single large crystal.

Detectors also can be solid state semiconductors rather than crystal. This allows direct conversion of the absorbed gamma ray energy into an electronic signal rather than going through the scintillation process. Materials that can operate at room temperatures include cadmium telluride and cadmium zinc telluride. These provide better energy resolution but have the disadvantages of low intrinsic efficiency for high energy gamma rays and cost of production. As a result, their use has been primarily limited to small field of view cameras.

Photon Transducers

A photomultiplier tube (PMT) converts a light pulse into an electrical signal of measurable magnitude. An array of these tubes is situated behind the sodium iodide crystal and may be placed directly on the crystal, connected to the crystal by light pipes, or optically coupled to the crystal with a silicone-like material. A scintillation event occurring in the crystal is recorded by one or more PMTs. Localization of the event in the final image depends on the amount of light sensed by each PMT and thus on the pattern of PMT voltage output. The summation signal for each scintillation event is then formed by weighing the output of each tube. This signal

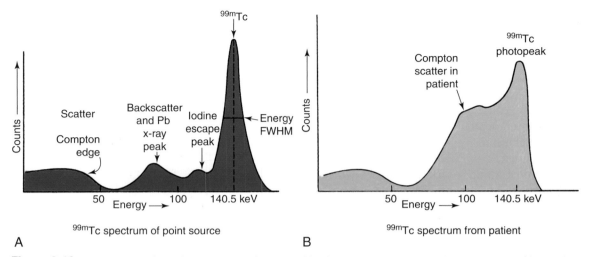

Figure 2-12. Energy spectra for technetium-99m when viewed by the gamma camera as a point source (A) and in a patient (B). Note the marked amount of Compton scatter near the photopeak that occurs as a result of scatter within the patient's body. *FWHM,* Full width at half maximum.

has three components: spatial coordinates on x- and y-axes as well as a signal (z) related to intensity (energy). The x- and y-coordinates may go directly to instrumentation for display on the CRT or may be recorded in the computer. The signal intensity is processed by the pulse height analyzer (PHA).

The light interaction caused by a gamma ray generally occurs near the collimator face of the crystal. Thus although a thicker crystal is theoretically more efficient, the PMT is farther away from the scintillation point with a thick crystal and is unable to determine the coordinates as accurately. Therefore spatial resolution is degraded. The number of PMTs is also important for the accurate localization of scintillation events; thus for spatial resolution, the greater the number of PMTs, the greater the resolution. Most gamma cameras use about 40 to 100 hexagonal, square, or round PMTs.

Some newer commercial imaging systems have used position sensitive PMTs (PS-PMT) and avalanche photodiodes (APD). PS-PMTs are usually used with small field of view devices that have pixilated detectors rather than a large single crystal. APDs are solid state photon converters that can be thought of as a light sensitive diode and are being used in PET/MRI applications because they are less sensitive to magnetic fields.

Pulse Height Analyzer

The basic principle of the PHA is to discard signals from background and scattered radiation and/or radiation from interfering isotopes,

so that only primary photons known to come from the photopeak of the isotope being imaged are recorded. The PHA discriminates between events occurring in the crystal that will be displayed or stored in the computer and events that will be rejected. The PHA can make this discrimination because the energy deposited by a scintillation event in the crystal bears a linear relation to the voltage signal emerging from the PMTs.

A typical energy spectrum from a PHA is shown in Figure 2-12. The photopeak is the result of total absorption of the major gamma ray from the radionuclide. If the characteristic K-shell x-ray of iodine (28 keV) escapes from the crystal after the gamma ray has undergone photoelectric absorption, the measured gamma-ray energy for ^{99m}Tc would be only 112 keV (140 minus 28 keV). This will cause an *iodine escape peak.*

A *backscatter peak* may result when primary gamma rays undergo 180-degree scatter and then enter the detector and are totally absorbed. This can occur when gamma rays strike material behind the source and scatter back into the detector. It may also occur when gamma rays pass through the crystal without interaction and Compton scatter from the shield or PMTs back into the crystal.

The *lead x-ray peak* is caused by primary gamma rays undergoing photoelectric absorption in the lead of shielding or the collimator; as a result, characteristic x-rays (75 to 90 keV) are detected. The effect of Compton scattering in the detector gives a peak from 0 to 50 keV. The sharp edge at 50 keV is called the *Compton edge*. If the source of radiation is within a patient, Compton scattering occurs within the patient's tissue, and some of these scattered gamma rays travel toward the detector with an energy from 90 to 140 keV. These scattered photons from within the patient cause imaging difficulties because the Compton scatter overlaps with the photopeak distribution.

Signal intensity information is matched in the PHA against an appropriate *window,* which is really a voltage discriminator. To allow energy related to the desired isotope photopeak to be recorded, the window has upper and lower voltage limits that define the window width. Thus a 20% symmetric window for 140 keV photopeak means that the electronics will accept 140 ± 14 keV (i.e., 140 keV ± 10%) gamma rays. Any signals higher or lower than this, particularly those from scattered radiation, are rejected. Most cameras have multiple PHAs, which allow several photopeaks to be used at once. This is particularly useful for radionuclides with multiple gamma emissions of different energies, such as indium 111 (^{111}In) and gallium-67 (^{67}Ga). On newer cameras, the signal processing circuitry, such as preamplifiers and PHAs, is located on the base of each PMT, so that there is little signal distortion between the camera head and the console.

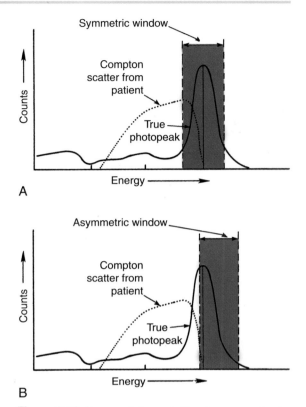

Figure 2-13. Energy windows. **A,** Use of a symmetric window allows some of the Compton scatter to be counted and displayed. **B,** Theoretically, use of an asymmetric window obviates this problem.

Console Controls

Most gamma cameras allow for a fine adjustment known as *automatic peaking* of the isotope. This essentially divides the photopeak window into halves and calculates the number of counts in each half. If the machine is correctly peaked, each half of the window has the same number of counts from the upper and lower portions of the photopeak. Occasionally, an *asymmetric window* is used to improve resolution by eliminating some of the Compton scatter (see Fig. 2-13).

Image exposure time is selected by console control and is usually a preset count, a preset time, or preset *information density* for the image accumulation. Information density refers to the number of counts per square centimeter of the gamma camera crystal face. Other console controls are present for orientation and allow the image to be reversed on the x- and y-axes.

In addition, the CRT image may be manipulated by an intensity control, which simply affects the brightness of the image, or by a

persistence control, which regulates the length of time the light dots composing the image remain on the screen. Hard copy images on film may be obtained directly from the computer, although most institutions now display digital images on monitors and store the images in a picture archiving system.

Resolution

Resolution is one of the common performance parameters for gamma cameras. Resolution usually refers to either spatial or energy resolution. *Energy resolution* is the ability to discriminate between light pulses caused by gamma rays of differing energies. *Spatial resolution* refers to the ability to display discrete but contiguous sources of radioactivity. The spatial resolution of various gamma camera systems is usually given in terms of either inherent or overall resolution. *Inherent spatial resolution* is the ability of the crystal PMT detector and accompanying electronics to record the exact location of the light pulse on the sodium iodide crystal. Gamma cameras have an inherent resolution of about 3 mm.

Statistical variability is particularly important in resolution. An event occurring exactly between two PMTs does not always give the same number of photons to each tube; thus for any single event, the distribution of photons is statistically variable. Statistical variation is relatively greater when fewer light photons are available. In other words, the inherent resolution of a system or its ability to localize an event is directly related to the energy of the isotope being imaged. When radioisotopes with low energy gamma rays or characteristic x-rays are used, the camera has less inherent spatial resolution.

Overall spatial resolution is the resolution capacity of the entire camera system, including such factors as the collimator resolution, septal penetration, and scattered radiation. The simplest method of examining overall spatial resolution is to determine the full width at half maximum (FWHM) of the line spread function. This refers to the profile response of the gamma camera to a single point source of radioactivity and reflects the number of counts seen by the crystal at different lateral distances from the source (Fig. 2-14, *A*). The source is often placed 10 cm from the crystal for these measurements. The FWHM is expressed as the width in centimeters at 50% of the height of the line spread peak. The narrower the peak, the better the resolution. When state-of-the-art cameras and ^{99m}Tc are used, the position of scintillation events can be determined to within 3 to 5 mm. A typical high resolution collimator has three times better resolution than does a representative high sensitivity collimator but allows only one tenth as many counts per minute for a given activity.

Although spatial FWHM is useful for comparing collimators, it often does not give other desirable information and does not necessarily relate to the overall clinical performance of the collimator. More difficult but perhaps more encompassing measurements of collimator performance are modulation transfer functions, which take other factors for optimizing collimator design, such as the presence of scattering material and septal penetration, into account. The value of this can be seen in Figure 2-14, *B*, which illustrates that the septal penetration occurring in the collimator may be completely undetected by the measurement of FWHM alone.

When the overall spatial resolution of the system with high energy isotopes is considered, the limiting resolution is that of the collimator.

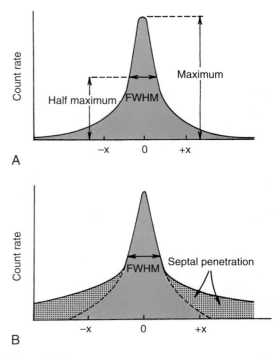

Figure 2-14. Full width at half maximum A, The full width at half maximum (FWHM) is the response in count rate to a single point source of radioactivity at different lateral distances from the point source. **B,** With septal penetration, the image may be significantly degraded even though FWHM is unchanged.

When low energy isotopes are imaged, the inherent resolution becomes more important than the collimator resolution. As the energy of the incident gamma ray decreases, the inherent resolution of the crystal decreases markedly because the lower energy gamma rays provide less light for the PMTs to record; thus there is more statistical uncertainty regarding the origin of the gamma ray. Although the inherent resolution of cameras is often championed by salespeople, the overall resolution determines the quality of the image because it is a combination of the resolutions of each of the components in the imaging chain, including the collimator, the inherent resolution, septal penetration, and scatter. The overall system resolution (R_s) is

$$R_s = \text{square root of the sum of } R^2_i + R^2_c$$

where R^2_i is inherent resolution and R^2_c is collimator resolution.

Another category of resolution is *energy resolution,* or the ability of the imaging system to separate and distinguish between the photopeaks of different radionuclides. If the energy resolution is good, the photopeaks are tall and narrow; if energy resolution is poor, the photopeaks appear as broad bumps in the energy spectrum. The FWHM concept is also used to examine energy resolution and is usually quoted for the relatively high energy (662 keV) photon of cesium-137 (^{137}Cs). With lower energy photons, the energy resolution is worse. Most gamma cameras have an energy resolution of 10% to 15%, allowing use of 15% to 20% energy windows to encompass all of the photons of interest.

Count Rate and Dead Time

As with any detection system, it is important that scintillation events do not occur so fast that the electronic system is unable to count each as a separate event. If two equal light pulses occur too close together in time, the system may perceive this as one event with twice the energy actually present. Such an occurrence of primary photons would be eliminated by the energy window of the PHA, and none of the information from the two events would be imaged; thus the sensitivity of the system would be diminished. A more significant problem is loss of spatial resolution when several scattered (low energy) photons strike the crystal at the same time, so that their light production is summed and mimics a primary photon of interest. The time after an event during which the system is unable to respond to another event is referred to as *dead time*. Dead time can be important in high count rate dynamic studies (in the range of 50,000 counts/second), particularly with single crystal cameras. An example is a first-pass cardiac study.

Field Uniformity

Despite the efforts of manufacturers to produce high quality collimators, crystals, PMTs, and electronics, nonuniformity inevitably occurs. Acceptable field nonuniformity is on the order of 2% to 5%. Much of this can be corrected by the computer system. Analysis of field uniformity is discussed later in the chapter.

Image Acquisition: Memory and Matrix Size

Data may be acquired either by *frame mode* or by *list mode*. In the frame mode, incoming data are placed in a spatial matrix in the memory that is used to generate an image. In the list mode, all data are put in the memory as a time sequence list of events. At regular intervals, a special code word is inserted into the list. This list is flexible and can be sorted or divided into images at a later time. The list mode has the disadvantage of a low acquisition rate and a large memory requirement. Frame mode uses much less memory than does the list mode and is more commonly used, except for gated cardiac studies. All data for images that are collected in the frame mode are acquired in a matrix. The usual image matrix sizes are 64 × 64 and 128 × 128, although 32 × 32 and 256 × 256 matrix sizes are occasionally used. The main disadvantage of frame mode is that the identity of individual events within a time frame is lost.

Matrix size refers to the number of picture elements along each side of the matrix. These elements may be either bytes or words. In an 8-bit computer, both a byte and a word are composed of 8 bits. In a 16-bit computer, a byte is 8 bits and a word is 16 bits. The maximum number of counts that can be represented by an 8-bit picture element (pixel) is 2^8, or 0 through 255 (256 different values). Ordinarily, 16-bit collections are used; the maximum size is 2^{16}, or 0 through 65,535 (65,536 different values) per pixel.

The matrix size determines the image resolution. Although the matrix size and the number of counts desired have a significant impact on memory required, the ultimate memory requirements depend on what the computer system is being used for and how many cameras it is interfaced with simultaneously. The matrix size has nothing to do with the final size of the displayed image. A 32 × 32 matrix has relatively few pixels; therefore the final image is coarse. An image obtained in a 256 × 256 acquisition matrix is much more detailed. Remember that an image resolution of 256 × 256 may refer to either the memory acquisition matrix or the CRT display matrix. Some manufacturers take a 64 × 64 matrix image from the memory and display it on the CRT in a 256 × 256 or 1024 × 1024 matrix, using interpolation methods.

The 32 × 32 matrix occupies less memory and therefore less disk space. In addition, it can be acquired faster than can a finer matrix. Thus there is a trade-off between spatial and temporal resolution. In a 32 × 32 matrix, the spatial resolution is poor, but, because it can be acquired rapidly, the temporal resolution is excellent. For a given computer system, the matrix size desired for acquisition and the read–write speed of the hard disk dictate the maximum framing rate that is possible.

The amount of memory determines the number of frames that can be collected in the electrocardiographic R-R interval on electrocardiogram gated cardiac studies. For optimum measurement of ejection fraction, at least 25 frames/second are needed. If peak ejection or peak filling rate is to be measured, 50 frames/second are needed.

Image Display and Processing

Image display and processing is necessary in all nuclear medicine computer systems. The computer plays an extremely important role in lesion detectability, and it can perform this function in a number of ways, including reduction of noise, background subtraction, construction of cine loops, and production of tomographic images. Data are normally collected in 64 × 64 byte images. Although a 32 × 32 byte mode can be used, the decrease in spatial resolution is usually intolerable. Even in 64 × 64 pixel images, there is a noticeable saw-toothed appearance to the image edges. Because the pixel matrix achieved on a display video is 1024 × 1024 with 256 levels of gray, the data are usually processed to use all of the pixels. The simplest method to fill in the extra pixels is linear interpolation.

To reduce the effects of statistical variation, particularly in low count images, the image can be smoothed. Smoothing is accomplished through the use of filters, which may be either spatial or temporal. Temporal filters are used for dynamic acquisition, and spatial filters are used on static images. Spatial filters attempt to remove statistical fluctuations of the image by modifying values of data points within various pixels.

Spatial Filters

The processing performed by spatial filters is done according to the spatial frequencies of the information. By attenuating or augmenting parts of the spatial frequency spectrum, an image should be obtained that is easier to interpret or that has more diagnostic value. The simplest smoothing method is nine-point smoothing. This takes 9 pixels of information and, by taking weighted averages of the 8 pixels on the edge of a central pixel, changes the value of that central pixel.

Other kinds of filters that are commonly used are low-pass, high-pass, and band-pass filters.

A low-pass filter selectively attenuates high frequencies and smoothes the image by removing high-frequency noise. This filtering improves the statistical quality of an image but degrades the sharpness and spatial resolution. Figure 2-15, *A*, shows an example of low-pass filtering applied to data from a SPECT liver scan. High-pass filtering enhances edges to some extent but also augments the noise (see Fig. 2-15, *B*). This type of filtering is important in cardiac nuclear medicine when locating the edge of the ventricle is needed. A band-pass filter is a combination of low-pass and high-pass filters that effectively suppresses high-frequency and low-frequency signals and transmits only signals that are in a given spatial frequency window.

A simple way of performing low-pass filtering is by the addition of dynamic images. Remember that dynamic images have a low number of counts in each pixel and are therefore usually in the byte mode. Thus the highest number of counts that can be stored in a pixel is 255. When adding images, it is necessary to change from the byte mode to the word mode so that the maximum number of counts that can be accommodated in each pixel is expanded. If the computer is in the byte mode and the number of counts per pixel exceeds 255, the computer begins counting at 0 again for that pixel. This results in a negative defect (rollover artifact) in areas that would normally have a high count rate. An example of this is seen in Figure 2-15, *A*.

Temporal Filters

Temporal filters are used on dynamic images and involve a weighted averaging technique between each pixel on one image and the same pixel from the frames before and after. Temporal filtering causes a loss of spatial resolution but allows a cine loop to be viewed without flicker. Remember that temporal filtering of dynamic studies does not preclude spatial filtering of the same study, and, in fact, the two processes are frequently performed together.

Frame Manipulation

Another common computer image-processing application is frame subtraction. This method may be used for background subtraction and for subtraction of studies performed simultaneously with two different radionuclides. Although less commonly used, additional computer capabilities include frame multiplication

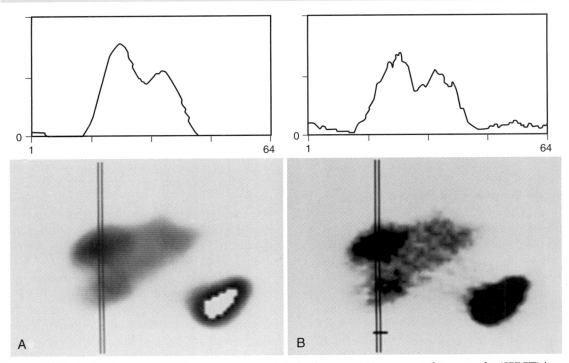

Figure 2-15. Application of spatial filtering to a coronal single-photon emission computed tomography (SPECT) image of the liver and spleen. Histograms of the activity defined in a linear region of interest are shown in the upper portions of **A** and **B**. The reconstructed tomographic images are shown in the lower portions (*left*, liver; *right*, spleen). **A**, A low-pass filter removes high frequencies and smoothes the image. Rollover artifact is seen as the white area in the central portion of the spleen. **B**, With a high-pass filter, the image appears noisier, but edges are enhanced.

and division. Combinations of the maneuvers may be used to produce the so-called functional parametric images obtained from radionuclide ventriculography.

Operator Interaction

The operator interacts with the computer in one of two ways, either by selecting from a menu or by using a command structure. The menu system requires sequential choices from a list or menu presented on the video terminal. Although the menu system is somewhat slower than is the command system, the operator does not need to be familiar with all of the possible commands (usually about 100 commands that are chosen through use of a two- or three-letter mnemonic).

Interaction of the operator with the computer also occurs when a region of interest is selected. This can be done by moving a cursor, light pen, trackball, mouse, or joystick. Once a region of interest is defined, the operator can perform various functions: the most common of which is determining the total number of counts within the region of interest. A region of interest can be maintained over multiple frames to produce a dynamic time-activity curve.

SINGLE-PHOTON EMISSION COMPUTED TOMOGRAPHY

The successful application of computer algorithms to x-ray imaging in computed tomography (CT) has led to their application to radionuclide techniques and to the advent of single-photon emission computed tomography (SPECT) and positron emission tomography (PET). Although planar radionuclide organ imaging in multiple views is sufficient for many clinical settings, tomography offers several readily apparent advantages over two-dimensional planar images. The most obvious advantage of tomography is improved image contrast because it focuses on a thin slice of an organ, thus minimizing overlying and underlying activity that may obscure a lesion or area of interest. In addition, SPECT and PET permit absolute three-dimensional localization of radiopharmaceutical distribution, with the possibility of quantification and three-dimensional cinematic representation of the organ imaged.

Emission CT can be accomplished by one of two main techniques: (1) transverse or rotational tomography (usual for SPECT) or (2) fixed-ring detector (usual for PET). Although both approaches have been clinically applied with

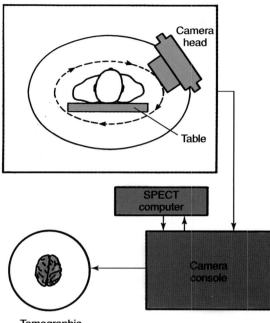

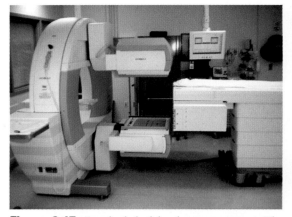

Figure 2-17. Standard dual head gamma camera. The detector heads are in the common opposed configuration. The rod in between the heads contains radioactive sources and is part of the automated quality control program.

Figure 2-16. Schematic representation of a single-photon emission computed tomography (SPECT) system using a single camera head. The camera detector usually rotates around the patient in a noncircular orbit while acquiring data to be fed to the computer. The tomographic computer-reconstructed images are subsequently displayed.

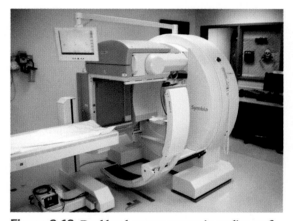

Figure 2-18. Dual head gamma camera in cardiac configuration with attenuation correction. The large rectangular camera heads have been moved to a perpendicular configuration. The gadolinium sources used for attenuation correction are contained in the crescentic structures opposite each camera head.

success, rotational techniques have enjoyed widespread application. The purpose of this section is to describe SPECT instrumentation and principles. Clinical applications of each technique are discussed later in the organ system chapters. Most modern gamma cameras have rotating detector heads and thus are SPECT capable.

Instrumentation

In its simplest form, rotational SPECT is accomplished by using a conventional gamma (Anger) camera detector head and a parallel hole or hybrid collimator fitted to a rotating gantry. The detector is capable of orbiting around a stationary patient on a special imaging table, with the camera face continually directed toward the patient. The camera head rotates around a central axis called the *axis of rotation* (AOR). The distance of the camera face from this central axis is referred to as the *radius of rotation* (ROR). The orbit may be circular, with a 360-degree capacity, although elliptical (Fig. 2-16) or body contour motions are also used. Rotational arcs of less than 360 degrees may be used, particularly for cardiac studies. The detector electronics

are coupled with a computer capable of performing acquisition and processing of the image data according to preselected parameters. The gamma camera is capable of acquiring data from a large volume of the patient during a single orbit, and multiple slices (sections) are produced from just one data acquisition sequence. More complex systems using multiple camera heads are also in widespread use. The various camera head configurations are shown in Figures 2-17 and 2-18.

Minor artifacts and inconsistencies can be tolerated in planar imaging, but they cause major problems with SPECT. As the principal component of the SPECT imaging system, the gamma camera must be state of the art, with an intrinsic resolution of at least 3 to 4 mm, an absolute linearity deviation of less than 1 mm, and a basic uncorrected uniformity deviation of 3% to 5% or less across the useful field of view of the detector. A system with excellent energy resolution is needed to permit adequate rejection of scattered radiation, a major degrader of contrast in SPECT images. This is enhanced by an autotune feature, which continually tunes and balances the PMTs of the detector during the operation. Although count rate capacity of the camera is not critical in SPECT, the system should be able to handle significantly high count rates to avoid any field uniformity distortion caused by high–count-rate effects.

The rotation of the detector on the gantry subjects the camera head to thermal, magnetic, and gravitational forces not experienced by planar instruments, and the system construction must take these factors into consideration. This includes shielding of the PMTs with a mu metal to protect against changing magnetic fields during rotation.

Several manufacturers have introduced dedicated cardiac SPECT cameras. These typically have a 180-degree detector array directed at the anterior and lateral left chest. Some are designed for small spaces and one can scan the patient in the sitting position. They use either sodium iodide or cadmium zinc telluride (CZT) detectors. By optimizing the collimator, detector design and by imaging only the cardiac area they are able to increase count sensitivity, shorten imaging time, and somewhat improve spatial resolution. There is also the possibility to reduce administered activity. In studies comparing these devices with conventional SPECT the agreement rate for presence or absence of perfusion defects was 92% to 96%. The main advantage appears to be shorter imaging time or, alternatively, the possibility of employing lower administered doses of radiopharmaceuticals. The downside of these devices is that they are limited to cardiac studies and cannot be used for most other types of examination.

Data Acquisition

The data required to produce diagnostic SPECT images are usually acquired as a series of multiple planar images collected at discrete angular intervals or in continuous acquisition as the detector head moves around the patient. In the step-and-shoot technique, the orbit of the camera is interrupted at regular angular intervals, referred to as azimuth *stops*, so that an image may be recorded for a specified period of time at each of the stops. For example, a 360-degree acquisition orbit using 60 stops yields 60 planar images obtained at 6-degree intervals. If each image is acquired for 20 seconds, then the entire scanning time will require 20 minutes plus the small amount of time needed to move the detector head from each stop to the next. For practical reasons, a compromise must be reached regarding the number of stops and the scanning time at each stop needed to produce tomographic images of good statistical quality. These factors are largely dictated by the type of study, amount of radiopharmaceutical used, patient motion considerations, and specific resolution requirements.

A 360-degree arc is usually required for most SPECT acquisitions. An arc of 180 degrees may be preferred, however, for certain studies such as cardiac perfusion imaging. With any given arc, the more individual projections or views obtained, the better the quality of the reconstructed images. Because the time allotted for obtaining each projection multiplied by the number of projections (usually about 15 to 20 seconds per stop in most studies) essentially determines the length of the study, an increase in the number of projections typically results in a decrease in the time at each stop. Each planar view obtained, however, must be statistically significant (sufficient counts per pixel) for adequate reconstructed images. Therefore fewer views obtained at longer times are generally used in count-poor studies, such as perfusion brain imaging, whereas a greater number of images at shorter times may be used for count-rich examinations, such as sulfur colloid liver scans. In typical clinical applications, about 32 stops per 180 degrees of rotation (64 stops per 360 degrees) are obtained to produce acceptable images.

In general, the smaller the orbital ROR or the closer the camera head is to the patient, the greater the potential resolution of the tomographic images. Thus RORs should be kept as small as feasible. Standard circular orbits are frequently not ideally suited for imaging noncircular body parts, such as the chest or abdomen, because the camera distance varies significantly according to its orbital position. Furthermore, unless the detector head is small, imaging smaller body parts such as the head may be compromised by the need for a larger-than-desired ROR dictated by the shoulders and upper torso. Noncircular orbits and body contour orbits have the potential to solve these problems.

Specific parameters for acquisition of clinical SPECT images are presented in more detail in chapters concerning specific organ systems and procedures and in Appendix E. However, a few generalizations may prove helpful. Optimally, a clinical imaging department seeks the highest-quality images with the best resolution achievable in the shortest time. Practically, the usual trade-offs between resolution and sensitivity must be made, which require the selection of a specific set of acquisition parameters for each study.

Attenuation Correction

Photons attenuated by overlying soft tissue are a major source of artifactual defects on both planar and SPECT radionuclide images. This is particularly true in SPECT myocardial perfusion imaging, in which artifacts produced by breast and diaphragmatic attenuation are a primary cause of false-positive examinations. Thus some form of correction to prevent these artifacts is desirable.

More recent methods solve this problem by obtaining a patient-specific transmission map of body thickness and contour. This is usually accomplished by using an external line source of an isotope with a long half-life, such as gadolinium-153 (^{153}Gd) or americium-241 (^{241}Am), that rotates on the opposite side of the patient from the camera detector during SPECT imaging, producing a transmission image as the external photons pass through the patient. This image resembles a poor-quality CT scan, but the data are good enough to perform attenuation correction when applied to the emission image of the organ of interest, such as the heart. Depending on the difference between the photon energies of the radioisotopes used, the emission and transmission images may be obtained simultaneously by using two different pulse-height windows. SPECT-CT hybrid instruments that obtain statistically rich x-ray transmission scans in a very short time solve many of the issues associated with radioisotope–based attenuation correction methods and afford better anatomic localization of abnormal radiopharmaceutical accumulations.

Acquisition Time

An acquisition time that allows adequate image statistics is mandatory for the production of diagnostic images. This is in large part determined by count rate, matrix size, and number of projections per orbit. Obviously, the longer the acquisition, the more counts collected and the better the image resolution. Typical patient tolerance for acquisition times, however, makes 30 to 45 minutes a realistic maximum. Thus times per projection (stop) must be predicated on an appraisal of the patient's ability to remain still. Any significant motion by the patient during acquisition may render the results unusable.

Image Matrix Size

The two matrix sizes commonly used in SPECT images are 64 × 64 and 128 × 128. With increased matrix size, however, come the trade-offs of substantial increases in acquisition time, processing time, and contiguous disk storage space. Selection of a 128 × 128 matrix over a 64 × 64 matrix requires a fourfold increase in most acquisition aspects of the study, including time, which may not be worth the added spatial resolution. Furthermore, the count density in tomographic slices acquired in a 128 × 128 matrix is reduced by a factor of 8, which adversely affects perceived image contrast. In most clinical studies, the 64 × 64 matrix may be the best compromise.

Number of Views

Generally, the more views obtained, the better the image resolution possible. A compromise with total imaging time must be reached, however, so that use of 64 views over a 360-degree orbit commonly produces adequate tomograms.

Tomographic Image Production
Image Reconstruction

The data available in the multiple digitized images are combined and manipulated by the computer using mathematic algorithms to reconstruct a three-dimensional image of the organ scanned. One method to accomplish this is known as *back projection*, which produces a transaxial view of the organ by applying the technique to the data in each of the planar views acquired. Unfortunately, simple back projection produces a composite image with significant artifacts (principally the "starburst" artifact) that seriously degrade the quality of the image, rendering it clinically unusable. For this reason, a refined technique called *filtered back projection* was developed.

As modern computers have become more computationally powerful, *iterative* algorithms for reconstruction have been used in place of filtered back projection. Such processing can give better image quality compared with that of the filtered back-projection algorithm. Further, the streak artifact observed when an area of the body is significantly more radioactive relative to its surroundings (e.g., the bladder on bone scans) is often severe with filtered back projection but is markedly improved by using iterative techniques for bone SPECT studies. Once reconstructed, the tomographic views are still in need of further filtering to produce acceptable images for interpretation.

Image Filtering

Image filtering of raw data has become a standard nuclear technique for producing processed images that are visually pleasing and yet preserve the integrity of the acquired data. Essentially, filtering algorithms improve image quality by reducing noise.

Filters are mathematic operations designed to enhance, smooth, or suppress all or part of digital image data, ideally without altering their validity. In SPECT, however, image filtering not only enhances the data presentation but also is a basic requirement for the production of the reconstructed sections.

Filters used in SPECT are usually expressed in terms of their effect on spatial frequencies; hence, the term *frequency filtering*. Filters can be described by the frequencies that they allow to pass through into the final image. Noise in such images is generally predominant at high spatial frequencies. High-pass filters (passing more relatively high frequencies) generally produce sharper, but noisier, images with enhanced edge definition; low-pass filters (passing fewer high frequencies) render smoother, less noisy images with less distinct edges. When applied, filtering may be performed in one, two, or three dimensions. Three-dimensional filtering allows filtering between transaxial slices and is commonly applied in SPECT image processing.

In SPECT image production, filtering can be done before, during, or after transaxial reconstruction. To avoid artifacts, accurate back-projection reconstruction requires correction of all spatial frequencies through the use of a *ramp filter*. Many different filters are usually available in the SPECT software, and selection depends on a number of factors, including the study being performed, the statistical character of the acquired images, and operator bias. The default filter commonly used for filtering SPECT images is the Butterworth filter.

Image Display

After being processed, the acquired data may be displayed visually as a three-dimensional representation of the part of the body imaged. This is usually presented cinematically as an image of the body turning continually in space, the so-called rotating-man image. This view is useful in three-dimensional localization and also in determining whether any significant patient motion occurred during the acquisition. In addition to the transaxial tomographic slices provided, the data can also be easily manipulated to render tomographic sections of the body in standard coronal and sagittal planes, as well as in any oblique planes required by the organ being imaged. Oblique reconstructions are frequently used in cardiac perfusion imaging.

Although current methodology allows the production of high-quality diagnostic images for qualitative interpretation, the inherent problems of photon attenuation with depth and the imperfect attenuation methods available render absolute quantitation of radionuclide distribution difficult. Semiquantitative methods of comparing image data with normal distribution, as defined by large series of normal patients, have met with some success.

SPECT/CT

The success of PET/CT systems has prompted an interest in SPECT/CT systems. The typical system involves two rotating gamma camera SPECT heads combined with a CT scanner (Fig. 2-19). The gamma camera portion has the same characteristics as the SPECT cameras just discussed. A SPECT/CT system has several advantages, including accurately co-registered SPECT and anatomic CT images as well as data-rich attenuation correction using CT transmission images. CT attenuation correction allows for better quantification of radiotracer uptake than with other methods. The incorporated CT scanners are typically less expensive versions of standard multidetector helical CT scanners. Most

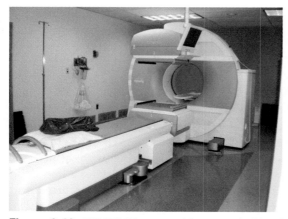

Figure 2-19. SPECT/CT scanner. There is a dual head gamma camera located in front of the CT scanner gantry and bore. *CT*, Computed tomography.

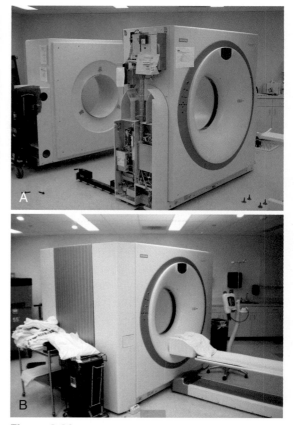

Figure 2-20. PET/CT scanner. The machine is essentially a CT scanner placed adjacent to a PET scanner. Here the machine is shown at installation (**A**) and operational (**B**) with a CT scanner in the front and PET scanner behind.

have only 1 to 16 rows of detectors, which has limited their usefulness for gated cardiac scans.

The CT scanners can be operated as "low dose nondiagnostic" scans or in regular diagnostic mode. Low dose CT has an effective dose in the range of 1 to 4 mSv whereas a diagnostic scan has an effective dose of up to 14 mSv. Using the diagnostic mode provides more accurate interpretation and is often more convenient for the patient, eliminating the need to return for a dedicated CT scan. Examples of SPECT/CT scans are provided later in the various chapters.

POSITRON EMISSION TOMOGRAPHY

All commercially available PET cameras now come as hybrid PET/CT scanners (Fig. 2-20, *A* and *B*). The CT specifics are discussed later in the chapter. The relatively limited integration of the PET and CT hardware allows easy upgrades when advances occur in either modality. Primary integration has occurred in the software to reduce complexity and to present similar menu appearances. The following section refers to the PET detection system of a PET/CT scanner.

Overview of PET Cameras

PET cameras contain multiple rings of detectors consisting of scintillation crystals coupled with photomultiplier tubes (PMTs). The ring design takes advantage of the fact that two photons detected in close temporal proximity by two opposed detectors in the ring are likely to be from a single annihilation event. Such a simultaneous detection event is called a *coincidence*.

The near simultaneous detection of two photons provides localizing information in that the annihilation event can be assumed to have occurred somewhere on a line between the two detectors (the line of response, or LOR). The many coincidence events recorded by the PET scanner constitute a raw data set representing projections of the distribution of the positron radiopharmaceutical in the body. These data are then reconstructed by using a filtered back projection algorithm or an iterative algorithm to produce cross-sectional images.

Because photons travel at the speed of light, PET cameras require very fast electronics to determine whether two detected photons were likely produced by a single annihilation event. In a PET scanner, each annihilation photon reaching a detector generates a single electronic pulse in the detector. For this photon to be accepted and used in the PET image, it must be in a specific energy range (ideally approaching 511 keV) and be paired with another photon reaching another detector simultaneously. Coincidence circuitry connecting the many detectors in the rings determines whether two such single pulses (representing the captured photons in opposing detectors) fall within a short *coincidence time window,* typically 6 to 12 nanoseconds. If so, they are deemed to constitute a coincidence event and are recorded in the resultant image. The actual coincidence time is typically about 1 nanosecond. However, the time window for coincidence detection varies with different camera systems and depends in large part on the speed of the electronic circuitry and detector scintillation crystal type. It is about 12 nanoseconds for bismuth germanium oxide (BGO), 8 nanoseconds for gadolinium oxyorthosilicate (GSO) and sodium iodide (NaI), and 6 nanoseconds for lutetium oxyorthosilicate (LSO) systems. Because the energy resolution of the various crystal detectors is not precise, photons within a broad energy range ($\approx$250 to 600 keV) are counted as valid annihilation photons.

Because of detector ring geometry and photon attenuation through scatter and absorption, many annihilation events result in only one of the two 511 keV photons interacting with the PET camera detectors (single event). Consequently, a very large number of such single events are incident on the PET detectors. Because PET scanners use only photon pairs meeting the coincidence criterion in constructing PET images, single counts can be identified and discarded. In practice, about 99% of detected photons are rejected by the coincidence circuitry of the PET system. However, this principle of coincidence detection provides a virtual electronic collimation of the events and makes PET scanners inherently more efficient than are traditional gamma cameras, which use parallel hole lead collimators.

Events detected by PET scanners include true, scattered, and random events, all of which may be recorded as coincidences, provided that both annihilation photons are actually detected and fall within the coincidence window. True coincidences are those that result when both 511 keV photons from an annihilation reaction are detected within the coincidence time window, neither photon having undergone any form of interaction before reaching the detector. These true coincidence events provide the desired information for constructing accurate images of the distribution of a PET radiopharmaceutical in clinical imaging.

When a positron is emitted, it travels for a short distance from its site of origin, gradually losing energy to the tissue through which it moves. When most of its kinetic energy has been lost, the positron reacts with a resident electron in an annihilation reaction. This reaction generates two 511 keV gamma photons, which are emitted in opposite directions at about (but not exactly) 180 degrees from each other. In a PET scanner, these photons interact with the detector ring at opposite sites, which defines a line along which the annihilation reaction occurred and permits localization of the reaction (Fig. 2-21). By using many such events, an image can be reconstructed.

It is important to remember that the site of origin of the positron and the site of the annihilation reaction occur at slightly different locations. Positrons are not all emitted with the same energy, and, therefore the distance the positron travels before annihilation varies for each specific radionuclide (Fig. 2-22). For example, the positrons from fluorine-18 (^{18}F; 640 keV) and carbon-11 (^{11}C; 960 keV) have a range in water of about 1 to 1.5 mm and 2.4 mm in tissue, whereas rubidium 82 ([82]Rb; 3.35 MeV) has a range of about 14 mm in water and 16 mm in tissue before annihilation. The fact that the positron travels a distance before annihilation causes some uncertainty in determining the original location of the positron (range-related uncertainty). Further, the two resultant annihilation photons may actually be emitted up to $\pm$0.25 degrees from the theoretical 180 degrees (Fig. 2-23). This variation in emission angles (noncolinearity) also generates some uncertainty in the original location of the annihilation reaction.

Scattered coincidences occur when one or both annihilation photons undergo Compton interaction in body tissues and are deflected away from their expected path but still reach the detectors within the time window and are recorded as a coincidence event (Fig. 2-24). Because the direction of the scattered photon has changed during the Compton interaction, the resulting coincidence event is likely to be assigned an inaccurate LOR that no longer passes though the point of annihilation, leading to erroneous localization information and decreasing image contrast.

Random coincidences arise when two photons, each originating from a different annihilation reaction, reach any detector within the

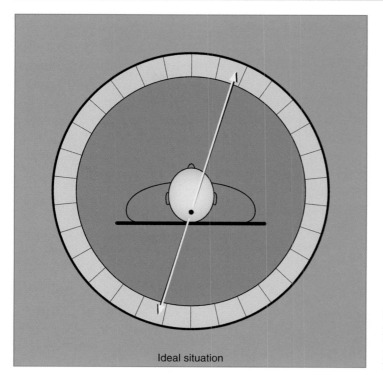

Ideal situation

Figure 2-21. Positron emission tomography. In the ideal situation, annihilation photons would be emitted at exactly the same point as the positron emission occurred and would travel in exactly opposite directions.

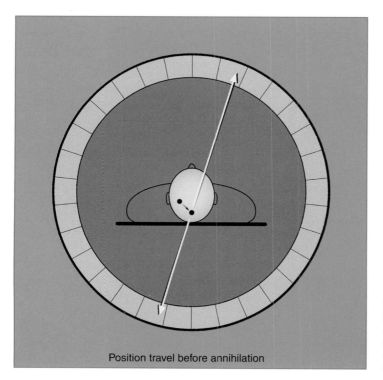

Position travel before annihilation

Figure 2-22. Image degradation caused by positron travel. Positron travel after emission and before interacting with an electron results in the scanner localizing the event at some distance from the actual site of the positron emission.

time window and thus appear to represent a true coincidence (Fig. 2-25). Using detectors that allow very precise timing permits the recognition and exclusion of random events with a resultant improvement in image quality. If left uncorrected, both scattered and random coincidences add background to the true coincidence distribution, thereby increasing statistical noise, decreasing contrast, and causing the radioisotope concentrations to be overestimated.

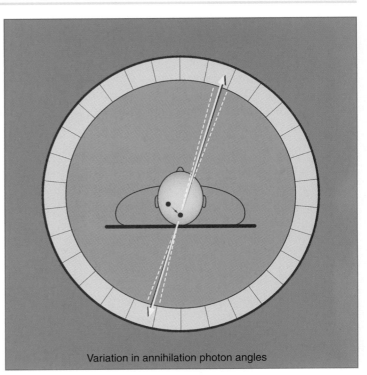

Figure 2-23. Image degradation caused by angle of photon emission. Slight variation in angle of emission of the annihilation photons results in the scanner placing the event at some distance from where the annihilation actually occurred, causing additional loss of spatial resolution.

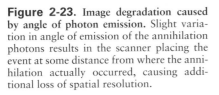

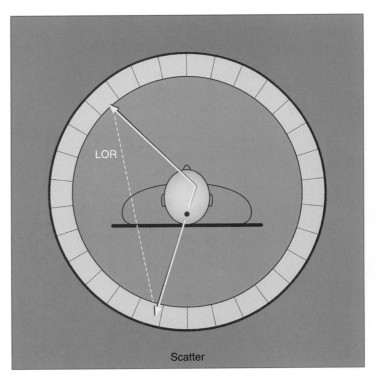

Figure 2-24. Image degradation caused by scatter of photons. Scatter of an annihilation photon after emission can result in the scanner assuming that the positron emission took place on a line of response (LOR) very far from the actual event.

There are a number of methods available to reduce the image degrading impact of scattered coincidences. Most scattered photons are not detected because they are absorbed in tissues of the body, are scattered away from the detector rings, or have lost significant energy during Compton scattering. These lower energy scattered events can be rejected by using an energy window designed to exclude photons of certain energies. The success of such rejection depends

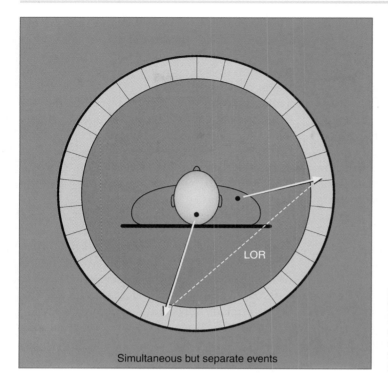

Figure 2-25. Image degradation caused by simultaneous separate events. Photons being recorded from separate but almost simultaneous events will result in the scanner assuming that the positron emission took place on a line of response (LOR) very far from the actual event.

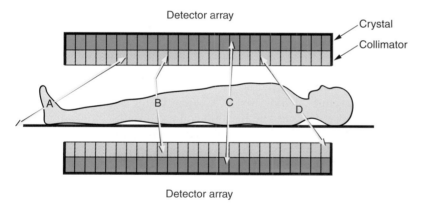

Figure 2-26. Two-dimensional acquisition. Two-dimensional acquisition is essentially slice acquisition performed with septa or collimation in place. *A*, The collimation results in annihilation photons occurring outside opposing detector elements and *B*, scattered photons being unable to reach the detector. *C*, Photons occurring in the "slice" seen by opposing detectors are recorded, whereas *D*, photons emitted at steep angles are not able to reach the detector elements.

on the energy resolution characteristics of the detectors being used. Because crystal detectors have only a finite energy resolution, if one were to measure only photons approaching 511 keV and exclude scattered photons of slightly different energies, a large number of true events would also be excluded, thereby either reducing image statistics or increasing image acquisition times unacceptably. Therefore a rather broad energy window is used that allows some scattered events to be recorded as true events.

Another method to reduce scatter from outside the plane of a detector ring is to use thin lead or

tungsten septa positioned between the detector elements. Imaging with lead septa is called two-dimensional (or slice) imaging because most of the photons counted originate in the plane of a single detector ring. Two-dimensional imaging improves image quality by reducing image noise (Fig. 2-26). It also minimizes count losses related to system dead time by incidentally reducing the very large numbers of photons reaching the detectors that may occur at high count rates. However, although this reduces the number of scattered events originating outside of the field of view (FOV), it also significantly reduces the true counts and increases imaging times.

Faster detector crystals and faster electronics in new PET instruments have made imaging without septa, so-called three-dimensional (or volume) imaging possible (Fig. 2-27). This allows imaging from the volume defined by the entire FOV of the multiple detector rings of the camera and permits detection of true coincidence events that occur in different detectors on different rings. Compared with two-dimensional imaging, three-dimensional acquisitions increase sensitivity of the system by fivefold or more. However, because both true coincidence and scatter rates are increased, better temporal and energy resolutions are needed to accurately eliminate scatter and random events.

PET Scintillation Detectors

All positron systems use the principle of scintillation whereby the photon interacting with a crystal produces a flash of light, which is then detected and localized by photomultiplier tubes (PMTs) coupled to the scintillation crystal. The ideal PET crystal detector would have (1) high stopping power for 511 keV photons providing high efficiency and optimum spatial resolution; (2) fast, intense light output with rapid decay of the light for decreased system dead time; and (3) good energy resolution for accurate scatter rejection. Stopping power is best for crystalline materials with high density and high effective atomic number (Z value). There are several types of crystalline detector materials used for PET imaging. These include sodium iodide (NaI), bismuth germinate (BGO), lutetium oxyorthosilicate (LSO), and gadolinium oxyorthosilicate (GSO).

BGO has the poorest energy resolution, whereas NaI has the best energy resolution as a result of the highest light output. The energy resolution of BGO crystals requires that a wide energy window (≈250 to 600 keV) be used to avoid rejecting true events and reducing the detected count rate. The use of a wide energy window means that a BGO detector system will accept more scattered events than will the other systems with better energy resolution. NaI systems use a narrower energy window than do BGO, LSO, or GSO systems.

The light signal produced by scintillation detectors is not discrete in time but occurs over a short time interval (scintillation decay time, 10 to 300 nanoseconds), which includes the period over which the light fades to background. Along with the speed of processing electronics, this decay time is an important determinant of system dead time. Dead time is the brief period during which a crystal-PMT detector is busy producing and recording a scintillation event and having the scintillation light decay so that the next distinct scintillation event can be recognized and recorded. During this time, additional arriving events cannot be processed and are lost. This limits the rate at which events may be detected. High count rate capability of PET instruments is particularly important in three-dimensional acquisitions and in settings requiring high activities of very short-lived radionuclides (e.g., oxygen 15). Current count rate capabilities are about 500,000 counts/second.

The relatively long decay times of both BGO and NaI crystals limit count rate capability. The shorter decay time of light output for LSO crystals can reduce scan times for comparable

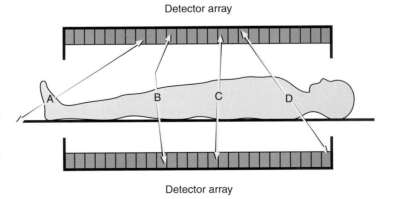

Detector array

Detector array

Figure 2-27. Three-dimensional acquisition. Three-dimensional acquisition is essentially volumetric acquisition, and collimation or septa are not used. As a result, many more events are detected per unit of time than with two-dimensional acquisition. *A,* Although events occurring outside of the volume are not recorded because the second photon is not interacting with a detector, *B,* scattered, *C,* central, and *D,* steep angle events are all recorded.

images to about half of the time required for BGO systems. LSO crystals probably have the best combination of properties for optimizing PET imaging, especially in three-dimensional imaging systems (without septa) with the potential for very high count rates.

PET Detector Geometry

State-of-the-art PET scanners are multidetector full ring (circular or polygonal) systems that axially surround the patient (360 degrees). These cameras have multiple adjacent detector rings that significantly increase the axial FOV of the patient. A larger FOV allows more counts to be detected for a standardized administered radiopharmaceutical dose and a fixed scan time by allowing more time at each table position.

The most common detector arrangement used in dedicated PET cameras consists of rings of individual detector modules of small crystal arrays or cut block scintillation crystals (usually BGO or LSO) coupled with PMTs (Fig. 2-28). In crystal arrays, multiple separate, very small (≈4 mm front surface edge) scintillation crystals are grouped together in blocks, often arranged in 6 × 6 or 8 × 8 blocks (36 to 64 "crystals" per detector block). This concept is more

economically achieved by using a single crystalline block onto which deep channels have been cut, forming a matrix (8 × 8 or 64 elements) on the face of the block. The channels in the crystal are filled with opaque material so that the light from scintillation events cannot spread between sections but travels toward the PMTs only. This achieves the effect of multiple small crystalline detectors.

Many such blocks (hundreds) are then assembled to form a crystal ring. The light from each block is collected by PMTs (about four per block) servicing the entire block of crystals. Even though the number of PMTs per block is far less than the number of individual crystal elements, it is still possible to attribute each light pulse to a particular crystal for localization by comparing pulse heights in each of the PMTs. Current full multi-ring PET scanners have 10,000 to 20,000 "crystals" arranged in about 200 to 400 blocks and with about 500 to 1000 PMTs. For multicrystal PET cameras, the intrinsic spatial resolution is a function of the crystal size; thus the small sizes of the crystal faces allowed by block design permits optimization of intrinsic resolution. Further, a large number of small independent detectors in a PET system significantly

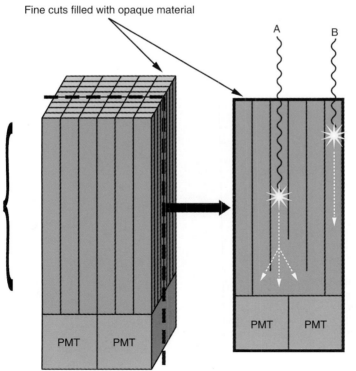

Fine cuts filled with opaque material

Crystal detector block

A   B

PMT   PMT

PMT   PMT

Figure 2-28. PET scintillation block detector. Many crystal detectors are made from a single block of material and have cuts made to different depths and filled with opaque material. There are often 8 × 8 detector elements made, and the different depths of cuts allow localization with only four photomultiplier tubes *PMTs. A,* If a photon interacts with a central detector element, the shallow cut allows the light from the scintillation to be localized by several PMTs. *B,* A photon interacting with a detector element near the edge of the block may have light that is seen by one PMT only.

reduces dead time count losses and allows camera operation at higher count rates.

With ring detectors of any sort, resolution varies with location in the FOV. As an annihilation event gets closer to the edge of the FOV, more image blurring occurs because the path of an annihilation photon may traverse more than one detector element and is capable of producing a scintillation in any of them (Fig. 2-29).

Alternative detector arrangements to the small "multi-crystal" complete ring design have been available. These include a hexagonal array or a ring of large curved thallium-doped sodium iodide (NaI[Tl]), crystals, and dual opposed arcs of small detectors that rotate around the axis of the patient to acquire data. There are advantages and disadvantages to these alternative configurations. Because septa are not typically used with these systems, only three-dimensional imaging is used.

Attenuation Correction

Attenuation is the loss of true events through photon absorption in the body or by scattering out of the detector FOV. Attenuation problems are significantly worse with PET imaging than with SPECT. Even though the energy of the annihilation photons is greater than for single-photon imaging, with PET, two photons must escape the patient to be detected and the mean photon path is longer, increasing the likelihood of attenuation. In a large person, the loss of counts attributable to attenuation can exceed 50% to 95%.

Loss of counts through attenuation increases image noise, artifacts, and distortion. Significant artifacts may occur on whole-body PET images obtained without attenuation correction. These include the following: (1) distortions of areas of high activity (such as the bladder) as a result of variable attenuation in different directions, (2) a prominent body surface edge ("hot skin"), and (3) apparently high count rates (increased activity) in tissues of low attenuation, such as the lungs. As a result, attenuation correction of these images is necessary before the true amount of radionuclide present at various locations in the body can be accurately determined. This is true both for accurate qualitative assessment of activity distribution on regional or whole-body images and for precise quantitative measurements of tracer uptake, such as standardized uptake values (SUVs).

Methods of attenuation correction include the following: (1) calculated correction, based on body contour assumptions and used primarily

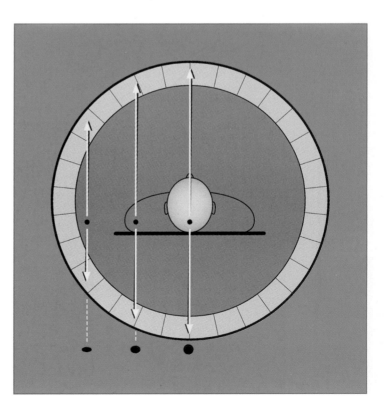

Figure 2-29. Radial blurring. As the annihilation reaction and source of the photon emission gets closer to the edge of the field of view, the photon is more likely to traverse more than one detector element, which results in more uncertainty as to the actual location of the original event and subsequent blurring of the image.

for imaging the head/brain where attenuation is relatively uniform; and (2) measured correction using actual transmission data, used for imaging the chest, abdomen, pelvis, and whole body where attenuation is variable. Transmission attenuation correction is performed by acquiring a map of body density and correcting for absorption in the various tissues. The amount of positron-emitting radionuclide at a specific location can then be determined. Once the correction is performed, the information is reconstructed into cross-sectional images.

In PET/CT scanners, x-rays from the computed tomography (CT) scan are used for attenuation correction and for providing localizing anatomic information. Because the x-rays used are less than 511 keV, the transmission data are adjusted to construct an attenuation map appropriate for annihilation photons. Attenuation maps can be obtained quickly (during a single breath-hold) with a PET/CT scanner, achieving high quality attenuation maps. However, because the attenuation map obtained with CT is obtained much more quickly than is the PET scan to which it is applied, artifacts in regions of moving structures such as the diaphragm may occur.

Attenuation is more likely when the annihilation reaction occurs in the center of the patient and less likely when the event occurs at the edge of the body. Thus in a nonattenuation-corrected image, there is less activity in the center of the body and more activity at the skin surface. Typically both attenuation-corrected and nonattenuation-corrected images are provided for interpretation. Images without attenuation correction can be recognized by the surface of the body (or "skin") and the lungs appearing to contain considerably increased activity (see Fig. 2-29). On attenuation-corrected images, the lungs have less activity than do structures nearer the surface and appear photopenic. Some lesions located near the surface of the body are more obvious on the uncorrected images, but most will be seen on the corrected images. A misalignment artifact can occur when a patient moves in between the transmission and emission scans. This can result in overcorrection on one side of the body and undercorrection on the other. Further, very high density (high Hounsfield units) contrast on the CT scan can cause overestimation of tissue ^{18}F-FDG concentrations, producing areas of apparent increased activity. Thus

an artifact may occur as a result of the bladder filling with radionuclide during the PET scan acquisition. This results in a hot area appearing around the bladder on the attenuation-corrected images but not on the nonattenuation-corrected images. A similar effect occurs if there are significant metallic objects (implants or dental work) in the patient.

A specific problem may occur when using bolus injection of intravenous contrast for a CT scan of the neck or chest. The attenuation-corrected images may show foci of artifactually increased ^{18}F-FDG activity in the region of venous structures first accepting the undiluted bolus. If co-registration is not perfect, this may be misinterpreted as abnormal activity in a lymph node or other structure. However, for practical purposes, most oral or intravenous contrast regimens do not cause significant artifacts, and, because the high-density source of any artifacts can be recognized on the CT portion of the study, there is usually little problem in interpretation. Further, because these artifacts are the result of attenuation correction, their specious nature can be substantiated by their absence on review of the nonattenuation-corrected images. The artifacts from oral and intravenous contrast administration as well as those from metal implants have diminished as attenuation-correction algorithms have become more sophisticated and as more appropriately designed diagnostic CT protocols have become available. In addition, recent studies have shown no statistically or clinically significant spurious elevation of SUVs which may potentially interfere with the diagnostic value a PET/CT resulting from the use of intravenous iodinated contrast.

System Sensitivity and Resolution

The sensitivity is defined as the recorded true coincidence rate (i.e., without scatter and random events) divided by the activity concentration (the true emitted events from the source). Sensitivity of a PET camera is determined by multiple factors, including, but not limited to, scanner geometry, crystal efficiency, and photon attenuation in tissue. Most photons emitted from the patient (98% to 99%) are not detected because they are emitted in all directions from the patient and the detector rings cover only a fraction of the patient's body surface. When attenuation by absorption or scatter is considered, current systems record substantially less than 0.1% of the true events. However, because state-of-the-art PET scanners typically image in three-dimensional mode (without collimators or septa), their efficiency for detecting emitted radiation is still considerably greater than that for SPECT imaging. Further, the sensitivity of PET is such that picomolar concentrations of PET radiopharmaceuticals can be detected.

Spatial resolution in PET scanners is, in large part, a function of detector size, with smaller detectors increasing the resolving capability of the system. Because of inherent physical limitations on positron localization imposed by their movement from the site of their emission (range) and the noncolinearity of annihilation photons, submillimeter resolution, such as possible with magnetic resonance imaging (MRI), is not achieved. The ultimate limit of spatial resolution when using ^{18}F-fluorodeoxyglucose (^{18}F-FDG) is about 1 mm. However, the practical spatial resolution for clinical imaging is about 4 to 6 mm.

Conventional PET scanners create images by observing annihilation radiation produced by positron-emitting radioisotopes injected in the body. Although these conventional scans track where the rays go, they do not consider the time it takes for each ray to reach the detector. Time-of-flight (TOF) PET systems, on the other hand, do measure the difference in the arrival times of the annihilation photons. These systems provide a better signal-to-noise (S/N) ratio and annihilation localization than that in conventional PET images. TOF systems detectors must have extreme resolution of timing and use lanthanum bromide (LaBr$_3$) and LYSO detectors with an intrinsic timing resolution as short as 600 ps. TOF PET is advantageous for whole-body imaging because the improvement with TOF increases with the size of the patient, and PET image quality degrades noticeably for large patients because of increased attenuation. Clinical TOF PET improves the image quality most in heavy patients.

PET Image Acquisition and Processing

PET systems are most commonly used in a whole-body scanning mode. This usually entails obtaining sequential segmental views of the body by moving the scanning table stepwise to acquire multiple contiguous views. There is a need to overlap the views to get uniform counting statistics, because in multiple detector ring systems, the detector rings at the edge of the FOV have less sensitivity than do those in the middle. A whole-body scan in a dedicated PET scanner usually extends from the base of the brain to the mid-thighs using a two- or three-dimensional acquisition. Depending on the size of the patient and the scanner, overlapping images are usually obtained every 15 to 22 cm for several minutes per position.

Images on a PET scanner can be acquired by using either two-dimensional (slice) or three-dimensional (volume) technique. With two-dimensional imaging, there are thin lead or tungsten septa (axial collimators) between the detectors and the adjacent rings of detectors such that each ring of detectors accepts coincidences only between detectors in the same ring or in closely adjacent rings. This defines a single plane (slice), eliminating out-of-plane scatter. Although sensitivity is reduced, image quality is enhanced. Two-dimensional imaging is usually performed when imaging small portions of the body (such as the heart) or obese patients, when using respiratory gating or short scan times with high activity, or when obtaining higher resolution or accurate quantification.

The current trend is to acquire data in a 3-D rather than a 2-D mode. When three-dimensional acquisition is performed, septa are not present or are retracted. This allows acquisition of a large volume defined by the FOV with coincidences recorded between the multiple detector rings in any combination. Sensitivity is about 5 to 10 times higher than with two-dimensional acquisition because of absence of the septa and the increased FOV of each crystal. However, although the number of recorded true coincidences is increased, out-of-plane scatter and random events are also considerably increased reducing image contrast and quality. With three-dimensional acquisition, as much as 30% to 60% of recorded events will be the result of scatter. To compensate for increased scatter and random count rates and to minimize dead time count losses, faster detectors with significantly better energy resolution (such as LSO and GSO) are needed. Three-dimensional imaging is typically used for low-scatter studies such as imaging the brain, small patient size (pediatrics), and attempts to shorten scan times when there is low administered activity. As improvements in hardware and three-dimensional algorithms are made, the use of three-dimensional imaging, with its increased sensitivity for true coincidences, is likely to become more commonly used.

Disadvantages of three-dimensional acquisition include the following: (1) an increased number of bed positions is required; (2) more random and scatter events are detected; and (3) if too much activity is administered, the count rate limit of a three-dimensional system can be overwhelmed. Three-dimensional imaging detects more random events because, in a high count rate environment, the true counting rate increases linearly with activity in the FOV, whereas the random rate increases as the square of activity in or near the FOV. More bed positions are needed because the scanner has maximum sensitivity in the center of the FOV with a rapid fall in sensitivity at the edges of the FOV. As a result, there needs to be a decrease in the axial FOV to maintain a uniform count profile and hence more bed positions to cover a given length of the patient. As a general rule, if there is sufficient activity and counts to perform a study in two-dimensional mode, that is the preferred image acquisition mode.

The emission data acquired by either two- or three-dimensional technique are converted to an image format by using filtered back projection or iterative reconstruction. Filtered back projection can be used with two-dimensional reconstruction and when the data are relatively noise free. The method is simple and fast. Because of the complexity of the data from three-dimensional acquisition, iterative algorithms are used. The iterative technique involves use of several analytic processes (iterations) to reach the desired result. Compared with filtered back projection, iterative reconstruction requires substantially more time and computer power. When appropriate, iterative algorithms can also be used to reconstruct two-dimensional acquisition data.

PET/CT

Interpretation of dedicated PET scans is hampered by difficulty in determining the anatomic location of an area of increased activity within the body. The addition of contemporaneous CT imaging to PET instruments yields several distinct advantages, depending on the CT protocols used. These include more efficient and accurate attenuation correction, shorter imaging times, more precise anatomic localization of lesions, and acquisition of diagnostic CT and PET scans in one effort. Recent studies have shown that PET/CT scans produce more accurate results than does CT or PET alone or side-by-side visual correlation of PET and CT scans. The primary improvement has been a reduction of equivocal interpretations.

Current PET/CT scanners may appear to be a single machine, but most are simply a CT and PET scanner placed together within a single cover. The patient table traverses the bore of both machines. These systems obtain diagnostic quality studies with 4- to 16-slice CT devices. Most oncology applications use a multidetector 16-slice scanner, although 64 (or higher) slice scanners are used for cardiac studies.

Most current PET/CT scanners can produce excellent whole-body fused or co-registered PET/CT images in less than 30 minutes. When fusing the data, matching CT and PET images is possible to within a few millimeters. However, there may still be slight differences because of the limited spatial resolution of the PET scanner as well as patient movement and/or differences in positioning occurring between the CT scan and completion of the PET scan. Because PET images are acquired over minutes and CT images are acquired over seconds, there are still some minor alignment problems related to the position of the diaphragm.

In addition to providing precise anatomic localization, the CT scan data are also used to perform PET attenuation correction (Fig. 2-30) as discussed above.

At most institutions, the CT scan is performed before the PET scan. A typical protocol with good results uses 500 to 750 mL of oral contrast (1.3% to 2.1% barium sulfate, glucose free) 60 to 90 minutes before ^{18}F-FDG injection. High-density barium should be avoided. Another 100 to 200 mL of oral barium is given 30 minutes after the ^{18}F-FDG injection. The patient then rests quietly for an additional 30 minutes, and the CT scan is performed just before the PET scan. The CT scan uses 80 mL of intravenous contrast (300 mgI/mL) at 3 mL per second to achieve arterial contrast, followed by another 60 mL at 2 mL/second for venous and parenchymal enhancement.

Typical diagnostic CT parameters for normal weight adult patients are as follows: 80 mAs and 140 kVp, 512 × 512 matrix and a slice width

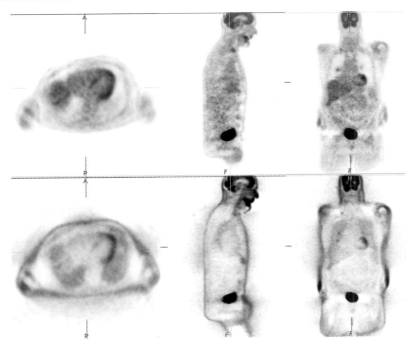

Figure 2-30. Attenuation-corrected and uncorrected PET images. Attenuation corrected mages (*upper row*) from an ^{18}F-FDG scan show activity in the deep structures, including the brain, heart, liver, bladder, and a right lung cancer. The uncorrected images (*lower row*) are easily recognized by the apparent activity in the skin and lungs. *FDG,* Fluorodeoxyglucose.

of 5 mm, a pitch of 1.6 for diagnostic scans, and reconstruction increments of 2.5 mm. The mA can be reduced to 40 to 60 mA in smaller patients, and the mA can be increased to 120 to 160 for very large patients. If the CT scan is only being done for attenuation correction purposes, an mA of only 10 to 40 is necessary. The CT scan time is usually very short (≈30 seconds), and the PET acquisition is much longer (20 to 30 minutes). For most purposes, the CT scan is usually performed from the meatus of the ear to the mid-thigh during shallow breathing. It is important to obtain the CT and PET images in the same manner, that is, with the arms up or down on both, and with shallow breathing or partial breath-hold, rather than obtaining the CT in maximum inspiration breath-hold mode. Even so, co-registration of small pulmonary, diaphragmatic, or superiorly located liver lesions, which may vary with even slight changes in position or respiration, may not be perfect.

PET/CT scanners are now commonly used in radiation therapy treatment planning, particularly with conformal and intensity modulated radiotherapy, which requires more precise target volume definition.

PET/MRI

PET/MRI scanners have been hindered in their development because the combination of the modalities required four significant changes to the previously available PET and MRI scanners. One major problem was that the PET phototubes are sensitive to even low magnetic fields and needed to be replaced by avalanche photodiodes that required expensive cooling systems. Second, the presence of PET detectors interfered with MR field homogeneity, gradients and frequency, causing artifacts on MR images. This required development of detectors invisible to MRI. Third, the MRI radiofrequency coils interfered with the PET electronics, and special shielding around the PET electronics was needed. Finally, PET attenuation correction methods needed to be developed based on MRI data. With these problems solved, it has been possible to get simultaneous data acquisition (which is not truly possible with PET/CT).

There are three possible designs for a PET/MRI system. One design is to have the systems in tandem as with a PET/CT scanner. Putting a separate PET and CT gantry about 2.5 m apart but with a common patient table requires the least system modifications. This method, however, means that there cannot be simultaneous imaging causing co-registration errors because of physiologic motion such as peristalsis. Imaging time will likely be longer, and the room must be bigger than with other systems.

Another design has a PET detector inserted into the bore of a MRI scanner. This requires few MRI modifications but significant modifications to the PET system. The system must use detectors that do not interfere with the magnetic field, and the PET electronics must be somewhat removed from the MR bore The biggest problem is that with the PET inside the MRI bore there is not much room for the patient and thus these approaches will likely be used for brain or limb scanning.

A third approach is to put the PET within the MR system itself; however, this is technically most difficult.

Presently, PET/MRI instruments with the tandem and insert design are just beginning to enter clinical use, and their efficacy and indications remain unclear. It can be expected that they would be useful for brain pathology (stroke and tumors) and for whole body oncologic applications (such as liver metastases). Obvious benefits of PET/MRI are the reduction in radiation dose compared with PET/CT, superior soft-tissue contrast of MRI, and the ability of MRI to assess tissue chemistry.

INSTRUMENTATION QUALITY CONTROL

Before any equipment is installed, it is important to ensure that there is a suitable environment to house it; otherwise, attempts at quality control will be ineffective. Most nuclear medicine equipment and computers generate a tremendous amount of heat, and all aspects of ventilation and temperature control need to be examined. Consoles should never be placed close to a wall, and dust and smoke also cause serious problems, especially for computers. In addition, shutting down newer imaging and computer systems at night prolongs the useful life of many components.

The frequency of recommended quality control tests varies among manufacturers and different models of equipment. The NRC requires that at a minimum, one must follow the manufacturer's recommendation. The frequency may be shorter if problems have been encountered recently, repairs have been performed, or if institutional written policies require more frequent testing. Tests typically performed are listed in Table 2-2. In the following text, essential concepts related to quality control of imaging equipment are presented. For detailed information on how each test is performed, the manufacturer's operating manual should be consulted. There are a number of accreditation organizations,

including the American College of Radiology (ACR) and the Intersocietal Commission on the Accreditation of Nuclear Medicine Laboratories (ICANL), that have quality control standards for nuclear medicine equipment. Essentially, all of the manufacturer's operating manuals take such standards into consideration.

Gamma Cameras

Scintillation camera systems are subject to a variety of detector and associated electronic problems that can cause aberrations of the image and may not be detected by the casual observer. Thus quality control procedures are especially important to ensure high-quality, accurate diagnostic images. The three parameters usually tested are (1) spatial resolution, or the ability to visualize an alternating, closely spaced pattern of activity; (2) image linearity and distortion, or the ability to reproduce a straight line; and (3) field uniformity, or the ability of the imaging system to produce a uniform image from the entire crystal surface. In general, these determinations can be made with (extrinsic) or without the collimator (intrinsic). Radioactive sources used for these tests are typically a cobalt-57 sheet or point source or a ^{99m}Tc point source. Less commonly a Lucite phantom filled with water and ^{99m}Tc is used.

Spatial Resolution and Linearity Testing

Historically, to test for spatial resolution, several phantoms have been used. In general, they are either Lucite sheets embedded with lead bars or a sheet of lead with holes in it. The phantom is placed between the camera or collimator face and a radioactive flood or sheet source, and a transmission image is then obtained. The most common four-quadrant bar phantom has four sets of lead bars of different widths and spacing in each quadrant, which are arranged at 90-degree angles to each other. The four quadrants test a spectrum of resolution ranging from relatively coarse to fine. Spatial resolution measurements require that the phantom be rotated 90 degrees or turned over and re-imaged to check the spatial resolution in all areas of the crystal (Fig. 2-31). Linearity and distortion problems are manifested when the otherwise straight bars are depicted as wavy lines. A number of new gamma cameras have automated daily, weekly, and monthly quality control routines,

TABLE 2–2	Typical Quality Control Procedures*	
PERFORMANCE PARAMETER	**QUALITY CONTROL PROTOCOL**	**FREQUENCY†**
Survey meter	Battery check Background check Constancy (with long-lived reference source) Calibration	Before each use Before each use Before each use Annually
Well counter and organ uptake probe	Background adjustment Constancy (with long-lived reference source) Energy resolution (FWHM) Efficiency (cpm/Bq) ref. source ± 5%	Daily Daily Quarterly Annually
Intraoperative probe	Battery check Background check Constancy (with long-lived reference source)	Before each use Before each use Before each use
Dose calibrator	Constancy (reference source ± 5%) Linearity (shielding or decay method ± 5%) Accuracy (2 radionuclides ± 5%) Geometry ± 5%	Daily Quarterly Quarterly After repair, recalibration, or relocation
Sealed sources	Wipe test for leaks	6 months
Gamma Camera		
Uniformity	Intrinsic or extrinsic flood evaluated qualitatively	Daily (~4-10 million counts)
High count uniformity	Same	1-6 months (100-200 million counts)
Energy spectrum	Radionuclide photopeak peaking	Daily; automatic on many new cameras
Collimator damage	Visual inspection unless doing extrinsic daily floods	Daily
Spatial resolution and linearity	Resolution phantom (quadrant bar phantom)	Weekly; not required by manufacturer on some newer cameras
Energy resolution	Full width at half-maximum of technetium-99m photopeak expressed as percentage	Annually
Energy linearity	Multiple radionuclide photopeaks within ± 5% of true value	Annually
Count rate response	20% data loss, resolving time, maximum count rate for 20% window	Annually
Sensitivity	Count rate per microcurie with 15% window; calculate absolute sensitivity for a collimator	Annually
Collimator integrity	10 million count floods through each non-pinhole collimator for evaluation of collimator defects	Quarterly or when suspect damage
Formatter performance	Flood images at all locations and for all image sizes	Annually
Whole-body accessory	Scan bar phantom along diagonal, and compare with stationary image; calibrate speed	Annually
Energy window setting	Confirm energy window for specific radionuclide used	For each patient
Multiple window spatial registration	Point source (^{67}Ga/medium energy collimator or ^{201}Tl low energy collimator)	Annually
Crystal hydration	Image each ½ photopeak (^{133}Xe,^{201}Tl, or ^{99m}Tc)	Annually
Spect Gamma Cameras (In addition to above)		
Center of rotation	1 or more point sources or line source	1-4 weeks
Head tilt angle	Bubble level	Quarterly; not needed on some newer cameras

TABLE 2–2	Typical Quality Control Procedures*—cont'd	
PERFORMANCE PARAMETER	**QUALITY CONTROL PROTOCOL**	**FREQUENCY†**
System performance	SPECT phantom	Quarterly
Spatial resolution in air	Point or line source reconstructed	6-12 months
PET Scanners		
Ambient environment	Temperature	Daily
Attenuation correction	Blank scan (transmission sources but nothing in the FOV)	Daily
Tomographic uniformity	^{68}Ge cylinder or rod source	Daily
Detector calibration	Normalization scan (positron source in FOV)	1-3 months
Image plane	Uniform cylinder with positron emitter	Weekly or monthly
Sensitivity	Sleeved rod sources	6-12 months
Spatial resolution	Spatial resolution of point source in sinogram and image space	Annually
Count rate performance	Line source in polyethylene cylinder	Annually
Scatter fraction	Line source in polyethylene cylinder	Annually
System performance	Uniformity "hot sphere" contrast using ACR or IEC phantom	Annually
CT Scanner		
Tube warm-up	Manufacturers procedures (tube cooling temperature, etc.)	Daily
Air calibration	Manufacturer's procedures	Daily
Constancy	Water, noise, uniformity, CT number (water/air/acrylic) artifacts	Daily
CT/NM 3-D vector alignment	Alignment phantom	Annually
Dose check	Per regulatory and industry standards	Annually or after tube replacement or repair
Slice thickness, contrast resolution CT number linearity, radiation profile MTF	Per regulatory and industry standards	Annually or after major repair/recalibration

ACR, American College of Radiology; *CT*, computed tomography; *FOV*, field of view; *FWHM*, full width at half maximum; ^{67}*Ga*, gallium; *IEC*, International Electrotechnical Commission; *ME* medium energy; *MTF*, modulation transfer function; *NM*, nuclear medicine.

*The frequency of recommended tests varies among manufacturers and different models of equipment. At a minimum, one must follow the manufacturer's recommendations. Other tests may be required at acceptance testing or annually by a physicist.

†The frequency may be shorter if problems have been encountered recently.

some of which do not specifically test for spatial resolution.

Field Uniformity Assessment

For intrinsic uniformity evaluation, either a planar or a point source can be used after the collimator has been removed. The point-source method may use a small volume of ^{99m}Tc or a point cobalt-57 source (see Fig. 2-17). Most current gamma cameras use the point source method. Field uniformity is tested extrinsically (with the collimator) or intrinsically (without the collimator). Extrinsic field uniformity is sometimes evaluated by using a flood-field image obtained by presenting the collimator–crystal combination with a uniform planar source of activity. The planar source is usually a ^{57}Co solid plastic sheet source or a plastic tank filled with ^{99m}Tc in liquid. Covering the detector head with a plastic cover is an excellent way to avoid collimator and crystal contamination if a liquid source is used. If the flood field is

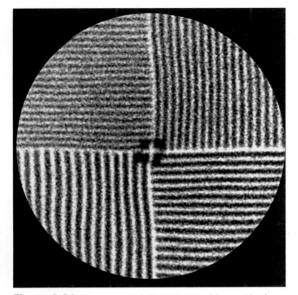

Figure 2-31. Linearity and distortion problems. The four-quadrant bar phantom demonstrates wavy lines seen particularly in the left lower quadrant.

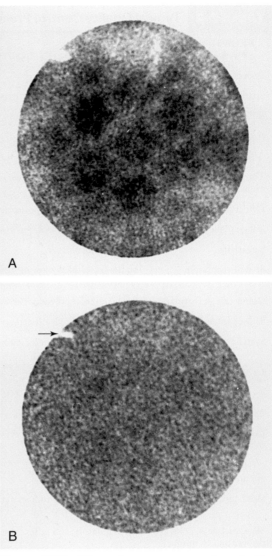

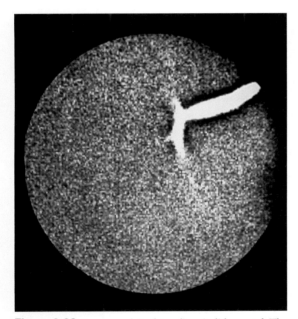

Figure 2-32. Large crack in the sodium iodide crystal. The branching white pattern is caused by a crack and because no scintillations are occurring in this region. The dark edges are due to the edge-packing phenomenon.

Figure 2-33. Effect of computer correction. A, The extrinsic flood-field image was obtained without computer correction. **B,** The lower image was done with computer correction and demonstrates a much more homogeneous flood field. A defect (*arrow*), however, remained. This was because of a deformity of the lead septa of the collimator.

obtained by mixing ⁹⁹ᵐTc and water in a plastic flood tank, there must be adequate mixing. After mixing, all air bubbles must be removed to prevent inhomogeneity.

A daily flood image should be placed in a logbook to assess any changes in uniformity and for accreditation inspections. A variety of abnormalities can be identified on flood-field images,

including cracks in the crystal (Fig. 2-32), collimator defects (Fig. 2-33), electronic or photomultiplier abnormalities (Fig. 2-34) and poor source preparation (Fig. 2-35). Most cameras have microprocessor and computer circuits to correct for image nonuniformity. An initial flood-field image is obtained and stored in the computer memory. Field uniformity is then obtained by adjusting subsequent clinical images based on the initial image in its memory. A flood field should also be obtained without the use of the computer correction so that the operator can see

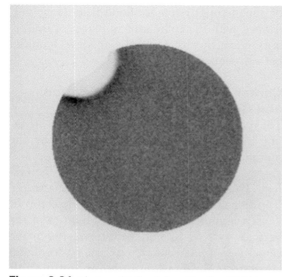

Figure 2-34. Photomultiplier defect. The flood field image shows a peripheral crescentic defect resulting from a nonfunctioning photomultiplier tube *PMT*.

the status of the detectors and whether there is degradation over time or need for adjustment. If this is not done, data losses of up to 50% may result in prolonged imaging times. Other computer correction systems are also available.

Historically, there needed to be assurance that the correct energy window for the imaged radionuclide was selected and that the photopeak is included in the energy window. Centering the energy window too high or too low resulted in nonuniform or blurry images (Fig. 2-36). Current gamma cameras automatically detect the spectrum of the radionuclide being used and set the energy window, and, as a result, it has become virtually impossible to obtain off-peak images.

SPECT Quality Control

To ensure high performance standards of SPECT cameras, routine detector quality control procedures should be performed weekly, as with any gamma camera, including tests of intrinsic uniformity, extrinsic uniformity (collimator in place), resolution, and linearity. Regular meticulous quality control of SPECT imaging systems is absolutely essential for the production of clinically useful, artifact-free images. Although even significant deviations from optimum performance can be tolerated in routine planar imaging, more minor departures from performance standards in SPECT imaging may produce unacceptable or even misleading images.

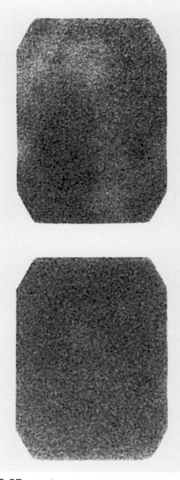

Figure 2-35. Inadequate mixing of technetium in the flood-field phantom. *Top,* This panel demonstrates an inhomogeneous appearance because the technetium was not adequately mixed with the water in the phantom. *Bottom,* This panel demonstrates a much better homogeneity and was obtained after the phantom was shaken several times.

Field Uniformity Assessment and Correction

Because rotational SPECT images are produced from planar views and because that process amplifies any suboptimal characteristics introduced by the instrumentation, quality control of SPECT imaging begins with assurances that the imaging system is operating at the highest intrinsic performance standards. This is especially true of system uniformity, which is governed by multiple factors in the imaging chain: principally, detector uniformity of response (intrinsic uniformity), collimator integrity (extrinsic uniformity), and the quality of the analog/digital signal conversions at the camera–computer interface. Significant camera field nonuniformities can result in image

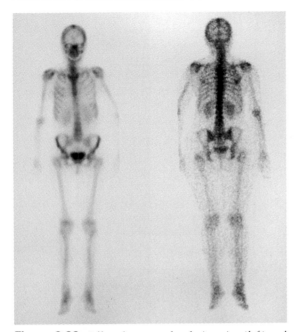

Figure 2-36. **Off-peak camera head.** Anterior (*left*) and posterior (*right*) images from a bone scan were obtained with a moving dual-headed gamma camera and a fixed table. The camera head anterior to the patient was properly peaked for the radionuclide energy, whereas the posterior camera was improperly peaked, resulting in poor spatial resolution. Current scanners automatically detect the radionuclide energy and peak the camera.

artifacts, the most common of which is the *ring artifact.*

In ordinary planar imaging, system uniformity variation of 3% to 5% may be acceptable. Nonuniformities that are not apparent in planar images, however, can give rise to significant errors in the reconstructed tomographic views, which may appear as full or partial ring artifacts. A 5% detector or collimator nonuniformity on the axis of rotation (AOR) can produce a 35% cold or hot spot on the reconstructed image. The farther the nonuniformity is from the AOR, the less intense is the artifact. In addition, use of noncircular orbits minimizes nonuniformity artifacts. Because the back-projection process used in SPECT amplifies nonuniformities inherent in the imaging system, a uniformity deviation in SPECT imaging must be 1% or less to produce artifact-free images. This is significantly less than that achievable because of inherent system inhomogeneity, so system nonuniformity must be corrected.

To correct system nonuniformity, a superior uniformity correction is needed. This is attained by the weekly acquisition and computer storage of a high-count reference flood-field image performed with the collimator in place for uniformity correction of each planar view acquired before reconstruction.

Center of Rotation Determination and Correction

The center of rotation (COR) of the imaging system is superficially determined by the mechanical construction of the camera and gantry, as well as by the electronics of the system. Thus the apparent COR may be affected by mechanical aberrations in the detector or gantry alignment, electronic instabilities in the detector system, or nonlinearities between the camera–computer coupling analog-to-digital converter (ADC). In fact, the apparent COR as perceived by the computer may differ from the actual mechanical COR because of conditions affecting the system electronics. Thus it is necessary to align the electronic center (center of computer matrix) with the mechanical COR (camera COR) properly to prevent COR misalignment artifacts. Any significant misalignment (>0.5 pixel for a 64 × 64 matrix) results in increasing losses of contrast and resolution in the reconstructed images, and often gross image distortion (Fig. 2-37). The maximum acceptable uncorrected error in the COR is 0.5 pixel.

Evaluation of the COR of the system is a relatively simple procedure, typically consisting of placing a ^{99m}Tc or ^{57}Co point or line source near the COR of the camera and performing a SPECT scan of the source. With a small COR misalignment, the point source appears blurred; but with a large misalignment, it has a doughnut appearance. Most commercial SPECT systems have software programs capable of calculating the apparent COR and any offset from the computer matrix center and storing these data for later COR correction as needed in clinical acquisitions. If a misalignment is found, a correction can be made by the computer software to realign the rotation and matrix centers by shifting the rotational axis of the camera to the center of the computer matrix.

COR calibration must be performed for each collimator, zoom factor, and usually matrix size used for clinical imaging. Furthermore, COR calibration factors based on ^{99m}Tc may be valid only for other radionuclides if energy registration circuits have been properly calibrated. With a newly installed camera, COR calibration

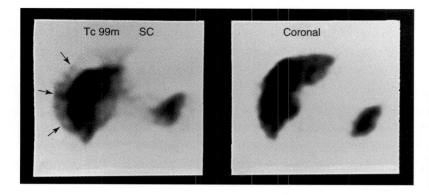

Figure 2-37. Center of rotation artifact demonstrated on a coronal sulfur colloid liver-spleen scan. *Left,* Image obtained with a 1-pixel center-of-rotation misalignment, resulting in blurring and halo artifact. *Right,* With correction, the image is markedly improved.

should probably be performed frequently (perhaps daily) until system stability is established and then every 1 to 2 weeks. Frequent fluctuations in COR values suggest a problem requiring professional servicing of the instrument.

Detector Head Alignment with the Axis of Rotation

To produce accurate back-projected images without loss of resolution or contrast, the planar images must be acquired in planes perpendicular to the AOR of the camera. This requires the camera face to be level and untilted from the AOR. A 1% tilt at a distance of 14 cm produces a shift of about 1 pixel in a 64 × 64 matrix. Head tilt may be assessed by using the camera and computer to collect a set of 36-point source images over 360 degrees and adding selected frames together. If no tilt is present, the images describe a straight line parallel with the x-axis.

Alternatively, a simple check independent of system electronics may be performed by using a carpenter's (bubble) level to evaluate camera face position at the 12-o'clock and 6-o'clock positions on the gantry. The latter test presumes that the crystal face, detector housing, and AOR are all parallel with the earth's surface in the above positions. Camera head tilt should be assessed quarterly and corrections made as necessary.

Collimator Evaluation

For optimum image production, the collimator should be as close to the manufacturer's specifications as possible and free of obvious defects. Damaged collimator septa may introduce significant field nonuniformity, which can degrade image quality. Various methods have been described to evaluate collimator integrity and may be used when a serious problem is suspected. Routinely, collimator inspection should be performed through the actual visual examination of the collimator and inspection of high-count extrinsic flood images. Defective collimators should be replaced.

System Performance

Overall system performance under different acquisition parameters can be assessed by using a variety of commercially available ^{99m}Tc-filled phantoms, including the Jaszczak or Carlson phantoms. These are best used according to the manufacturer's protocols but usually are performed monthly. Parameters evaluated may include object contrast and image noise, field uniformity, and accuracy of attenuation correction. Each view should contain at least 200,000 counts in a 64 × 64 or 128 × 128 matrix. The angular sampling (number of views) should match the matrix size. System evaluation using phantoms can be repeated and compared with previous acquisitions to check system performance over time and after hardware or software upgrades or major repairs. The same radius of rotation, filter, and cutoff frequency should be used each time.

PET/CT Quality Control

There are a few specific quality control tests for dedicated PET systems. These procedures are intended to monitor system stability and maintain consistency and accuracy of performance.

Ambient Temperature

The scanning room temperature should be checked daily because the sensitivity of the system changes with temperature. As the temperature rises, fewer visible photons are produced by the crystals. The pulse height analyzer spectrum in BGO crystals also changes with temperature, with the energy range varying inversely with room temperature (e.g., appearing lower as the temperature rises and vice versa).

Normalization Scan

Because a state-of-the-art PET camera may have thousands of crystal elements coupled to hundreds of PMTs, there are inevitable small variations in axial sensitivity among the detector units. To produce uniform images, these discrepancies must be corrected. A normalization scan is accomplished by scanning a uniform calibrated positron-emitting source placed in the FOV. This data set measures the response of each detector pair and is used to obtain a calibration factor to "normalize" the lines of response that pass through the source. These stored calibration factors can be applied to patient data sets to correct for differences in detector response so that accurate images of tracer distribution are produced. Normalization scans should be performed at least monthly, but they may be obtained weekly or more frequently as needed.

Blank Scan

This is accomplished by performing a scan by using the system transmission radiation sources with nothing in the FOV. This usually takes an hour or less. The data acquired are used with the patient transmission data to compute attenuation correction factors. Blank scans should be performed daily and, as such, are also an excellent method to monitor system stability, including significant discrepancies in individual detector sensitivities. Some PET instruments will perform this function automatically at a specified time during the night and even compare the results to previous blank scans.

Image Plane Calibration

Calibration of each image plane by using a radioactive source is also required on multiring detectors. This can be done with a uniform cylinder filled with a positron-emitter and may be done weekly or monthly. This procedure is essential for the production of accurate whole-body scans.

CT Scanner

Daily calibration begins with manufacturer's warm-up and automatic monitoring program. This checks a number of parameters, including tube coolant temperature, kVp and mA settings, and detector response. A phantom is then used to check that water measures 0 Hounsfield units and air measures minus 1000 units with a standard deviation of 2 to 3 units. The water image is evaluated for standard deviation to assess for image noise. The image quality is usually assessed by assuring that the Hounsfield units have a standard deviation of 1 to 5 across the phantom image. Many of these procedures are automated, but, if the images are evaluated visually, they should be inspected to see that there are no arc or ring artifacts.

TECHNICAL ARTIFACTS
Areas of Decreased Activity

There are really no problems in radiopharmaceutical preparation or administration that lead to a focal area of decreased activity. In gamma cameras, decoupling of the gel between the crystal and the photomultiplier tubes, malfunctioning or off-peak photomultiplier tubes (see Fig. 2-36) cause "cold" defects. They also can be produced by computer processing errors. One of the most common of these is caused by setting the color or gray scale in too narrow a range, producing so-called scaling artifacts. If, for example, circumferential activity of a perfusion agent in the myocardium ranges from 19% to 30% and the technician sets the scale to show the color scale from 20% to 30%, the small area that is 19% appears as a defect even though it is not statistically different from the rest of the myocardium. On the more technically demanding SPECT images, ring, COR, patient motion, and attenuation artifacts may produce cold defects. The COR artifacts can sometimes be recognized by a tail of activity extending out from the defect (see Fig. 2-37).

If there is something between the radiopharmaceutical and the gamma camera that causes attenuation of the photons, however, this appears as an area of focal photopenia. The key to recognition of these artifacts is that they do not persist in the same location with respect to the organ on differing or orthogonal projections. Attenuation can be the result of something within the patient. Examples of this include residual barium from a radiographic gastrointestinal study (Fig. 2-38), a metallic prosthesis, a large calcification or stone, a subcutaneous pacemaker, or metallic fixation rods or plates. Soft tissue can be a problem as well.

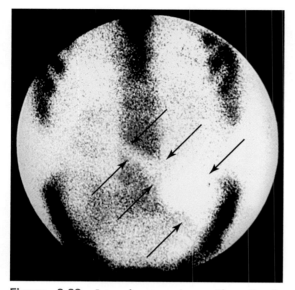

Figure 2-38. **Internal attenuation artifact.** Focally decreased activity is seen (*arrows*) on a bone scan because of internal attenuation of photons from residual barium after an upper gastrointestinal examination.

Diaphragmatic attenuation can cause inferior defects on myocardial scans, and pendulous breast tissue can cause problems on both cardiac and liver scans. Attenuation artifacts caused by objects external to the patient are usually due to metallic jewelry, coins in pockets, metallic belt buckles, snaps, zippers, and external breast prostheses (Figs. 2-39 and 2-40).

Cold defects can also be caused by problems in the imaging chain of the gamma camera. In general, these artifacts can be recognized because they stay in the same relative location on each image regardless of the patient projection. Such artifacts may include a cracked crystal (usually seen as a linear or branching white defect with dark edges) (Fig. 2-41). A PMT artifact is typically a round or hexagonal cold defect (Fig. 2-42).

Some problems with radiopharmaceutical preparation can cause poor labeling and therefore decreased activity in the organ of interest. Examples of these include inadequate

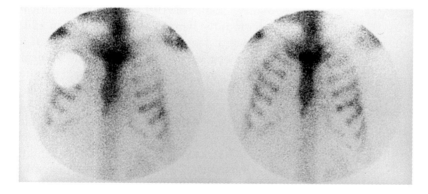

Figure 2-39. **External attenuation artifact.** *Left,* An external breast prosthesis has caused a round area of decreased activity over the upper right chest wall on a bone scan. *Right,* The image was repeated after the prosthesis was removed.

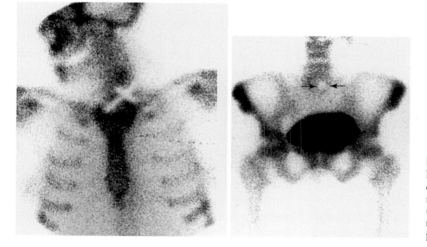

Figure 2-40. **External metallic artifacts.** *Left,* A bone scan clearly shows a "cold" cross on a necklace. *Right,* The "501" sign (*arrows*) of small round photopenic defects caused by snaps on blue jeans.

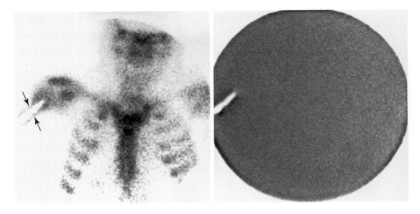

Figure 2-41. Cracked crystal artifact. *Left,* A linear area of decreased activity is seen over the upper right humerus (*arrows*). This was due to a cracked crystal in the gamma camera, as evidenced by the linear defect seen on the flood-field image (*right*).

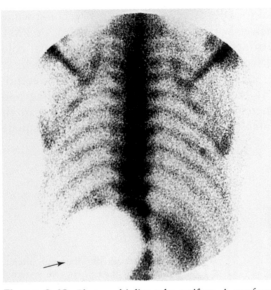

Figure 2-42. Photomultiplier tube artifact. A nonfunctional PMT caused a round, focal defect (*arrow*) on this posterior image from a bone scan.

incubation time of bone radiopharmaceuticals, problems with red blood cell labeling kits, and decreased labeling of hepatobiliary compounds resulting from low pH or low ligand concentration. Competition with nonradioactive compounds or medication can also cause generalized decreased activity. A classic example of this is nonvisualization of the thyroid on an iodine-123 (^{123}I) scan in a patient who recently received intravenous iodinated contrast.

Only a few instrumentation problems can result in generalized decreased activity. The most common is an off-peak camera that does not allow the most abundant photons to be recorded. This causes an image with few counts and poor spatial resolution. Inappropriate intensity settings on the hard copy imaging device or use of a high-energy instead of a low-energy collimator also can cause images that appear to have generally decreased activity.

Areas of Increased Activity

Perhaps the most common problem with radiopharmaceutical preparation and administration that results in focal hot spots is extravasation of the radiopharmaceutical at the injection site (Fig. 2-43). When this happens in an upper extremity, some of the radiopharmaceutical may get into the lymphatics and be seen in axillary or supraclavicular lymph nodes. When a significant arm extravasation site is placed near to the body during imaging, scatter from the site may produce an apparent hot spot in the adjacent truncal soft tissues. Urine contamination on a bone scan is common. Another example is when blood is drawn back into the syringe or the radiopharmaceutical is injected through an indwelling catheter while a perfusion lung scan is being performed. This often results in focal hot spots in the lungs secondary to injected small, labeled clots.

Differences in soft-tissue attenuation can occasionally cause what looks like focally increased activity in the less attenuated areas. For example, a bone scan of a patient who has had a mastectomy may appear to show increased activity over the chest wall on the mastectomy side because of less soft-tissue attenuation of the photons emanating from the ribs. A liver–spleen scan performed on an obese patient may show a horizontal band of apparently increased activity; however, this is the result of more photons reaching the gamma camera through the creases in the fat (or conversely, more attenuation of photons by folds of fat).

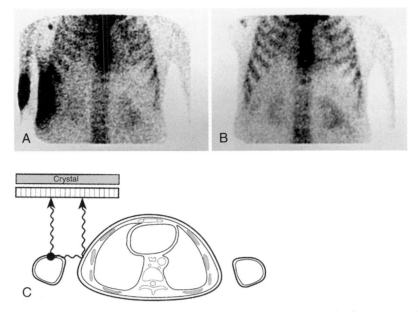

Figure 2-43. **Effect of soft-tissue scatter. A,** A focal area of increased activity is seen on this bone scan in the right antecubital region and along the right chest wall. This is due to extravasation of radiopharmaceutical at the injection site and scatter of photons from this site in the soft tissues of the chest wall (narrow angle scatter). **B,** By lifting the arm up and away from the chest wall, the scatter artifact disappears. **C,** Diagrammatic representation of the effect seen in *A.*

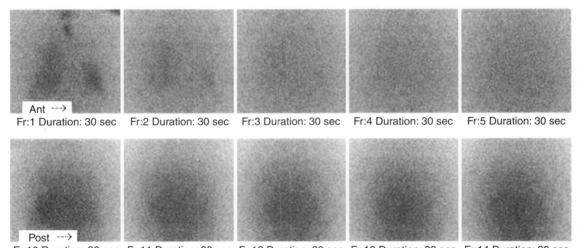

Figure 2-44. **Artifact caused by recent radionuclide examination.** Multiple images from a xenon-133 ventilation scan are of very poor quality because of residual activity from a ^{18}F-FDG scan performed 6 hours earlier.

As with cold lesions, gamma camera or instrumentation problems causing focal hot spots can be recognized because they appear in the same place on the field of view regardless of projection of the images. Increased focal activity as a result of instrumentation is usually the result of camera or collimator contamination with radionuclide or of an off-peak camera or voltage problems with the photomultiplier tubes.

There are a number of artifacts that occur because of either prior recent nuclear medicine examinations or to radioactivity in another nearby patient. This can be difficult to discern from quality control problems especially if the energy of the radionuclides is different (Fig. 2-44). A patient who was injected with 740 MBq (20 mCi) of ^{18}F-FDG who is within several meters of another patient being scanned can cause significant background interference.

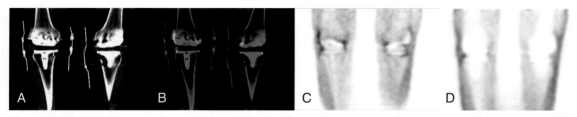

Figure 2-45. **PET/CT attenuation correction artifact.** An ^{18}F-FDG scan performed on a patient with knee pain and bilateral total knee replacements. **A,** The CT scan shows the metallic prostheses. **B,** The PET/CT scan and **C,** the attenuation corrected PET image show increased activity medial near the prostheses. However, the nonattenuation corrected images (**D**) do not show any abnormality indicating that the apparent increased activity was artifactual.

VOI Results:	
Parameter	Value
CT 1	
Max	129.00 HU
Min	−60.00 HU
Avg.	44.21 HU
Std. Dev.	23.78
Vol.	8.21 cm³
X size	39.46 mm
Y size	19.24 mm
Z size	20.65 mm
Recon Tomo 1	
Max	3.28 SUV
Min	1.73 SUV
Avg.	2.52 SUV ←
Std. Dev.	0.32
Vol.	8.21 cm³
X size	39.46 mm
Y size	19.24 mm
Z size	20.65 mm

Figure 2-46. **Standardized uptake value (SUV artifact).** An image from an ^{18}F-FDG scan in a patient with widespread metastatic disease shows markedly increased activity in the liver and to a lesser extent in the bone marrow, lungs, and bones. However, the calculated SUV in the liver was very low at 2.52 (*arrow*). A number of factors can cause errors in the calculation of the SUV—in this case, as a result of an error in calibration after machine servicing.

Artifactually increased activity is also seen on PET/CT scans as a result of attenuation correction problems when there is material on the CT scan that is very dense, such as metallic prostheses (Fig. 2-45) or dense barium. These can be identified as artifacts by examining the nonattenuation corrected image. The increased activity will not be present on the latter images. There also can be attenuation correction artifacts in PET/CT (and to a lesser extent in SPECT/CT) which result in decreased apparent activity as a result of respiratory and cardiac motion causing misregistration of the data sets. In cardiac studies, polar maps show decreased activity in the right upper quadrants as a result of cardiac position mismatch and decreased activity on the left lateral portion from chest wall motion, diaphragm contraction, or mismatch in overlap between the liver and heart.

Artifacts can also occur in evaluation of the standard uptake value (SUV) on PET/ CT scans (Fig. 2-46). Either high or low false values can occur as a result of incorrect calibration of the reference gadolinium source, errors in entry of the radionuclide half-life, or injection time. Partial volume effects can also cause underestimation of activity concentration in a lesion. With PET scanning partial volume issues mostly affect lesions less than three times the size of the PET resolution (4 to 7 mm) and thus partial volume effects start to occur with lesions 1.2 to 2.0 cm.

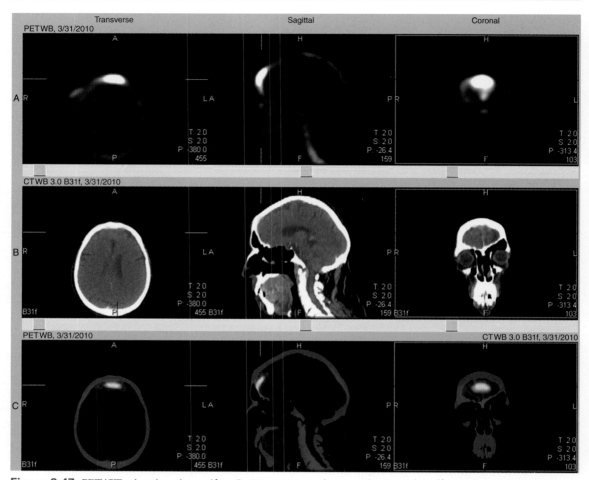

Figure 2-47. PET/CT misregistration artifact. Patient movement between the time of the ^{18}F-Na fluoride PET bone scan and the CT acquisitions caused a frontal bone prostate metastasis to appear intracranial.

The shape of the lesion, presence of sharp borders, and relation to background activity also affect partial volume issues but to a lesser extent. Inaccurate SUVs are also obtained when there is a mismatch in registration between the CT and PET scans.

Misregistration of CT and PET scan images by more than 1 cm can occur for peripheral or basal lung lesions or for lesions in the upper portion of the liver, if there is a difference in breathing during the two scans or if the patient moves between scans. If shallow breathing is used to obtain both CT and PET scans, lesions in the chest are usually registered within about 1 cm of each other, but near the diaphragm and within the superior portion of the liver, the lesions may be misregistered by up to 2 cm. When the CT scan is acquired at full inspiration and the PET image is obtained over many breathing cycles, there is a curvilinear cold artifact at the lung bases. In addition, if there is a liver lesion near the dome of the liver and the CT is performed with deeper inspiration than the PET scan, the lesion can erroneously appear to be in the lung base. Misregistration may be minimized by performing the CT scan during a breath-hold at normal tidal expiration and the PET scan during normal tidal breathing. A "cold" curvilinear artifact above the liver can be seen on PET scans because of respiratory motion, and this particular artifact is unique to CT attenuation-corrected scans. Significant misregistration can also occur if the patient moves during the 20- to 30-minute PET scan (Fig. 2-47). Many of the interpretative errors caused by these and other artifacts can be avoided by examining the nonattenuation-corrected PET images.

PEARLS & PITFALLS

- A "survey" meter usually has a Geiger-Mueller detector filled with pressurized gas on the end of a cable. It is used to detect and measure low levels of activity or radiation. It cannot measure high levels.

- An ionization chamber usually has the detector inside the device housing. It is used to measure high levels of activity or radiation. It is less efficient for detecting low levels of activity when compared to a Geiger counter.

- A well counter is a cylindrical sodium iodide crystal with a hole drilled in it and a photomultiplier tube (PMT) on the end.

- A thyroid probe has a single sodium iodide crystal, a PMT on the end, and a single hole collimator.

- The dose calibrator is a gas-filled ionization chamber.

- Most dose calibrators have a digital readout that indicates the amount of activity in millicuries or Becquerels when the specific radionuclide being measured has been specified. Because not all radionuclides generate the same number of photons per radioactive decay, the radionuclide must be specified on the dose calibrator

- A gamma camera detector usually has a single large, flat sodium iodide crystal and multiple PMTs.

- SPECT reconstruction uses the same basic Fourier transformation back-projection method as does CT. It is usually an iterative method rather than back filtered.

- Gamma cameras localize the source of activity by using collimators. In contrast, PET scanners use coincidence registration.

- Gamma cameras typically have large flat crystal detectors while PET scanners have multiple rings of many small crystalline detectors situated around the patient. In some cases, the detectors may be semiconductors.

- All instruments require some quality control and calibration. Many have different required tests and frequency. The U.S. Nuclear Regulatory Commission requires that, at a minimum, the manufacturer's recommendations be followed.

- Quality control on newer gamma cameras is often done automatically. Flood fields for uniformity on newer cameras are usually performed daily using a point source of technetium-99m or cobalt-57.

- Intrinsic flood-field images are performed without the collimator. Extrinsic images are performed with the collimator in place.

- If required, spatial resolution can be tested weekly with a bar phantom.

- In corrected flood-field images, any inhomogeneities have been adjusted by the computer system so that the resulting image is homogeneous.

- A defect seen only on the extrinsic flood-field image, and not on the intrinsic image, is caused by a defective collimator.

- Poor spatial resolution can result from an insufficient amount of injected activity (inadequate counts), use of a high-energy or a particularly low-energy radionuclide, poor background clearance of the radiopharmaceutical, a patient too distant from the detector face, or very rarely an off-peak energy window.

- For SPECT cameras, uniformity and center of rotation (COR) checks are done weekly, and gantry and table alignment is checked quarterly. COR artifacts usually cause cold defects and blurring. When extreme, ring artifacts may be caused. Negative defects caused by COR artifacts on SPECT images may have a tail of activity extending peripherally.

- A rounded or hexagonal negative defect on an image is likely the result of a photomultiplier tube problem. Other round defects include metallic objects such as pacemakers.

- A linear or branching negative defect with dark borders on an image is likely the result of a cracked crystal.

- A very dense object can cause an attenuation correction artifact on PET scans. This is seen on the attenuation corrected images as an area of increased activity. It is absent on the nonattenuation corrected images.

SUGGESTED READINGS

Buck A, Nekolla S, Ziegler S, et al: SPECT/CT. J Null Med 2008;49:1305-19.

Bushberg JT, Seibert JA, Leidholdt EM,et al. The Essential Physics of Medical Imaging, 2nd ed. Baltimore: Williams & Wilkins; 2002.

European Association of Nuclear Medicine Physics Committee: Routine quality control recommendations for nuclear medicine instrumentation. Eur J Nucl Med 2010;37:662-71.

Madsen MT: Recent advances in SPECT imaging. J Nucl Med 2007;48:661-73.

Mawlawi O, Townsend D: Multimodality imaging: An update on PET/CT technology. Eur J Nucl Med 2009;36(Suppl 1): S15-S29.

Patton J, Turkington T: SPECT/CT physical principles and attenuation correction. J Nucl Med Technol 2008;36: 1-10.

Pichler BJ, Kolb A, Nagele T, et al: PET/MRI: Paving the way for the next generation of clinical multimodality imaging applications. J Nucl Med 2010;51:333-6.

Ranger NT: The AAPM/RSNA Physics Tutorial for Residents: Radiation detectors in nuclear medicine. Radio-Graphics 1999;19:481-502.

Zanzonico P: Routine quality control of clinical nuclear medicine instrumentation: A brief review. J Nucl Med 2008;49:1114-31.

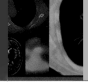

3 Central Nervous System

RADIONUCLIDE BRAIN IMAGING
  Planar Brain Imaging
  SPECT and PET Brain Imaging
  Clinical Applications

CEREBROSPINAL FLUID IMAGING
  Radiopharmaceuticals and Technique
  Normal Examination
  Clinical Applications

RADIONUCLIDE BRAIN IMAGING

Nuclear medicine imaging of the central nervous system has been largely eclipsed by the widespread availability of computed tomography (CT) and magnetic resonance imaging (MRI). In certain clinical settings, however, radionuclide planar, single-photon emission computed tomography (SPECT) or positron emission tomography (PET) brain imaging can provide valuable functional and perfusion information about suspected cerebral abnormalities or cerebrospinal fluid (CSF) dynamics that is not obtained through anatomic imaging. For this reason, an understanding of the techniques and principles involved in radionuclide brain imaging remains important.

In the normal cerebrum, passage of most substances from the cerebral capillaries into the extravascular space is severely restricted, constituting what has been referred to as the *blood-brain barrier*. The degree of permeability of this barrier varies with the nature of the material attempting to pass and with the numerous complex carrier mechanisms used to facilitate or hinder passage through the cell membranes involved.

The most common nuclear medicine imaging procedures of the brain can be divided into three different approaches relative to this principle:

Planar brain imaging, which uses radiopharmaceuticals that are perfusion agents. Planar imaging is usually performed for brain death studies only.

SPECT brain perfusion imaging, which uses lipophilic radiopharmaceuticals that routinely cross the blood-brain barrier to localize in normal brain tissue and pathologic processes in proportion to regional cerebral blood flow.

PET metabolic brain imaging, which uses functional positron-emitting radiopharmaceuticals, such as radiolabeled fluorodeoxyglucose (a glucose analog which reflects regional glucose metabolism) and neuroreceptor agents.

Planar Brain Imaging
Technique

Planar radionuclide cerebral imaging generally consists of two phases: (1) a dynamic or angiographic study composed of rapid sequential images of the arrival of the radioactive bolus in the cerebral hemispheres, which essentially constitutes a qualitative measure of regional brain perfusion; and (2) delayed static images. The most common application of planar technique is in the setting of suspected brain death. Most brain scans are performed with either a transient perfusion agent (technetium-99m [^{99m}Tc]–diethylenetriamine pentaacetic acid [DTPA], ^{99m}Tc-pertechnetate) or a lipophilic perfusion agent that is extracted by the brain on the first pass (^{99m}Tc–hexamethylpropyleneamine oxime [HMPAO], ^{99m}Tc–ethylene l-cysteinate dimer [ECD]). A sample protocol giving details of the technique and associated radiation doses are given in Appendix E-1.

Normal Planar Brain Scan

Normally, there is prompt symmetric perfusion that in the anterior projection looks similar to a trident. The middle cerebral arteries are seen to the right and left, and the anterior cerebral arteries are seen as a single midline vertical line of activity. Perfusion should extend to the calvarial convexities bilaterally (Fig. 3-1). Although symmetry is the hallmark of the arterial-capillary phase of a normal perfusion scan, asymmetry in the venous phase is common because of variations in venous anatomy. Care should be taken not to overinterpret lack of symmetry in the venous phase in the absence of an arterial abnormality.

On the static images of a ^{99m}Tc-DTPA or ^{99m}Tc-pertechnetate scan, radioactivity does not normally lie within the brain itself because of the integrity of the blood-brain barrier, but rather is located in the overlying scalp soft tissues, calvarium, and subarachnoid spaces that outline the cerebral hemispheres. Activity is also seen in the larger blood pool accumulations, such as the sagittal and transverse sinuses. Thus, the normal static brain images include a number of consistent landmarks (Fig. 3-2). On the posterior view, the transverse sinuses are generally symmetric, although it is not uncommon for the right sinus to be dominant. On the

lateral views, activity in the suprasellar and sylvian regions is noted, although it is less constant and less well defined than activity in the venous sinuses.

In contrast to ^{99m}Tc-DTPA or ^{99m}Tc-pertechnetate imaging, normal static planar images obtained with a first-pass extraction perfusion agent (^{99m}Tc-HMPAO, ^{99m}Tc-ECD) will demonstrate activity in the brain substance (primarily gray matter) (Fig. 3-3).

SPECT and PET Brain Imaging Radiopharmaceuticals

Although planar brain perfusion imaging is usually limited to compounds that enter the brain substance only when there is disruption of the normal blood-brain barrier, SPECT brain perfusion imaging uses several groups of lipophilic radiopharmaceuticals. These radiopharmaceuticals cross the intact blood-brain barrier and are retained by the brain tissue in proportion to regional cerebral blood flow (rCBF). They thus map the distribution of brain perfusion in

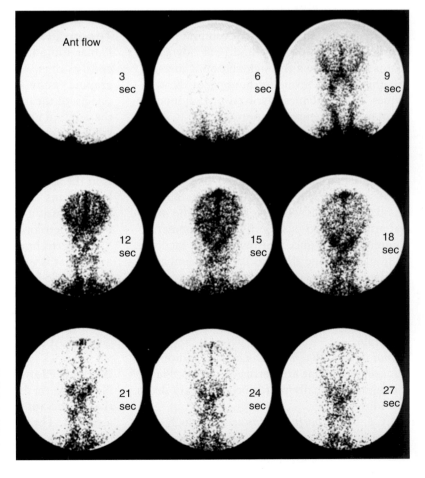

Figure 3-1. Normal anterior radionuclide angiogram (^{99m}Tc DTPA). The anterior and middle cerebral arteries are clearly visualized on the 9-second frame. The sagittal sinus is easily seen by 15 seconds. *DTPA,* Diethylenetriamine pentaacetic acid.

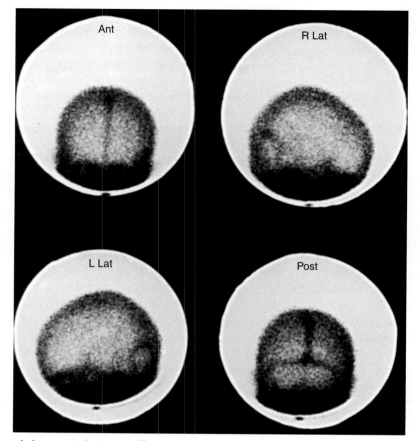

Figure 3-2. Normal planar static brain scan (^{99m}Tc-DTPA). A large amount of activity is normally seen in the face and base of the skull. The sagittal and transverse sinuses are normally prominent.

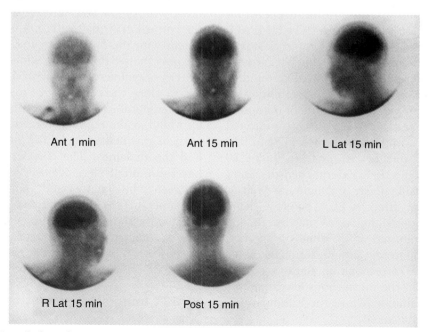

Figure 3-3. Normal planar brain images. Planar images of the brain done after administration of a first-pass extraction agent (^{99m}Tc-HMPAO). The images show activity primarily in the gray matter. *HMPAO*, Hexamethylpropyleneamine oxime.

both normal and pathologic brain tissue. These agents include the following:

^{99m}Tc-HMPAO (exametazime)

^{99m}Tc-ECD (bicisate)

Technetium-99m HMPAO (^{99m}Tc exametazime or Ceretec) is a lipophilic agent that crosses the blood-brain barrier with rapid first-pass uptake. Once in the brain substance, HMPAO is metabolized to a hydrophilic form that cannot diffuse out of the brain. Uptake in the brain peaks several minutes after injection. About 5% of the injected activity localizes in the brain, with no significant late redistribution. Activity of ^{99m}Tc-HMPAO is highest in gray matter and is proportional to rCBF. Because it may be unstable in vitro, ^{99m}Tc-HMPAO should be injected within 30 minutes after its preparation, although a stabilized form is available that can be used up to 4 hours after preparation.

Technetium-99m ECD (bicisate or Neurolite) has uptake and redistribution properties similar to HMPAO. ^{99m}Tc-ECD is rapidly localized in a normal brain in proportion to rCBF, with slow clearance. It is retained in the brain tissue by rapid de-esterification to a polar metabolite that does not recross the blood-brain barrier and therefore maintains residence within the brain tissue. Thus there is no intracerebral redistribution. A high ratio of gray to white matter that persists over time is identified. Intracerebral activity peaks several minutes after administration, with about 6% of the dose localizing within the brain. Although similar to ^{99m}Tc-HMPAO, ^{99m}Tc-ECD demonstrates more rapid clearance from the blood pool, thus reducing background activity and increasing target to background. It also demonstrates better chemical stability with a longer post preparation shelf life of 6 hours.

^{99m}Tc-ECD and ^{99m}Tc-HMPAO are injected intravenously using 10 to 20 mCi (370 to 740 MBq). SPECT images are obtained 15 to 20 minutes after injection. External sensory stimuli, such as pain, noise, and light, as well as patient motion, affect rCBF. Therefore these, along with cognitive functions such as reading, should be minimized at the time of injection and localization to prevent interfering increased activity in the corresponding sensory cortex. For like reason, the intravenous access should be placed 5 minutes before the radiopharmaceutical is administered.

Thallium-201 chloride is used for SPECT imaging in the differential diagnosis of recurrent tumors versus radiation necrosis. Very little thallium is concentrated in normal brain tissue, and an increase in thallium often indicates the presence of viable tumor.

The major PET radiopharmaceutical for brain imaging used in the United States is ^{18}F-fluorodeoxyglucose (FDG). Uptake is reflective of regional glucose metabolism and not regional blood flow. Areas of the brain stimulated by activity during ^{18}F-FDG injection and uptake show relatively increased metabolism. These include the visual (occipital) or auditory cortical areas in visually (eyes open) or auditorally (sound) stimulated patients, language centers in talking patients, and the motor cortex in moving patients. Thus injection and uptake of ^{18}F-FDG are best accomplished in silent, motionless patients in a quiet, darkened room. Various disease states can cause either an increase or decrease in FDG accumulation (Table 3-1). Certain drugs may alter global and/or relative regional brain metabolism, including sedatives, antiepileptic and neuroleptic drugs, and barbiturates. Other amyloid plaque and neuroreceptor PET agents are in use in Europe.

Details of suggested techniques and radiation doses are shown in Appendix E.

Normal SPECT Brain Scan

The normal distribution of lipophilic brain perfusion agents is proportional to regional blood flow, with significantly greater activity seen in the cortical gray matter (Fig. 3-4). This is consistent with the fourfold greater blood flow in the gray matter than in the white matter. Thus activity is symmetric and greatest in the strip of cortex along the convexity of the frontal, parietal, temporal, and occipital lobes. Activity is also high in the regions corresponding to subcortical gray matter, including the basal ganglia and the thalamus. The cortical white matter has substantially less activity, and the border between white matter and ventricles may be indistinct. Although high-resolution images obtained with dedicated multidetector cameras display greater anatomic detail, the primary purpose of SPECT imaging is to evaluate relative rCBF rather than structural detail.

SPECT Image Interpretation

The cerebral perfusion images should be inspected for symmetry of radiopharmaceutical distribution and for continuity of perfusion in

TABLE 3–1	Accumulation of ^{18}F-FDG in Abnormal Conditions	
TISSUE/ ORGAN	**ACTIVITY LEVEL**	**COMMENTS**
Brain		
Ictal seizure focus	High	Very rarely done because of need to remain still and poor temporal resolution of PET
Interictal seizure focus	Low	Review temporal lobes
Radiation necrosis	Low	
Recurrent tumor	Variable	If increased activity suspect recurrence
Dementia— Alzheimer	Low posterior temporoparietal cortical activity	Often identical pattern to Parkinson dementia
Dementia— Pick	Low frontal lobes	
Dementia— Multi-infarct	Scattered small areas of decreased activity	
Cerebellar diaschisis ("crossed")	Low area in one hemisphere	Low activity in cerebellum contralateral to supratentorial stroke, tumor, trauma, etc.
Huntington disease	Low activity in caudate nucleus and putamen	

the rim of cortical gray matter. In general, local perfusion is measured as increased, similar, or decreased relative to the perfusion in the identical area in the contralateral cerebral hemisphere. Pathologic processes that alter local brain perfusion produce areas of increased or decreased activity, depending on the changes in blood flow relative to the normal adjacent brain tissue. Because the anatomic detail of the images is limited, more precise localization of an abnormality may be facilitated by visual comparison or superimposition (fusion) of the SPECT images with corresponding CT or MRI slices.

PET Image Interpretation

PET with ^{18}F-FDG permits the noninvasive in vivo quantification of local cerebral metabolism and, unlike CT or MRI, provides a physiologic test that may illustrate pathologic conditions *before* morphologic manifestations are discernible. PET metabolic imaging has significant usefulness in certain discrete clinical settings and has been used to evaluate refractory seizure disorders, dementia, and recurrent brain tumors.

The normal distribution of ^{18}F-FDG in the brain is highest in the gray matter of the cortex, basal ganglia, and thalami (Fig. 3-5). This pattern changes with aging, and significant variations in cortical uptake have been noted. Relatively decreased frontal lobe metabolism with normal aging is not uncommon. Metabolism in the thalami, basal ganglia, cerebellum, and visual cortex is generally unchanged with normal aging.

Certain areas of the cerebral cortex can normally be focally hypermetabolic compared with the remainder of the cortex. These include the posterior cingulate cortex (anterior and superior to the occipital cortex), a focus in the posterior superior temporal lobe (Wernicke region), the frontal eye fields (anterior to the primary motor cortex and may be asymmetric), and a symmetric area of increased activity in the posterior parietal lobes. The degree of uptake in the cerebellar gray matter is significantly less on an FDG PET study than on a SPECT perfusion scan.

Clinical Applications
Brain Death

The planar radionuclide angiogram is a simple, noninvasive method of determining the presence or absence of intracerebral perfusion and thereby of confirming a clinical diagnosis of brain death. To prevent mistaking scalp perfusion for intracerebral blood flow, an elastic band can be placed around the head just above the orbits. This may diminish blood flow to the superficial scalp vessels.

In the presence of cerebral death, the injected activity typically proceeds through the carotid artery to the base of the skull, where the radioactive bolus stops (Fig. 3-6). As with all radionuclide arteriograms, injection of a good bolus is important. If distinct activity in the common carotid artery is not identified, the injection should be repeated. The absence of intracerebral flow is strong corroborative evidence of cerebral demise. Generally, a single anterior or lateral cerebral view is obtained within 5 to

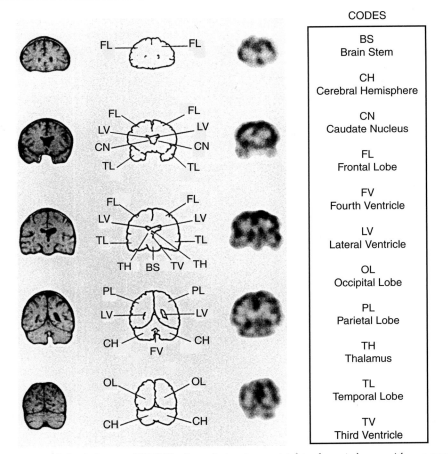

CODES

BS
Brain Stem

CH
Cerebral Hemisphere

CN
Caudate Nucleus

FL
Frontal Lobe

FV
Fourth Ventricle

LV
Lateral Ventricle

OL
Occipital Lobe

PL
Parietal Lobe

TH
Thalamus

TL
Temporal Lobe

TV
Third Ventricle

Figure 3-4. Tomographic brain images. SPECT brain perfusion images (*right columns*) shown with comparable magnetic resonance images (*left columns*) and anatomic diagrams (*middle columns*). (IMP Incorporated, Houston.)

10 minutes of the completion of the angiographic portion of the study to determine the presence of any sagittal sinus activity. The significance of such activity without an obvious arterial phase is somewhat controversial, but it may represent a small amount of intracerebral flow. Most of these patients have a grave prognosis. The presence of slight dural sinus activity does not contradict the diagnosis of brain death.

When intracranial carotid blood flow ceases in the setting of brain death, increased or collateral flow through the maxillary branch of the external carotid artery may produce markedly increased perfusion projecting over the nasal area in the anterior view, as seen on the radionuclide angiogram and subsequently on static images. This so-called "hot-nose" sign cannot be used specifically to indicate brain death, but it may be used as a secondary sign when intracerebral perfusion is absent. This sign may also occur with a generalized decrease of cerebral perfusion from various causes, including

severe cerebrovascular or carotid occlusive disease or increased intracranial pressure of any cause.

If clinical evaluation of the patient suggests brain death and no cerebral perfusion is demonstrated on the radionuclide study, brain death is virtually certain. Although an actual diagnosis of brain death should not be made by using nuclear imaging techniques alone, these techniques are important supportive evidence of such a diagnosis in the proper clinical settings.

Radiopharmaceuticals used for SPECT brain perfusion imaging (^{99m}Tc-ECD and -HMPAO) may also be used for cerebral angiography in the same manner as conventional brain imaging agents. Absence of perfusion on the angiographic phase and lack of cerebral activity on subsequent static planar or SPECT images confirm brain death. Advantages over conventional ^{99m}Tc-pertechnetate or ^{99m}Tc-DTPA imaging are conferred by the ability to perform static planar or SPECT imaging, which renders the

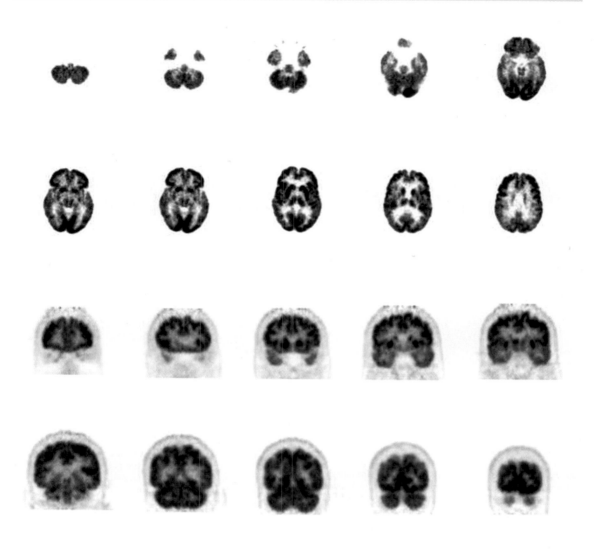

FIGURE 3-5. Normal ^{18}**F-FDG PET brain scan.** Axial images inferior to superior (*upper rows*) and coronal images anterior to posterior (*lower rows*). *FDG,* Fluorodeoxyglucose; *PET,* positron emission tomography.

examination less dependent on the radionuclide angiographic phase, including bolus adequacy and the problems associated with interfering superficial scalp blood flow and sagittal sinus activity.

Cerebrovascular Disease

SPECT brain perfusion imaging has been demonstrated to be of value in the diagnosis and prognosis of cerebrovascular disease manifested by TIAs, acute cerebral infarction, and intracranial hemorrhage.

Cerebral Infarction. SPECT brain perfusion imaging is more sensitive than CT and MRI in detecting cerebral ischemia during the first hours of stroke. Only about 20% of CT scans are positive 8 hours after cerebral infarction, whereas 90% of SPECT brain perfusion images show deficits. By 72 hours, however, the sensitivity of the two examinations is about equal. Sensitivity of SPECT brain perfusion imaging is significantly affected by the size of the infarct. Small infarcts, particularly those in the white matter (lacunar infarcts), may not be detected with SPECT or PET. Acute infarcts are usually identified on noncontrast MRI within 4 to 6 hours. In addition, SPECT and PET brain imaging cannot distinguish between hemorrhagic and ischemic infarction, which is critical in the early stages of evaluation and treatment.

During the *acute phase* of stroke (first hours to 2 to 3 days after vascular insult), a reduction

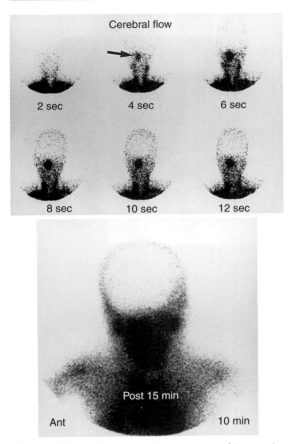

Figure 3-6. Brain death. *Top,* Angiographic anterior images (⁹⁹ᵐTc-DTPA) of the head demonstrate flow in both carotid arteries at 4 seconds. Throughout the remainder of the images, the normally expected trident appearance of the intracerebral vessels is not seen. In addition, the "hot nose" sign is present (*arrow*). *Bottom,* A delayed image at 10 minutes fails to demonstrate any evidence of intracerebral or sagittal sinus activity.

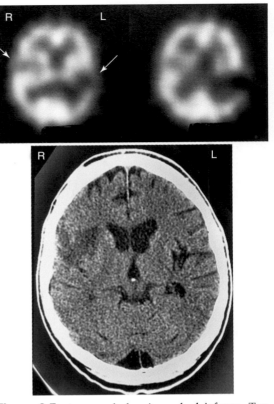

Figure 3-7. Acute and chronic cerebral infarcts. *Top,* Two ⁹⁹ᵐTc-HMPAO transaxial SPECT images demonstrate an area of decreased activity in the region of the right middle cerebral artery (*small arrow*). A much larger area of decreased activity is seen in the posterior distribution of the left middle cerebral artery (*large arrow*). *Bottom,* Computed tomographic scan obtained at the same time demonstrates low density in the area of the older infarction on the right, but very little abnormality is visible in the area of the recent infarction on the left.

in blood flow to the affected area is identified (Fig. 3-7). The area of decreased perfusion on SPECT imaging may be greater than that seen with CT imaging, suggesting tissue at risk (ischemic penumbra) surrounding the infarct.

In the *subacute phase* of stroke (1 to 3 weeks after onset), the brain SPECT perfusion pattern is complicated by the phenomenon of increased, or "luxury," perfusion; that is, the blood supply is greater than is metabolically required because the cells are already dead or dying (Fig. 3-8). This phenomenon may decrease the sensitivity of SPECT perfusion imaging in the subacute phase of stroke.

Prognostically, patients displaying improvement of perfusion during the first week after infarction display a greater chance of recovery of neurologic function than do those whose perfusion improves at a later time.

In the *chronic phase* (≥1 month after symptom onset), luxury perfusion has generally subsided, and the perfusion deficits seen on SPECT imaging stabilize. Except for monitoring improvement and serving as comparisons for future studies, SPECT brain imaging is of limited use in the chronic phase of stroke.

During the acute and subacute phases of stroke, crossed-cerebellar diaschisis (seen primarily with cortical strokes) is a common phenomenon and should not be confused with primary cerebellar ischemia or other pathology (see following).

Transient Ischemic Attacks. The sensitivity for detecting localized cerebral ischemia

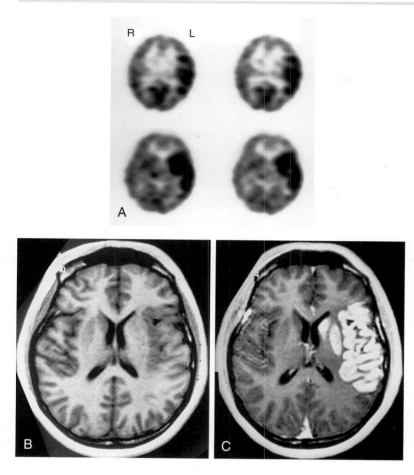

Figure 3-8. Infarction with "luxury" perfusion. **A,** Four transaxial ^{99m}Tc-HMPAO SPECT images obtained 7 days after infarction demonstrate a large area of increased perfusion in the left middle cerebral artery distribution. **B,** A noncontrasted T^1-weighted magnetic resonance imaging scan demonstrates a small amount of decreased density in the left middle cerebral artery region. **C,** A gadolinium-enhanced magnetic resonance imaging scan shows the marked increase in perfusion.

associated with TIA is time sensitive; 60% of these perfusion deficits are detected in the first 24 hours, but less than 40% are detected 1 week after the insult. In addition, hypoperfusion duration is variable and may persist even after symptoms have resolved. Most patients with TIAs or carotid stenoses do not display cortical perfusion defects without pharmacologic intervention. A simple method for evaluating the adequacy of cerebrovascular reserve is to assess brain perfusion response to pharmacologic cerebrovascular vasodilatation using acetazolamide (Diamox), a carbonic anhydrase inhibitor, in conjunction with SPECT brain perfusion imaging. In normal patients, cerebral blood flow increases threefold to fourfold with use of Diamox. In areas in which regional perfusion reserve is diminished because autoregulatory vasodilatation is already maximal, a relative Diamox-induced regional perfusion defect is identified on SPECT brain perfusion images compared with the surrounding normal regions,

which increase in perfusion (and thus activity) compared with baseline images obtained without Diamox intervention (Fig. 3-9).

Brain Tumors

Both primary and metastatic brain lesions present on SPECT brain perfusion imaging as localized defects that correspond to the mass lesions. This technique alone is of limited value in the primary diagnosis or evaluation of intracranial mass lesions. In conjunction with Thallium-201 (201Tl), however, SPECT brain perfusion imaging may be valuable in distinguishing between radiation necrosis and tumor recurrence in patients with malignant gliomas treated with high-dose radiation. The study may also localize suspected recurrences for biopsy.

In the differentiation of recurrent malignant glioma from radiation necrosis, ^{99m}Tc-HMPAO images generally show a focal defect in the region of abnormality, whether containing necrotic tissue, recurrent tumor, or both.

Post-Diamox

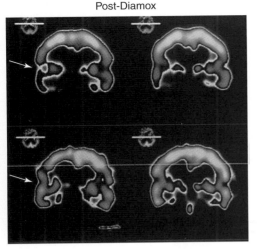

Pre-Diamox

Figure 3-9. Diamox challenge study. Post- and pre-Diamox coronal SPECT brain perfusion images show decreased vascular reserve (decreased perfusion) in the right temporal region (*arrows*) after Diamox administration. (Case courtesy B. Barron, MD, and Lamk Lamki, MD.)

Thallium-201 activity, however, is a marker of viability, localizing in living tumor cells but not in nonviable tumor cells or necrotic tissue. Thallium-201 activity may be graded as low (less than scalp activity), moderate (equal or up to twice scalp activity), or high (greater than twice scalp activity) (Fig. 3-10). A high degree of increased thallium activity in the region of a ^{99m}Tc-HMPAO defect is indicative of tumor recurrence, whereas a low degree is consistent with postradiation necrosis. Careful attention to study acquisition and processing is needed to compare identical areas between the two SPECT studies and with correlative CT or MRI scans.

PET/CT may play a role in the evaluation of brain malignancies. The degree of ^{18}F-FDG uptake in primary brain tumors generally correlates inversely with patient survival. Tumors with high FDG uptake are likely to be high-grade aggressive lesions with poor patient survival, whereas relatively hypometabolic neoplasms generally represent lower-grade tumors. FDG PET imaging is limited, however, because many low-grade tumors (and some high-grade tumors) show uptake similar to normal white matter. High uptake in a tumor previously known to be low grade is likely to represent anaplastic transformation. Lymphoma is typically very hypermetabolic.

After therapy, FDG PET scanning can help differentiate recurrent tumor (increased activity) (Fig. 3-11) from radiation necrosis (decreased activity) (Fig. 3-12). A flare response after chemotherapy of brain neoplasms has been described, occurring a few days after treatment. This FDG increased activity may be related to an influx of inflammatory cells in response to tumor cell death. The study may occasionally be affected by therapy with corticosteroids because steroids have been shown to decrease glucose metabolism in the brain.

Detection of brain metastases with FDG PET is usually poor because of the high background activity normally present in gray matter, poor uptake of FDG (Fig. 3-13), and the limited spatial resolution of PET instruments. Occasionally, very hypermetabolic metastases (such as those from melanoma) and incidental pituitary adenomas (Fig. 3-14) can be detected. Regardless, contrast-enhanced MRI remains the preferred imaging technique in these settings.

Cerebellar Diaschisis

A benign, asymptomatic phenomenon known as *diaschisis* may cause focal areas of hypoperfusion and hypometabolism in areas of the brain remote, but connected by neural pathways, from the location of a lesion, including neoplasm, stroke, and trauma. The phenomenon is manifested on FDG PET or SPECT perfusion imaging by diminished activity in the cerebellar hemisphere contralateral to the supratentorial abnormality. This reduced metabolism is often seen in the cerebellar hemisphere contralateral to a supratentorial lesion (*crossed cerebellar diaschisis*). The cerebellar metabolic depression is typically asymptomatic, and the effect frequently resolves when occurring with stroke but may persist when associated with brain tumors. It is important to recognize these phenomena and not to mistake it for a concomitant cerebellar lesion. Subcortical-cortical cerebral diaschisis also occurs, such as when small thalamic strokes are associated with ipsilateral depression of cortical metabolism.

Epilepsy

Patients with partial (focal) epilepsy refractory to therapy may benefit from surgical ablation of the seizure focus. The most common pathology at these foci is mesial temporal sclerosis (gliotic

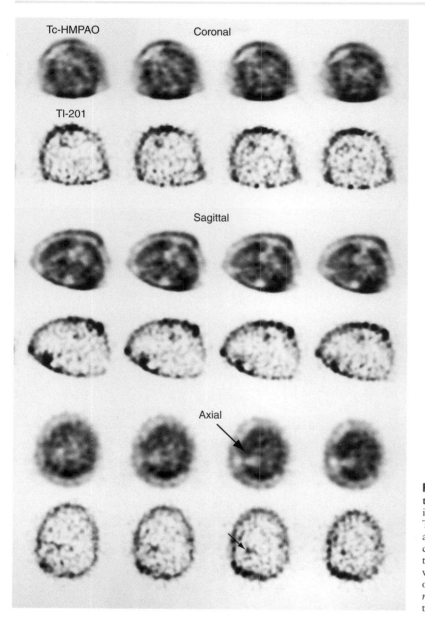

Figure 3-10. Recurrent brain tumor. Sets of paired coronal, sagittal, and axial Tc-HMPAO and Tl-201 images are shown. The axial 99m Tc HMPAO images best demonstrate decreased activity in the right parietal region (fifth *row*) while the thallium-201 images demonstrate increased activity (sixth *row*) differentiating this recurrent tumor from radiation necrosis.

temporal scarring). Although most complex partial seizures arise from epileptic foci in the temporal lobes, they also may arise from other cortical areas. If seizure foci can be localized to the temporal lobes, about 70% of patients undergoing partial temporal lobectomy experience amelioration or eradication of seizures. The value of SPECT and PET imaging in this setting is well established.

The primary nuclear imaging techniques used for seizure localization have been those that attempt to localize the seizure foci based on their metabolic or perfusion status. Seizure foci may exhibit hyperperfusion and

hypermetabolism during seizures (ictal studies) and hypometabolism and hypoperfusion between seizures (interictal studies). PET imaging using ^{18}FDG is the method of choice for evaluating metabolism, whereas SPECT imaging with ^{99m}Tc perfusion agents, such as ECD or HMPAO, appears to be the method of choice for evaluation of perfusion status. In general, ictal studies are more sensitive in the detection of temporal lobe seizure foci than are interictal studies, with a sensitivity of 85% to 95% ictally and about 70% interictally. The positive-predictive values of PET and interictal SPECT are comparable.

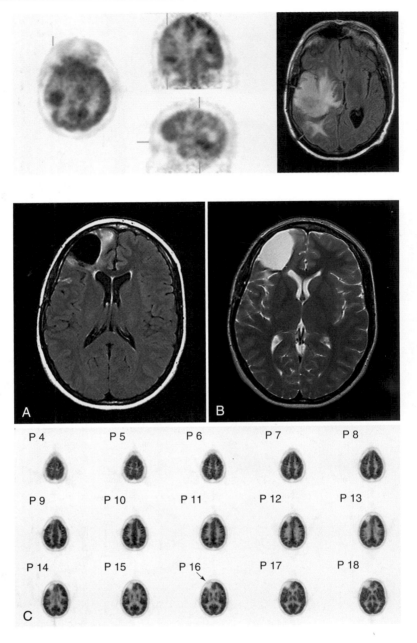

Figure 3-11. Recurrent glioma. *Right,* A post-treatment magnetic resonance imaging scan shows a large right hemisphere lesion. *Left,* ^{18}F-FDG PET images show a focus of intense metabolic activity because of a recurrent tumor. (Case courtesy William Spies, MD.)

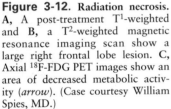

Figure 3-12. Radiation necrosis. **A,** A post-treatment T[1]-weighted and **B,** a T[2]-weighted magnetic resonance imaging scan show a large right frontal lobe lesion. **C,** Axial ^{18}F-FDG PET images show an area of decreased metabolic activity (*arrow*). (Case courtesy William Spies, MD.)

Ictal Imaging. By using ^{99m}Tc-HMPAO or ^{99m}Tc-ECD, which do not significantly redistribute, patients can be injected during the seizure or within 30 seconds after its completion. To obtain ictal studies, the patient may be hospitalized and monitored with electroencephalography. The radiopharmaceutical is kept at the bedside until a seizure occurs, at which time it is injected. Other times the studies are obtained inadvertently while an intended interictal study is being performed. Epileptogenic foci appear as areas of increased activity (hyperperfusion) and may involve the entire temporal lobe or a small mesial focus only (Fig. 3-15).

Ictal studies with PET are usually not technically feasible. It is very rare to obtain scans during the ictal phase, and this usually occurs if a patient has an unexpected seizure during an intended interictal study. During and shortly after a seizure, a focus of increased activity should be demonstrated (Fig. 3-16). Because uptake of FDG occurs over many minutes, the area of increased activity is often diffuse and is not very reliable in precisely localizing the seizure focus. Further, unrecognized seizure

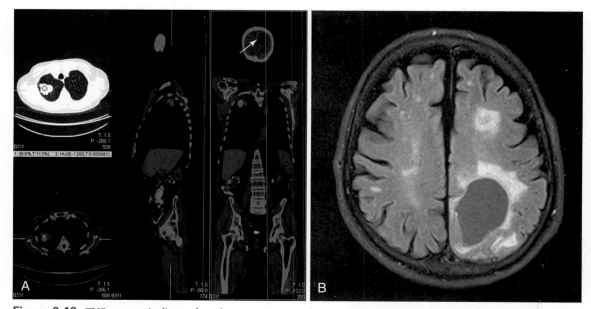

Figure 3-13. CNS metastatic disease from lung cancer. **A,** In this patient who was being staged for a lung cancer with an ^{18}F-FDG PET/CT scan, a hypometabolic area (*arrow*) is seen in the posterior aspect of the brain. **B,** MRI reveals the lesion much more clearly. *CT,* Computed tomography; *MRI,* magnetic resonance imaging.

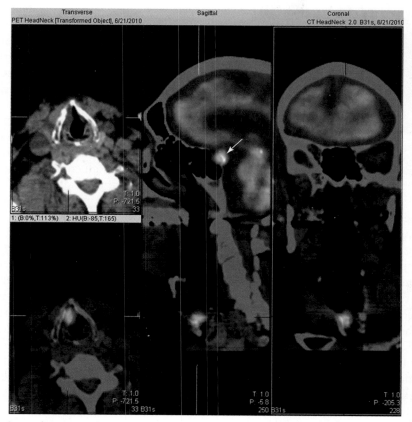

Figure 3-14. Pituitary adenoma. In this patient who was having an ^{18}F-FDG PET/CT scan for staging of a right vocal cord cancer, an incidental pituitary adenoma is seen (*arrow*).

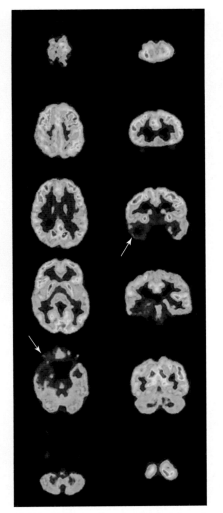

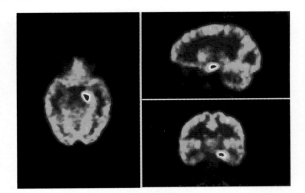

Figure 3-16. Epilepsy ictal study. An intense focus of metabolic activity is seen in the left temporal lobe on this ^{18}F-FDG PET scan. (Case courtesy William Spies, MD.)

Figure 3-15. Epilepsy (interictal). Axial and coronal SPECT brain perfusion images obtained with the radiopharmaceutical ^{99m}Tc-HMPAO between seizures show decreased activity in the right temporal lobe (*arrows*).

activity during the FDG-uptake period may produce a relative increase on the side of the lesion, making the contralateral normal temporal lobe appear spuriously hypometabolic. Thus, EEG during administration and uptake of FDG to detect subclinical seizures may aid in preventing false localization of a presumed interictal focus in this setting. PET imaging has not proved as accurate or helpful in the localization of extratemporal seizure foci.

Interictal Imaging. Because interictal SPECT perfusion studies are performed between seizures, blood flow to epileptic foci is normal or reduced. To be detected on SPECT imaging, these must be seen as areas of decreased activity (hypoperfusion). There are several interictal patterns that can be seen. Most often, decreased activity in the temporal lobe is noted,

which is usually more pronounced laterally than mesially. With mesial temporal lobe epilepsy, there can be asymmetrically decreased perfusion of both temporal lobes, or there can be decreased activity in a temporal lobe with ipsilateral decrease in frontal lobe perfusion. Foci with normal interictal blood flow escape detection. PET scanning is helpful in patients with complex partial seizures. Mesial temporal lobe epilepsy is the most common form. There is often an area of unilateral interictal temporal lobe hypometabolism in the seizure focus (Fig. 3-17), similar to the hypoperfusion seen with SPECT brain perfusion agents.

Extratemporal Lobe Epilepsy. Localization of partial seizure foci outside of the temporal lobe is more difficult than in the temporal lobe. Interictal glucose hypometabolism and hypoperfusion, the hallmarks of temporal lobe epilepsy, are uncommon in extratemporal lobe epilepsy when lesions are not identifiable on CT or MRI. Ictal SPECT may be more sensitive and accurate. Focal cortical dysplasia is a common cause of epilepsy in children. FDG-PET demonstrates areas of hypometabolic activity in regions of the cortex involved by FCD. FDG-PET scans show hypometabolic activity in areas of seizure caused by tuberous sclerosis.

Dementia

Considerable experience with SPECT brain perfusion imaging of dementias has corroborated its use in the early diagnosis and differentiation of the various types of dementia that may permit the identification of treatable causes, such as vascular dementia. In dementia, metabolic distribution patterns demonstrated on ^{18}F-FDG PET scans are broadly comparable to those seen

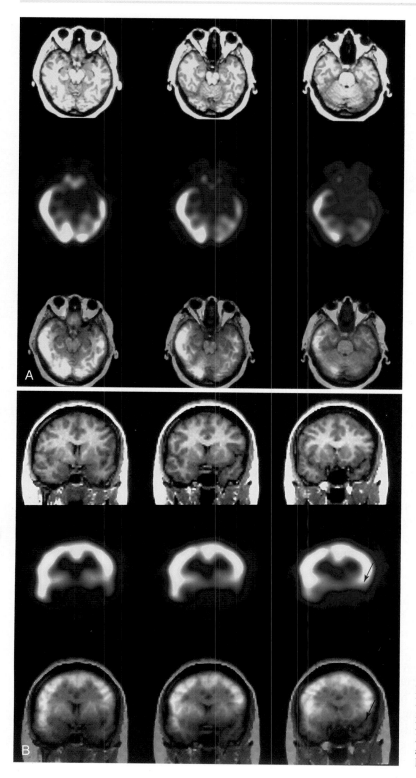

Figure 3-17. Epilepsy interictal PET/MRI study. **A,** Transaxial and **B,** coronal magnetic resonance imaging (MRI) (*upper row*), ^{18}F-FDG PET images (*middle row*), and PET/MRI images (*lower row*) show an area of decreased metabolism in the left temporal lobe (*arrows*).

by using SPECT brain perfusion agents, generally with greater sensitivity and overall accuracy. Despite the patterns mentioned in the following, there remains considerable overlap in the patterns seen in various dementias (Table 3-2).

Alzheimer Disease (AD). The most common and highly suggestive finding of Alzheimer disease on SPECT brain perfusion images using ^{99m}Tc-HMPAO or ^{99m}Tc-ECD is symmetric bilateral posterior temporal and parietal

TABLE 3–2	¹⁸F-FDG PET Imaging in Dementia		
DIAGNOSIS	**EARLY METABOLIC DEFICITS**	**LATE METABOLIC DEFICITS**	**RELATIVE SPARING**
Alzheimer disease	Often asymmetric parietal, temporal, posterior cingulate, cortical deficits	Bilateral involvement common	Primary sensorimotor and visual cortices typical Thalamus, basal ganglia, and cerebellum sparing
Multi-infarct dementia	Scattered cerebral, cortical, subcortical, cerebellar defects		
Pick disease (fronto-temporal dementia)	Frontal, anterior, temporal, and mesiotemporal cortices	Parietal and lateral temporal cortices	Primary sensorimotor and visual cortices
Parkinson disease	Similar to Alzheimer disease	Similar to Alzheimer disease	More mesiotemporal and less visual cortical sparing than in Alzheimer disease
Huntington disease	Caudate and lentiform nuclei	Diffuse cortical lesions	
Dementia with Lewy bodies	Similar to Alzheimer disease	Similar to Alzheimer disease	Less sparing of occipital cortex than in Alzheimer disease

Adapted from Silverman DHS: Brain F-18-FDG PET in the diagnosis of neurodegenerative dementias: comparison with perfusion SPECT and with clinical evaluations lacking nuclear imaging. J Nucl Med 2004;45:594-607.

perfusion defects (posterior association cortex), with a positive predictive value of more than 80% (Fig. 3-18). Although characteristic, however, this imaging appearance is not pathognomonic and has been described in patients with vascular dementia, Parkinson disease, and various encephalopathies. About 30% of Alzheimer patients have asymmetrically decreased cortical activity. Other patterns, including unilateral temporal parietal hypoperfusion, which may be seen in 15% to 20% of patients, and frontal hypoperfusion, have been described but are less predictive of Alzheimer disease. Depending on the clinical setting, the negative predictive value of a normal SPECT perfusion scan is generally high, and other causes for dementia should be sought.

PET studies using ¹⁸FDG demonstrate hypometabolism patterns similar to those seen with SPECT brain perfusion agents; the most common of these is a typical pattern of posterior temporal parietal glucose hypometabolism (Fig. 3-19). Again, this finding is not pathognomonic, although it is highly predictive. In Alzheimer dementia, there is development of intracerebral senile plaques and neurofibrillary tangles with related abnormal deposition of proteins (amyloid and tau). The plaques destroy neurons by lysis of cell membranes, and the tangles fill the cytoplasm of axons and dendrites, preventing glucose transport. Thus, ¹⁸F-FDG scans in patients with Alzheimer dementia may reveal regionally decreased glucose metabolism as a result of both decreased glucose transport and neuronal loss. With Alzheimer dementia, decreased glucose metabolism is most commonly seen in the posterior temporal and parietal association cortices bilaterally with sparing of the primary sensorimotor and visual cortex, the basal ganglia, thalamus, brainstem, and cerebellum. However, in early stages it can be significantly asymmetric or even unilateral. One of the earliest findings is focal metabolic decrease in the posterior cingulate cortex, and frontal cortical involvement may become prominent with advanced disease. Similar findings of parietotemporal hypometabolism can be seen in dementia because of Parkinson disease, but often with some metabolic reduction in the occipital (visual) cortex. However, ¹⁸F-FDG scans cannot be used to differentiate these entities with certainty. If Parkinson dementia patients are excluded, the sensitivity and specificity for ¹⁸F-FDG imaging in Alzheimer dementia are about 90% and 70%, respectively. At present, PET scanning for Alzheimer dementia is being used in conjunction with MR hemodynamic imaging, MR spectroscopy, and sensitive volumetric techniques.

An investigational PET tracer, fluoro-ethyl, methyl amino-2 napthyl ethylidene malononitrile (¹⁸F-FDDNP) crosses the blood-brain barrier and binds to senile plaques and neurofibrillary tangles. Another approach has been

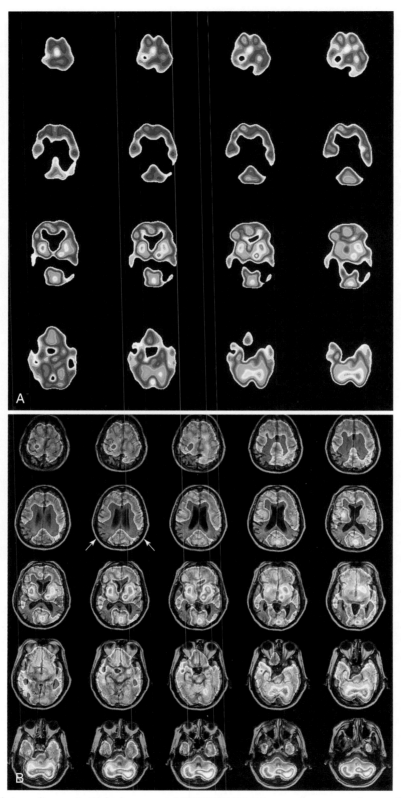

Figure 3-18. **Alzheimer disease. A,** Multiple transaxial SPECT HMPAO images demonstrate decreased perfusion in both temporal parietal regions. **B,** Fusion images of the SPECT and MRI scans help with anatomic localization of the abnormalities.

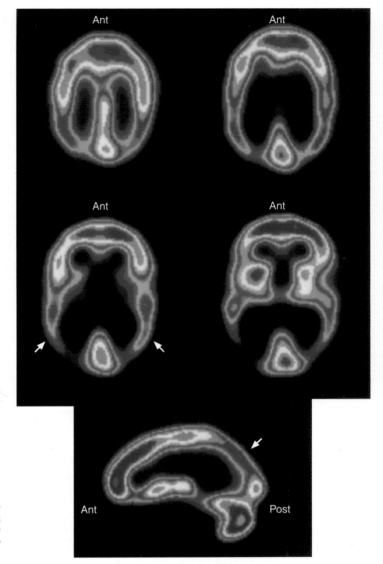

Figure 3-19. Alzheimer dementia. Multiple transaxial and one sagittal image from a ^{18}F-FDG PET scan show symmetrically decreased metabolic activity in the posterior tempoparietal regions (*arrows*).

the development of ^{11}C-nicotine to show nicotinic (cholinergic) receptor loss in Alzheimer disease. PET scans done by using H$_2$^{15}O can also show reduced blood flow in areas of hypometabolism. New PET amyloid ligands such as N-methyl [^{11}C]2-(4' methylaminophenyl)-6-hydroxy-benzothiasole (Pittsburgh compound B) have revealed high retention in the association cortex in Alzheimer patients even at prodromal stages (Fig. 3-20). Another promising agent is ^{18}F-florbetapir (E-4-(2-(6-(2-(2-(2-(^{18}F-fluoroethoxy)ethoxy)ethoxy)-pyridin-3-yl)vinyl)-N-methyl benzeneamine E)-4-(2-(6-(2-(2-(2-([18 F]-fluoroethoxy)ethoxy)ethoxy)- pyridin-3-yl) vinyl)-N-methyl benzenamine. Also known as AV-45 or Amyvid, it has been shown to correlate with the presence and density of beta-amyloid in the brain and is being studied in some

patients with dementia. How well the scan findings correlate with clinical Alzheimer disease or how the scan findings may affect patient management remains uncertain.

Multi-Infarct Dementia. Unlike patients with Alzheimer disease, patients with multi-infarct dementia usually present with multiple bilateral asymmetric areas of hypoperfusion and hypometabolism scattered throughout the cortex and deep structures. These are typically manifested as scattered defects of varying sizes on SPECT perfusion and PET metabolic brain images. This presentation generally distinguishes vascular dementia from the typical scan appearance of Alzheimer disease.

Frontotemporal Dementia (Pick Disease). Frontotemporal dementia (FTD) is rare and presents earlier in life than Alzheimer disease.

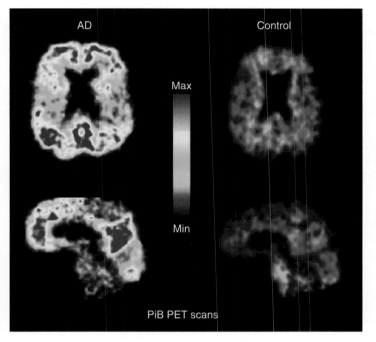

AD Control

Max

Min

PiB PET scans

Figure 3-20. Amyloid plaque imaging. On the left are PET scans of a patient with mild Alzheimer disease (AD) viewed as if looking from the top of the head down (*top left*) and from the side of the head (*bottom left*). The images on the right show similar PET scans from a healthy elderly person (control) with no memory impairment. The images were obtained by using a carbon-11 labeled marker for amyloid plaques, called Pittsburgh Compound-B *PIB*. The red, orange, and yellow areas show brain regions with heavy amyloid plaque loads in the AD patient (*red* indicating the highest levels). These plaques form the basis for the definitive diagnosis of AD at autopsy. (Case courtesy C. Mathis, MD, and the University of Pittsburgh PET Amyloid Imaging Group.)

Clinically, personality and mood changes often appear before memory loss. On SPECT perfusion imaging, FTD presents with bilateral frontal or frontotemporal perfusion defects. Bilateral frontal abnormalities have also been reported in the early phase of Alzheimer disease and in patients with schizophrenia, depression, and progressive supranuclear palsy. On ^{18}F-FDG PET imaging, FTD is classically characterized by hypometabolism in the frontal and frontotemporal regions.

Lewy Body Dementia. Dementia with Lewy body (DLB) disease is the second most common cause of dementia after Alzheimer disease. On SPECT perfusion and FDG PET imaging, it demonstrates patterns similar to Alzheimer, but with less sparing of the occipital (visual) cortex and greater involvement of the posterior parietal and occipital cortices.

Huntington Disease.

In patients with Huntington disease, there is often loss of ^{18}F-FDG activity in the basal ganglia, particularly the caudate and lentiform nuclei. Cortical perfusion defects and areas of hypometabolism may also be present.

Parkinson Disease (PD). Parkinson disease is a neurodegenerative disorder characterized by the progressive loss of dopaminergic neurons in the substantia nigra and with both motor and cognitive deficits. SPECT and PET scanning can show a decrease in dopamine transporter density in the striatum when compared to healthy controls.

Compounds used have been [123]I N-omega-fluoro propyl-2β-carbo methoxy-3β(-4-iodophenyl) nortropane (^{123}I FP-CIT) for SPECT and 6-[^{18}F] fluoro-L-3,4-dihydroxyphenylalanine (F-DOPA) for PET scanning. Approval by the FDA of the SPECT brain imaging agent ^{123}I-phenyltropane (ioflupane ^{123}I-DaTscan), which has a high binding affinity for presynaptic dopamine transporters (DAT), provides a means to map spatial distribution of the transporters in the brains of adult patients with suspected parkinsonism. Parkinson patients also show decreases in regional blood flow when scanned with ECD (Neurolite) or HMPAO. Decreases are seen initially in the frontal cortex, then in the prefrontal and parietal lobes, and, finally, hypoperfusion in all cortical areas.

Acquired Immunodeficiency Syndrome Dementia Complex. Up to half of patients with acquired immunodeficiency syndrome (AIDS) demonstrate neurologic involvement. The study may be useful in distinguishing subtle AIDS dementia complex from depression, psychosis, or focal neurologic disease. Because these findings may occur even in the presence of normal CT and MRI scans, SPECT imaging may constitute the only objective evidence of AIDS dementia complex. The SPECT perfusion pattern is that of multifocal or patchy cortical and subcortical hypoperfusion deficits. Lesions are most frequent in the frontal, temporal, and parietal lobes and basal ganglia. These perfusion abnormalities may resolve with therapy, and SPECT may provide a role in monitoring improvement. Because the brain perfusion patterns seen in AIDS dementia complex may also be seen in chronic cocaine or multidrug users, interpretation in this setting should be made with caution.

Head Trauma

Although SPECT brain perfusion imaging in the setting of brain trauma appears to be more sensitive and able to detect abnormalities earlier than CT can, its clinical utility is less clear. The size and number of perfusion abnormalities may have prognostic value in predicting the amount of permanent damage and may suggest patients who will develop post-traumatic headache.

Substance Abuse

Both acute and chronic cocaine use result in alterations in cerebral blood flow. Chronic cocaine use frequently presents as multifocal alterations in rCBF without underlying structural damage on CT or MRI scans. On SPECT perfusion imaging, typical findings include multiple perfusion defects of small and moderate size in the cerebral cortex (especially the frontal lobes), diminished blood flow to the basal ganglia, and generalized reduction in cerebral blood flow. The findings may occur in asymptomatic patients and may be partially reversible with abstinence or opioid antagonist (buprenorphine) therapy. The SPECT imaging patterns are not specific and are often indistinguishable from those of early AIDS-related dementia.

Neuropsychiatric Disorders and Behavioral Dysfunction

Various neuropsychiatric disorders have been evaluated by using PET and SPECT imaging, but clear-cut diagnostic or prognostic functional abnormalities have not been consistently described, and the clinical utility of such imaging techniques in this setting remains uncertain. There are a few studies of children with attention-deficit hyperactivity disorder (ADHD) that show increased perfusion in the motor, premotor, and anterior cingulate cortex when the children were withdrawn from their medication, methylphenidate, and effective treatment with methylphenidate was associated with increases in perfusion in the prefrontal cortex and caudate nucleus.

Neuroreceptor Imaging

Imaging of neuroreceptor distribution in the brain is possible by using a number of receptor-specific radiopharmaceuticals designed to map receptors such as muscarinic cholinergic receptors, Dopamine D_2 receptors, and the benzodiazepine and serotonin-2 receptors. These agents, including the dopamine receptor seeking radiopharmaceutical ^{11}C-N-methylspiperone, permit the mapping of neuromediator distribution in a number of disease states; however, the assessment of neurotransmitter function is complex, and the technique plays a limited role in clinical practice.

CEREBROSPINAL FLUID IMAGING

About 400 to 500 mL/day of CSF is formed in the normal adult, largely in the choroid plexus of the cerebral ventricular system. CSF is essentially an ultrafiltrate of plasma with an actively secreted component added by the choroid plexus. The total CSF volume ranges between 120 and 150 mL, of which about 40 mL are contained within the ventricular system. After exiting the ventricles by way of the fourth ventricular foramina, the CSF flows cephalad through the subarachnoid spaces to the cerebral convexities, where primary resorption occurs in the arachnoid villi. Absorption also occurs across the meninges of both the brain and the spinal cord as well as through the ependymal lining of the ventricular system. These latter pathways are probably of great importance in pathologic states in which there is blockage of normal absorption through the arachnoid villi.

The principle involved in imaging the CSF consists of intrathecal administration of a substance that is miscible with and diffusible in the CSF and that remains in the CSF compartment until it is absorbed through the normal pathways. Any such substance must be nontoxic and nonpyrogenic. Strict pyrogen testing of all intrathecally administered agents should be routinely performed.

Radiopharmaceuticals and Technique

The most widely used agent for studies of CSF dynamics is indium-111 (^{111}In)–labeled DTPA, with a physical half-life of 2.8 days. The administration of ^{111}In DTPA is accomplished by lumbar puncture with a small-bore

(22-gauge) needle into the subarachnoid space. To minimize leakage from the puncture site, it is wise to postpone such procedures for about 1 week after the most recent diagnostic lumbar puncture.

Initial posterior images over the thoracolumbar spine may be obtained at 2 to 4 hours to discern the success of injection. For evaluation of CSF dynamics, anterior, posterior, and lateral gamma camera images of the head are obtained at 6, 24, and 48 hours, and at 72 hours or longer, if necessary. For CSF leaks, early imaging at 1 to 24 hours is preferred in projections that are most likely to demonstrate the site of the leak and/or position that provokes or encourages flow at the leakage site.

For CSF shunt patency studies, 1 to 3 mCi (37 to 111 MBq) of ^{99m}Tc-DTPA or 500 μCi (18.5 MBq) of ^{111}In-DTPA may be injected into the shunt reservoir or tubing.

A sample technical protocol is presented in Appendix E-1.

Normal Examination

After injection of ^{111}In-DTPA into the lumbar subarachnoid space, the activity ascends in the spinal canal and reaches the basal cisterns at 2 to 4 hours in adults (Fig. 3-21). Subsequent images obtained during the next 24 hours demonstrate ascent of the radiopharmaceutical through the intracranial subarachnoid spaces, with identification of activity in the sylvian and interhemispheric cisterns. At 24 hours, there should be complete ascent of the radiopharmaceutical, which consists of distribution of the activity over the cerebral convexities and the parasagittal region, with relative clearance from the basilar cisterns.

The presence of radioactivity in the lateral ventricles at any point in the examination should be viewed as abnormal. However, transient entry noted at 4 hours and disappearing by 24 hours is of questionable pathologic significance and is considered by some to be a normal variant flow pattern. Failure of the radionuclide to achieve complete ascent over the cerebral convexities or activity in the ventricles at 24 hours is an indication for further evaluation at 48 hours and/or 72 hours.

Clinical Applications

The major indications for radionuclide imaging of the CSF are the following:
■ Investigation of suspected communicating hydrocephalus (normal-pressure hydrocephalus),
■ Evaluation of suspected CSF leaks.
■ Verification of diversionary CSF shunt patency.

Communicating Hydrocephalus

Normal-pressure hydrocephalus characteristically presents as a clinical triad of ataxia, dementia, and urinary incontinence. By definition, hydrocephalus without significant atrophy

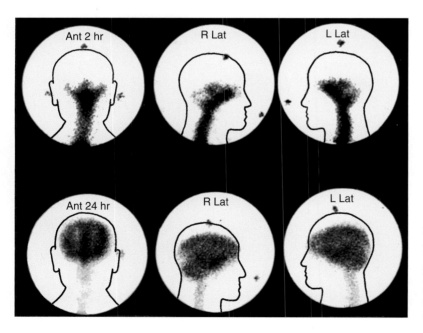

Figure 3-21. Normal cisternogram. The images obtained at 2 hours demonstrate activity in the basal cisterns as well as some activity in the sylvian and interhemispheric cisterns. The images obtained at 24 hours demonstrate that there has been normal ascent of activity over the convexities.

is noted on CT scans, with a normal CSF pressure determination. If the diagnosis of normal-pressure hydrocephalus can be established, CSF shunting from the ventricular system may provide prompt relief of symptoms in selected patients. CSF imaging may provide corroborative evidence of the diagnosis and aid in selecting patients most likely to benefit from shunt therapy.

Hydrocephalus with normal lumbar pressures often presents a problem of differentiation between cerebral atrophy and normal-pressure hydrocephalus. CT or MRI studies can generally provide the answer. In some patients with mild degrees of atrophy and dilated ventricles, radionuclide CSF imaging provides additional differential information. The classic pattern of scintigraphic findings in normal-pressure hydrocephalus (Fig. 3-22) consists of the following:

- Early entry of the radiopharmaceutical into the   lateral ventricles at 4 to 6 hours
- Persistence of lateral ventricular activity at 24, 48, and even 72 hours
- Considerable delay in the ascent to the parasagittal region, with or without delayed clearance of activity from the basilar cisterns

In general, patients who demonstrate these characteristic findings are among those most likely to benefit from diversionary shunting. Although varying degrees of ventricular entry and persistence, with or without delay in convexity ascent, may be noted, these so-called mixed patterns are of questionable value in establishing a firm diagnosis of normal-pressure

hydrocephalus or in predicting therapeutic success.

Noncommunicating Hydrocephalus

Because the radiopharmaceuticals injected into the lumbar space normally do not enter the ventricular system, a radionuclide cisternogram cannot be used to distinguish communicating from noncommunicating hydrocephalus. By injecting the material directly into the lateral ventricles, however, communication between the ventricles and the subarachnoid space can be discerned. This method may rarely be of value in the investigation of enlarged lateral ventricles noted on CT when noncommunicating disease is suspected.

Cerebrospinal Fluid Leaks

Radionuclide cisternography is frequently used to substantiate the presence of a CSF leak from the nose or ear or to localize more precisely the site of a leak. The most common sites of CSF fistulas are in the region of the cribriform plate and ethmoid sinuses, from the sella turcica into the sphenoid sinus, and from the sphenoid ridge into the ear (Fig. 3-23). Because these leaks are frequently intermittent, the results of the radionuclide cisternogram greatly depend on whether the leak is active at the time of the examination.

The radionuclide evaluation of CSF leaks should consist of (1) imaging the site of the leak and (2) measuring differential activity in pledgets placed deep into each nostril or ear,

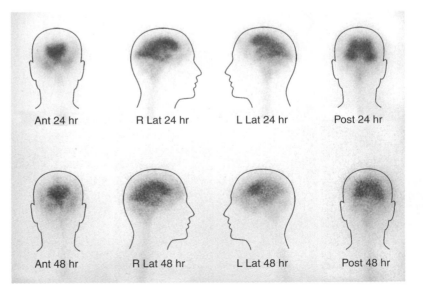

Figure 3-22. Normal-pressure hydrocephalus. Anterior, lateral, and posterior images of the head performed at 24 and 48 hours. The images do not show the usual trident pattern but rather a central, heart-shaped structure representing activity in the lateral ventricles. The activity more laterally and lower represents activity in the sylvian fissures. Even at 48 hours, activity has not ascended over the superior aspect of the convexities as would normally be expected by 24 hours, and there is persistence of activity within the lateral ventricles centrally.

Ant 24 hr   R Lat 24 hr   L Lat 24 hr   Post 24 hr

Ant 48 hr   R Lat 48 hr   L Lat 48 hr   Post 48 hr

as appropriate. It is important to image for a CSF leak at the time the radioactivity reaches the suspected site of origin of the leak. Because most of these leaks develop near the basilar cisterns, imaging between 1 and 3 hours is typical. Imaging at half-hour intervals after lumbar puncture may better allow determination of the optimal time to detect a leak. Likewise, if any position or activity is known by the patient to provoke or aggravate the leak of CSF, such should be accomplished immediately before or during imaging.

Pledgets placed before lumbar injection of the radiopharmaceutical are removed 4 to 24 hours after placement and counted in a well counter. Concurrent blood serum samples should be obtained and counted. Sample counts should be expressed in terms of counts per gram to normalize for differences in pledget size and amounts of absorbed fluid. Pledget-to-serum ratios of more than 1.5 may be interpreted as evidence of CSF leak.

Shunt Patency

Malfunction of diversionary CSF shunts is a common complication of ventriculoatrial or ventriculoperitoneal shunts used to treat obstructive communicating and noncommunicating hydrocephalus. The clinical presentation of a malfunctioning shunt is often nonspecific,

especially in young children. A number of methods of determining shunt patency have been devised by using radionuclide techniques. These studies are frequently helpful in confirming the presence of shunt malfunction or obstruction when clinical indicators and conventional radiologic examinations are equivocal.

Because of the relatively short duration of the radionuclide examination, ^{99m}Tc-labeled radiopharmaceuticals (1 to 3 mCi) (37 to 111 MBq), especially ^{99m}Tc-DTPA, are usually used, although ^{111}In-DTPA may also be used. The procedure consists of injecting the radiopharmaceutical into the shunt reservoir or tubing under strict antiseptic conditions.

In the presence of distal shunt patency, serial gamma camera images demonstrate rapid passage of the radiopharmaceutical through the distal limb of the shunt; activity is noted in the peritoneal cavity or right atrium within minutes of shunt injection. If the distal limb of the shunt is manually occluded during injection of the reservoir, some reflux of the radiopharmaceutical may be found in the ventricular system. This procedure may give information regarding the patency of the proximal limb of the shunt. It also may permit subsequent evaluation of rate of ventricular clearance of the radiolabeled CSF from the ventricular system by using serial images. Failure to obtain reflux in the

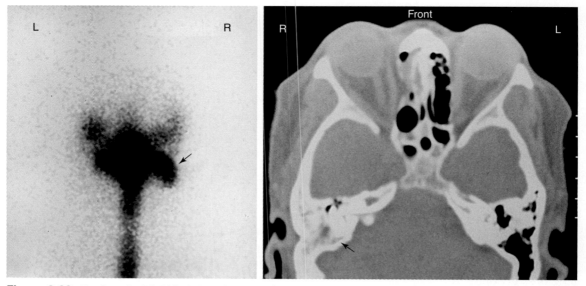

Figure 3-23. Cerebrospinal fluid leak in right ear. *Left,* Posterior image of the head obtained 6 hours after intrathecal administration of ^{111}In-DTPA shows asymmetry with an abnormal area of increased activity on the right (*arrow*). *Right,* Computed tomographic scan performed on the same patient shows that the right mastoid air cells (*arrow*) are filled with cerebrospinal fluid because of a sphenoid ridge fracture.

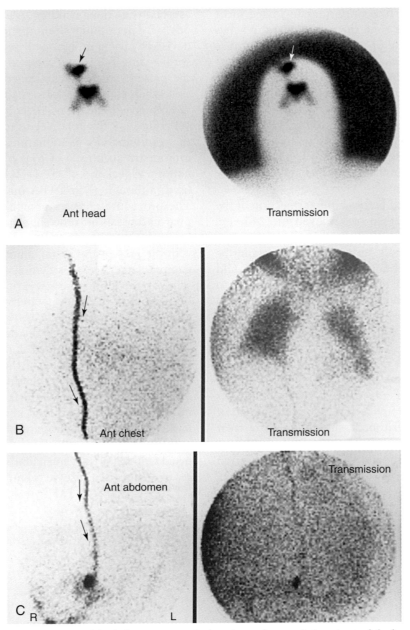

Figure 3-24. Normal cerebrospinal fluid shunt patency. A, Anterior and transmission views of the head were done with injection of the shunt reservoir (*arrows*). Manual occlusion of the distal limb has allowed reflux into the lateral ventricles. The transmission scan was done by using a ^{99m}Tc planar source behind the patient to outline the head and shoulders. **B,** Anterior and transmission views over the anterior chest after the manual occlusion of the distal limb was released to show activity progressing inferiorly (*arrows*). **C,** Anterior and transmission views over the anterior abdomen demonstrate activity at the end of the catheter (*arrows*) but also diffusing normally throughout the abdomen and collecting in the regions of the right and left pericolic gutters.

ventricular system or failure of the radiopharmaceutical to clear from the ventricles after several hours may be indicative of partial proximal limb obstruction.

Partial or complete distal limb obstruction frequently can be inferred from delayed clearance of the injected radiopharmaceutical from the shunt reservoir, with a region of interest placed over the reservoir and a time-activity curve generated. The clearance half-time from a reservoir with a patent distal shunt limb is generally several minutes, usually less than 10 minutes (Fig. 3-24). The value of reservoir clearance evaluation in proximal limb obstruction is less clear.

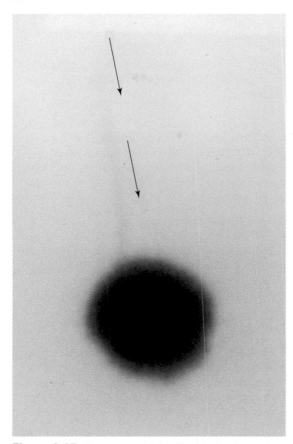

Figure 3-25. Entrapment of the distal limb of a cerebrospinal fluid shunt. An anterior image of the abdomen demonstrates activity progressing inferiorly (*arrows*) but then collecting in a loculation at the end of the shunt secondary to adhesions.

In ventriculoperitoneal shunts, the activity reaching the peritoneal cavity must be seen to diffuse throughout the abdomen for the study to be considered normal. If the radiopharmaceutical collects focally in a closed pool at the tip of the catheter, obstruction of the distal limb by entrapment in adhesions is likely (Fig. 3-25). Because the CSF does not resorb properly in the abdomen under these circumstances, relative obstruction of the shunt flow develops because of increased pressure in the loculation.

In examining CSF diversionary shunts, it is important to determine the type of shunt used and to understand the mechanics of its operation before proceeding with the shunt patency examination. In many cases, the technique can be tailored to the particular clinical problem suspected and to the type of shunt in place.

Even though the sensitivity and specificity of a normal shunt study are high, the possibility of shunt obstruction or malfunction should be considered in patients with persistent symptoms and normal examinations, especially children.

PEARLS & PITFALLS

Brain Imaging

- The common indications for brain imaging are perfusion abnormalities (stroke), dementia (Alzheimer or multi-infarct), epilepsy, brain death, and distinguishing recurrent tumor from radiation necrosis.

- The radiopharmaceuticals ^{99m}Tc-ECD (SPECT), ^{99m}Tc-HMPAO (SPECT), and nitrogen-13 (^{13}N) ammonia (PET) are perfusion agents.

- The radiopharmaceuticals ^{99m}Tc-HMPAO and ^{99m}Tc-ECD are lipophilic, extracted on the first pass, and reflect regional perfusion. Their uptake is highest in the cortical and subcortical gray matter. FDG represents regional metabolic activity.

- On most SPECT perfusion and FDG PET metabolic imaging, the central area of decreased activity is primarily white matter and should not be mistaken for dilated lateral ventricles.

- The radiopharmaceuticals ^{201}Tl (SPECT) and ^{18}FDG (PET) show activity in viable recurrent or persistent tumors but not in areas of radiation necrosis.

- Brain death can be diagnosed with either ^{99m}Tc-DTPA (which is cheaper) or ^{99m}Tc-HMPAO or ECD (which do not require a flow study). The diagnosis is a clinical one and often includes other tests such as EEG. Radionuclide imaging improves certainty. A "hot-nose" sign may be present on flow images.

Continued

PEARLS & PITFALLS—cont'd

- Multi-infarct dementia presents with multiple asymmetric cortical perfusion defects and decreased perfusion to basal ganglia and thalamus. Multiple small perfusion defects can also occur from cocaine abuse or vasculitis.

- Glucose metabolism patterns seen in dementias are nonspecific, although symmetrically decreased activity in temporoparietal regions should suggest Alzheimer disease, decreased frontal activity Pick disease, and scattered decreased areas multi-infarct dementia.

- Alzheimer dementia classically presents with symmetrically decreased activity in the posterior parietal-temporal lobes with preserved activity in the calcarine cortex and basal ganglia. This is not pathognomonic and can be seen in other entities, including Parkinson and Lewy body dementia. About 30% of Alzheimer patients have asymmetrically decreased activity.

- AIDS dementia is associated with multifocal or patchy areas of decreased cortical uptake in frontal temporal and parietal lobes.

- Herpes encephalitis can be seen as increased activity in the temporal lobe on SPECT perfusion imaging.

- Epileptic seizure foci show increased perfusion (^{99m}Tc-HMPAO or ^{99m}Tc-ECD) and metabolism (^{18}FDG) during seizure activity but decreased or normal activity interictally.

- A normal radionuclide angiographic examination of the brain presents a trident appearance of intracranial flow in the anterior cerebral and right and left middle cerebral territories. In brain death, there is no obvious arterial phase (the trident is absent) and only scalp activity is seen, which is often accompanied by a hot-nose sign. These studies can also be performed by using ^{99m}Tc-HMPAO or ^{99m}Tc-ECD (SPECT or planar).

- A Diamox challenge study evaluates cerebral vascular reserve. It is analogous to the use of dipyridamole in myocardial perfusion studies. In areas of vascular disease, regional perfusion worsens after Diamox, compared with perfusion without Diamox.

Cerebrospinal Fluid Imaging
- Common indications for CSF imaging are for evaluation of a CSF leak or for differentiating normal-pressure hydrocephalus from other causes of hydrocephalus. These studies are done with intrathecal administration of ^{111}In-DTPA.

- Most CSF leaks occur in the ear, paranasal sinuses, or nose. Substantial leaks can be imaged by noting asymmetric activity around the region of the ears on the frontal view or activity in the nose on the lateral view. Some leaks are detected only by removing and counting cotton pledgets that were placed in the area of concern.

- Cisternography images are usually obtained anteriorly. Six hours after injection, these images normally show a trident appearance of activity produced by labeled CSF in the anterior interhemispheric and right and left sylvian cisterns. Any abnormal entry into the lateral ventricles is seen as heart-shaped activity. Early ventricular entry with stasis, accompanied by the lack of activity over the superior surface of the brain after 24 to 48 hours, supports a diagnosis of normal-pressure hydrocephalus.

- The classic clinical triad of normal-pressure hydrocephalus includes ataxia, incontinence, and dementia.

SUGGESTED READINGS

Bonte FJ, Devous MD Sr. SPECT brain imaging. In Sandler MP, Coleman RE, Patton JA, et al. (eds): Diagnostic Nuclear Medicine, 4th ed. New York: Lippincott Williams & Wilkins; 2003. p. 757-82.

Chen W. Clinical applications of PET in brain tumors. J Nucl Med 2007;48:1468-81.

Conrad GR, Sinha P. Scintigraphy as a confirmatory test of brain death. Semin Nucl Med 2003;33:312-23.

Henry TR, Van Heertum RL. Positron emission tomography and single photon emission computed tomography in epilepsy care. Semin Nucl Med 2003;33:88-104.

Kadir A, Nordberg A. Target specific PET probes for neurodegenerative disorders related to dementia. J Nucl Med 2010;51:1418-30.

Lawrence SK, Delbeke D, Partain CL, et al. Cerebrospinal fluid imaging. In: Sandler MP, Coleman RE, Patton JA, et al, editors. Diagnostic Nuclear Medicine. 4th ed. New York: Lippincott Williams & Wilkins; 2003. p. 835-50.

Matsuda H. Role of neuroimaging in Alzheimer's disease with emphasis on brain perfusion: SPECT. J Nucl Med 2007;48:1289-1300.

Minoshima S, Frey KA, Cross DJ, et al. Neurochemical imaging of dementias. Semin Nucl Med 2004;34:70-82.

Nordberg A. Amyloid plaque imaging in vivo: current achievement and future prospects. Eur J Nucl Med 2008;35(Suppl 1):S46-S50.

Norfray JF, Provenzale JM. Alzheimer's disease: neuropathic findings and recent advances in imaging. AJR Am J Roentgenol 2004;182:3-13.

Paschali A, Messinis L, Kargiotis O, et al. SPECT neuroimaging and neuropsychological functions in different stages of Parkinson's disease. Eur J Nucl Med Mol Imaging 2010;37:1128-40.

Rastogi S, Lee C, Salamon N. Neuroimaging in pediatric epilepsy: a multimodality approach. RadioGraphics 2008;28:1079-95.

Waxman A, Herholz K, Lewis D, et al. Society of Nuclear Medicine Procedure Guideline for FDG PET brain imaging. Version 1.0, 2009, http://www.SNM.org. Accessed June 28, 2011.

4

Thyroid, Parathyroid, and Salivary Glands

THYROID IMAGING AND UPTAKE

The use of iodine-131 (^{131}I) for measuring thyroid functional parameters and imaging the gland has historically served as the nucleus of the evolution of the field of nuclear imaging. Although significant changes have taken place in the radionuclide approach to thyroidology, the essential principles remain unchanged. Therefore, a basic understanding of these principles is necessary before interpretation of the functional data should be attempted.

Most thyroid imaging techniques capitalize on some phase of hormone synthesis within the thyroid gland. Iodides or iodide analogs are actively transported into the thyroid gland, a process called *trapping*. The iodides are then oxidized by thyroid peroxidase and originally bound to tyrosyl moieties (organification) to form mono- and di-iodinated tyrosine (MIT and DIT). These are then coupled to form tri-iodothyronine (T_3) and thyroxine (T_4). Technetium-99m (^{99m}Tc) pertechnetate, however, does not undergo organification to form thyroid hormone; instead, after trapping, it slowly "washes" from the gland.

Radiopharmaceuticals

The radioactive iodine (^{123}I) and technetium (^{99m}Tc) constitute the radionuclides used in imaging the thyroid gland. Both ^{123}I and ^{131}I are used for iodine uptake tests. Only ^{131}I is used for thyroid therapy.

Iodine-131

Iodine-131 decays by beta emission and has a half-life of 8.04 days. The principal gamma emission of 364 keV is considerably higher than the ideal for imaging with gamma cameras. A ½-inch-thick sodium iodide crystal has only a 30% efficiency for these photons.

The major advantages of ^{131}I are its low price and ready availability. Its major disadvantages are its long physical half-life and high beta emission, which cause a relatively high radiation dose to be delivered to the thyroid, although the whole-body dose is acceptable. The high thyroid dose makes ^{131}I undesirable for routine imaging of the thyroid. The high thyroid dose and relatively low whole-body dose of ^{131}I, however, make it an ideal radiotherapeutic agent for treating certain thyroid disorders. Also, its long half-life is of advantage in scanning for the detection of functioning metastatic thyroid carcinoma because imaging can be done over several days to allow for optimum concentration by the metastatic deposits.

Iodine-123

Iodine-123 has excellent physical properties for an imaging agent. Like ^{131}I, its biochemical behavior is identical to that of stable iodine. Iodine-123 decays by electron capture, with a photon energy of 159 keV and a half-life of 13 hours. The gamma emission of ^{123}I allows excellent imaging (≈80% efficiency for a ½-inch-thick crystal) with low background activity. It provides considerably lower doses of radiation to the thyroid with comparable activity than does ^{131}I. Iodine-123 is the iodine of choice for thyroid imaging (Fig. 4-1).

Technetium-99m

Technetium-99m pertechnetate is trapped by the thyroid in the same manner as iodides but is not organified; therefore, it is released over time as unaltered pertechnetate (^{99m}TcO4–) ion. Its short physical half-life of 6 hours and principal gamma energy of 140 keV are ideal for gamma camera imaging (greater than 90% efficiency with a ½-inch-thick crystal). These physical characteristics and its ready availability are distinct advantages for thyroid scanning. In addition, the low absorbed dose to the thyroid permits administration of higher doses and therefore allows for more rapid imaging of the gland with minimal motion artifact. Only 1% to 5% of administered ^{99m}Tc-pertechnetate is normally trapped by the thyroid, so image background levels are higher than those with radioiodine. On a ^{99m}Tc-pertechnetate scan, the salivary glands are usually well seen in addition to the thyroid. As a result, unless a patient is hyperthyroid, a ^{99m}Tc scan can usually be distinguished from an ^{123}I scan by excellent visualization of the salivary glands. Technetium-99m pertechnetate is preferred over radioiodine when the patient has recently received thyroid-blocking agents (such as iodinated contrast agents) or is unable to take medication orally or when the study must be completed in less than 2 hours.

Dosimetry

Radiation doses to the adult thyroid and whole body for the radioiodines and ^{99m}Tc-pertechnetate are presented in Appendix E with imaging protocols. With the usual administered activities for scanning, the radiation to the thyroid gland is comparable for ^{123}I and ^{99m}Tc, and the whole-body dose is only slightly greater with ^{99m}Tc. Both agents provide considerably less radiation dose to the thyroid and to the total body than does ^{131}I. The dose to the thyroid from ^{131}I is about 100 times greater than that from ^{123}I for the same administered activity (≈1 rad/µCi [10mGy/0.037 MBq] versus 1 rad/100 µCi [10 mGy/3.7 MBq]). The absorbed

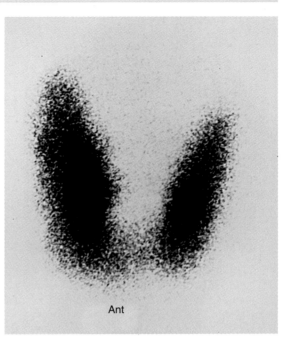

Figure 4-1. Normal iodine-123 scan of the thyroid. The normal bilobed gland with an inferior isthmus is easily appreciated. Note that no salivary gland activity is seen.

thyroid dose from ^{99m}Tc-pertechnetate is about 1 rad/5000 µCi (10 mGy/185 MBq).

Because both ^{99m}Tc and the various radioiodines cross the placenta and because the fetal thyroid begins accumulation of iodine at about the 12th week of gestation, care must be taken when administering these radiopharmaceuticals during pregnancy. They are also secreted in breast milk in lactating women and may be transferred to nursing infants. Nursing can usually be resumed 12 to 24 hours after the administration of ^{99m}Tc-pertechnetate and about 2 to 3 days after ^{123}I administration. When ^{131}I is administered in any form, nursing should be stopped and any pumped breast milk discarded, because the Nuclear Regulatory Commission (NRC) recommends that nursing should be discontinued entirely if administered activities of ^{131}I exceed about 1 µCi (0.04 MBq).

On an administered activity basis, the dose to the thyroid is greater in infants and children than in adults, and considerably smaller scanning and uptake doses should be administered to pediatric patients (see Appendixes D and E). In addition, because the radiation dose to the pediatric thyroid from ^{131}I nears the level shown to increase the incidence of thyroid carcinoma,

^{131}I is not recommended for scanning children and is contraindicated for therapy in pregnant women.

Many physicians incorrectly assume that a radiation dose to the thyroid from ^{131}I can be accurately determined by knowing the administered activity and the thyroid uptake. A complex of less easily determined factors (thyroid size, biologic half-life of iodine in the gland, size of the iodine pool, and spatial distribution of iodine in the gland) for a specific administered activity can change the absorbed dose by up to a factor of 10 in any given patient.

Iodine Uptake Test

The iodine uptake test is easily performed and gives a useful clinical index of thyroid function. The main purposes of an uptake examination before radioiodine therapy are to ensure that the thyroid will take up iodine and to determine how much activity to administer as a treatment dose. The diagnosis of hyperthyroidism or hypothyroidism, however, is not made by using radioactive iodine uptake but should be made by serum measurements of thyroid hormone and thyroid-stimulating hormone (TSH). However, the thyroid uptake can be used to differentiate Graves disease from subacute thyroiditis or factitious hyperthyroidism.

Principle and Technique

Thyroid uptake is based on the principle that the administered radiopharmaceutical is concentrated by the thyroid gland in a manner that reflects the gland's handling of stable dietary iodine and therefore the functional status of the gland. The higher the uptake of the radiopharmaceutical, the more active the thyroid; conversely, the lower the uptake, the less functional the gland. Uptake is conventionally expressed as the percentage of the administered activity in the thyroid gland at a given time after administration (usually at 4 to 6 hours and 24 hours). Normal range for both children and adults is about 10% to 30% for 24-hour uptake determinations. The normal range for a 4- to 6-hour uptake is about 6% to 18%.

To aid absorption, it is advisable for patients to be NPO beginning at midnight the day before oral administration of the radionuclide. It is also helpful to determine the functional status of the gastrointestinal tract before administering the radiopharmaceutical because vomiting or diarrhea may hinder adequate absorption.

To begin the test, about 5 μCi (0.2 MBq) of ^{131}I-sodium or 10 to 20 μCi (0.4 to 0.7 MBq) of ^{123}I-sodium in either liquid or capsule form is administered. ^{123}I uptakes may also be performed in conjunction with an ^{123}I thyroid scan using the scanning dosage. An identical amount of activity, called a *standard,* is placed in a neck phantom, and the activity is compared with that in the patient's thyroid, using a single-crystal counting probe with a flat-field collimator. Such standards obviate the use of decay constants or geometric corrections in calculating uptakes.

The distance from the face of the probe crystal to the anterior aspect of the neck (about 25 to 30 cm) and the method of counting the ^{131}I standard are the same for all patients. It is usually unnecessary to correct measurements for body blood pool activity in the neck at 24 hours, but this correction is used, especially when uptakes before 24 hours are desired. Correction is approximated by measuring the activity in the patient's thigh in the same manner as the neck measurements are performed. The number of counts obtained may then be subtracted from the neck reading to estimate counts isolated in the thyroid gland.

All measurements are usually performed twice, for 1 to 2 minutes each, and are then averaged to calculate the percentage uptake, using the following formula:

$$\% \text{ thyroid uptake} = \frac{\text{neck counts-thigh counts}}{\text{counts in standard}} \times 100\%$$

It is occasionally advantageous to perform a 4- or 6-hour radioiodine uptake in addition to the 24-hour determination, particularly for abnormalities in which the iodine turnover is rapid (Graves disease) or in which organification of the trapped iodine is defective (congenital, antithyroid drugs, Hashimoto thyroiditis). Occasionally, the uptake obtained at 6 hours may be significantly higher than that at 24 hours, owing to rapid uptake and secretion or enhanced washout from the gland.

A sample technical protocol for performing radioiodide uptakes can be found in Appendix E-1.

Factors Affecting Iodine Uptake

Increased circulating iodides compete with administered radioiodines for trapping and organification by the thyroid gland. An increase in the body iodide pool is most frequently caused by an increase in dietary intake of iodine, which may significantly reduce the uptake values obtained. Conversely, a decrease in ambient iodine produces an "iodide-starved gland," which traps and binds greater amounts of radioactive iodide, producing elevated uptake values. Some authors suggest a low-iodine diet for 3 to 10 days before the test, but this practice is not widespread. In addition, regional differences in dietary iodide intake give rise to local variations in the normal range. These factors, along with differences in technical aspects of the procedure among laboratories, make it necessary for each facility to determine its own range of normal values.

Good renal function is essential to normal radioiodine uptake. In patients with chronic renal failure, iodides usually excreted by the kidneys are retained, producing an increase in the stable iodide pool. This dilutes the percentage of radioiodine taken up by the gland, resulting in low uptake determinations. Large meals shortly before or after oral administration of radioiodine can slow or decrease absorption and interfere with uptake measurements.

Numerous medications and iodinated contrast agents also affect radioiodine uptake (Table 4-1 and Box 4-1). To perform a radioiodine uptake successfully, these medications must be withheld for appropriate periods before the uptake procedure is attempted. Also, careful interviewing of patients undergoing the uptake test is necessary to determine whether there is a history of antithyroid drugs, thyroid hormones, iodide preparations, or iodinated radiographic contrast agents used in computed tomography scans, and angiographic procedures. Notably, β-blockers, such as propranolol, which are commonly used to combat the clinical manifestations of hyperthyroidism, do not affect the function of the gland and therefore do not interfere with thyroid uptake of the radioactive iodine.

Clinical Considerations

Radioiodine uptake is used to estimate the function of the thyroid gland by measuring its avidity for administered radioiodine. In the absence of exogenous influences, glands demonstrating a poor avidity for iodide are generally considered to be hypofunctioning, and the converse is true for hyperfunctioning glands.

TABLE 4-1	Compounds That May Decrease Thyroid Iodine Uptake	
MEDICATION		**TIME***
Carbimazole Methimazole (Tapazole) Propylthiouracil		3 days
Multivitamins† Nitrates Perchlorate Salicylates (large doses) Sulfonamides Thiocyanate		1 week
Iodine solution (Lugol's or SSKI)† Iodine-containing antiseptics† Kelp† Some cough medicines and vitamin preparations		2-3 weeks
Tri-iodothyronine (Cytomel) Thyroid extract (Synthroid, Proloid)		3-4 weeks
Intravenous contrast agents (water soluble)		1 month
Amiodarone		3-6 months

SSKI, Saturated solution of potassium iodide.
*Time that patient should wait after medication is discontinued in order to obtain an accurate uptake.
†These relate to hyperthyroid patients. For hypothyroid patients, a 6-week interval is recommended.

Elevated Radioiodine Uptake

Primary hyperthyroidism (Graves disease or toxic nodular goiter) and secondary hyperthyroidism commonly produce elevated iodine uptakes. These uptakes are useful in determining the level of therapeutic ^{131}I doses for the treatment of Graves disease. On the other hand, hyperthyroidism produced by toxic nodular goiters (Plummer disease) may yield uptake values in the high, normal, or mildly elevated range. Therefore, a normal or borderline elevated radioiodine uptake alone cannot be used to exclude the diagnosis of hyperthyroidism when it is clinically suspected.

Elevated uptakes also may be produced by a variety of other conditions (see Box 4-1), including any state of the gland characterized by increased avidity of the organ for iodine. The so-called iodine rebound phenomenon may result from the release of TSH by the pituitary after sudden withdrawal from thyroid hormone suppression therapy. It may also result from hormone synthesis rebound after withdrawal of antithyroid drugs, such as propylthiouracil.

Box 4-1 Factors Affecting Iodine Uptake

Increased Uptake
Hyperthyroidism (diffuse or nodular goiter)
Early Hashimoto thyroiditis
Recovery from subacute thyroiditis
Rebound after abrupt withdrawal of
    antithyroid medication
Enzyme defects
Iodine deficiency or starvation
Hypoalbuminemia
Thyroid-stimulating hormone
Tumor-secreted stimulators (gonadal and
    chorionic origin)
Pregnancy

Decreased Uptake
Hypothyroidism (primary or secondary)
Iodine overload (especially radiographic
    contrast)
Medications (see Table 4-1)
Subacute or autoimmune thyroiditis
Thyroid hormone therapy
Ectopic secretion of thyroid hormone from
    tumors
Renal failure

High uptakes can also be the result of abnormally increased production of TSH by the pituitary or secretion of TSH-like hormones by gonadal or chorionic tumors (secondary hyperthyroidism), or may occur in the recovery phase of subacute thyroiditis.

Reduced Radioiodine Uptake

Primary or secondary hypothyroidism may produce decreased radioiodine uptake. Primary hypothyroidism is a failure of the gland to respond to TSH, whereas secondary hypothyroidism is caused by insufficient pituitary secretion of TSH. Because of the prevalence of iodine in the American diet, it has become increasingly difficult to use reduced radioiodine uptake as an indicator of hypothyroidism. Serum TSH and thyroid hormone assays are necessary to establish the diagnosis.

Of note in considering the causes of decreased radioiodine uptake are the numerous medications outlined in Table 4-1. Again, withdrawal of the medications for the times given in the table is necessary to obtain accurate measures of thyroid function. Rarely, well-differentiated thyroid cancers, teratomas, and struma ovarii

can be sites of ectopic secretion of thyroid hormone and cause low thyroidal uptake.

Thyroid Gland Imaging

Although ^{131}I or ^{123}I may be used for obtaining thyroid uptakes, ^{99m}Tc-pertechnetate and ^{123}I-sodium remain the agents of choice for obtaining maximum morphologic detail of the thyroid gland with the gamma camera. Either radionuclide, however, provides images of excellent quality, although the higher energy photons of ^{131}I may be preferable for imaging deep ectopic tissue. Even though ^{123}I is more expensive than ^{99m}Tc, it has the advantage of being able to provide concurrent radioiodine uptake and images with relatively low radiation dose. In addition, ^{123}I images reflect both trapping and organification in the gland.

The indications for scintigraphic thyroid imaging include:

- To relate the general structure of the gland to function, particularly in differentiating Graves disease from toxic nodular goiter. This distinction is important in determining therapeutic radioiodine dose.
- To determine function in a specific area, for example, to see if a palpable nodule is functional.
- To locate ectopic tissue, such as a lingual thyroid.
- To assist in the evaluation of congenital hypothyroidism or organification defects.
- To determine that a cervical or mediastinal mass is thyroid tissue.
- To differentiate among the causes of thyrotoxicosis, that is, Graves disease from subacute, silent, postpartum, or factitious hyperthyroidism. In the latter entities, there are symptoms of mild hyperthyroidism with elevated serum levels of thyroid hormone, but radioiodine studies reveal that the radioiodine uptake in the gland is low and visualization is poor.

Imaging with ^{99m}Tc-pertechnetate or radioiodine requires no prior preparation of the patient. As with uptake studies, a brief screening of patients for a possible history of recent medication or iodinated contrast administration is advisable. In addition, before imaging is begun, palpation of the thyroid gland, with the patient sitting upright, is recommended to assess any enlargement or nodules. The prior localization of palpable nodules within the gland makes it much easier to relocate these abnormalities with the patient in the supine scanning position, when marker localization may be required.

Even with a history of recent radioiodinated contrast or suppressive medication administration, it is frequently possible to obtain reasonably good anatomic assessment of the thyroid gland with ^{99m}Tc when it is not possible with radioiodine. This, in part, is related to the significantly greater allowable activity for pertechnetate scanning than for radioiodine. When feasible, however, the patient should return after an appropriate interval of withdrawal from the interfering drug for a more definitive examination.

Technique and Clinical Protocol
Technetium-99m
The thyroid is imaged 20 minutes after the intravenous administration of 5 to 10 mCi (185 to 370 MBq) of ^{99m}Tc-pertechnetate, using a scintillation camera with a pinhole collimator. Anterior and left and right anterior oblique images are then obtained for 100,000 to 300,000 counts (or 5 minutes) each, with the patient supine and neck extended. In addition, the position of palpable nodules under investigation should be documented and a view obtained with a radioactive marker placed on the lesion. This aids in an accurate correlation of the physical and scan findings. The oblique images are essential for the identification of laterally and posteriorly placed nodules that might be missed with simple anterior imaging.

In some laboratories, the static images are preceded by a blood-flow study of the thyroid. If this is to be done, at least 10 mCi (370 MBq) of ^{99m}Tc-pertechnetate should be injected as an intravenous bolus using a parallel-hole collimator. The field of view is from the level of the salivary glands to the upper sternum.

Iodine-123
Imaging with ^{123}I may be performed after the oral administration of 200 to 600 µCi (7.4 to 22.2 MBq) to a fasting patient. Imaging can be performed at 3 to 4 hours, but the images are better when done at 16 to 24 hours. Images of high quality are obtained using 50,000- to 100,000-count or a 10-minute acquisition. Imaging 24 hours after administration may give a more accurate indication of the distribution of organified iodine within the gland than earlier images.

The complete technical protocols for performing thyroid scintigraphy using ^{99m}Tc-pertechnetate and ^{123}I can be found in Appendix E-1.

Normal Images
The normal thyroid gland is a bilobed organ with reasonably homogeneous distribution of activity in both lobes (see Fig. 4-1). The normal gland weighs 1.3 g at birth and about 4.0 g by 5 years of age. In adults, the entire gland weighs between 15 and 20 g, and each lobe measures about 2 × 5 cm. Slight asymmetry in the sizes of the lobes is common, with the right lobe generally dominating. The lobes are usually joined inferiorly and medially by the thyroid isthmus, which may demonstrate relatively decreased activity compared with the adjacent lobes. In some instances, complete absence of activity is noted in this region. In a small number of patients, a pyramidal lobe is identified that arises from the isthmus or medial aspect of one lobe and extends superiorly and medially. Although this is a common variation, it may be accentuated in partial thyroidectomy patients and in patients with diffuse thyroid abnormalities such as Hashimoto thyroiditis or Graves disease. Less common variants of thyroid configuration include congenital absence of one lobe, substernal extension of the gland, or a sublingual thyroid with functioning tissue at the base of the tongue.

The most common artifact of ^{99m}Tc-pertechnetate studies of the thyroid is produced by activity secreted by the salivary glands and swallowed by the patient. This usually presents as a linear area of esophageal activity in the midline of the image. If this complicates interpretation or causes confusion with an enlarged pyramidal lobe, repeat imaging should be performed using oblique images or after clearing the esophagus by drinking water.

Clinical Applications
Ectopic Thyroid Tissue. Ectopic thyroid tissue may occur in the neck, in the base of the tongue (lingual thyroid) (Fig. 4-2), in the pelvis (struma ovarii), or retrosternally in the region of the mediastinum (substernal goiter). When ectopic sites deep within the body are suspected, 24-hour imaging with ^{131}I-sodium

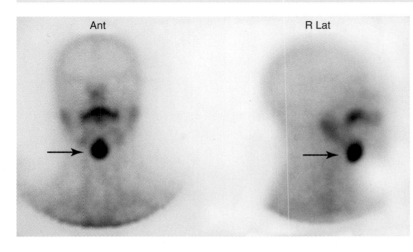

Ant

R Lat

Figure 4-2. Lingual thyroid. Anterior and lateral views of the cervical region from a technetium-99m pertechnetate study demonstrate no activity in the region of the thyroid bed, but a focal area of increased activity is seen high in the midline of the neck near the base of the tongue (*arrows*), compatible with a lingual thyroid. The patient was clinically hypothyroid.

is the method of choice (although ^{123}I also can be used). Because of interfering salivary gland activity in the neck, attenuation of 140-keV gamma rays by the sternum or soft tissues, and considerable blood pool activity, ^{99m}Tc-pertechnetate is generally not as useful.

Identification of an anterior mediastinal mass on chest radiograph is the most frequent benign indication for ^{123}I or ^{131}I imaging of the chest. Intrathoracic thyroid tissue most commonly presents as a substernal extension of a cervical thyroid goiter (Fig. 4-3). This occurs most commonly on the left, displacing the trachea to the right. Less commonly, it presents as a mediastinal mass anatomically unrelated to the thyroid gland. Thoracic thyroid tissue is most frequently found in middle-aged women but may occur in either sex at any age. Thyroid tissue in the chest may not demonstrate radioiodine uptake as intensely as that in the neck, and some mediastinal thyroid tissue may not function at all. Therefore, although uptake in a mediastinal or substernal mass indicates that the tissue is thyroid related, lack of concentration of radioiodine does not necessarily exclude that diagnosis.

Aberrant functioning thyroid tissue, struma ovarii, is rarely identified in some ovarian teratomas. Even more rarely, this tissue may hyperfunction, producing symptoms of hyperthyroidism with suppression of function in the normal thyroid.

Congenital Organification Defect. Congenital organification defects become apparent in the first months of life. The typical presentation is an infant with low serum thyroid hormone levels and a high TSH level. A 24-hour radioiodine scan usually shows no activity in the thyroid because without organification, the trapped iodine washes out of the gland and it is not possible to distinguish this from an absent thyroid. A ^{99m}Tc-pertechnetate, or 2- to 4-hour ^{123}I scan, on the other hand, clearly shows the presence of the thyroid because the trapping mechanism of the gland is intact (Fig. 4-4).

Thyroid Nodules. Although fine-needle aspiration biopsy has largely supplanted radionuclide imaging as the initial investigative procedure for palpable thyroid nodules, imaging can be useful in selected patients. In patients with suppressed TSH levels or with nodules with indeterminate cytology results, imaging provides information regarding the functional status of the nodule and may indicate the presence of additional nodules. Because hyperfunctional nodules are almost always benign, they can be managed medically with radioactive iodine therapy.

Conventionally, nodules are classified at imaging with respect to the relative amount of activity present. Cold nodules demonstrate an essential absence of activity, whereas hot nodules are identified by focally increased activity compared with the normal thyroid parenchyma. Nodules that are neither hot nor cold but contain activity comparable to that of the surrounding gland are frequently termed *warm* nodules.

Cold Nodule. A nonfunctioning thyroid nodule is essentially a nonspecific finding and may be the result of any of numerous pathologies (Table 4-2), the most common of which is a colloid cyst. Although most cold nodules

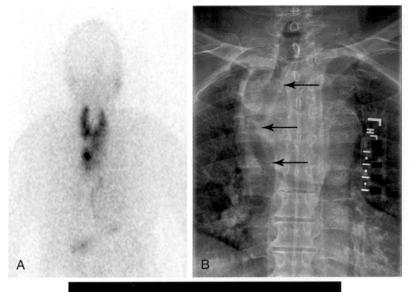

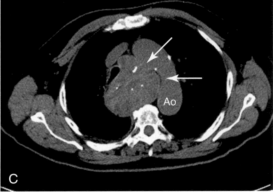

Figure 4-3. Substernal thyroid. **A,** A radioiodine scan shows the thyroid extending inferiorly into the chest. **B,** Chest radiograph demonstrates a large soft-tissue mass at the thoracic inlet, deviating the trachea (*arrows*) to the right. **C,** Axial CT scan shows the goiter with a few calcifications interposed between the trachea and aortic arch.

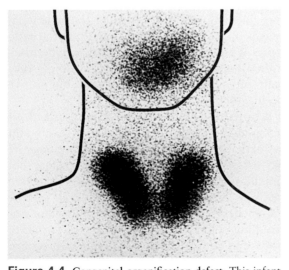

Figure 4-4. **Congenital organification defect.** This infant was clinically hypothyroid and had a thyroid-stimulating hormone concentration in excess of 400 mU/mL; a 24-hour iodine-123 scan showed no thyroid activity. This technetium-99m pertechnetate scan clearly shows the thyroid to be present and trapping. Normal activity in the mouth and salivary glands is seen superiorly.

TABLE 4-2	Pathologies of Solitary Cold Thyroid Nodule
PATHOLOGY	**INCIDENCE (%)**
Colloid cyst or adenoma	70-75
Carcinoma	15-25

Miscellaneous
  Focal area of thyroiditis
  Abscess
  Hemorrhage
  Lymphoma, metastases
  Parathyroid adenoma
  Lymph nodes
	<15

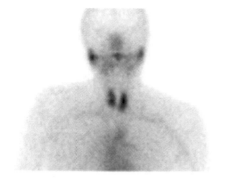

Ant

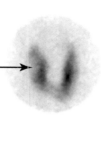

Ant pinhole

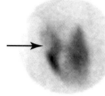

LAO pinhole

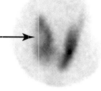

RAO pinhole

Figure 4-5. Nonfunctioning thyroid adenoma. A technetium-99m pertechnetate scan shows a "cold" area in the superior lateral aspect of the right lobe (*arrows*). A thyroid carcinoma may present an identical appearance.

are benign (Fig. 4-5), the small percentage that prove to be cancerous are sufficient to warrant further investigation or therapy, depending on the clinical circumstances. The reported percentage of solitary cold nodules harboring thyroid cancer varies, depending on the clinical bias of the particular study but is generally thought to be about 20%. The likelihood of carcinoma significantly increases if the patient is young. Suspicion is further increased if associated lymphadenopathy is identified or if the nodule fails to decrease in size after a trial of thyroid hormone suppression. If a history of previous head and neck radiation therapy is elicited, a cold nodule has about a 40% chance of being malignant (Box 4-2).

Ultrasound may be of value in distinguishing between a benign cystic abnormality and a solid lesion, which may harbor a neoplasm. Ultrasound is not useful in differentiating malignant from benign solid nodules. An anterior radionuclide thyroid blood flow study performed with ^{99m}Tc-pertechnetate may also provide information regarding the perfusion status of the lesion. Definite evidence of perfusion in the region of a cold nodule is compatible with a solid lesion in need of further investigation or biopsy.

Box 4-2 Clinical Factors Influencing Treatment of Cold Thyroid Nodule*

Factors Tending Toward Benign
Older patients
Female sex
Sudden onset
Tender or soft lesion
Multiple nodules
Shrinkage on thyroid hormone

Factors Tending Toward Malignant
Young patients
Male sex
History of radiation to head or neck
Hard lesion with palpation
Other masses in neck
No shrinkage on thyroid hormone
Familial history of thyroid carcinoma

*None of these factors is absolute.

Hot Nodule. Most nodules that demonstrate increased radionuclide concentration are benign, although thyroid carcinoma has been described in a small percentage (less than 1%). Hot nodules almost always represent hyperfunctioning adenomas, of which up to half are

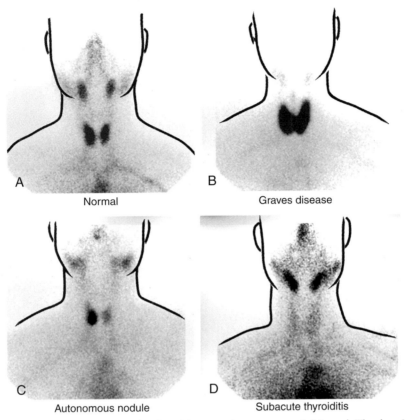

Figure 4-6. Appearance of the thyroid on technetium-99m pertechnetate scans. **A,** Normal. The thyroid is clearly visible, and the salivary glands are also seen but are somewhat less intense in activity. **B,** Graves disease. The thyroid is enlarged and has accumulated much of the activity, so that the salivary glands are harder to see. **C,** Hyperfunctioning "hot" nodule. The nodule is seen as an area of intense activity, and its autonomous hormone production has suppressed the remainder of the thyroid gland, so that the normal thyroid is hard to see. **D,** Subacute thyroiditis. In this case, the inflammation has caused the thyroid to have difficulty trapping, and the amount of activity in the thyroid is lower than normally expected, whereas the salivary gland activity is normal.

autonomous. Autonomous nodules function independently of the thyroid pituitary axis feedback mechanism; thus, they are not suppressible with exogenous thyroid hormone. Autonomous hyperfunctioning nodules may produce enough thyroid hormone to inhibit pituitary secretion of TSH and secondarily to suppress function in the surrounding normal thyroid tissue (Fig. 4-6, C).

Discordant Thyroid Nodule. By use of iodine imaging, a small number of cases of hot nodules on ^{99m}Tc-pertechnetate imaging have subsequently proved to be cold or "discordant," and a small number of those lesions have been shown to be thyroid carcinoma. Theoretically, the discordant images are produced either by the preservation of technetium trapping, but not of organification of iodine within the nodules, or by rapid turnover of organified iodine so that the nodule presents as a "cold" on a 24-hour radioiodine scan. Because the ^{99m}Tc-pertechnetate

scan is performed at 20 minutes, the avid trapping of pertechnetate by the nodules renders a focal area of increased activity. With radioiodine imaging, however, which is normally performed at 24 hours, the trapped radiopharmaceutical has either not been organified or has been organified and rapidly secreted and has thus washed out of the nodule, giving rise to a cold area on the scan (Fig. 4-7). It has been recommended that patients demonstrating solitary hot nodules on pertechnetate scans be reimaged using an iodine agent to determine whether the lesion represents a discordant nodule or a true hyperfunctioning adenoma. If the lesion proves to be discordant, further investigation may be warranted, depending on the clinical status of the patient.

Warm Nodule. Although some warm nodules do function normally, many are actually cold nodules deep within the thyroid gland,

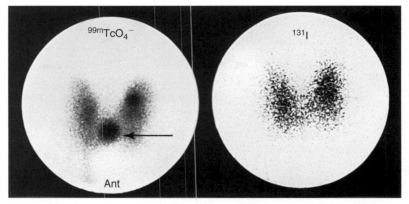

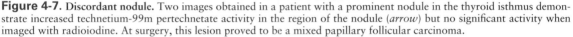

Figure 4-7. Discordant nodule. Two images obtained in a patient with a prominent nodule in the thyroid isthmus demonstrate increased technetium-99m pertechnetate activity in the region of the nodule (*arrow*) but no significant activity when imaged with radioiodine. At surgery, this lesion proved to be a mixed papillary follicular carcinoma.

with overlying normally functioning tissue. Oblique views often disclose the true nature of these abnormalities; however, frequently, the abnormality can be classified only as warm even after thorough imaging. Because of the risk of carcinoma in a cold nodule obscured by overlying tissue, it is probably prudent to classify these abnormalities as cold and in need of further investigation.

Multinodular Gland

Multinodular goiter typically presents as an enlarged gland with multiple cold, warm, and hot areas, which give the gland a coarsely patchy appearance (Fig. 4-8). These nodules generally constitute a spectrum of thyroid adenomas ranging from hyperfunctioning to cystic or degenerating lesions. This type of gland is most frequent in middle-aged women but may occur in younger patients, who are usually female. In adults, the cold lesions identified in a multinodular goiter are significantly less likely to represent carcinoma than are solitary cold nodules. Dominant or otherwise suspicious cold nodules in a multinodular goiter warrant further characterization. Multinodular goiters with cold lesions are more likely to harbor malignant neoplasms in children than they are in adults, although the incidence is still low. In addition, any patient with a previous history of head and neck irradiation is also at higher risk for carcinoma.

Occasionally, multinodular goiter may be mimicked by thyroiditis with multifocal involvement of the gland (Fig. 4-9). However, differentiation on clinical and laboratory grounds is usually possible.

Diffuse Toxic Goiter (Graves Disease)

Diffuse toxic goiter is thought to be of autoimmune origin. It usually presents with varying degrees of thyromegaly, with notably uniform distribution of increased activity throughout the thyroid gland, and often with a prominent pyramidal lobe (Fig. 4-10). On ^{99m}Tc-pertechnetate scan of a patient with Graves disease, the thyroid has increased activity, and the salivary glands are difficult to identify (see Fig. 4-6, *B*). Because salivary glands are not normally seen on an ^{123}I scan, it is often difficult to differentiate Graves disease from a normal scan without knowing the iodine uptake value. Twenty-four-hour iodine uptakes in patients with Graves disease are usually in the range of 40% to 70%.

Although cold nodules are sometimes found in patients with diffuse toxic goiter, carcinoma under these circumstances is exceedingly uncommon. It is still prudent, however, to further evaluate any solitary cold nodules occurring in this setting.

Thyroiditis

Chronic thyroiditis (Hashimoto thyroiditis) is the most common form of inflammatory disease of the thyroid. The disease is thought to be autoimmune in origin and is much more common in female patients. Thyromegaly is usually the presenting finding, although occasionally symptoms of mild hyperthyroidism or hypothyroidism may be present, depending on the stage and severity of the disease.

The scan appearance of the thyroid varies from diffusely uniform increased activity

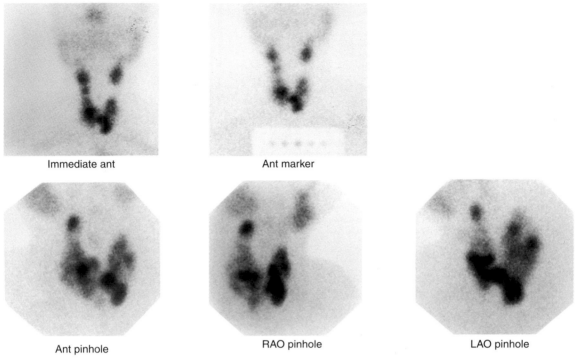

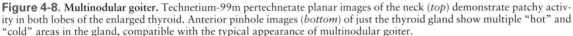

Figure 4-8. Multinodular goiter. Technetium-99m pertechnetate planar images of the neck (*top*) demonstrate patchy activity in both lobes of the enlarged thyroid. Anterior pinhole images (*bottom*) of just the thyroid gland show multiple "hot" and "cold" areas in the gland, compatible with the typical appearance of multinodular goiter.

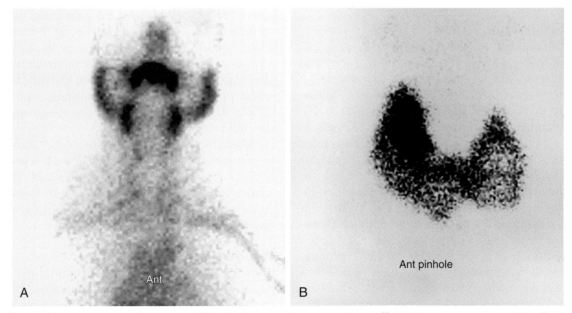

Figure 4-9. Subacute and chronic thyroiditis. A, Anterior planar image from a ⁹⁹ᵐTcO4- scan in a patient with subacute thyroiditis shows little, if any, activity in the region of the thyroid. B, A pinhole image of the thyroid from an iodine-123 scan in a different patient with chronic thyroiditis shows patchy or inhomogeneous activity throughout the gland. This pattern is also seen with multinodular goiter.

in the gland early in the disease (which may resemble Graves disease) to a coarsely patchy distribution of activity within the gland later in the disease (which may mimic multinodular goiter).

The more uncommon diseases of acute (bacterial) and subacute (viral or autoimmune) thyroiditis have such typical clinical features that they are usually diagnosed on physical and clinical grounds, and scanning generally plays

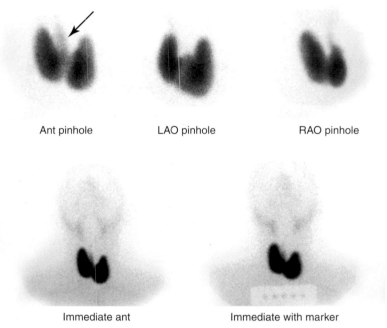

Ant pinhole   LAO pinhole   RAO pinhole

Immediate ant   Immediate with marker

Figure 4-10. Diffuse goiter in a patient with Graves disease. *Upper row,* The pinhole collimator images (technetium-99m [^{99m}Tc]- pertechnetate) demonstrate a large gland with increased activity and a pyramidal lobe arising from the right lobe (*arrow*). *Lower row,* Images obtained with the parallel-hole collimator demonstrate the relatively increased trapping of ^{99m}Tc-pertechnetate in the thyroid compared with the almost nonexistent salivary gland activity.

little role in their evaluation. Subacute thyroiditis usually presents as a painful swollen gland with elevated circulating thyroid hormone levels but with markedly depressed radioiodine uptake. Attempts at imaging with radioiodine or ^{99m}Tc-pertechnetate (see Fig. 4-6, *D*) usually show little or no localization of radiopharmaceutical in the gland. In some patients having ^{18}F-FDG PET scans for cancer or cardiac viability studies, there may be diffusely increased activity in the thyroid. This occurs in about 3% of patients and is often associated with chronic lymphocytic (Hashimoto) thyroiditis. Increased focal thyroid activity on such scans should raise the suspicion of thyroid cancer.

Thyroid Carcinoma

Ninety percent of all thyroid cancers are well differentiated and have the ability to concentrate radioiodine; therefore, thyroid cancer is usually amenable to adjunctive radioiodine therapy. Between 80% and 90% of well-differentiated thyroid cancers are papillary. These occur twice as often in female as in male patients and over a wide age range, with a mean age of about 45 years. These tumors almost always are seen on a thyroid scan as a single cold nodule but often are histologically multifocal. Papillary carcinoma commonly metastasizes to cervical lymph nodes. Ten percent to 20% of well-differentiated cancers are follicular. These also occur over a wide age group, but with a mean age of 50 to 55 years. These tumors most commonly metastasize hematogenously to the lungs (Fig. 4-11) and bone (Fig. 4-12) and less commonly to the liver and brain.

The overall prognosis of patients with well-differentiated types of thyroid cancer is good, with a 5-year survival rate of more than 95% in properly treated patients. The metastases of either lesion may histologically present the characteristics of the other; that is, primary follicular lesions may give predominantly papillary metastases, or vice versa.

Clinically and scintigraphically, primary carcinomas of the thyroid may initially present as discrete thyroid nodules or as enlargement of one lobe with or without cervical nodal or distant metastases. When discrete, the lesions are almost invariably demonstrated as cold areas on the radionuclide images. By use of a gamma camera, ^{99m}Tc-pertechnetate with a pinhole collimator, 80% of lesions 8 mm in diameter are detected.

Because the metastatic lesions of well-differentiated thyroid carcinomas with follicular

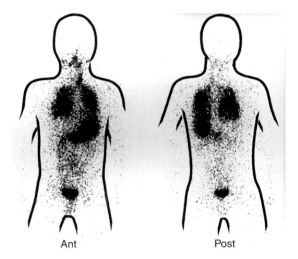

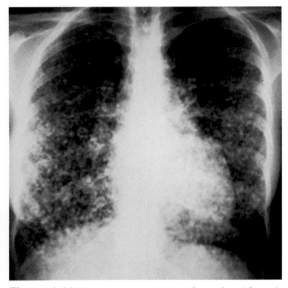

Figure 4-11. Pulmonary metastases from thyroid carcinoma. *Top,* Anterior and posterior images of a whole-body iodine-131 scan obtained 72 hours after injection. Normal physiologic activity is seen in the mouth and salivary glands, stomach, colon, and bladder. The activity in the lower neck represents functioning nodal metastases, and the activity in the lung is due to many tiny hematogenous pulmonary metastases, which are seen on the chest radiograph (*Bottom*).

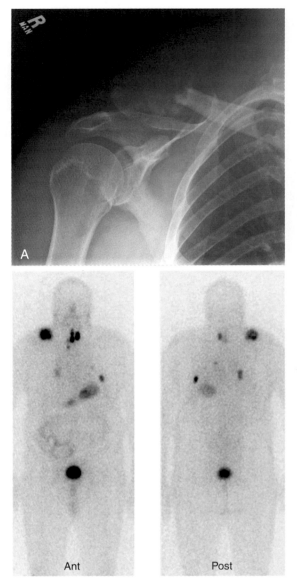

Figure 4-12. Osseous metastases from thyroid carcinoma. **A,** This 54-year-old patient presented with shoulder pain, and a radiograph showed an aggressive expansile destructive lesion of the distal clavicle. Biopsy indicated thyroid carcinoma. **B,** A whole body iodine-123 scan showed multiple lesions as well as the deformed thyroid. The stomach, bowel, and bladder activity is normal.

elements frequently (65% to 85%) concentrate radioiodine, whole-body imaging with ^{123}I or ^{131}I is of value in monitoring post-thyroidectomy patients to detect functioning metastases or to assess the results of treatment of known metastatic lesions.

Post-Thyroidectomy Imaging. Whole-body evaluation for metastatic thyroid disease is first performed within 1 to 2 months after total or subtotal thyroidectomy. Thyroid hormone replacement is withheld during this period to allow for endogenous TSH stimulation of any remaining normal tissue in the thyroid bed and any functioning metastatic lesions. This stimulation allows even poorly functioning or small amounts of tissue to be maximally visualized. A serum TSH value of greater than 30 μU/mL is desirable, and a level greater than 50 μU/mL is optimal. After the oral administration of about 3 to 5 mCi (111 to 185 MBq) of ^{131}I-sodium iodide, sequential whole-body images are obtained for the next several days, generally at 48, 72, and, if necessary, 96 hours or longer. When ^{131}I whole-body scanning is used, 1.5 mCi (55.5 MBq) is administered orally and imaging is optimally performed at 24 hours, although earlier imaging at 6 hours is possible.

A whole-body imaging device or large-field-of-view gamma camera may be used (optimally with a high-energy collimator, although a medium-energy collimator may be used). If gamma camera spot images are the method of imaging, it is important to include adequate neck, chest, abdominal, and pelvic views in the anterior position as well as appropriate posterior images.

Knowledge of the normal distribution of radioiodine before and after thyroid ablation is essential (Fig. 4-13). Activity is commonly seen in the stomach, bowel, and bladder. Mild diffuse activity in the liver is also normal and is caused by the clearance of bound iodine by the liver. Residual normal thyroid tissue in the neck may produce a star artifact when a medium-energy collimator is used. This is owing to septal penetration by the large number of high-energy gamma rays from the [131]I (see Fig. 4-13).

When whole-body radioiodine imaging using a diagnostic administration of ^{131}I is performed after thyroidectomy for detection of residual thyroid tissue or functioning metastases, some concerns have been raised regarding the possibility of stunning these tissues. "Stunning" results in a decreased ability to uptake a subsequent therapeutic dose of ^{131}I, leading to a less effective treatment. It has been postulated that this might result from a reduction in the number of functional cells or, more likely, a reduction in transport of radioiodine into the cells because of the beta radiation from the diagnostic dose. Because the severity of stunning is directly related to the amount of ^{131}I used, limiting the diagnostic dose to 3 to 5 mCi (111 to 185 MBq) for imaging before thyroid remnant ablation or treatment of functioning metastases has been recommended. If stunning is a major concern, imaging using 1.5 mCi (55.5 MBq) of orally administered ^{123}I can be performed at 24 hours. The only drawback is that ^{123}I is more expensive than is [131]I.

Postradioiodine Therapy Imaging. If significant functioning thyroid tissue remains in the neck, as is frequently the case even after "total" thyroidectomy, ablation of the remaining tissue

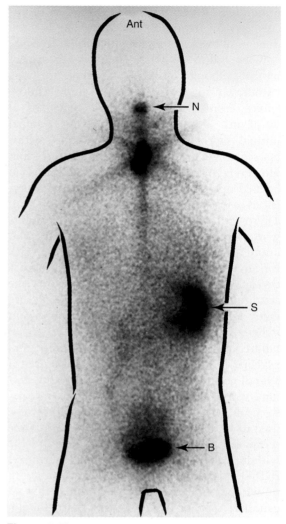

Figure 4-13. **Star artifact from iodine-131.** A residual thyroid remnant in this patient after thyroidectomy has accumulated a large amount of radioiodine. The high energy and activity of the radioiodine have caused a number of photons to penetrate the lead septa of the medium-energy collimator, causing a star pattern in the lower neck. Depending on the arrangement of the holes in the collimator, this pattern may be a six-pointed star or a cross pattern. Normal physiologic activity is seen in the nose (*N*), stomach (*S*), and bladder (*B*).

with high-dose ^{131}I therapy is indicated. Metastatic lesions are only infrequently visualized with ^{123}I or ^{131}I whole-body imaging when there is functioning thyroid in the neck. Ablation of residual tissue allows for sufficient TSH stimulation by the pituitary to permit functioning of distant metastatic sites, thus allowing their detection on follow-up ^{131}I imaging. Adequate endogenous TSH stimulation usually takes 4 to 6 weeks. Once all residual thyroid tissue in the neck has been ablated, follow-up whole-body imaging with ^{123}I or ^{131}I may be performed at

6-month to 1-year intervals. Although protocols vary by institution, such scanning is often done until the scans are negative for 2 years.

When follow-up ^{131}I imaging is performed, patients should undergo thyroid hormone withdrawal for 4 to 6 weeks to allow endogenous serum TSH levels to rise in excess of 30 µU/mL so that stimulation of any residual normal thyroid tissue or functioning metastases can enhance the likelihood of detection. However, because hormone withdrawal can be medically ill-advised in some patients, exogenous recombinant human thyrotropin (rhTSH, Thyrogen [Genzyme]) may be used in patients who continue on thyroid hormone but who are thought to be at significantly increased risk for adverse events related to withdrawal from thyroid hormone after a thyroidectomy. The conditions associated with adverse events are many and include history of stroke, transient ischemic attack, underlying heart disease, renal failure, history of past or active depression and psychiatric disorders, severe compromise of overall performance status, use of digoxin, lithium, warfarin, and age greater than 65 years. Recombinant human TSH (rhTSH) may also be used to supplement endogenous TSH when the serum levels fail to respond sufficiently to the withdrawal of replacement thyroid hormone; rhTSH is also approved for detection (with or without imaging) of differentiated thyroid cancer recurrence by stimulating thyroglobulin production before a serum test is performed.

The dosage for Thyrogen-assisted radioiodine imaging is 0.9 mg given intramuscularly every 24 hours for 2 doses, with diagnostic administration of ^{131}I given 24 hours after the last Thyrogen injection. Imaging is then performed 48 and/or 72 hours later. It should be recognized that the sensitivity of whole-body ^{131}I imaging after rhTSH is slightly less sensitive for both detection of residual thyroid tissue and tumor in the thyroid bed and for functioning metastases in 15% to 25% of patients compared with imaging after thyroid hormone withdrawal. Thus, in high-risk patients, hormone withdrawal may well be advised. Even though rhTSH is very expensive, and not as sensitive as thyroid hormone withdrawal, it is sometimes incorrectly prescribed as a matter of convenience for many patients who are simply unwilling to stop their thyroid hormone. Use of rTSH is not recommended for stimulation of radioiodine uptake for purposes of ablative radiotherapy for thyroid cancer.

After all functioning tissue within the thyroid bed has been ablated, subsequent identification of functioning tissue in the neck should be considered as tumor recurrence and treated appropriately. It is important not to mistake the physiologic excretion of radioiodine in the salivary glands, saliva, nose, stomach, colon, liver, and bladder for metastases. Most physiologic activity in the liver is diffuse, whereas hepatic metastases usually are focal.

In addition to whole-body ^{123}I or ^{131}I imaging, post-ablation thyroid cancer patients are also followed by monitoring serum thyroglobulin (Tg) levels. Serum Tg tests are the most accurate method of detecting recurrent thyroid cancer even if the patient is taking thyroid hormone. This glycoprotein is synthesized by follicular cells, and most well-differentiated thyroid cancers secrete Tg even if they do not concentrate radioiodine or if the patient is taking thyroid hormone. Measurement of Tg can vary from one laboratory to another, and it is best for the patient to have serial measurements performed by the same laboratory. Measurement of Tg before surgery and thyroid ablation is not useful. In addition, Tg levels can be high for the first 2 months after thyroidectomy, and tests should not be performed until after this period. A rising Tg level should raise serious concern about metastases or recurrence. A Tg level above 10 ng/mL is associated with metastases in more than 85% of patients. Whole-body radioiodine scans for follow-up are generally unnecessary in patients with negative serum Tg and no other signs of recurrent thyroid cancer.

In patients with suspected metastatic lesions to the skeleton, a radionuclide bone scan before the administration of a whole-body ^{123}I or ^{131}I scanning dose may be useful, although thyroid metastases to bone are not uncommonly photopenic and may go undetected on [99mTc]-diphosphonate bone scans (Fig. 4-14).

Imaging Noniodine-Avid Thyroid Cancers

Nonradioiodine-avid thyroid carcinomas are not visualized with radioiodine imaging but can be successfully imaged using either [99mTc]-sestamibi (Fig. 4-15) or more commonly, [18F]-fluorodeoxyglucose (18F-FDG) positron

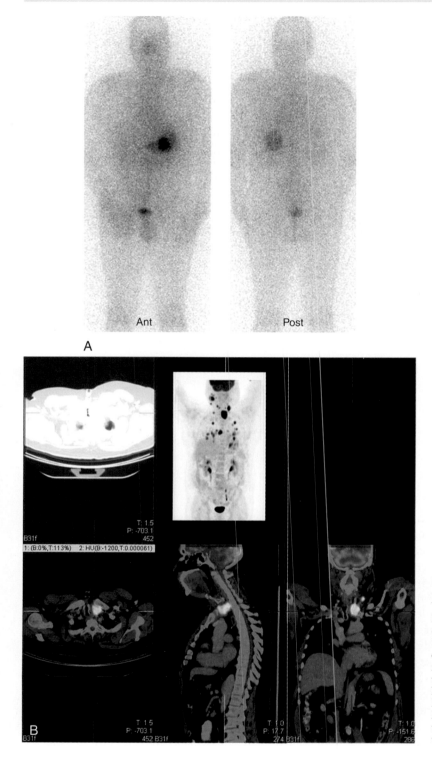

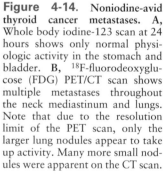

Figure 4-14. Noniodine-avid thyroid cancer metastases. **A,** Whole body iodine-123 scan at 24 hours shows only normal physiologic activity in the stomach and bladder. **B,** ¹⁸F-fluorodeoxyglucose (FDG) PET/CT scan shows multiple metastases throughout the neck mediastinum and lungs. Note that due to the resolution limit of the PET scan, only the larger lung nodules appear to take up activity. Many more small nodules were apparent on the CT scan.

emission tomography (PET) (see Fig. 4-14). Non-avid thyroid malignancies include anaplastic or poorly differentiated carcinomas (5%) which occur primarily in older patients. The prognosis is generally poor, and surgery is the only effective treatment. Medullary carcinoma of the thyroid parenchyma constitutes about 5% of malignant thyroid lesions and is not iodine avid. This cancer may be associated with other endocrine lesions, such as

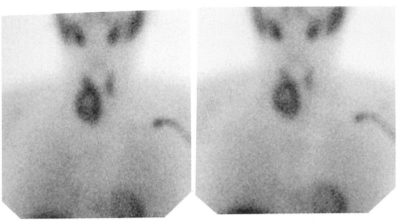

Ant 5 min   Ant 15 min

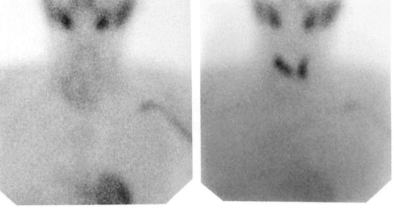

Figure 4-15. Thyroid carcinoma. Technetium-99m (^{99m}Tc) sesta-mibi scan (*top row* and *lower left*) shows a large area of increased uptake in the right lobe of the thyroid with a central cold area of necrosis. The activity decreases over 2 hours. ^{99m}Tc pertechnetate scan (*lower right*) shows the normal gland but no activity in this area because the cancer is unable to trap or organify.

Ant 2 hr   Ant TcO$_4$

pheochromocytoma; may actively secrete hormones (most notably thyrocalcitonin); and may be familial. Medullary carcinoma can be imaged with somatostatin receptor agents such as ^{111}In-pentetreotide (Fig. 4-16). The overall sensitivity of ^{18}F-FDG for medullary cancer is only about 60%. Hürthle cell carcinoma (5%) is an unusual variant of follicular cell carcinoma, which is generally more aggressive with early distant metastases. Most of these latter types of tumors do not concentrate iodine well and therefore are not usually amenable to metastasis localization or radioiodine therapy.

IODINE-131 THERAPY IN THYROID DISEASE

Iodine-131 plays an important role in the control and cure of certain thyroid diseases. Each institution should develop a protocol for patient care and personnel safety when patients are hospitalized or released for radioiodine

therapy. This needs to comply with relevant local, state, and NRC requirements. A sample protocol for hospitalized patients is provided in Appendix H-2 and issues related to patient release into the public are covered later in the chapter and in Chapter 13.

The primary therapeutic uses of ^{131}I are (1) the treatment of hyperthyroidism caused by either diffuse or nodular goiter, (2) the postsurgical ablation of the thyroid gland remnants, and (3) the treatment of functioning thyroid metastases.

Principle

Whether benign or neoplastic, any thyroid tissue capable of producing thyroid hormone will trap and organify stable iodine or its radioactive isotopes. Once a radioactive form of iodine has been taken up by the functioning tissue, therapeutic effects are made possible by the delivery of destructive ionizing radiation, primarily in the form of relatively high-energy beta

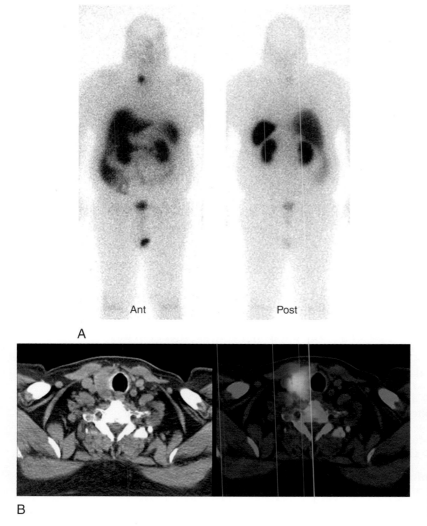

Ant   Post

A

B

Figure 4-16. Medullary carcinoma of the thyroid. **A,** Somatostatin receptor scan with ^{111}In-pentetreotide in patient with an elevated serum calcitonin level shows a focus of increased activity in the neck. The other activity is physiologic. **B,** SPECT/CT scan localizes the activity to the right lobe of the thyroid.

emissions. Subsequent to irradiation, cell death occurs over a period of weeks to months. The beta-emitting properties of ^{131}I have made this radioisotope the most useful for the elimination of unwanted benign or malignant thyroid tissue.

Several factors influence the dose of radiation delivered to functioning thyroid tissue by ^{131}I and therefore govern its effectiveness as a therapeutic agent. These include (1) the degree of uptake of ^{131}I, (2) the bulk of tissue to be destroyed, (3) the length of residence of ^{131}I within the tissue, (4) the distribution of ^{131}I within the tissue, and (5) the radiosensitivity of the particular cells. A pregnancy test should be performed on any woman of childbearing age for whom there may be a question of adequate birth control before radioiodine therapy.

Primary Hyperthyroidism

See Box 4-3 for major consideration involved in radioiodine treatment of hyperthyroidism. The three basic approaches to the therapy of primary hyperthyroidism are (1) antithyroid drugs, such as the thioamides, propylthiouracil, and methimazole; (2) surgery (3) and ^{131}I therapy. Iodine-131 is regarded as the treatment of choice for hyperthyroidism in patients older than 30 years and in patients of any age in whom hyperthyroidism is accompanied by medical complications or in whom other treatments have failed. Although antithyroid drugs are frequently used as an initial approach to the control of diffuse toxic goiter (Graves disease), such drugs are generally not used in the treatment of toxic nodules or multinodular goiter. In a significant number of patients with Graves disease, antithyroid drug therapy produces

Box 4-3 Factors to Consider for Radioiodine Therapy of Hyperthyroidism*

Patient Selection
Review patient record to confirm Graves disease, toxic or nontoxic multinodular goiter, or autonomously functioning nodule.
Review prior imaging reports and images.
Review recent TSH, free T_4, and free T_3 and thyroid iodine-123 or 131 uptake values.
Assess serum creatinine levels. Poor renal function will slow excretion of radioiodine from the body and increase absorbed dose to normal tissues.
Conduct directed physical examination.
Take prior radioiodine administration history.
Evaluate continence and mental status. If there is a problem, consider arranging for hospitalization with precautions.

Patient Preparation
Pretreatment with antithyroid drugs (methimazole or propylthiouracil) to deplete thyroid hormone stores may be helpful to reduce possibility of thyroid storm (especially in older and cardiac patients). Discontinue 3-5 days before therapy and resume 2-3 days after.
Beta blockers can be helpful for symptomatic control and do not need to be discontinued during therapy.
Recombinant TSH (rh-TSH) stimulation is not currently FDA approved for therapy but has been used off-label with nontoxic nodular goiter to maximize thyroid uptake.
For potentially pregnant females, do a pregnancy test 72 hours or less before treatment.
Discontinue breastfeeding. Breastfeeding may resume in the future after birth of another child.
Pregnancy should be avoided for 6 mo-1 year in case another treatment is needed.

Determination of Administered Activity
A number of methods are available, including using the 24-hour radioiodine uptake value to deliver 80-200 µCi (2.96-7.4 MBq) per gram of thyroid tissue. The higher administered activity is usually for nodular goiters, large diffuse toxic goiters, and repeat treatments.
Typical values are:
  10-15 mCi (370-555 MBq) for Graves disease
  20-30 mCi (740 MBq-1.11 GBq) for nodular goiters

Administration of Radioiodine
Patient should fast or, at a minimum, refrain from large meals 4 hours before and 1 hour after administration.
Informed consent should include:
  Purpose of treatment
  Additional treatments may be needed
  Side effects
    Early effects (salivary tenderness [30%], gastritis [30%], transient metallic taste, neck pain due to thyroiditis [10%-20%], late side effects (xerostomia [10%-20%], dental caries, reduced taste, dry eyes [rare], <1% possibility of radiation-induced neoplasms)
    Ophthalmopathy may worsen or develop after therapy for Graves disease.
    Long-term hormone replacement and follow-up will be required.
Written directive is prepared and signed.
Administration in capsule form is preferred.
Dose is verified in dose calibrator.
Patient is positively identified.
Patient report should include activity and route of administration.
Survey of administration area is made at the end of the day.

Release of Patient (see also Chapter 13)
Patient release is authorized by the NRC when a survey instrument at one meter reads ≤7 mrem/h (0.07 mSv/h); or when the oral I-131 dose is ≤33 mCi (1.2 GBq); or when a calculation indicates effective doses to other persons (such as family and caregivers) will be ≤500 mrem (5 mSv). With proper precautions and such calculations, hyperthyroid patients may be able to be released with administered activities in the range of 50 mCi (1.85 GBq).
Patient is provided with documentation of activity administered and radionuclide.
Patient is provided with written radiation safety and As Low As Reasonably Achievable precautions.
Release to a hotel is stongly discouraged.

Box 4-3 Factors to Consider for Radioiodine Therapy of Hyperthyroidism*—cont'd

For 5-7 days:
  Encourage hydration and frequent voiding.
  Refrain from kissing or sexual activity.
  Avoid pregnant women, infants, and children.
  Try to remain 1 meter from other persons.
  Avoid urine and sweat cross-contamination.

Follow-Up
The thyroid function will decrease over several months. Initial evaluation with thyroid function studies are recommended at 1 month. After this time, adjust hormone replacement levels as needed.

*For additional details, see Society of Nuclear Medicine: Procedure guideline for therapy of thyroid disease with iodine-131 (sodium-iodide), 9/17/2005. http://www.snm.org. Accessed September 16, 2011.

intolerable side effects, does not adequately control the disease, or results in patient compliance problems. In these patients and in patients with toxic nodular disease, ^{131}I therapy is of considerable value. Iodine-131 therapy is also of value in patients with recurrent hyperthyroidism after previous thyroidectomy, when repeat surgery would cause enhanced risks; in children who have experienced toxicity to antithyroid drugs; and in patients who refuse other therapy.

Although most children with hyperthyroidism have Graves disease, there is a certain amount of controversy regarding the treatment of children and adolescents with [131]I. The complication rate in children undergoing thyroid surgery is significantly higher than that in adults, and antithyroid therapy in children usually has poor compliance and carries a significantly higher risk of toxicity and relapse compared with that experienced in adults. As many as 80% of children and adolescents treated for Graves disease with antithyroid drugs eventually require ^{131}I therapy. Even though there is little evidence to indicate significant radiation carcinogenesis from therapeutic doses of ^{131}I in these patients, a few physicians still choose not to use ^{131}I therapy routinely in children and in adults younger than 30 years.

Proposed methods of calculating doses for treating hyperthyroidism are numerous and varied. Determination of dose follows one of two basic philosophies, commonly referred to as low-dose and high-dose therapy. Currently, low-dose therapy is rarely used. The difference in approaches is predicated on the likelihood of the induction of hypothyroidism. In low-dose therapy, there is an emphasis on reducing the resulting hypothyroidism in the first year after therapy and accepting any morbidity associated with the prolonged presence of hyperthyroidism. This method does not appear to alter the incidence of hypothyroidism after 1 year. The more commonly used high-dose therapy considers that hypothyroidism is an acceptable risk, indeed, almost an inevitable result, of ^{131}I therapy for Graves disease. Rapid reduction in thyroid function is the most important objective of high-dose therapy. With this approach, the patient is normally rendered hypothyroid and put on replacement hormone as soon as possible. High-dose therapy is especially appropriate for patients with underlying medical conditions worsened by hyperthyroidism, such as cardiac congestive failure.

Formulas for the calculation of actual administered activity generally take into account one or more of the following: (1) the size of the gland, (2) the presence or absence of nodularity in the gland, and (3) the results of the ^{131}I uptake test. Palpation used to estimate the mass of the thyroid gland often introduces a substantial subjective error into the calculation of dose, although assessment of thyroid images and the occasional use of ultrasonography may aid in improving the estimate of gland size. With experience, a reasonable estimate can be made by palpation alone. Rather than calculate a specific activity for a given patient, some laboratories simply use a fixed activity for patients with diffuse toxic goiter, often in the range of 10 to 15 mCi (370 to 555 MBq). Studies have shown that there is little difference in the success of therapy between calculated and fixed dose treatment.

Most institutions use high-dose therapy, and doses in the range of 8 to 30 mCi (296 to 1110 MBq) or higher may be initially administered to allow for definitive therapy. Administered doses are also selected at the higher end of the dose range if the patients are severely hyperthyroid or have large glands, significant nodularity, or cardiac disease aggravated by their thyrotoxic state. With high-dose therapy, retreatment is usually unnecessary. In general, for treatment of diffuse goiter, therapy may be in the range of 15 mCi (555 MBq) of ^{131}I in patients with no evidence of thyroid nodularity. These doses may be repeated at 3- to 6-month intervals as necessary for the control of hyperthyroidism.

Hyperthyroidism related to toxic nodular goiter (Plummer disease) is particularly resistant to radioactive iodine therapy and frequently requires doses two to three times larger than those applicable in diffuse toxic goiter. Thus, in addition to ^{131}I uptakes, thyroid imaging is usually used before ^{131}I therapy to distinguish toxic nodular goiter from Graves disease. Large multinodular goiters may require doses in excess of 30 mCi (1.11 GBq), and multiple treatments may be needed. Solitary toxic nodules generally can be successfully treated with administered doses in the 15- to 25-mCi (555 to 925 MBq) range. Even with such large doses, it is not usual to induce hypothyroidism when there is significant suppression of function in the remainder of the thyroid gland by the autonomous nodules.

Regardless of the type of dose regimen used, it is often difficult to predict accurately the outcome of radioactive iodine therapy in a given patient. Results are frequently significantly affected by a number of variables:
- Nodular thyroids (including those of nodular Graves disease) are usually more resistant and require larger doses.
- Bulkier thyroid glands demonstrate diminished response.
- Prior administration of antithyroid drugs increases resistance.
- Patients with severe hyperthyroidism may likewise be less responsive, possibly based on the rapid turnover of ^{131}I within the gland.

Although there is a clear correlation between the dose of radioiodine used and the onset of hypothyroidism in the first year after therapy, the incidence of hypothyroidism after that time shows less correlation with the dose used. At least half of patients exhibit hypothyroidism 10 years after therapy regardless of the ^{131}I dose regimen chosen. Therefore, careful follow-up is necessary in all patients who become initially euthyroid, to watch for the development of late hypothyroidism. In our experience, unless the gland is very large, a one-time orally administered activity of 15 mCi (555 MBq) is all that is needed to treat 90% to 95% of patients with Graves disease successfully, and 25 mCi (925 MBq) cures about 80% to 90% of patients with a toxic nodular goiter. Aside from latent hypothyroidism, other complications of radioiodine therapy for hyperthyroidism are rare. There is no evidence of increased incidence of radiation-induced malignancies, including thyroid cancer and leukemia, after radioiodine therapy for hyperthyroidism. No change in fertility rates or genetic damage in offspring has been found. Thyroid storm occurs in less than 0.1% of patients, and clinically significant radiation thyroiditis is uncommon. In patients with Graves disease and orbitopathy, the subsequent radiation-induced hypothyroidism confers an increased risk of exacerbation. This can be minimized by concurrent oral prednisone therapy or prompt T$_4$ replacement. Patients without orbitopathy are unlikely to develop it after radioiodine treatment.

Patient Preparation
Before the oral administration of a therapeutic dose of ^{131}I, the diagnosis of toxic goiter must have been firmly established on the basis of physical examination, history, and elevated circulating serum thyroid hormone levels and depressed TSH. An ^{131}I uptake should be routinely performed to exclude hyperthyroidism resulting from certain diseases, such as silent, painless thyroiditis, and to gauge the dose required. The patient should take nothing by mouth after midnight the evening before treatment. Female patients should be carefully screened for possible pregnancy, which is a contraindication for radioiodine therapy because of possible carcinogenic risk to the fetus and risk of injury to the fetal thyroid gland after the first trimester. In lactating mothers, therapy should be instituted only if the patient is willing to completely cease breastfeeding because the iodine is secreted in breast milk.

Severely hyperthyroid patients with marked symptoms may be pretreated with antithyroid drugs to avoid worsening the clinical status or causing thyroid storm, which results from the sudden release of hormone from the gland after radiation destruction of thyroid follicles. For most patients, however, this pretreatment is unnecessary.

If antithyroid drugs are already in use, they should be discontinued for 5 to 7 days before the ^{131}I treatment is administered, depending on the clinical status of the patient. If clinically necessary, these drugs may be readministered 7 to 10 days after therapy without adversely affecting the results of treatment. As an alternative, β-adrenergic blocking agents, such as propranolol, may be used throughout the therapy period because they do not affect thyroid function and therefore permit recirculation of ^{131}I in the gland for maximum radiation effect.

In the first week after a therapeutic dose of radioiodine, a patient may experience several symptoms, including sore throat, dysphagia, and an increase in hyperthyroid symptoms as a result of increased release of hormone from radiation-damaged follicles. Patients should drink as much fluid as possible and void often to reduce whole-body and bladder radiation doses.

Whichever dose regimen is used, there is generally no significant improvement in hyperthyroid symptoms for about 3 to 4 weeks after treatment. In adequately treated patients with diffuse toxic goiter, however, a significant shrinkage in the size of the gland is usually identified in the first month after therapy. If, after 3 to 4 months, the patient still has signs, symptoms, or laboratory evidence of hyperthyroidism, a repeat dose of ^{131}I may be administered.

Thyroid Carcinoma Therapy

Iodine-131 therapy is a valuable adjunct in thyroid carcinoma therapy for ablation of postsurgical residual thyroid tissue in the neck and for eradication of functioning local and distant thyroid metastases. Although most thyroid cancers are well differentiated and have an excellent prognosis when treated appropriately, 75% of the deaths from thyroid cancer occur from these initially well-differentiated lesions. Because thyroid cancer may undergo transformation into more aggressive forms with time, it is very important to detect and eradicate the lesions in their early stage while they are capable of concentrating radioiodine and thus can be successfully treated with ^{131}I. See Box 4-4 for major considerations involved.

Postsurgical Ablation

Radioiodine "ablation" typically refers to the destruction of functioning remnants of normal thyroid tissue remaining after subtotal thyroidectomy. Whole-body thyroid imaging is usually performed 4 to 6 weeks after thyroidectomy to detect residual functioning tissue in the thyroid bed and any possible distant metastases. The scan assists in determining the size of the ablation dose needed, depending on the amount of residual thyroid tissue and any unsuspected metastatic foci.

Surgery is seldom able to effect removal of all of the functioning thyroid tissue, even in the best hands. Residual tissue may be confused with local nodal metastatic disease when postsurgical scanning is performed. In addition, through suppression of endogenous TSH, residual thyroid tissue in the neck significantly reduces the likelihood that distant metastatic lesions will be visualized with follow-up whole-body ^{131}I scanning techniques. Therefore, ^{131}I ablation of remaining thyroid tissue in the neck is a convenient and relatively inexpensive method for obtaining the desired results of total thyroidectomy. Further, radioiodine ablation after surgical removal of the thyroid is associated with a deceased risk of recurrence and death in patients with well-differentiated thyroid cancer.

The amount of administered activity used after surgery to ablate residual normal thyroid is a matter of debate. In many hospitals, this depends on the particular characteristics of the tumor and the assumed risk level of recurrence. In lower-risk situations of residual postsurgical functioning tissue in which the primary tumor is less than 1.5 cm and has not invaded the thyroid capsule, ablation of a remnant can be done with 29.9 mCi (1.1 GBq) or less of ^{131}I. If needed, recombinant TSH (rhTSH) simulation of the thyroid remnant prior to I-131 ablation to increase uptake of the radioiodine may improve the efficacy of treatment.

In higher-risk patients, those with vessel, lymphatic, or capsular invasion, a primary lesion of greater than 1.5 cm, poorly differentiated cell types, metastasis, or multifocal lesions, high-dose therapy (greater than 30 mCi) in the range of 100 to 200 mCi (3.7 to 7.4 GBq), should be used. The rationales are that the residual normal thyroid remnant can be used as a source of radiation to nearby tissues and that the first chance at tumor cure will be the best chance.

Box 4-4 Factors to Consider for Radioiodine Therapy of Differentiated Thyroid Cancer*

Patient Selection
Review operative and histology reports. Make sure cancer is differentiated type.
Patient should have had total or near total thyroidectomy with neck dissection for T_3 and T_4 tumors.
Neck dissection may not be necessary for small T_1 or T_2 tumors.
Review prior imaging reports and images.
Radioiodine ablation is not recommended for intrathyroidal unifocal (<1 cm) or microscopic multifocal cancer without other high risk features. High risk features include metastases, thyroid capsule invasion, history of radiation therapy to head or neck, and unfavorable histology.
Conduct CBC, serum calcium tests (to exclude hypoparathyroidism post-thyroidectomy).
Assess serum creatinine level. Poor renal function will slow excretion of radioiodine from the body and increase absorbed dose to normal tissues.
Conduct iodine-123 (or I-131 [<4 mCi]) scan for residual thyroid tissue or disease status if this cannot be ascertained from the surgical report or neck ultrasonography.
Assess baseline serum thyroglobulin (obtained in hypothyroid state or after rhTSH).
Conduct directed physical examination.
Take prior radioiodine administration history.
Assess continence and mental status (if there is a problem, arrange for hospitalization with precautions).

Patient Preparation
Withhold hormone medications until TSH >30 μU/mL; this is usually 3 weeks after thyroidectomy or 4-5 weeks after discontinuing levothyroxine. Triiodothyronine can be substituted until 2 weeks before treatment. TSH may not rise if large volume of functioning tissue remains.
Patient should follow a low-iodine diet for 10-14 days (significant iodine is found in iodized salt, milk/dairy products, eggs, seafood, seaweed, many commercial breads, chocolate, many multivitamins, red dye #3).
Stop thyroid hormone for 5-7 days.
Recombinant TSH (rhTSH) stimulation is not currently FDA approved for therapy.
For potentially pregnant females, administer a pregnancy test 72 hours or less before treatment.
Discontinue breastfeeding. Breastfeeding may resume in the future after birth of another child.
Pregnancy should be avoided for 6 months to 1 year in case another treatment is needed.

Determination of Administered Activity
Postoperative thyroid remnants are usually ablated with 2.75-5.5 GBq (75-150 mCi).
For presumed thyroid cancer in neck or mediastinum, >7.4 GBq (200 mCi) is usually administered.
For distant metastases, 5.55-7.4 GBq (150-200 mCi) is usually administered.
Cumulative activity from repeated treatments above 29.6 GBq (800 mCi) should be done with extreme caution only, due to possible bone marrow depression.

Administration of Radioiodine
Patient should fast or, at a minimum, refrain from large meals 4 hours before and 1 hour after administration.
Informed consent should include:
   Purpose of treatment
   Additional treatments may be needed
   Side effects
      Early effects (salivary tenderness [30%], gastritis [30%], transient metallic taste, neck pain due to thyroiditis [10%-20%], transiently decreased white cell count [rare], transient hypospermia [rare] mucositis, and transient nausea or vomiting [rare])
      Late side effects (xerostomia [10%-20%], dental caries, reduced taste, dry eyes [rare], temporary, <1% possibility of radiation-induced neoplasms, pulmonary fibrosis [with multiple high administered activities with iodine-avid pulmonary metastases], permanent bone marrow depression [rare])
   Long-term hormone replacement and follow-up are required.
Written directive is prepared and signed.

> ## Box 4-4 Factors to Consider for Radioiodine Therapy of Differentiated Thyroid Cancer*—cont'd
>
> Administration in capsule form is preferred.
> Dose is verified in dose calibrator.
> Patient is positively identified.
> Patient report should include activity and route of administration.
> Survey of administration area is made at the end of the day.
>
> ### Release of Patient (see also Chapter 13)
> Patient release is authorized by the NRC when a survey instrument at one meter reads ≤7 mrem/h (0.07 mSv/h); or when the oral I-131 dose is ≤33 mCi (1.2 GBq); or when a calculation indicates effective doses to other persons (family and caregivers) will be ≤500 mrem (5 mSv).
> With such calculations and proper precautions, thyroid cancer patients may be able to be released with administered activities somewhat in excess of 200 mCi (7.4 GBq).
> Release to hotel is strongly discouraged but not prohibited.
> Patient is provided with documentation of activity administered and radionuclide.
> Patient is provided with written radiation safety and ALARA precautions.
> For 5-7 days:
>   Encourage hydration and frequent voiding.
>   Avoid kissing.
>   Avoid pregnant women, infants, and children.
>   Try to remain 1 meter from other persons.
>   Avoid urine and sweat cross-contamination.
>
> ### Follow-Up
> Perform whole body imaging 3-14 days after treatment.
> Check that TSH suppression is below 0.1 mU/L for high- and intermediate-risk patients and 0.1-0.5 mU/L for low-risk patients.
> Make periodic determination (6-12 months) of serum thyroglobulin in hypothyroid state or after rhTSH.
> At 12 months, perform a diagnostic whole body iodine scan after hormone withdrawal or rhTSH may be appropriate for high or intermediate risk patients.

*For additional details, see Society of Nuclear Medicine: Procedure guideline for therapy of thyroid disease with iodine-131 (sodium-iodide), 9/17/2005. http://www.snm.org. Accessed June 26, 2011.

Because well-differentiated thyroid cancers tend to be more aggressive in older patients, high-dose therapy is also recommended for the treatment of patients older than 45 years of age.

In the uncommon case in which a surgeon has actually removed all of the normal thyroid tissue and in which the whole-body scan is negative, high-dose therapy can be used with some modifications. If the tumor was less than 1.5 cm, was well differentiated, and had no capsular invasion, the patient may be placed on thyroid hormone and monitored by serum Tg measurements. Whether a patient with no residual thyroid and no functioning metastases seen on imaging should be treated with ^{131}I remains a matter of controversy. In this setting, ^{131}I ablation may be desirable whether or not residual thyroid tissue or metastases are identified—the rationale being that such therapy may destroy undetectable, functioning micrometastases. On follow-up, patients with elevated Tg levels may show improvement with repeat high-dose ^{131}I therapy even in the presence of a negative ^{131}I scan. After ablation therapy, imaging may be performed 4 to 10 days after treatment by using the residual ^{131}I activity. Thyroid hormone replacement may be instituted 3 to 5 days after the administration of therapy. Reexamination after ablation in 6 to 12 months is typical, and therapy is repeated if residual thyroid tissue is found.

Functioning Metastases

Doses for the eradication of well-differentiated thyroid metastases are high, usually 100 to 200 mCi (3.7 to 7.4 GBq). Iodine-131 may be administered up to 5 or 10 times, usually at about 6-month to yearly intervals. Typically, if metastases persist after three treatments, future therapy is not likely to be curative, although it may be palliative. In some institutions, increased radiation dose from ^{131}I to the functioning tissue is achieved by depleting the extracellular iodide pool using pretherapy low-iodine diets or drug-induced diuresis. In any case, serum TSH levels should be in excess of 30 μU/mL after an appropriate period of thyroid hormone withdrawal to facilitate uptake of the therapy dose of ^{131}I by the functioning lesions. In preparing patients, rhTSH can be used at the physician's discretion to supplement endogenous serum TSH levels as needed.

When patients are treated for functioning pulmonary thyroid metastases, pulmonary fibrosis is a possible complication, especially as cumulative doses exceed 600 mCi (22 GBq). Further, repeat doses of ^{131}I may produce changes in salivary gland function, leading to the unpleasant and irreversible side effect of xerostomia (dry mouth). Thus, after each treatment, patients should be instructed to stimulate saliva flow over several days through the use of items such as hard candy (e.g., lemon drops) to reduce radiation to the salivary glands.

In patients with extensive metastatic lesions or in whom repeat therapeutic administrations are contemplated, monitoring of the hematologic status is desirable because bone marrow suppression may occur in patients with large absorbed radiation doses. Significant bone marrow depression is likely when cumulative administered activities exceed 800 mCi (29.6 GBq). Because of the high doses used in therapy, strict radiation protection procedures must be outlined and carefully followed. According to prior NRC regulations, any patient with ^{131}I activity in excess of 29.9 mCi (1.1 GBq) needed to be hospitalized. Current NRC regulations permit release based on (1) administered activity (less than 33 mCi or 1.2 GBq) for ^{131}I, (2) measured dose rate at 1 m from the patient (less than 7 mrem [less than 70 μSv]/h for ^{131}I), or (3) patient-specific dose calculations that indicate that the maximum likely dose to another individual (family or caregiver) is no greater than 0.5 rem (5 mSv) in any 1 year (see Appendix H). Regulations regarding disposal of the radioactive urine vary from state to state. Patients are usually given thyroid hormone replacement several days later. Follow-up scanning is then performed at 6-month intervals, with ^{131}I therapy repeated as needed until the disease is eradicated. Patients may then be followed with serum Tg levels as described earlier.

An increase in secondary tumors as a result of ^{131}I therapy has been extensively examined. Most studies do not show an increase, although there have been suggested increases in leukemia after therapy for thyroid cancer, with a rate of about 5 per 1000 patients. Bladder and breast cancer incidence also may be slightly increased. Almost all of these cases have occurred in patients who received cumulative activities in excess of 800 mCi (29.6 GBq).

Radiation Safety Aspects

As mentioned earlier, both ^{99m}Tc and the various radioiodines cross the placenta, and, because the fetal thyroid begins accumulation of iodine at about the 12th week of gestation, care must be taken when administering these radiopharmaceuticals during pregnancy. They are also secreted in breast milk in lactating women and may be transferred to nursing infants (Fig. 4-17).

Regulations regarding release of patients after nuclear medicine therapy are presented in Appendix H; however, a few important points are presented here. After diagnostic nuclear medicine procedures, precautions for the public are rarely required, but after some therapeutic procedures, doses to the public and family members and others may need to be limited. Because ^{131}I is a frequently used high-energy gamma emitter and has an 8-day physical half-life, it is the radionuclide that results in the majority of the dose to medical staff, the public, and family members after procedures involving therapeutic administration of unsealed radionuclides. Patients are strongly discouraged from staying at a hotel immediately after treatment. The major aspect of radiation therapy that needs to be controlled when releasing a patient with radioiodine is external exposure of others. However, the typical doses that occur to other persons from patients treated with radioiodine have only a very low risk of cancer induction. Approximate dose rates at 1.0 m from a patient treated for hyperthyroidism are 0.185 mrem/mCi (0.05 μSv/MBq) immediately after administration, 0.11 mrem/mCi (0.03 μSv/MBq) at 2 to 4 days after administration, and 0.07 mrem/mCi (0.02 μSv/MBq) at 5 to 7 days after administration. Patients treated for thyroid cancer metastases eliminate iodine more quickly, and approximate values at the same times are 0.185 (0.05), 0.011(0.003), and 0.007 mrem/ mCi (0.002 μSv/MBq), respectively.

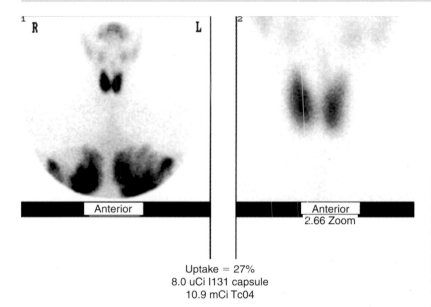

Uptake = 27%
8.0 uCi I131 capsule
10.9 mCi Tc04

Figure 4-17. Activity in lactating breasts. A planar parallel hole collimator anterior image of the neck and chest show activity in the thyroid and both breasts. In this case, the patient had a ^{99m}Tc-pertechnetate thyroid scan but also a radioiodine uptake. Both are secreted in the breast milk and would be transferred to the infant during nursing.

Internal contamination of family members from bodily fluids is most likely 1 to 7 days after treatment. The risks from internal contamination of other adults are less significant than are those from external exposure. Incorporation of large activities of ^{131}I in an adult caregiver or family member that might cause hypothyroidism is extremely unlikely. However, thyroid cancer as a result of radiation exposure appears to be a significant risk for unborn children, infants, and persons under the age of 20, and particular care should be taken to avoid internal contamination of infants and children. Contamination of infants and young children with saliva from a treated patient during the first several days could result in significant doses to the child's thyroid and potentially raise the risk of subsequent radiation-induced thyroid cancer.

In the United States, the NRC dose limit for adult caregivers and family members is 500 mrem (5 mSv) per I-131 treatment episode. For members of the public, pregnant women, and infants and small children, the dose limit is 100 mrem (1 mSv). Treating physicians must provide the released patient, or the patient's parent or guardian, with instructions, including written instructions, on actions recommended to maintain doses to other individuals as low as is reasonably achievable if the total effective dose equivalent to any other individual is likely to exceed 100 mrem (1 mSv).

Continuation of breastfeeding is absolutely contraindicated after radioiodine therapy.

Because the patient may need to be retreated with radioiodine, pregnancy is contraindicated until at least 6 months after radioiodine therapy.

Very low activities of ^{131}I are observed in the environment as a result of medical uses. Even with direct release to sewer systems, the relatively short physical half-life results in doses to the public or sewer workers well below public dose limits and low compared with other sources. No environmental effects have been linked to the levels of radionuclides released as a result of medical uses of unsealed radionuclides.

PARATHYROID IMAGING AND LOCALIZATION

Hyperparathyroidism occurs with a frequency of about 0.5 per 1000, with approximately half of the persons being asymptomatic and detected by serum calcium screening. Those with symptoms may have recurring nephrolithiasis, frank hypercalcemia with low serum phosphate, weakness, fatigue, and bone pain.

Because of the small size and location of the normal parathyroid glands, imaging with most modalities is difficult. Normally, there are two pairs of parathyroid glands usually located on the posterolateral surface of the upper and lower lobes of the thyroid. About 80% to 85% of parathyroid adenomas are found adjacent to the thyroid, but the remainder are ectopically placed and may be in the anterior or posterior superior mediastinum, within or next to the thymus, along the esophagus, along the carotid sheath, or even at the carotid bifurcation. This variation results in 5% of hyperfunctional parathyroid lesions being missed at the initial surgical procedure.

Hyperfunctioning glands, however, can be imaged by using nuclear medicine techniques. Eighty percent to 85% of cases of primary hyperparathyroidism are due to single or multiple hyperfunctioning adenomas. Hyperplasia accounts for 12% to 15% of cases and parathyroid carcinomas for about 1% to 3% of cases.

Technetium-99m sestamibi is the radiopharmaceutical of choice for imaging parathyroid adenomas because of its good energy characteristics for imaging and its avid localization in the mitochondria of parathyroid tissue. Technetium-99m sestamibi has yielded sensitivity rates of about 90% in primary hyperparathyroidism but significantly lower rates in secondary hyperparathyroidism. No special patient preparation is necessary before these scans, but it is important to perform a physical examination specifically to palpate for nodular thyroid disease and other masses.

The basis of the examination is predicated on the selective uptake of ^{99m}Tc-sestamibi by both the thyroid and parathyroid glands. With this method, 20 mCi (740 MBq) is administered intravenously, and images are obtained at about 15 minutes and again at 1 to 3 hours. The complete technical/clinical protocol can be found in Appendix E-1.

Technetium-99m sestamibi initially concentrates in normal thyroid tissue, thyroid adenomas, parathyroid adenomas, and hyperplastic parathyroid glands. Activity in the normal thyroid tissue significantly decreases with time (Fig. 4-18). Thyroid adenomas and hyperplastic parathyroid glands initially have more intense activity than does the thyroid but also typically fade with time (Fig. 4-19). Most parathyroid adenomas are more intense than is the thyroid on the early images but also retain much of their activity on the delayed images and become more visible. A majority of parathyroid adenomas greater than 500 mg can be detected with parathyroid scanning. Some

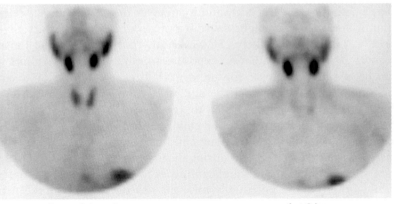

Figure 4-18. Normal parathyroid scan. An immediate technetium-99m sestamibi image of the chest and neck shows activity in the parotids, salivary glands, thyroid, and left ventricle. On the 2-hour image, the thyroid activity has faded almost completely, whereas the other areas remain mostly unchanged. The individual normal parathyroid glands are not seen.

Immediate ant   Ant 2 hr

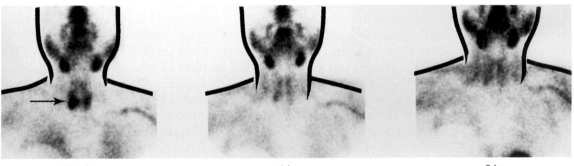

15 min   1 hr   3 hr

Figure 4-19. Thyroid adenoma on early and delayed technetium-99m sestamibi images. The thyroid adenoma (*arrow*) is initially seen as an area of increased activity relative to the thyroid. Both the normal thyroid and the adenoma fade significantly on the delayed images.

thyroid adenomas may not fade as much as expected on delayed images, and some parathyroid adenomas may behave atypically by fading somewhat on delayed images. If delayed sestamibi images are inconclusive in either of these respects, it may be helpful to reinject the patient with ^{99m}Tc pertechnetate to see if the equivocal focus hyperconcentrates pertechnetate, likely representing a thyroid adenoma, or presents as a relative defect, indicative of a parathyroid adenoma. It should be noted that ^{99m}Tc-sestamibi may also concentrate and persist in thyroid cancers producing a false-positive examination. Despite its established success in localizing hyperfunctioning parathyroid adenomas, ^{99m}Tc-sestamibi imaging is still unable to image hyperplastic or normal parathyroid glands consistently. At the present time, SPECT/CT is the standard of practice for these lesions. Parathyroid imaging is especially useful in patients with negative neck explorations and recurrent or persistent hypercalcemia (Fig. 4-20). Because of the possibility of ectopic parathyroid adenomas, a routine large-field

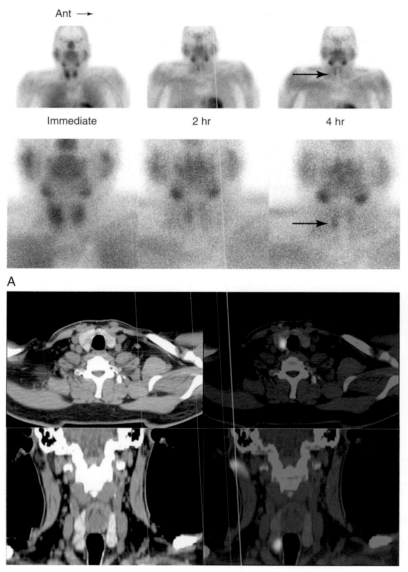

Figure 4-20. Parathyroid adenoma. A, Parathyroid adenoma (located at the inferior aspect of the right lobe of the thyroid) (*arrows*) is present as an area of increased activity relative to the thyroid on the delayed images. **B,** SPECT/CT scan precisely localizes the lesion.

view of the chest and mediastinum should be performed.

Many surgeons will routinely use either ultrasound or radionuclide parathyroid imaging before surgery. However, radionuclide methods also are useful to locate the adenoma during surgery. The technique for intraoperative parathyroid localization involves injection of the patient with ^{99m}Tc-sestamibi about 2 to 4 hours before surgery and use of a small gamma probe during the operation to localize the parathyroid adenoma. This procedure is typically reserved for patients with a solitary parathyroid adenoma and a normal thyroid gland (to exclude confusion caused by activity in a thyroid adenoma). After removal, the parathyroid adenoma should be counted and should be at least 20% and usually 50% higher than the thyroid background.

SALIVARY GLAND IMAGING

As noted in the discussion of thyroid imaging with ^{99m}Tc-pertechnetate, activity is seen in the parotid, submandibular, and sublingual glands.

Although activity in these glands and in the saliva can be a source of confusion when imaging the thyroid, the concentration of pertechnetate in the salivary glands can help in the diagnosis and assessment of some salivary and parotid disorders.

Evaluation of suspected mass lesions of the salivary glands is best done by using computed tomography. Use of ^{99m}Tc-pertechnetate scans is generally reserved for functional evaluation, although most mass lesions, including primary tumors and metastases, are seen as areas of decreased activity. The exception to this is Warthin's tumor, which usually appears as a focal area of increased uptake (Fig. 4-21). Warthin tumors are benign parotid gland lesions, which predominate in elderly men and are frequently bilateral.

Functional assessment is performed by administering 5 to 15 mCi (185 to 550 MBq) of ^{99m}Tc-pertechnetate intravenously and obtaining 1-minute images of the salivary glands over about 20 minutes. Computer-generated regions of interest are placed over the glands

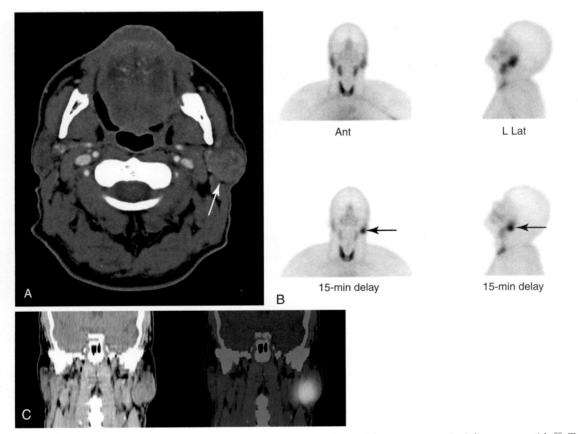

Figure 4-21. Warthin tumor. A, Axial CT scan demonstrates an L parotid mass (*arrow*). **B,** Salivary scan with ^{99m}Tc-pertechnetate shows focal retention in the left parotid gland (*arrow*). **C,** Coronal SPECT/CT scan clearly shows the anatomic relationship.

of interest, and time-activity curves are generated for accumulation and clearance of activity. Trapping in the glands usually begins at 1 minute and reaches a peak in about 5 to 10 minutes. Stimulation of the glands with lemon juice usually results in rapid diminution of activity as saliva and ^{99m}Tc-pertechnetate are secreted. In patients with Sjögren syndrome, there may be decreased accumulation of activity relative to the thyroid, as well as delayed clearance of activity from the glands. These findings may be asymmetric.

PEARLS & PITFALLS

- Common indications for radionuclide thyroid imaging are to differentiate between various types of hyperfunction (Graves disease, toxic multinodular goiter, or autonomous adenoma) and to assess nodularity (cold or hot) and ectopic tissue.

- Salivary glands are usually seen on ^{99m}Tc-pertechnetate scan unless the patient has Graves disease. They are not seen on an ^{123}I scan.

- ^{99m}Tc-pertechnetate is administered intravenously and a scan can be obtained 15 to 30 minutes post injection. Iodine-123 and 131 are administered orally and scans are obtained at 4 to 24 hours.

- A normal 24-hour iodine uptake in most laboratories ranges between 10% and 30% to 35%.

- ^{99m}Tc-pertechnetate is trapped (but not organified) by the thyroid. Iodine-123 and 131 are trapped and then organified.

- Oral administration of supersaturated potassium iodide (SSKI) or perchlorate can effectively block unwanted radioiodine from accumulating in normal thyroid tissue. Blocking efficacy approaches 100% if administered before the radioiodine, but it retains some effectiveness even if administered up to 12 hours later.

- A lingual thyroid is usually located in the midline at the base of the tongue, with no thyroid seen in the normal location. The ectopic gland is often hypofunctional.

- A thyroid gland with an organification defect is usually seen as a normal gland on a ^{99m}Tc-pertechnetate scan but manifests no activity on an iodine scan in a child with a high TSH level.

- A large gland with intense homogeneous activity is usually Graves disease. A pyramidal lobe is commonly associated with Graves disease.

- A large gland with patchy activity is usually a multinodular goiter but could also be chronic thyroiditis or an infiltrative process.

- Most hot nodules are benign hyperfunctioning adenomas. They can be single or multiple and can suppress the normal portions of the gland.

- Chronic thyroiditis can mimic numerous thyroid conditions but on imaging is usually patchy and decreased in activity.

- Subacute thyroiditis classically presents with a markedly depressed radioiodine uptake and nonvisualization of the gland in a patient with thyrotoxicosis and a tender, swollen thyroid.

- Thyroid cancer is usually a single focal cold lesion and only rarely is seen to be diffuse or multifocal on thyroid scans.

- Thyroid cancers may concentrate ^{99m}Tc-sestamibi and persist on delayed images. They are typically "cold" on ^{99m}Tc-pertechnetate scans.

- If there is a rising serum Tg and a negative whole-body iodine scan, thyroid cancer can often be visualized on a 18F-FDG PET scan with 80% to 85% sensitivity, and sometimes on a ^{99m}Tc-sestamibi scan.

- Activity in the bladder, stomach, and bowel and mild diffuse activity in the liver is usually normal on a whole-body iodine scan and is very unlikely to represent metastatic disease.

- Whole-body thyroid scans may be performed with ^{123}I rather than ^{131}I. The ^{123}I scans have better resolution and may cause less stunning.

- Most patients with Graves disease are treated with about 10 to 15 mCi (370 to 555 MBq) of ^{131}I, and most with toxic multinodular goiter are given about 15-29 mCi (555 MBq to 1.1 GBq) of ^{131}I. Cancer treatment doses depend on the

Continued

PEARLS & PITFALLS—cont'd

size and stage of disease, but most patients receive about 100 to 150 mCi (3.7 to 5.5 GBq) of [131]I.

- After successful radioiodine ablation of residual thyroid tissue, serum thyroglobulin (Tg) measurements are a sensitive method to detect recurrent thyroid cancer.

- Recombinant human TSH (rhTSH) is commonly used to enhance I-131 imaging diagnosis of recurrent thyroid cancer It is also approved for enhancing radioiodine uptake in post surgical thyroid remnants prior to I-131 ablation-therapy. FDA approved rTSH for pre ablation stimulation of thyroid remnants in 2007.

- Iodine-131 treatment doses for thyroid cancer have been shown to be effective when using the following schedule:
  - Functioning tissue in the thyroid bed: 75 to 100 Ci (2.75 to 5.55 GBq) of [131]I.
  - Known or suspected cervical node or mediastinal metastases: 100 to 200 mCi (3.7 to 7.4 GBq) of [131]I.
  - Lung or skeletal metastases: 200 or more mCi (7.4 or more GBq) of [131]I.

- Undifferentiated or non radioiodine-avid thyroid cancers can often be imaged using ^{18}F-fluoro-deoxyglucose PET/CT. This includes anaplastic cancers and Hurthle cell variants.

- Medullary thyroid cancers are most effectively imaged using the somatostatin receptor agent ^{111}In-octreotide. ^{18}F-fluorodeoxyglucose PET/CT is less useful in this setting.

- The most common indication for parathyroid imaging is to localize the hyperfunctioning gland (adenoma) either in the thyroid bed or in an ectopic location (lower neck or mediastinum).

- Parathyroid adenomas are usually single.

- Parathyroid imaging is usually performed by using ^{99m}Tc-sestamibi with sequential images over 2 hours. Normal thyroid tissue and thyroid adenomas usually fade over 2 hours, whereas parathyroid adenomas usually hyperconcentrate ^{99m}Tc-sestamibi and persist over time. The most common false positive is related to atypical thyroid adenoma.

- Decreased salivary uptake on a ^{99m}Tc-pertechnetate scan can be caused by the thyroid taking most of the activity (e.g., Graves disease) or by a salivary problem (Sjögren disease). Increased focal activity can occur in salivary tumors, especially Warthin tumors.

SUGGESTED READINGS

Cooper DS, Doherty GM, Haugen BR, et al. Revised American Thyroid Association management guidelines for patients with thyroid nodules and differentiated thyroid cancer. Thyroid 2009;19(11):1167-214.

Eslamy HK, Ziessman HA. Parathyroid scintigraphy in patients with primary hyperparathyroidism: ^{99m}Tc-sestamibi SPECT and SPECT/CT. RadioGraphics 2008;28:1461-76.

Iagaru A, McDougall IR. Treatment of thyrotoxicosis: continuing education. J Nucl Med 2007;48:379-89.

Intenzo CM, Capuzzi DM, Jabbour S, et al. Scintigraphic features of autoimmune thyroiditis. RadioGraphics 2001;21:957-64.

Intenzo CM, dePapp AE, Jabbour S, et al. Scintigraphic manifestations of thyrotoxicosis. RadioGraphics 2003;23:857-69.

International Commission on Radiological Protection. Release of patients after therapy with unsealed radionuclides. Publication 94, Annals of the ICRP 2004;34(2).

Luster M, Clarke SE, Dietlein M, et al. Guidelines for radiotherapy of differentiated thyroid cancer (European Association of Nuclear Medicine). Eur J Nucl Med Mol Imaging 2008;35:1941-59.

Mariani G, Gulec SA, Rubello D, et al. Preoperative localization and radioguided parathyroid surgery. J Nucl Med 2003;44:1443-58.

Siegel JA, Silberstein EB. A closer look at the latest NRC patient release guidance. J Nucl Med 2008;49(7):N17-N20.

Smith JR, Oates ME. Radionuclide imaging of the parathyroid glands: patterns, pearls, and pitfalls. RadioGraphics 2004;24:1101-15.

Society of Nuclear Medicine. Procedure guideline for therapy of thyroid disease with iodine-131 (sodium-iodide). 9/17/2005. http://www.snm.org. Accessed June 26, 2011.

Society of Nuclear Medicine. Procedure guideline for scintigraphy for differentiated papillary and follicular thyroid cancer. 9/5/2006. http://www.snm.org. Accessed June 26, 2011.

5 Cardiovascular System

Clinical nuclear medicine studies play a pivotal role in the noninvasive evaluation of cardiac physiology and function. The widespread use of nuclear cardiovascular examinations permits the sensitive detection and diagnosis of numerous cardiac abnormalities as well as the determination of the functional consequences of disease.

Two general types of radionuclide imaging procedures constitute the primary thrust of cardiovascular nuclear imaging. These are designed to assess:

- Myocardial perfusion and viability
- Regional and global ventricular function

Extensive experience with these procedures in their appropriate clinical settings has proved them to be valuable noninvasive tools for the clinical assessment of cardiac disease with application to a broad spectrum of patients. Notably, gated single-photon emission computed tomography (GSPECT) allows evaluation of coronary perfusion and left ventricular (LV) function in a single study, while PET imaging provides quantitative enhancements to myocardial perfusion and viability assessments at lower patient doses. Further, hybrid imaging with SPECT/CT and PET/CT has permitted image attenuation correction, eliminating many common artifacts and increasing the specificity of results.

ANATOMY AND PHYSIOLOGY

Because the heart functions predominantly as a pump, it is important to examine the physiology and anatomy related to this function. The volume of each chamber may be expressed as *end-diastolic volume* (EDV), which is the volume of the chamber after it is completely filled with blood at the end of diastole. Although the EDVs of the left and right ventricles are different, under normal circumstances, the *stroke volumes* (volume of blood ejected by each ventricle during systole) must be equal and normally range from 80 to 100 mL. *Cardiac output* is the volume of blood pumped by either ventricle over a period of 1 minute. It can be obtained by multiplying stroke volume by heart rate. The *ejection fraction* of a chamber is the measurement commonly used clinically because it takes into account the EDV and the stroke volume. The ejection fraction is the percentage of EDV that is ejected by a ventricle during systole.

During systole, the LV normally shortens at least 20% along its long axis and 40% along the short axis as the various walls of the LV move inward. The apical portion of the LV moves inward the least, and the anterior wall moves the most and is the largest contributor to LV pump function. The septum thickens and moves slightly toward the center of the LV. Assessment of wall motion by nuclear medicine techniques depends largely on viewing ventricular wall segments in tangent. When identified, regional wall motion abnormalities are generally classified as *hypokinetic* (diminished wall motion), *akinetic* (absent wall motion), or *dyskinetic*. Dyskinesia indicates that a particular segment moves paradoxically outward rather than contracting inward during systole. It is associated with prior myocardial injury and usually indicates the presence of a cardiac aneurysm.

In the diastolic phase of the cardiac cycle, the myocardium first relaxes without a change in volume but with an exponential decline in LV pressure. This is referred to as *isovolumic relaxation*. As the ventricular pressure falls below that of the left atrium, the mitral valve opens, and the early, rapid-filling phase is initiated. This is followed by diastasis, the third and final phase of diastole, which begins with the decline of passive filling and ends with the onset of an atrial "kick" that concludes diastole (Fig. 5-1).

The heart muscle is supplied by the right and left coronary arteries. The major branches of the left coronary artery are the left anterior descending (LAD) and circumflex coronary arteries (Fig. 5-2). The LAD branch supplies the interventricular septum anteriorly, primarily through the first septal perforator branch, and the anterolateral wall of the LV, primarily by multiple diagonal branches. The left circumflex branch supplies the left atrium and the posterolateral wall of the LV, primarily through its obtuse marginal branch. The right coronary artery has an acute marginal branch and often terminates as the posterior descending artery. It supplies the right atrium, the right ventricle, the inferior wall of the LV, and a variable portion of the interventricular septum. In 80% of people, the right coronary artery is dominant even though it is usually smaller. Dominance is determined by which main coronary artery, right or left, gives rise to the posterior descending coronary artery, which supplies the inferior wall of the heart.

The normal coronary blood flow is about 0.6 to 0.8 mL/min/g of myocardium. With exercise or

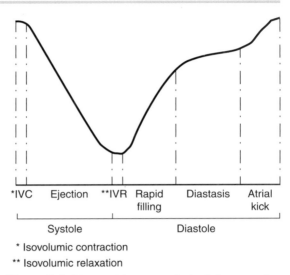

* Isovolumic contraction

** Isovolumic relaxation

Figure 5-1. Time-activity curve obtained from a region of interest placed over the left ventricle. The curve reflects changes in left ventricular volume over one cardiac cycle.

pharmacologic stress, however, both the coronary flow and the cardiac output may increase fourfold to sixfold. Myocardial blood flow is greatest during diastole because, at this time, the blood flows fastest through vessels that are not being constricted by the surrounding cardiac muscle. These flow changes with the cardiac cycle are much more prominent in the left coronary artery than in the right, owing to the larger mass and higher pressure achieved by the LV muscle. When the narrowing of a coronary artery diameter is less than 50% of the diameter of the vessel, the effect on blood flow generally is clinically insignificant. As diameter narrowing approaches 70%, the lesions become much more hemodynamically significant, particularly during exercise. To be significant at rest, 90% or greater narrowing is usually required.

SPECT MYOCARDIAL PERFUSION IMAGING

Imaging of myocardial perfusion with radiopharmaceuticals is the most commonly performed cardiac examination in clinical nuclear medicine practice. Its primary goal is to determine the adequacy of blood flow to the myocardium, especially in conjunction with exercise or pharmacologic stress for the detection and evaluation of coronary artery disease (CAD). Although the basic principles are similar, protocols for imaging vary among the radiopharmaceuticals used. SPECT myocardial perfusion

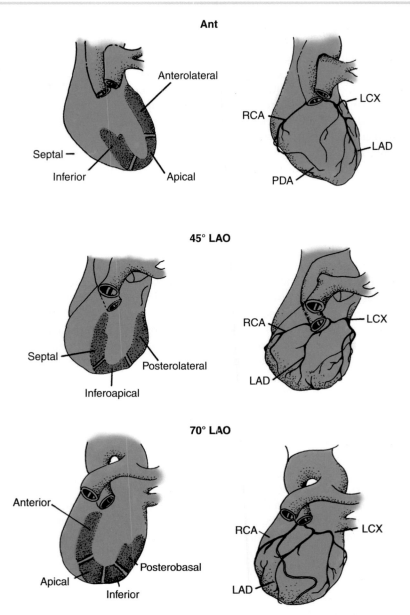

Figure 5-2. Schematic representation of the left ventricular walls and the associated blood supply. *LAD,* Left anterior descending artery; *LAO,* left anterior oblique view; *LCX,* left circumflex artery; *PDA,* posterior descending artery; *RCA,* right coronary artery.

imaging may be performed by using one of several technetium-99m (^{99m}Tc)-labeled agents, thallium-201 (^{201}Tl) chloride, or positron-emitting radiopharmaceuticals. The state of the art for myocardial perfusion imaging is SPECT with electrocardiogram (ECG) gating (GSPECT). This procedure is capable of producing excellent tomographic images of the myocardium reflective of regional perfusion in addition to LV functional parameters, which, taken together, provide enhanced physiologic assessment of the heart. For purposes of discussion, the technical and interpretative aspects of perfusion and functional GSPECT are presented separately.

Principle

The diagnosis of occlusive coronary disease using radionuclide imaging is made by detection of relatively decreased myocardial perfusion distal to the site of vascular obstruction, compared with the more normally perfused surrounding myocardium. The success of imaging depends on a number of factors, especially the degree of stenosis and its hemodynamic significance under conditions of increased myocardial metabolic demand, such as exercise. Because even severe stenosis may not produce detectable blood flow abnormalities at rest, some form of stress, either exercise or pharmacologic stress, is usually needed to render a flow differential that can be seen on myocardial perfusion imaging.

The myocardium is so efficient in extracting oxygen from the blood to meet metabolic demands that there is little room for improvement in extraction as metabolic demands increase during exercise. Thus the heart satisfies increased oxygen requirements primarily by augmenting coronary blood flow, through the rapid dilatation of the vessels in response to oxygen deficit. This ability to increase blood flow from resting baseline to maximal levels is termed *coronary reserve*. In the presence of a fixed coronary stenosis, the ability of the vessel to dilate and thus the coronary reserve are diminished during conditions of stress. Under such circumstances, the myocardium supplied by the stenosed artery becomes apparent as a relative defect on myocardial perfusion images because perfusion to the involved area increases less than in the neighboring, relatively normally perfused tissue. Although stenoses of up to 90% of the arterial diameter may not produce a decrease in blood flow significant enough to be detected at rest (Fig. 5-3), stenoses of 50% or more are reliably detected with myocardial perfusion imaging under conditions

of maximal myocardial stress. By comparing myocardial perfusion at rest (baseline perfusion) to perfusion under conditions of stress (maximal perfusion), areas of reduced coronary reserve indicative of stenoses and resultant stress-induced ischemia can be identified. These principles are the same regardless of the radiopharmaceutical or method of stress used.

Radiopharmaceuticals

Although ^{201}Tl was the first clinically successful myocardial perfusion imaging agent and is still used in many clinical settings, ^{99m}Tc labeled radiopharmaceuticals are now generally preferred. Because there are significant biokinetic differences among these radiopharmaceuticals, protocols for imaging vary, although the basic underlying physiologic principles and rationale for interpretation remain the same. A major determinant of protocol design is whether the administered radiopharmaceutical remains fixed in the myocardium, washes out, or redistributes in the myocardium over time. Because of these differences, the choice of radiopharmaceutical influences almost every aspect of the approach to imaging, including the timing and acquisition of image sequences. Thus an understanding of the in vivo behavior of the radiopharmaceutical or combination of radiopharmaceuticals used to perform myocardial perfusion imaging is critical in determining the examination protocol and to the interpretation of the resulting images.

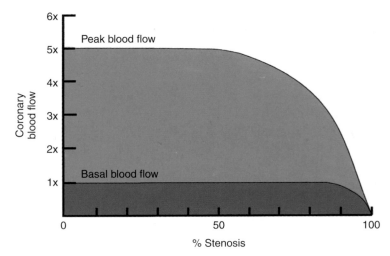

Figure 5-3. Coronary blood flow. Relationship of coronary blood flow at exercise (peak blood flow) and rest (basal blood flow) relative to the percentage diameter of coronary artery stenosis (diameter narrowing).

Thallium-201

Physical Characteristics. Thallium-201 is a cyclotron-produced radionuclide that decays by electron capture, with a half-life of about 73 hours. On decay, the major emissions are characteristic x-rays of the daughter product, mercury-201 (^{201}Hg), with an energy range of 69 to 81 keV. These are the primary photons used in myocardial imaging. Thallium-201 also emits smaller numbers of gamma rays at energies of 135 keV and 167 keV. The relatively long physical half-life of ^{201}Tl is advantageous, providing convenient shelf storage and successful imaging over a period of hours. The long half-life, however, also increases absorbed dose to the patient and limits the amount that can be administered. The relatively low administered activity requires longer imaging acquisition times and results in lower-count densities with inferior contrast resolution compared to ^{99m}Tc-labeled radiopharmaceuticals. Further, soft-tissue absorption of the low-energy emissions of ^{201}Tl increases the likelihood of attenuation artifacts from overlying breasts and diaphragm, producing spurious defects that decrease the specificity of the study.

Biokinetics. Thallium has biokinetic properties similar but not identical to potassium. Like potassium, thallium crosses the cell membrane by active transport mechanisms, especially the adenosine triphosphate (ATP)-dependent Na^+-K^+ pump. After intravenous administration, it ultimately has a mainly intracellular distribution. Thallium localizes in the myocardium in two phases: (1) initial distribution based on blood flow and cellular extraction by viable myocardium, and (2) delayed redistribution in the myocardium mediated by a dynamic equilibrium based on the continued extraction of thallium from the blood and ongoing washout of previously extracted thallium from the cells.

The extraction of thallium from the blood by viable myocardial cells is rapid, approaching 90% extraction efficiency. However, the total amount of thallium ultimately accumulating in the normal heart is limited by the concentration of thallium circulating through the coronary blood supply. Therefore, only about 3% to 5% of the total injected dose is localized in the heart.

Under resting and normal stress conditions, regional myocardial uptake of ^{201}Tl is linearly related to the regional coronary perfusion. Decreased perfusion to an area of myocardium results in a decrease in thallium accumulation in that region, compared with adjacent areas of relatively normal activity. A flow differential between normally perfused and poststenotic ischemic myocardium of about 2:1 is required before a definite defect is noted on thallium imaging.

After the rapid initial uptake of ^{201}Tl by the normal myocardium, there begins a slower process of washout of the thallous ion from the myocardial intracellular compartment back into the vascular compartment. At the same time, however, there is representation of additional bloodborne thallium to the myocardial cells for reextraction provided by the large pool of the injected radioisotope that was initially held by other organs of the body. These simultaneous processes of thallium washout and reextraction across the cell membrane provide a means for a dynamic equilibrium between intracellular and extracellular thallium, which defines the phenomenon known as *redistribution*. The washout component of redistribution depends strongly on coronary perfusion, with ischemic areas demonstrating much slower washout than normal regions.

Because of the more rapid washout of thallium from normally perfused tissue and the slower washout from myocardium that became ischemic at stress, the delayed redistribution images show an ultimate equalization of activity between the normal and ischemic tissue under most circumstances. Thus, on post-exercise thallium images, a defect indicative of relatively decreased perfusion should disappear on later redistribution images if the initial defect was caused by transient reversible stress-induced ischemia. A nonreversible defect carries other implications and frequently indicates an area of scarring.

Technetium-99m Labeled Radiopharmaceuticals

The development of several classes of ^{99m}Tc-labeled radiopharmaceuticals that overcome the technical limitations of ^{201}Tl has led to their widespread use in myocardial perfusion imaging. These include principally isonitriles and diphosphines. Compared with ^{201}Tl, the technetium label confers the favorable characteristics of ready availability; larger administered activity for better statistics, with reduced radiation dose to patients; and advantageous photon energy, producing higher-resolution SPECT images. The larger administered activity leading to higher myocardial count rates allows shorter acquisition times, with resultant decrease in patient motion and improved patient tolerance for the examination. The higher 140-keV photon of ^{99m}Tc also helps minimize attenuation artifacts from the breast or diaphragm. In addition, good statistics and reasonably long retention in the myocardium of ^{99m}Tc-labeled radiopharmaceuticals optimizes GSPECT acquisition for evaluation of LV function and wall motion. Thus, myocardial perfusion and function can be assessed by using a single tracer.

In addition to the technetium label, a major distinction between the most commonly used ^{99m}Tc agents and ^{201}Tl is that, unlike thallium, the technetium agents do not undergo clinically significant redistribution and remain in a fixed myocardial distribution, reflecting regional perfusion at the time of injection. Thus, diagnostic evaluation comparing resting and post-stress imaging requires two separate injections, one at rest and one at peak stress. In addition, whereas thallium localizes in the myocardium by active transport through the cell membrane, these lipophilic technetium agents enter the cells by passive diffusion. Nevertheless, like thallium, their deposition in the myocardium is proportional to regional blood flow, with regions of lower blood flow accumulating less of the radiopharmaceutical and thus presenting as areas of decreased activity (defects) compared with adjacent normal areas of relatively higher flow.

Whichever ^{99m}Tc agent is used, the overall sensitivity for the detection of CAD is comparable to that of thallium imaging, and the specificity may be improved, resulting in part from fewer attenuation artifacts.

Technetium-99m Sestamibi

Technetium-99m sestamibi (Cardiolite) is a lipophilic cationic isonitrile that is extracted by the myocardium with a first-pass efficiency of 60% and with lengthy myocardial retention (myocardial clearance half-time of >6 hours), primarily through binding to cytoplasmic mitochondria. Unlike thallium, there is minimal redistribution (<20%) over time in the myocardium. Advantages to this fixed distribution include the convenience of delaying imaging when necessary, without loss of sensitivity, and the ability to reimage in case of equipment malfunction, positioning error, or patient motion. However, lack of significant redistribution also

means that imaging of myocardial perfusion under stress and rest conditions requires two separate injections of radiopharmaceutical.

After intravenous injection, initial concentration of sestamibi is highest in the heart and liver. Approximately 1% to 2% of the activity localizes in the heart at rest. Accumulation of sestamibi in the myocardium is directly proportional to blood flow at physiologic levels. However, at high flow rates (greater than about two to three times baseline flow), such as those achieved during pharmacologic stress, blood flow may be underestimated. Although there is minimal change in concentration in the heart, there is progressive clearance of liver activity through biliary excretion ($\approx$35%) into the bowel and ultimately into the colon, which receives the highest absorbed dose. There is also some ($\approx$25%) renal excretion (Fig. 5-4). Because adjacent or overlapping liver activity may interfere with cardiac imaging, enhanced clearance of activity from the liver and gallbladder may be accomplished by having the patient drink 8 ounces of milk or eat a fatty meal about 15 minutes after sestamibi injection. However, this may result in an increase in interfering bowel activity, especially when imaging is sufficiently delayed to allow passage of the radiopharmaceutical into the transverse colon and splenic flexure. When sestamibi is administered with the patient at rest, hepatobiliary clearance is slower but usually sufficient to permit imaging about 45 to 90 minutes after injection. Accumulation of sestamibi in the liver and gallbladder is relatively less with maximal exercise than at rest, so post-exercise imaging may generally be obtained 30 to 45 minutes after injection.

Technetium-99m Tetrofosmin

Technetium-99m tetrofosmin (Myoview) is a cationic diphosphine with good myocardial uptake (1% to 2% of the injected dose with a first-pass extraction efficiency of $\approx$50%) and retention with little redistribution from the myocardium over time. Tetrofosmin underestimates myocardial blood flow at high flow rates (about two times baseline flow). There is rapid clearance of background activity from the blood pool. Similar to sestamibi, its cellular localization involves binding to cytoplasmic mitochondria. Its biokinetics are also in many ways similar to those of ^{99m}Tc-sestamibi. Less hepatic uptake and more rapid clearance from

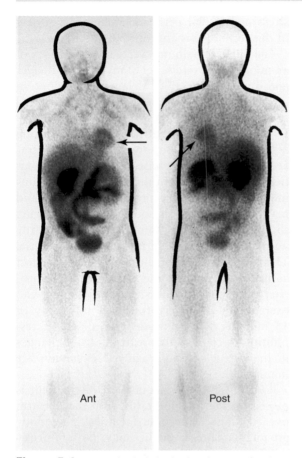

Figure 5-4. Normal whole-body distribution of technetium-99m sestamibi. Post-exercise anterior (*Ant*) and posterior (*Post*) planar images demonstrate left ventricular (*arrow*) and skeletal muscle activity. There is also a large amount of activity in the liver, gallbladder, and bowel, as well as in the kidneys and bladder because of hepatobiliary and renal excretion routes.

the liver after exercise, however, make imaging possible within 30 minutes of intravenous injection and minimizes the likelihood of artifacts associated with overlapping hepatic activity.

New Radiopharmaceuticals

Emerging radiopharmaceuticals labeled with Tc-99m and other radioisotopes suitable for SPECT imaging hold promise of providing more specific information regarding regional and global myocardial perfusion and viability status. This is true of I-123 BMIPP, a labeled fatty acid.

Dedicated Cardiac SPECT Cameras

The widespread use of myocardial perfusion imaging, the notable radiation doses from administered activity needed using decades-old

SPECT technology, and the recognition of opportunities for imaging improvements with cardiac-specific devices has led to the development of innovative cameras dedicated to cardiac imaging. These have the potential to provide increased count sensitivity, allowing dose reduction or increased patient throughput using standard doses, in some cases with improved resolution. Fast imaging also decreases patient discomfort and movement, thus avoiding many motion-related image artifacts. In many cases designs have departed from the traditional orbiting SPECT cameras to introduce arrays of detectors which may be fixed (as in PET cameras) or with limited rotation, with curved sodium iodide detectors or solid state detectors such as cadmium zinc telluride (CZT) and using specialized collimators. Scan times may be reduced from 10 to 15 minutes per acquisition to 2 to 5 minutes. In addition to new hardware, advances in image reconstruction software specific to the properties of camera design, known as resolution recovery algorithms, have allowed reduction in image noise and an improvement in spatial resolution. These programs use iterative reconstruction techniques, instead of traditional filtered back projection, to correct for the factors in SPECT imaging which inherently degrade image quality, especially in settings of shorter imaging times and reduced counting statistics. While more complex and time-consuming, iterative back projection may allow for production of transaxial images of equal or superior quality to those of traditional SPECT imaging.

Imaging Protocols

SPECT, with or without gated acquisition, is the standard for myocardial perfusion imaging with both ^{201}Tl- and ^{99m}Tc-labeled radiopharmaceuticals. As expected, SPECT imaging acquisition and processing protocols differ significantly depending on the radiopharmaceutical used. However, regardless of the specifications, SPECT imaging is a technically demanding procedure. Strict compliance with SPECT quality-control measures and familiarity with study protocols established in each laboratory are essential for the standardization of the procedure and for achieving consistently accurate results. Some technical sources of error are listed in Box 5-1.

Box 5-1 Stress Myocardial Perfusion Scintigraphy

Sources of False-Positive Examinations

True Defects
Coronary anomaly
Coronary spasm (variant angina)
Noncoronary disease
  Mitral valve prosthesis
  Cardiomyopathies
  Aortic stenosis
  Myocardial bridge
  Idiopathic hypertrophic subaortic stenosis
  Conduction defects
  Left bundle-branch block (LBBB)
  Long-distance runners
  Ischemia of noncoronary origin

Apparent Defects
Artifacts
  Chest wall artifacts
  Breast tissue or pectoral muscles
  Breast prosthesis
  Electrocardiogram leads
  Braces
  Items in pockets, pendants, etc.
  Obesity
  High left hemidiaphragm
  Excess patient motion (deep respiration)
  Misinterpretation of normal variants
  Overappreciation or underappreciation of
    apical defects
  Variant activity at cardiac base, proximal
    septal area, and posterolateral walls
  Papillary muscle attachments
  Small ventricular cavity

Sources of False-Negative Examinations
Early or delayed redistribution
Submaximal exercise
Noncritical stenoses (<50%)
Small ischemic area
Isolated right coronary lesion
Coronary collaterals
Multivessel disease (balanced)
Overestimation of stenosis on angiogram
Interfering medication

Exercise Thallium SPECT Imaging Protocol

Exercise is the most common form of stress for most patients undergoing myocardial perfusion imaging.

Because ^{201}Tl is the prototypical exercise myocardial perfusion radiopharmaceutical and because the protocol elucidates the principles of stress myocardial perfusion imaging, a review of this technique is appropriate.

The SPECT thallium exercise test consists of an initial post-exercise set of myocardial images and an identical set of delayed redistribution images. An outline of the procedure is presented in Figure 5-5.

Initial Post-Exercise Imaging. When using ^{201}Tl, 2 mCi (74 MBq) are administered intravenously at peak exercise. Because redistribution of thallium within the myocardium begins immediately at the termination of exercise and may be very rapid in some patients, imaging should commence as soon as possible, ideally within the first 10 to 15 minutes after exercise. This helps ensure that the initial images reflect as nearly as possible the distribution of coronary perfusion at peak stress. In patients who exercise especially vigorously, a full delay of 15 minutes may be prudent to allow for respiration to calm so that artifacts from changes in the extent of diaphragmatic excursion are minimized.

For SPECT image acquisition, the patient is placed on the imaging table with the left arm over the head. In some facilities, potentially attenuating breast tissue may be uniformly compressed over the chest or elevated to minimize potential attenuation artifacts. Specific SPECT acquisition protocols vary among laboratories and depend largely on available instrumentation and the preferences of the imaging physician. When using a single-detector SPECT camera, a rotational arc of 180 degrees is commonly used, frequently beginning at the 45-degree right anterior oblique (RAO) position and ending at the 45-degree left posterior oblique (LPO) position. When using a 64 × 64 computer matrix, 64 images are obtained over the 180-degree arc for a total study recording time of about 30 minutes. Although high-sensitivity or high-resolution collimators may be used, a low-energy, all-purpose collimator provides an adequate compromise between sensitivity and image resolution.

If available, multidetector cameras are preferable for SPECT acquisitions because they allow increased counts over the same imaging time or, alternatively, the same number of counts over a shorter acquisition than do single detector systems. Because the position of the patient during cardiac SPECT imaging is somewhat uncomfortable, and patient motion during image

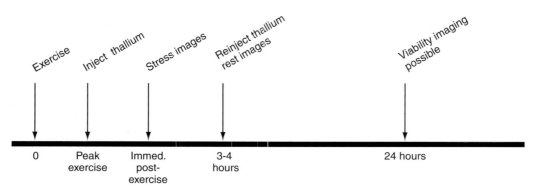

Figure 5-5. Schematic representation of thallium stress–redistribution (rest) imaging protocol.

acquisition may severely compromise image quality, preference may be given to shortening acquisition times. Specific protocols vary with respect to the number of detectors used. After the completion of post-exercise imaging and before the redistribution imaging, the patient is instructed to eat sparingly and to avoid strenuous exercise, even climbing stairs. In some laboratories, if the stress images are normal, the study is terminated; in others, a redistribution study is done routinely.

Redistribution SPECT Imaging. Redistribution images are obtained 3 to 4 hours after the initial set and reflect the status of myocardial perfusion at rest. Ideally, these are performed on the same instrument that was used to perform post-exercise imaging. Care is taken to reproduce the positioning of the patient so that it is as similar as possible to that used during post-exercise imaging, especially with regard to breast and arm location. To ensure that adequate ambient thallium is available for redistribution, the administration of an additional dose of 1 mCi (37 MBq) of thallium before the second set of images (ranging from 1 hour before to immediately before reimaging) is helpful. In some laboratories, 24-hour repeat imaging may be performed in patients who exhibit nonreversible defects on the 4-hour redistribution images to determine with greater certainty any degree of reversibility of the post-exercise defects.

Exercise Technetium-99m Radiopharmaceutical SPECT Imaging Protocol

The requirement of separate stress and rest injections of ^{99m}Tc sestamibi or ^{99m}Tc tetrofosmin to differentiate fixed from reversible defects

has given rise to several different imaging protocols. These may be summarized as 1- and 2-day protocols (Fig. 5-6). The simplest approach is to perform the stress and rest examinations on two separate days. This allows the use of a full imaging dose of 15 to 30 mCi (555 MBq to 1.11 GBq) for each study and avoids interference in the subsequent study by residual myocardial activity from the first. When the stress study is performed first, the rest study may be omitted if the stress images are entirely normal. This stress-only imaging strategy has the added benefit of decreasing patient dose.

For reasons of patient convenience and timeliness of results, however, a 1-day protocol is the most frequently used. In this setting, either the stress or the rest study may be performed first, although the rest–stress sequence is the more widely used. Because of the long retention of sestamibi/tetrofosmin in the myocardium, it is necessary to adjust the administered doses so that activity from the first study does not interfere with the second. In the rest–stress, same-day protocol, 8 to 10 mCi (296 to 370 MBq) of ^{99m}Tc-sestamibi/tetrofosmin is administered at rest, with imaging performed about 30 to 60 minutes after injection, followed 1 to 4 hours later by stress imaging by using 25 to 30 mCi (925 MBq to 1.11 GBq), for a total administered dose of about 30 to 40 mCi (1.11 to 1.48 GBq). The patient should be encouraged to void frequently to decrease absorbed dose to the bladder and adjacent pelvic structures.

Because hepatobiliary or other splanchnic activity may be a larger problem than with thallium imaging, any interfering activity should be taken into account when evaluating the myocardial images, especially the inferior wall. In addition, because GSPECT is often performed with

^{99m}Tc sestamibi or tetrofosmin, the myocardial perfusion findings must be correlated with the LV wall motion and functional information obtained.

Dual Isotope Imaging: ^{201}Tl–^{99m}Tc Sestamibi/Tetrofosmin Protocol

Dual-isotope, 1-day, rest–stress imaging using separate ^{201}Tl and ^{99m}Tc sestamibi/tetrofosmin SPECT acquisitions is an efficient alternative to single isotope protocols. In this protocol (Fig. 5-7), a rest ^{201}Tl (2.5 to 4.0 mCi [92.5 to 148 MBq]) study is first obtained, followed shortly by a stress ^{99m}Tc sestamibi or tetrofosmin study (25 to 30 mCi [925 MBq to 1.11 GBq]), so that the entire examination can be completed within 90 minutes. The rest study is performed first with the lower-energy ^{201}Tl (68 to 80 keV) to prevent interference from the higher-energy ^{99m}Tc (140 keV). Because attenuation defects are generally more prominent on thallium imaging than with technetium agents, stress imaging is subsequently performed with ^{99m}Tc sestamibi or tetrofosmin to minimize false-positive

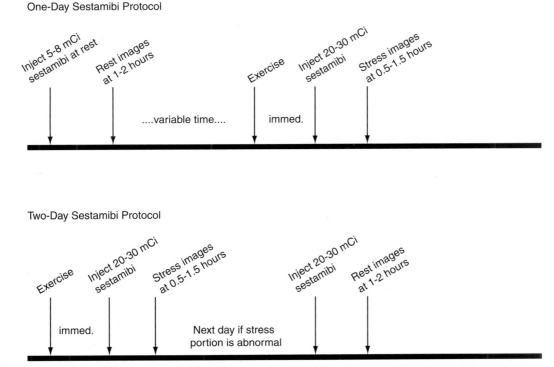

Figure 5-6. Schematic representation of 1- and 2-day technetium-99m (^{99m}Tc) sestamibi myocardial exercise protocols. The protocol using ^{99m}Tc-tetrofosmin is similar, except that rest images may be obtained as early as 30 minutes after injection of the radiopharmaceutical.

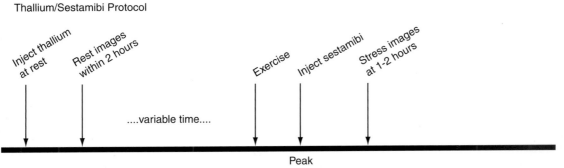

Figure 5-7. Schematic representation of 1-day thallium-201-technetium-99m (^{99m}Tc) sestamibi exercise imaging protocol. A similar protocol may be used followed ^{99m}Tc tetrofosmin.

examinations caused by such artifacts. Further, post-stress GSPECT using ^{99m}Tc radiopharmaceuticals may increase the specificity of any perfusion defects. Extra care should be taken in processing the two different sets of images because different parameters need to be used to optimize the image quality of each data set.

Patient Absorbed Dose Considerations

While justification for myocardial perfusion imaging in an individual patient may be present, imaging physicians should be aware that these studies impose a relatively high radiation dose. Collectively, these studies have typically accounted for approximately one quarter of cumulative effective population dose from medical sources. Given the rapid growth in myocardial perfusion scan volume in the last 20 years, estimates suggest that they contribute about 10% of the entire cumulative effective dose to the U.S. population from all sources, excluding radiotherapy.

Patient doses from myocardial perfusion imaging may be lowered by selection of the protocol used. The relative patient effective doses for the commonly used protocols are given in Table 5-1. Dual-isotope, rest-stress imaging, using Tl-201 and Tc-99m sestamibi may increase patient throughput, but they are associated with notably greater radiation doses than other protocols. Protocols using only Tc-99m radiopharmaceuticals characteristically cut doses to half that of dual-isotope imaging. Further, protocols limited to stress-only acquisitions, such as foregoing the rest study if the stress images are normal, offer a significant dose reduction as may lowering the administered doses used in standard rest-stress protocols. In the future, PET myocardial perfusion imaging and SPECT studies using recent innovations in camera and image reconstruction technologies may offer even lower dose alternatives.

Strategies for reducing patient doses from myocardial perfusion imaging include:

- Use Tc-99m radiopharmaceuticals.
- Use lower administered dose protocols, especially in smaller patients.
- Use stress-only protocols in patients with normal post-stress images.
- For SPECT-CT and PET-CT, use lower x-ray tube current protocols.
- Hydrate patients and encourage frequent bladder emptying.
- Consider advanced, dedicated cardiac camera and reconstruction technologies.

TABLE 5-1 Myocardial Perfusion Imaging: Patient Dose* by Protocol

RADIOPHARMACEUTICAL	PROTOCOL	DOSE IN MCI (MBQ)		EFFECTIVE DOSE $(E_1)^†$ (MSV)
		Rest	Stress	
Tc-99m sestamibi	Rest-stress	10 (370)	27.5 (1018)	11.3
	Stress only	0	27.5 (1018)	7.9
	2-day	25 (925)	25 (925)	15.7
Tc-99m tetrofosmin	Rest-stress	10 (370)	27.5 (1018)	9.3
	Stress only	0	27.5 (1018)	6.6
	2-day	25 (925)	25 (925)	12.8
Tl-201	Stress-redistribution	0	3.5 (130)	22.0
	Stress-reinjection	1.5 (55.5)	3.0 (111)	31.4
Tl-201/Tc-99m sestamibi	Rest-stress	3.5 (130)	25 (925)	29.2
Rb-82 PET		50 (1850)	50 (1850)	13.5
N-13 ammonia PET		15 (555)	15 (555)	2.4
F-18 FDG PET		10 (370)	0	7.0

*Published values of effective dose vary somewhat and the main purpose for use of effective doses is to roughly compare the radiation from various examinations.

†Using ICRP Publication 60 weighting factors. Adapted from Einstein AJ, Moser KW, Thompson RC, et al: Radiation dose to patients from cardiac diagnostic imaging. Circulation 2007;116(11):1290-1305.

Myocardial SPECT Image Processing and Display
Image Processing

After acquisition, the post-stress and rest (redistribution) images are reformatted in oblique planes. For structures with an oblique axis of symmetry in the body, such as the heart, the standard reconstructed cross-sectional views referencing the body are inadequate. Thus image reconstruction of cardiac tomograms is performed in three planes that are perpendicular or parallel with the long-axis of the heart and oblique to the axis of the body; these include (1) short-axis (SA), (2) vertical long-axis (VLA), and (3) horizontal long-axis (HLA) images (Figs. 5-8 to 5-10). Generally, the primary operator input required for reconstruction is the identification of the long axis of the heart. This allows the computer to reconstruct tomographic images in three orthogonal planes relative to the orientation of the heart in the chest. Typically, the reconstructed slices are 1 to 2 pixels in thickness when a 64 × 64 matrix is used.

The quality of SPECT images is greatly enhanced by computer processing and display. The most frequent maneuvers applied to the raw data are background subtraction, contrast enhancement, and image filtering. These processes are meant to make the images more pleasing to the eye and to improve contrast by removing distracting, unwanted activity, and statistical noise. A wide choice of image filters is available for image manipulation, commonly including Butterworth, Hamming, and Hanning filters. The specific filtering processes used vary greatly among laboratories and depend on the preferences of individual interpreters. Care must be taken not to overprocess images such that the data are distorted and artifacts are induced (Fig. 5-11).

SPECT Image Display

After processing is completed, the myocardial slices must be displayed in a fashion that facilitates comparison of the stress and redistribution/rest image sets. It is attendant on the interpreter to ensure that corresponding slices between the two sets of images are displayed so that an accurate comparison is made. The orientation of the images obtained in each reconstruction plane is standardized to the generally accepted convention (Fig. 5-12). This is usually automatically performed by using the user software supplied by the equipment manufacturer. Generally, only tomographic sections that represent slices through both the myocardium and the cavity of the heart are used to avoid partial-volume artifacts. Subsequent interpretation is best performed by manipulation of the image intensity and contrast on the computer screen or the viewing station of a picture archiving system.

Bull's Eye (Polar Map) Display

In addition to the conventional display of tomographic slices, the entire three-dimensional perfusion distribution of a set of exercise or rest images may be condensed into one two-dimensional

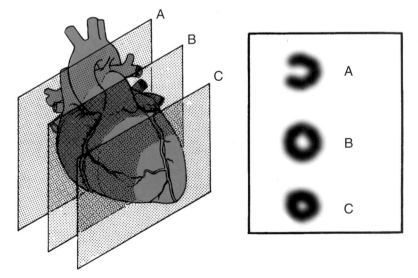

Figure 5-8. Short-axis anatomy and images. Short-axis sections through the left ventricle from the base of the heart to the apex are shown with corresponding single-photon emission computed tomography (SPECT) slices of the myocardium. Note the considerable thinning of the proximal septal wall in plane *A* (the base of the heart) as a result of the membranous septum.

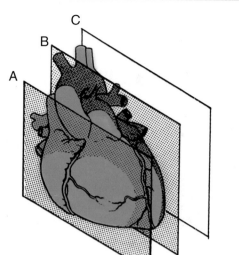

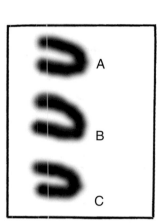

Figure 5-9. Vertical long-axis anatomy and images. Vertical long-axis sections through the left ventricle from septum to free (lateral) wall are shown with corresponding single-photon emission computed tomography (SPECT) slices of the myocardium.

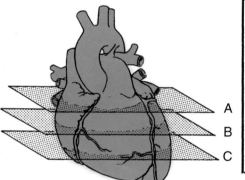

Figure 5-10. Horizontal long-axis anatomy and images. Horizontal long-axis sections through the left ventricle from the anterior to the inferior wall are shown with corresponding single-photon emission computed tomography (SPECT) slices of the myocardium.

0.3 Cutoff

0.45 Cutoff

1.0 Cutoff

4.0 Cutoff

Figure 5-11. Effect of the cutoff value of a filter applied to a single short-axis image of the left ventricle. Sharpness of the image is improved with an increasing cutoff value, but artifactual defects may be created. The image becomes fuzzy with a low cut-off value, which may mask true defects. Obviously, the choice of filter may have great effect on the quality of the images and, if not properly chosen, can produce false-positive or false-negative interpretation.

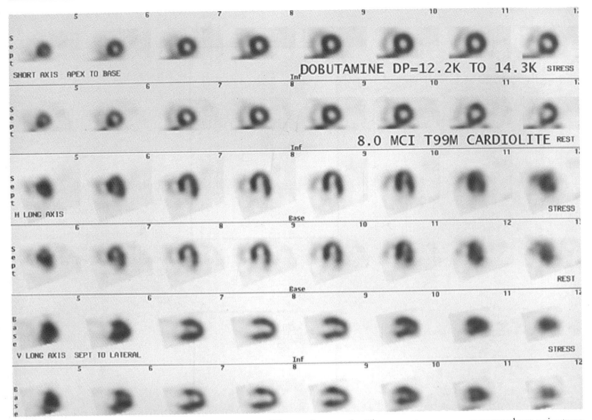

Figure 5-12. Normal SPECT technetium-99m sestamibi stress/rest study. The upper two rows represent short-axis stress and short-axis rest images. These "slices" progress from the apex on the left to the base of the heart on the right. The next two rows show horizontal long-axis stress and rest images, from the inferior to the anterior left ventricular wall. The lower two rows are the vertical long-axis stress and rest images, from the septum on the left to the lateral wall on the right.

display by using a so-called polar or bull's eye map (Fig. 5-13). This display may be thought of as the heart viewed from its apex and opened up like an umbrella. Semiquantitative methods are applied to this bull's eye display of the SPECT perfusion data that compare the radiopharmaceutical distribution for each patient to a gender-matched normal database of distribution. Thus regional activity less than that expected in a normal population identifies a perfusion deficit and is displayed as such on the polar map. The actual visual appearance of this deficit based on its severity is determined by the gray or color scale used. When using this display, however, the interpreter should be aware that perfusion defects at the base of the heart (outer circumference of the polar map) tend to be overemphasized, whereas centrally located defects, such as the LV apex, tend to be underrepresented. The bull's eye representations of stress and rest (redistribution) myocardial perfusion can easily be visually compared in a third

bull's eye display that shows the differences in activity. This defines the reversibility or fixed nature of a perfusion defect. These bull's eye plots are a convenient tool to be used as an adjunct to standard visual image interpretation and to summarize a patient's perfusion pattern in a single image.

Interpretation
Approach to Interpretation

Image interpretation principles are virtually the same as for qualitative interpretation of thallium and Tc-99m labeled agents, with a few exceptions. Consistent interpretation of SPECT myocardial perfusion images is best ensured by a systematic approach that includes the following elements:

- Proper alignment (co registration) of the post-stress and rest tomographic slices
- Perusal of the images for obvious motion and attenuation artifacts, with review of sinogram or rotating cine images as needed

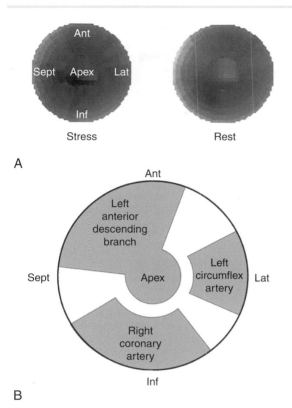

A

B

Figure 5-13. Normal polar (bull's eye) display of myocardial perfusion. **A,** Both the stress and rest images demonstrate relatively uniform activity without significant deviation from perfusion in age-matched controls. **B,** Approximate coronary artery distribution relative to the polar plot. The unshaded regions are areas of variable arterial supply. *Ant,* Anterior; *Inf,* inferior; *Lat,* lateral; *Sept,* septum.

■ Evaluation of the LV myocardium for the presence of perfusion defects and classification regarding size, severity, location, and degree reversibility, if any
■ Estimation of LV cavity size and any transient enlargement
■ Assessment of lung activity on thallium scans
■ Assessment of right ventricular activity
■ Assessment of interfering adjacent splanchnic (liver, spleen, or bowel) activity
■ Correlation with stress ECG findings and adequacy of stress
■ Correlation of findings with ancillary patient information, including history and clinical findings, prior coronary angiography or revascularization procedures, and previous myocardial perfusion studies
■ On GSPECT studies: evaluation of LV ejection fraction (LVEF) and correlation of LV wall motion with any perfusion abnormalities noted on the tomographic slices

Alignment of Images

An initial task of the interpreter is to assess the two series of processed images consisting of reconstructed stress and rest (redistribution) slices to ensure that they are properly aligned. Such coregistration of the slices in all three planes is essential for accurate comparison of perfusion in corresponding regions of the myocardium. Misalignment of the image sets may lead to a false impression of the fixed or reversible nature of areas of relative hypoperfusion and significantly reduce the accuracy of the examination.

Artifacts

Because tomographic images are composed of highly processed data, the interpreter should ascertain that the acquisition and resulting processed images are artifact free. If an artifact is suspected, careful examination of the raw data in a rotating cine display of the sequential planar projections aids in detecting gross patient motion, areas of significant soft-tissue attenuation, and any superimposed liver or spleen activity. Other means for detecting patient motion, such as a sinogram (an abrupt break in the otherwise continuous sinogram stripe signifies patient motion), or a summed display of all the projections, may be generated and viewed as needed. A thorough knowledge of SPECT imaging artifacts is critical in SPECT image interpretation (Table 5-2).

Attenuation Artifacts. Significant soft-tissue attenuation by large breasts or breast implants may produce spurious fixed anterior or lateral wall defects (Fig. 5-14), and considerable accumulation of adipose tissue in the lateral chest wall in obese patients may give rise to fixed lateral wall myocardial defects if the patient is imaged identically in the post-exercise and subsequent rest (redistribution) studies. Changes in positioning of the patient or of the patient's breasts in the rest (redistribution) images that make the attenuation defect less apparent than on the post-exercise images, however, may give rise to apparent reversible abnormalities.

Patients with left hemidiaphragmatic elevation may have spurious inferior wall defects because of focal attenuation. In addition to attenuation, intense liver, spleen, or bowel activity overlying the inferior wall of the LV may mask areas of decreased perfusion or may paradoxically produce an inferior wall defect (Fig. 5-15).

TABLE 5-2	SPECT Myocardial Perfusion Imaging: Common Artifacts		
ARTIFACT	**CAUSE**	**APPEARANCE**	**PREVENTION/ RESOLUTION**
Scaling artifact	Suppression of normal activity respresentation as a result of scaling image to a very hot pixel	Apparent defects in myocardium–often adjacent to or between papillary muscles–best seen on short-axis views	Defects are not substantiated other planes. Rescale images.
Breast attenuation	Photon attenuation by overlying breast tissue	Fixed or sometimes reversible defects (if breast overlies on the myocardium only on the post-stress view); usually anterior, anterolateral, or anteroseptal walls.	Review rotating raw images to confirm offending breast tissue. Review gated SPECT cine to determine whether a fixed defect shows wall motion and thus is not a scar. Use Attenuation Correction Program.
Diaphragmatic attenuation	Photon attenuation by overlying diaphragm	Fixed inferior wall defect	Review rotating raw images to confirm attenuation by diaphragm. Review gated SPECT cine to determine whether the fixed defect shows wall motion and thus is not a scar. Use Attenuation Correction Program.
Chest wall attenuation (obesity)	Photon attenuation by fat in chest wall	Fixed lateral wall defect	Review rotating raw images to confirm offending chest wall fat. Review gated SPECT cine to determine whether the fixed defect shows wall motion and thus is not a scar.
Left bundle branch block	Altered septal perfusion proportional to elevated heart rate	Reversible septal or anteroseptal defect	Use pharmacologic stress instead of treadmill exercise stress. Review ECG prior to study.
Wall thinning: apex, base of inferior wall or septum	Anatomic variants	Fixed defects in areas of thinning	Review gated SPECT cine to determine whether the fixed defect shows wall motion and is thus not a scar.
Reconstruction/ramp filtration artifact	Focus of increased abdominal activity adjacent to inferior LV wall	Inferior wall defect in post-stress and/or rest image; usually reversible, but may be fixed	Reimage patient after clearance of activity away from inferior wall.
Abdominal activity (liver, gallbladder, spleen, bowel, including reflux into stomach)	Activity in the liver or refluxed into the stomach which overlaps the inferior wall	Can mask an inferior wall defect and make a fixed defect appear reversible if overlap present only on resting images.	Perform prone imaging (which may produce an anterior wall defect), or reimage patient after activity is cleared away from inferior wall.
Upward creep of the heart	Increased post-stress lung volumes diminishing during imaging	Reversible inferior or inferolateral wall defect	Delay post-stress imaging until normal respiration is restored (15-20 min). Reimage patients suspected of upward creep artifact.
Patient motion artifact	Patient movement during imaging: vertical, horizontal, or rotational	Vertical: anterior and/ or inferior defects; others variable Image blurring with "tails" of activity extending from myocardial walls	Review rotating raw planar images or static sonogram to confirm motion. Use motion correction algorithm to realign planar images.

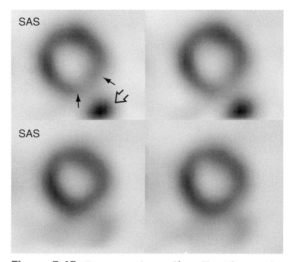

Figure 5-15. Reconstruction artifact. *Top,* Consecutive short-axis post-stress images from a technetium-99m tetrofosmin myocardial perfusion study demonstrate a focal defect in the inferolateral wall of the left ventricle (*short arrows*) adjacent to a focus of intensely increased bowel activity (*open arrow*). *Bottom,* Repeat images after the bowel activity has passed from the area show the defect to have resolved. Such artifactual myocardial defects adjacent to areas of nearby extracardiac increased activity are a result of filtered back-projection using ramp filtration. *SAS,* Short-axis stress.

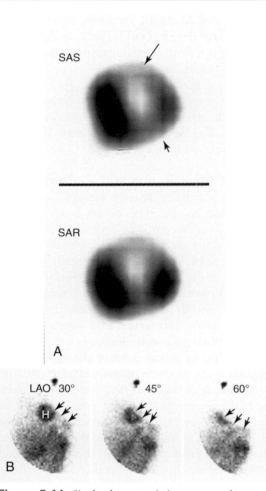

Figure 5-14. Single-photon emission computed tomography (SPECT) breast attenuation artifact. A, Both the short-axis stress (*SAS*) and short-axis rest (*SAR*) myocardial perfusion images demonstrate an anterior wall (*large arrow*) defect attributable to breast attenuation. The apparent defect is fixed because the breast position is similar on both the stress and rest images. There is a true defect in the inferior wall (*small arrow*). **B,** Soft-tissue attenuation of breast tissue can easily be appreciated on three-dimensional rotating views of the thorax. Here, selected planar image frames from the SPECT acquisition at different angles show the overlying breast tissue (*arrows*) having progressively more attenuation of the myocardial (*H*) activity as the SPECT camera rotates around the patient during acquisition. *LAO,* Left anterior oblique view.

This latter artifact is thought to be related to an inherent effect of filtered back projection on myocardial segments immediately adjacent to such areas of intense activity.

In addition to indirect approaches, such as review of the raw data as a rotating display of frames in a cine loop format, regional wall motion data available with GSPECT often allow differentiation of true fixed defects, substantiated by locally diminished wall motion, from attenuation artifacts with regionally preserved wall motion.

Attenuation Correction Issues. Direct attenuation correction methods can greatly improve the specificity of SPECT imaging by eliminating or minimizing soft-tissue attenuation artifacts (Fig. 5-16). Although becoming more available, these technologies are not widely used. With SPECT/CT hybrid scanners, however, this maneuver has become routine.

Interpretation of attenuation corrected myocardial perfusion images requires an appreciation of the potential differences between the corrected and uncorrected images. Attenuation-corrected images often have mildly decreased activity in the distal anterior wall and apex, similar to that seen with PET myocardial perfusion studies. This is more prominent the larger the heart. Thus the finding is more prominent in men because of anatomically larger hearts, compared to women. In addition, it should be noted that causes of image artifacts commonly seen in uncorrected SPECT, such as patient motion, respiration differences, and extracardiac activity, as well as misregistration, are amplified by the attenuation correction process. It is not uncommon for artifactual defects to

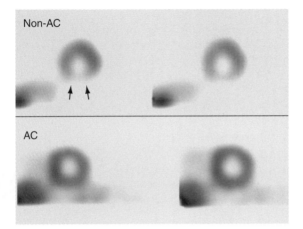

Figure 5-16. Attenuation correction. *Top,* Consecutive nonattenuation-corrected, short-axis, post-stress myocardial perfusion images show an inferior wall defect (*short arrows*). Review of the rotating display of SPECT image frames suggested diaphragmatic attenuation. *Bottom,* Repeat imaging using an attenuation correction program corrects for the diaphragmatic attenuation and the defect is no longer seen. *AC,* Attenuation-corrected; *Non-AC,* nonattenuation-corrected.

occur in the anterior and lateral LV walls when the SPECT emission and transmission (attenuation map) images are misregistered. Additionally, apparent myocardial defects may occur when the transmission and emission images are performed sequentially rather than simultaneously with patient movement between the two image sets. Thus it is advised that both corrected and uncorrected images be displayed for comparison during interpretation.

Motion Artifacts. Patient motion is a significant cause of artifactual myocardial defects, and the appearance of the scan artifact depends on the direction and degree of motion and whether it is abrupt or gradual. Motion-correction software may be used in many instances to salvage studies in which motion is not extreme. In patients who exercise vigorously, exaggerated diaphragmatic respiratory motion that persists after exercise and subsequently returns to normal may induce an artifact that mimics inferior wall ischemia if the patient is imaged during this interval. This is produced as the diaphragm and thus the heart subsequently "creep" upward during image acquisition. To avoid this *cardiac creep artifact,* a delay in acquisition of immediate post-exercise images for about 15 minutes to allow for hyperventilation to subside and the depth of respiration to return to normal is recommended.

Technical Artifacts. Artifacts during image reconstruction may occur if the long axis of the LV is incorrectly selected during processing. This generally results in overestimation or underestimation of activity at the apex. As expected, breaches in quality control of the imaging system, such as center of rotation malalignment and flood-field nonuniformity, may also produce significant image artifacts.

Normal Appearance and Variants

After myocardial perfusion images have been determined to be free of obvious artifacts or after any recognized artifacts have been accounted for and/or corrected, visual interpretation of SPECT images may proceed.

In the normal myocardial perfusion study, there is often slightly diminished activity at the LV apex, and in areas of anatomic thinning at the base of the intraventricular septum (membranous portion) and in the base of the inferior wall. Thinning at the base of the septum and inferior walls may be distinguished from true perfusion defects in that they are limited to the base of the heart and do not extend distally to the apex. These anatomic variants should not be mistaken for fixed perfusion defects. Defects that extend from the base to the apex should be considered abnormal. Furthermore, the lateral myocardium normally demonstrates more activity than do other myocardial territories, especially when compared with the septum in the short-axis slices. This likely results from the lateral wall being closest to the camera during much of the usable acquisition.

Areas of focally increased activity in and at the insertions of the papillary muscles frequently can be seen, especially on the short-axis images at about the 2-o'clock and 7-o'clock positions. These hot spots may give a false impression of a defect adjacent to or between them, owing to relative differential in activity, when in actuality the intervening activity is normal. The apparently diminished perfusion is often accentuated by the scaling of relative intensities in the displayed images based on the most intense pixel in the images (the markedly increased activity in the papillary muscles). This may artifactually suppress activity in the normal but relatively less intense regions. These apparent differences in relative activity must be interpreted with caution. Generally, review of these areas in the long-axis slices, in which the papillary muscles are not as well seen, will demonstrate a homogeneous normal distribution in these regions, confirming a *scaling artifact* rather than a real perfusion deficit. However, significant perfusion defects which are also evident on the long-axis slices and are not attributable to artifact may be viewed as a positive finding.

Abnormal Scans
Visual Analysis.

Myocardial Activity. Two distinct patterns of abnormal radiopharmaceutical distribution in the myocardium provide the basis for the detection and differential diagnosis of stress-induced ischemia and permanent myocardial damage. These patterns are referred to as (1) *reversible (transient) defects* and (2) *nonreversible (fixed) defects.* Defects may also be partially fixed with a reversible component. A third pattern, called *reverse perfusion defects,* is well documented, but its significance is less well defined.

True defects usually are visible on at least two of the three standard sets of reconstructed slices. In addition to the short-axis views, defects are often best seen on the long-axis image set in which the axis of the slices is perpendicular to the involved wall (i.e., the anterior or inferior wall on VLA images and the septum or posterolateral wall on HLA images).

Reversible (Transient) Defects. A reversible defect is virtually synonymous with stress-induced ischemia in patients with CAD. The abnormality is identified on the initial post-stress images as an area of relatively decreased radiopharmaceutical activity that disappears or becomes significantly less apparent on the rest or redistribution views (Fig. 5-17).

Nonreversible (Fixed) Defects. Fixed defects demonstrate no significant change in activity between the post-stress and rest or redistribution studies (Fig. 5-18). They most frequently indicate areas of scarring or fibrosis, usually after myocardial infarction, or areas of chronically ischemic, "hibernating" myocardium. Some fixed lesions identified on the initial post-stress images may be partially reversible. Ischemia associated with a previous myocardial infarction with scarring (peri-infarct or "flanking" ischemia) commonly presents in this manner.

This straightforward approach to exercise–rest scan interpretation is complicated by the recognition that nonreversible, fixed defects may actually represent primarily viable myocardium rather than postinfarction scarring. In patients with severe coronary stenoses, these defects frequently represent chronically ischemic, but viable, "hibernating" myocardium that remains poorly perfused at rest with loss of functional wall motion. Fixed defects in viable myocardium may also be caused by "repetitive stunning," a chronic process of repeated, but transient episodes of ischemia in regions with or without normal resting perfusion that also leads to prolonged regional contractile dysfunction. There is some evidence that these conditions may be related and coexist in the same patient, and if recognized, both may be reversed by revascularization intervention with restoration of regional contractile function.

To differentiate hibernating myocardium from scar in patients with fixed myocardial perfusion defects, PET imaging with fluorine-18 deoxyglucose (^{18}F-FDG) is the procedure of choice (described later in the chapter). However, thallium imaging also offers an effective method to confirm myocardial viability in this setting because thallium uptake in myocardial cells serves as an indicator of preserved cell membrane function. Thallium uptake in a fixed perfusion defect with accompanying myocardial dysfunction predicts improvement of function after revascularization. If a stress–redistribution thallium imaging protocol was initially used, providing additional thallium, additional time for redistribution, or both is required. Reinjection of patients with additional thallium (1 mCi [37 MBq]) before 4-hour redistribution imaging and/or further delayed 18- to 24-hour imaging are common approaches.

If the initial study was performed by using a technetium labeled agent, a thallium rest–redistribution protocol may be used on a separate day (to allow for radioactive decay). In this protocol, the patient is injected with thallium at rest and imaged immediately and again after a variable delay of 4 to 24 hours to image the chronically ischemic myocardium.

Reverse Perfusion Defect (Reverse Redistribution). In some instances, a scan appears normal or with only a slight defect on the post-stress views and shows a new or worsened defect on the rest or redistribution images (Fig. 5-19). The exact mechanisms that produce this pattern and its significance are uncertain. In many instances, the effect is simply related to

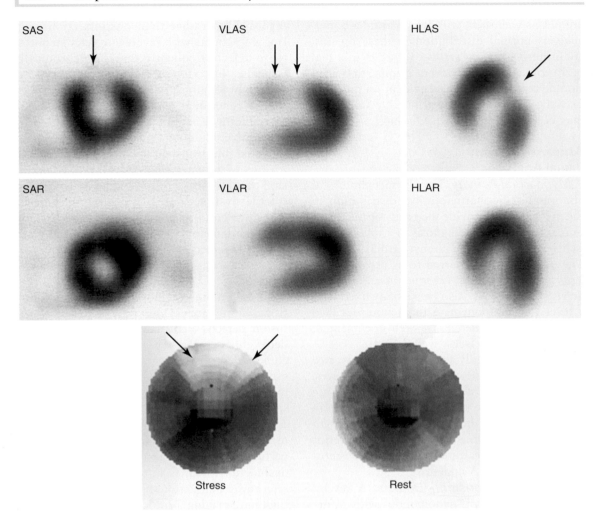

Figure 5-17. Anterior wall ischemia (reversible myocardial perfusion defect). SPECT images (*upper row*) in short-axis stress (*SAS*), vertical long-axis stress (*VLAS*), and horizontal long-axis stress (*HLAS*) stress images clearly demonstrate a perfusion defect (*arrows*). The rest images are seen on the *middle row,* and the perfusion defect has disappeared on the rest (redistribution) views. Bull's eye images (*lower row*) confirm the perfusion defect at stress (*arrows*) but not at rest. *HLAR,* Horizontal long-axis rest; *SAR,* short-axis rest; *VLAR,* vertical long-axis rest.

a worse attenuation artifact on the post-stress images than on the rest images. However, reverse redistribution has been associated with prior myocardial infarction, especially after revascularization or thrombolytic therapy. This is likely to be the result of some residual tissue viability and some postulate that the regional hyperemic response to exercise may mask resting hypoperfusion in these areas. The finding does not indicate stress-induced ischemia.

Description of Myocardial Perfusion Abnormalities. Once identified, myocardial perfusion defects should be described with reference to (1) the defect size (large, medium, or small), (2) severity of perfusion deficit (severe, moderate, or mild), (3) location (including the involved wall and expected coronary artery distribution, if possible), and (4) degree of reversibility, if any. Generally, with respect to defect size, small describes a defect that is less than 10% of the LV myocardium, medium represents 10% to 20%, and large greater than 20%. Regarding defect severity, mild may describe a defect that exhibits a decrease in counts compared to those in the adjacent wall without apparent thinning of the LV wall thickness; moderate, a decrease in counts with relative wall thinning; and severe, a decrease in counts approaching image background.

Lung Activity. The presence of excessive ^{201}Tl in the lungs should be noted as part of the routine interpretation of post-exercise and

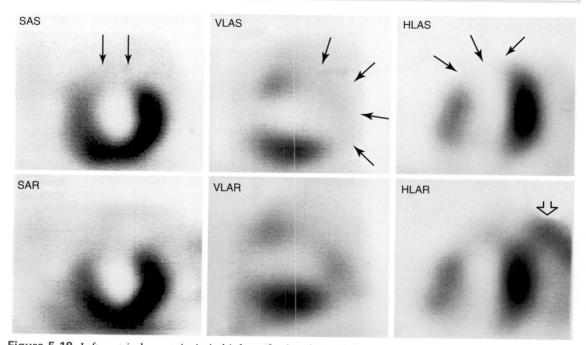

Figure 5-18. Left ventricular anterior/apical infarct (fixed perfusion defect). The *upper row* shows decreased perfusion (*arrows*) to the left ventricular anterior wall and apex on short-axis stress (*SAS*), vertical long-axis stress (*VLAS*), and horizontal long-axis stress (*HLAS*) technetium-99m sestamibi SPECT images. The *lower row* shows that the anterior/apical defect persists on rest images in all three projections. Of note is activity (*open arrow*) on the horizontal long-axis rest (*HLAR*) image owing to sestamibi in the colon after hepatic excretion. *SAR*, Short-axis rest; *VLAR*, vertical long-axis rest.

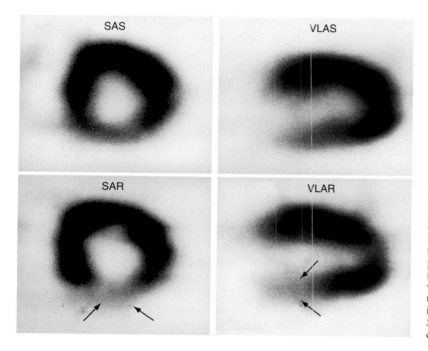

Figure 5-19. Reverse redistribution (reverse perfusion defect). The *upper row* shows SPECT myocardial perfusion stress images both in short-axis stress (*SAS*) and vertical long-axis stress (*VLAS*) projections that demonstrate slightly reduced perfusion of the inferior wall. However, rest (redistribution) images show that the defect is much more obvious (*arrows*). *SAR*, Short-axis rest; *VLAR*, vertical long-axis rest.

redistribution myocardial images. This activity may be visually assessed or quantified by calculating a ratio of lung-to-heart activity. This is performed by using counts from regions of interest created over the LV myocardium and the left mid lung field just above the heart. An anterior planar projection from a SPECT acquisition or a separately obtained anterior planar view of the thorax may be used. Abnormally increased lung activity (lung-to-heart ratio greater than 50%)

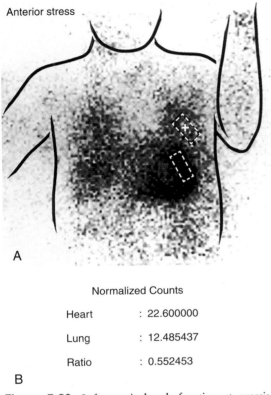

Anterior stress

A

Normalized Counts

Heart : 22.600000

Lung : 12.485437

Ratio : 0.552453

B

Figure 5-20. Left ventricular dysfunction at exercise. A, Anterior view of the chest demonstrates abnormally increased thallium-201 activity in the lungs. **B,** Calculation of lung-to-heart ratio using the regions of interest shown confirms an abnormally high lung-to-heart ratio of 55% during a ^{201}Tl exercise stress examination.

on post-exercise images has been consistently shown to be a marker of transient LV dysfunction at exercise (Fig. 5-20).

In the presence of CAD, the mechanism appears to be related to transient interstitial pulmonary edema caused by a rise in LV end-diastolic pressure secondary to stress-induced myocardial ischemia. Thallium leaking into the pulmonary interstitium appears as increased lung activity on the immediate post-exercise images. Abnormally increased thallium uptake in the lungs correlates anatomically with multivessel CAD or high-risk disease involving either a high-grade proximal LAD artery stenosis or a dominant left circumflex lesion. It correlates clinically with increased morbidity and mortality rates.

Because of differences in pharmacokinetics, increased lung activity is not generally seen under similar circumstances when ^{99m}Tc myocardial perfusion agents, such as sestamibi or tetrofosmin, are used.

Transient Ischemic Dilatation. Apparent transient LV cavity dilatation is present when the diameter of the LV cavity is visibly larger on post-stress images (either with exercise or with pharmacologic stress) than on images obtained at rest. This should be distinguished from fixed cavity dilatation, which is present to an equal degree on both sets of images and indicates preexisting cavity enlargement. The primary underlying mechanism for transient ischemic dilatation (TID) is transient stress-induced diffuse subendocardial ischemia producing an apparent cavity dilatation (Fig. 5-21) and not true cavity dilatation. In the presence of CAD, TID correlates with high-risk disease (left main or multivessel involvement) and a worse prognosis. However, in some cases, microvascular disease, such as in diabetes, or LV hypertrophy may be associated with TID in the absence of epicardial coronary disease.

Right Ventricular Activity. Right ventricular activity is a common normal finding on immediate post-stress images and is usually significantly less apparent on rest or redistribution views. Because of the greater administered activity and improved resolution on studies performed by using ^{99m}Tc radiopharmaceuticals, right ventricular activity may normally be more apparent compared with that on ^{201}Tl images. When the right ventricular myocardium is evident, any transient right ventricular defects should raise suspicion of right CAD. Significant right ventricular activity persisting on rest or redistribution imaging that approaches the intensity of the LV myocardium is abnormal and is often caused by either right ventricular wall hypertrophy (Fig. 5-22) or increased workload ("strain") of the right ventricle in response to increased pulmonary vascular resistance and pulmonary hypertension. An increase in LV cavity size may rarely indicate right heart volume overload, such as seen in atrial septal defects or tricuspid valve regurgitation.

Splanchnic Activity. Because splanchnic activity (liver and bowel) on post-exercise studies generally decreases with increasing success of stress, the amount of such activity is a rough estimate of the adequacy of exercise. A large amount of activity suggests submaximal exercise, whereas minimal or absent activity suggests that significant exercise was achieved. Good myocardial activity-to-background activity ratios are also usually seen in patients with

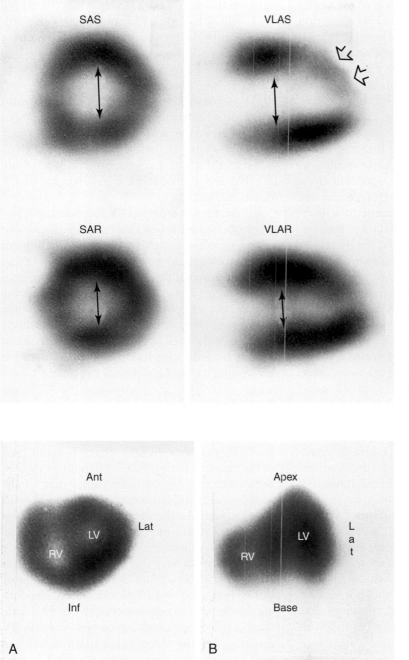

Figure 5-21. Left ventricular transient dilatation (TID) with exercise. Short-axis stress (*SAS*) and vertical long-axis stress (*VLAS*) images (*upper row*) show a much larger left ventricular cavity than seen at rest (*lower row*). This is a high-risk finding in this patient with coronary artery disease. Note the large reversible defect in the anterior wall consistent with stress-induced ischemia (*open arrows*). *SAR,* Short-axis rest; *VLAR,* vertical long-axis rest.

Figure 5-22. Right ventricular hypertrophy. On these SPECT myocardial perfusion rest images presented in **A,** short-axis and **B,** horizontal long-axis views, the right ventricle (*RV*) myocardial activity is markedly increased so that it is equal to that of the left ventricle (*LV*). *Ant,* Anterior; *Inf,* inferior; *Lat,* lateral.

adequate exercise. With any myocardial perfusion radiopharmaceutical, a perusal of liver and bowel activity aids in identifying interfering activity that may affect image interpretation. Because the commonly used technetium-labeled radiopharmaceuticals are excreted into bowel by the liver through the biliary system, problematic intense activity may be seen in the liver, biliary tract, stomach (with bile reflux),

transverse colon and splenic flexure, and occasionally the small bowel.

Quantitative Analysis. Visual interpretation of SPECT myocardial perfusion images is subject to considerable interobserver variability and depends markedly on the quality of the visual display. As an adjunct to visual assessment, computer quantitative analysis of myocardial perfusion images, primarily with the goal of exhibiting the relative distribution of the radio-pharmaceutical in the myocardium as a function of space or time, may be used. These techniques permit a more objective and reproducible assessment of any change in activity within a given segment of myocardium between the post-stress and rest images. This can be helpful in the documentation and quantitation of areas of scarring or ischemia, especially for comparison with future studies obtained to assess the progression of disease or success of medical or revascularization therapy. Protocols for quantitative analysis of images, as well as the display of the derived information, vary from department to department and with different manufacturer processing software. In general, however, the principles underlying such programs are the same. Quantified data may include assessment of defect size, severity, and reversibility. One frequently used semiquantitative approach uses a 17 myocardial-segment perfusion scoring system based on dividing three short-axis slices (distal, mid, and basal) selected to represent the entire LV into small regions, plus an additional apical segment.

As previously discussed, bull's eye or polar maps are frequently used to display the processed data and to compare the perfusion data from a particular patient with a pooled database of gender-matched normal controls. A difference of more than 2.5 standard deviations below the mean is usually considered abnormal.

SPECT with Gated Acquisition (GSPECT)

GSPECT is the state of the art for myocardial perfusion imaging and is the most common mode of data acquisition and display in clinical practice. It combines all of the information contained in myocardial perfusion tomography discussed previously in addition to relevant regional and global LV functional data. Nongated myocardial SPECT imaging is performed without respect to the cardiac cycle so that the images obtained represent data averaged during image acquisition by ventricular wall excursions of the beating heart. By synchronizing the collection of SPECT imaging data with the patient's ECG, the degrading effect of ventricular wall motion can be eliminated or reduced. In addition, cinematic display of the myocardial images is possible over the entire cardiac cycle, allowing the evaluation of wall motion and correlation with any evident perfusion

abnormalities. LV parameters easily measured by GSPECT include LVEF and LV absolute volumes (end-systolic and end-diastolic). Because the RV myocardium is not adequately seen on the perfusion images, GSPECT is not used to evaluate RV function. Although GSPECT with ^{201}TI is possible by using multidetector cameras, non redistributing ^{99m}Tc-labeled myocardial perfusion agents are preferred because of higher count statistics, better imaging characteristics for the gamma camera, and more reliable and reproducible measurement of LV functional parameters.

Recent data comparing LV functional parameters obtained by GSPECT using a variety of common software programs showed significant differences in LV volumes and LVEF which varied in magnitude between the software programs used. These findings may highlight the importance of using the same programs when performing sequential studies and certainly emphasize the need of each laboratory to obtain and be familiar with its own normal values for LV volumetric and functional parameters.

Technique

The technique of gating to the cardiac ECG cycle is similar to that used during gated blood pool ventriculography (described in detail later in the chapter) but produces a dynamic image of the contracting myocardium rather than of the blood pool chamber. Definition of the LV walls uses automated computer software for detection of the epicardial and endocardial edges of the myocardium. Once the endocardial margins are detected, this defines the LV cavity throughout the cardiac cycle so that changes in LV volume can be measured and LVEF calculated. Depending on the time of acquisition, the GSPECT cine images reflect either resting or post-exercise LV function. Because of the higher administered and thus higher myocardial activity, GSPECT is most frequently obtained during the post-exercise acquisition because the better imaging statistics permit more reliable definition of the LV wall. However, either or both the rest or post-stress studies may be acquired in gated mode.

A typical post-stress GSPECT acquisition requires 20 to 30 minutes. The study is usually acquired as 8 to 16 frames per cardiac cycle and is displayed in endless-loop cine format for visual analysis. Although 16-frame acquisition provides better temporal resolution, the increased number of frames requires a longer acquisition time. It should be noted that an 8-frame acquisition results in about a 5% lower calculated ejection fraction than that obtained with a 16-frame acquisition. Software accomplishing automated reformatting of the SPECT slices into a three-dimensional cine representation is usually rapid, accurate, and reproducible. However, precise determination of the LV walls may be hampered by the presence of adjacent areas of significantly increased activity, usually splanchnic in origin, which are mistaken by the edge detection algorithm for myocardium (Fig. 5-23). Large, severe perfusion defects, sizable LV aneurysms, or marked distortion of the LV for any reason may also create uncertainty for myocardial edge detection algorithms. These may lead to inaccurate results, especially when calculating LVEF and LV volumes. However, more focused operator input into the processing may overcome these problems in some instances.

Accuracy of the technique is also limited in patients with small hearts (often producing falsely high LVEF), such as some women and pediatric patients. Enlargement or zooming of the images may be helpful in these instances. In addition, post-stress LVEF determinations (the most common GSPECT LVEF measurement)

may be reduced from actual resting LVEF by the presence of stress-induced ischemia and accompanying wall motion abnormalities persisting into the post-stress acquisition period and temporarily impairing LV function. This problem does not occur with ejection fractions obtained from a true resting gated acquisition. Thus, in reporting a GSPECT LVEF, it is important to specify whether it was obtained after stress or at rest.

As with all ECG-gated studies, severe arrhythmias (atrial fibrillation, heart block, frequent ectopic beats) may preclude successful gating so that nongated myocardial perfusion imaging is more appropriate. However, for less significant variations in cardiac rhythm, application of one of several software methods for rejection of aberrant beats allows valid data to be collected. This is usually accomplished by comparing the R-R interval of each beat during imaging to the average R-R interval of cardiac cycles (calculated prior to image acquisition) and excluding those cycles that vary by more than ±10% from the patient's mean. Although arrhythmia filtering increases imaging times, it is necessary because the inclusion of "bad beats" in the data set can invalidate results for both wall motion and calculated parameters such as LVEF.

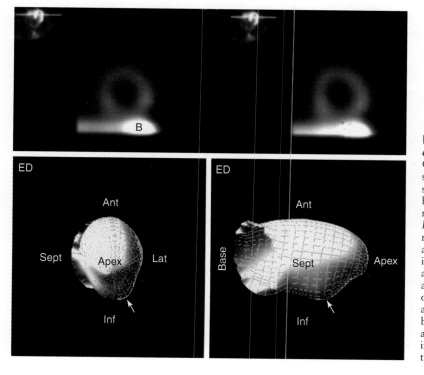

Figure 5-23. GSPECT edge detection uncertainty artifact. *Top,* Consecutive images from a ^{99m}Tc-sestamibi myocardial perfusion study show significantly intense bowel activity (*B*) near the inferior wall of the left ventricle (LV). *Bottom,* The three-dimensional representation of the LV shows a bulge deformity (*arrow*) of the inferior contour of the LV with an accompanying wall motion abnormality. This bulge is a result of the myocardial edge detection algorithm confusing the adjacent bowel activity for myocardial activity, which was mistakenly incorporated into the contour of the LV. *ED,* End diastolic.

Data Display and Interpretation

As expected, the routine display of coregistered sets of post-stress and rest slices of the myocardium identical to that produced by nongated studies of myocardial perfusion are produced. In addition, a closed cine loop of cardiac wall motion can be displayed as both individual contracting slices as well as a three-dimensional representation of the entire LV viewed from multiple directions, such that all LV walls can be scrutinized (Fig. 5-24). This allows correlation of segmental myocardial perfusion defects noted on the static slices with the presence or absence of wall motion abnormalities in the same region (Fig. 5-25). This permits more specific and accurate interpretation of suspected perfusion abnormalities.

Wall motion is visually assessed globally and regionally by the degree of endocardial excursion and by regional myocardial wall thickening during contraction. Wall motion abnormalities are categorized in the conventional manner as hypokinetic, akinetic, or dyskinetic. Because camera resolution and partial volume effect limit accurate measurement of actual wall thickness, wall thickening is inferred from local increases in count intensity or "brightening" during systole. Localized brightening has been shown to be proportional to regional wall thickening. To augment visual assessment, software programs supplying automated quantitative indices of regional wall motion and wall thickening are also available.

In addition to perfusion and wall motion, automated, user-friendly computer programs supply values for LVEF, LV volumes, and other ventricular parameters, which add further significance to the results. As with all computer quantitation programs, the specific definitions of normal limits and criteria for abnormalities of the program used are essential for the accurate interpretation of the processed data.

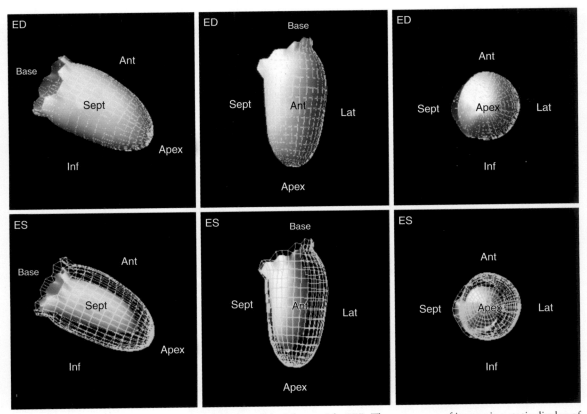

Figure 5-24. Normal GSPECT 3-D representation of the left ventricle (LV). The upper row of images is a static display of the LV in three of the projections of the LV normally reviewed in endless loop cine format to assess LV wall motion. These images are "frozen" at end-diastole (ED). The second row displays the same projections at end-systole (ES). The green mesh defines the endocardial surface at end-diastole as a reference to assess wall excursion during systole (between the two sets of images). In this case normal wall motion is implied and was also observed when these 3-D images were viewed in cine format.

GSPECT Clinical Applications

The information provided by GSPECT regarding LV wall motion and LV function adds powerful adjunctive data to myocardial perfusion imaging in several well-defined settings. These are further discussed as relevant in the "Clinical Application" section of "Myocardial Perfusion Imaging." However, in summary, GSPECT is especially helpful in the following clinical situations:

- Identification of suspected attenuation artifacts
- Enhanced detection of multivessel CAD
- Risk assessment of patients with known or suspected CAD
- Assessment of myocardial viability
- Follow-up of patients undergoing revascularization procedures to assess any LV wall motion improvement
- Distinguishing ischemic from nonischemic cardiomyopathy

Exercise Stress Protocol

In most patients, exercise is the most suitable method for stressing patients undergoing myocardial perfusion imaging. The basic exercise protocol used is the same regardless of the radiopharmaceutical used.

Patient Preparation

Patients should remain NPO for 4 to 6 hours before the exercise test. This allows for a decrease in splanchnic blood flow and, therefore, a reduction in uptake in the bowel and liver. Calcium-channel blockers and β-blockers should be discontinued, if possible, for a sufficient length of time before the examination to avoid any interference with obtaining an adequate stress examination by limiting heart rate response. Long-acting nitrates should also be withheld on the day of testing. It is also advisable to avoid caffeinated beverages for 24 hours or more before the examination, so that if necessary, the exercise stress can be converted to vasodilator pharmacologic stress using dipyridamole or adenosine/regadenoson without interference.

Exercise Protocol

The most common mode of stress used in myocardial perfusion imaging is a multistage treadmill exercise test based on a Bruce or modified Bruce protocol. Basically, this involves a consistent measured increase in the speed and grade (upward elevation) of the treadmill to provide gradually increasing levels of stress.

Once exercise has begun, timing is critical. Regardless of the radiopharmaceutical used, it should be injected at peak stress, through a previously established intravenous line or heparin lock. Ideally, the patient continues to exercise for about 30 seconds to 1 minute after the injection to allow sufficient time for the radiopharmaceutical to localize in the myocardium under

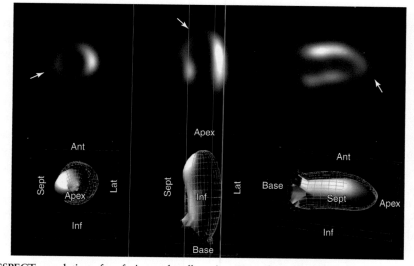

Figure 5-25. GSPECT correlation of perfusion and wall motion. *Top,* Short, horizontal long-axis and vertical long-axis post-stress images from a GSPECT myocardial perfusion scan show a prominent perfusion defect (*arrows*) at the left ventricular apex extending into the inferior and septal walls. The defect persisted on rest images. The differential diagnosis includes a postinfarct scar and hibernating myocardium. *Bottom,* Three-dimensional representation (*lower* row) of the left ventricle at end-systole shows diminished wall motion at the apex and septum with a focal area of dyskinesia in the distal septum consistent with a scar with aneurysm formation.

conditions of peak exercise. The determination of peak stress varies with the institution, but it is generally considered to be maximal when chest pain or significant ECG changes appear, when the patient's heart rate reaches 85% of predicted maximum heart rate (roughly equivalent to 220 beats/minute minus the patient's age in years), or when the heart rate-blood pressure product (maximum heart rate achieved multiplied by the maximum systolic blood pressure reached) exceeds a value of 25,000. If none of these conditions is met, the stress is generally deemed submaximal.

Maximal stress provides for optimal myocardial-to-background ratios for imaging as well as for the most sensitive evaluation of myocardial perfusion. The most common cause of a false-negative examination and reduced test sensitivity is failure of the patient to achieve maximal stress. Still, a submaximal exercise myocardial perfusion study is more sensitive than is stress ECG alone for the detection of CAD. In patients who have recently sustained acute myocardial infarction, an intentionally submaximal exercise test may be performed for predischarge evaluation of residual stress-induced ischemia (myocardium still at risk).

Alternatives to Exercise: Pharmacologic Stress

In patients who cannot perform or tolerate adequate exercise, whose heart rate response may be limited by β-blockers or calcium-channel blockers, who have a pacemaker rhythm, or in whom the presence of left bundle-branch block (LBBB) may produce spurious, reversible exercise-induced septal perfusion defects, pharmacologic stress allows a successful myocardial perfusion study to be performed. Test sensitivity and specificity are comparable to that of maximal exercise studies, in the range of 85% to 90%, and image interpretation criteria are essentially the same.

Commonly used intravenous agents are (1) the non nitrate vasodilators, dipyridamole (Persantine), adenosine, and regadenoson (Lexiscan) and (2) the inotropic drug, dobutamine. Although pharmacologic stress may be safely performed in most patients, it is a good idea to use the technique only in patients who would otherwise be candidates for an exercise study. Pharmacologic stress should be used advisedly in patients with unstable angina,

acute myocardial infarction (within 72 hours), hypotension, or refractive congestive heart failure, and is usually best avoided altogether. Because dipyridamole, adenosine, and regadenoson may exacerbate or induce severe bronchospasm, they should not be used in patients with asthma or reactive airway disease. In addition, adenosine and regadenoson should not be used in patients with second- or third-degree heart block or sinus node disease.

Dipyridamole Stress Imaging

Dipyridamole is an adenosine deaminase inhibitor that allows the accumulation of endogenous adenosine, a potent vasodilator, in the myocardium by preventing adenosine degradation. This produces selective vasodilatation of normal coronary arteries, predominantly in the small, resistance vessels of the coronary bed. At the commonly used dosages, intravenous dipyridamole increases coronary blood flow by three to five times resting levels, compared with a onefold to threefold increase with exercise.

Unlike normal coronary arteries, diseased stenosed vessels demonstrate no further dilatation because they are already maximally dilated secondary to autoregulatory mechanisms triggered by myocardial hypoperfusion. Therefore, although there is proportionally increased flow to the myocardium supplied by normal vessels, blood flow in the distribution of abnormal vessels is not increased as much, depending on the degree of stenosis. Thus, when dipyridamole is used in conjunction with myocardial perfusion imaging, there is radionuclide mapping of this discrepancy in perfusion, which results in a relative defect in the hypoperfused myocardium. For purposes of imaging, this accomplishes the effect of exercise on the coronary arteries with one important exception: there is minimal effect on cardiac work or myocardial oxygen demand, thus providing an additional margin of safety in patients with significant coronary stenosis.

Patient Preparation. Because they reverse the cardiovascular effects of dipyridamole, xanthine-containing medications, including theophylline (aminophylline), should be withheld for 48 hours, if tolerated by the patient, and caffeine-containing beverages should be withheld for 12 to 24 hours before the study. Stopping or altering any preexisting oral dipyridamole therapy is generally not necessary.

Dipyridamole Protocol. Dipyridamole may be administered orally or intravenously, although the intravenous route is preferred because of its more predictable blood levels. Intravenous infusion through a large (antecubital) arm vein is performed over 4 minutes at a concentration of about 0.5 mg per kg in 20 to 40 mL of normal saline (an infusion rate of 0.14 mg/kg/min), with a total dose of 0.56 mg/kg. ECG, heart rate, and blood pressure should be monitored throughout the study. Patients may be supine, standing, or sitting, and low levels of exercise, including walking or isometric hand grip, may be used adjunctively if desired. The myocardial perfusion imaging agent is administered intravenously 3 to 4 minutes after the dipyridamole infusion is completed (7 to 8 minutes into the study, when maximal coronary dilatation occurs). Imaging is started at a time appropriate to the radiopharmaceutical used.

As with many interventional pharmaceuticals, significant undesirable side effects may occur in about 50% of patients. Dipyridamole may cause chest discomfort, headaches, dizziness, flushing, and nausea. These side effects may be rapidly reduced by the intravenous administration of aminophylline (100 to 200 mg). This antidote should be readily available during the procedure. Because the plasma half-life of dipyridamole (30 to 40 minutes) is longer than that of aminophylline, careful patient monitoring even after aminophylline administration is prudent.

Image Interpretation. Myocardial uptake of ^{201}Tl or ^{99m}Tc sestamibi is greater with dipyridamole than with exercise stress. When thallium is used for dipyridamole imaging, the pattern of liver, spleen, and splanchnic activity is the reverse of that noted with maximal-exercise thallium imaging; that is, increased activity in these regions is seen on initial images, but activity decreases on the delayed views.

The cardiac findings are interpreted identically to exercise examinations, with comparable sensitivity and specificity. As expected, however, important physiologic information such as ECG response, exercise capacity, and heart rate and blood pressure product obtained during conventional exercise stress is not available. Because normal thallium lung activity is slightly higher with dipyridamole or adenosine stress than with maximal exercise, the threshold for abnormal accumulation is somewhat higher.

A lung-to-heart ratio of greater than 60% to 65% is generally considered abnormal and correlates with the presence of multivessel CAD.

Adenosine Stress Imaging

Because dipyridamole achieves coronary dilatation indirectly through the accumulation of adenosine in the coronary bed, an alternative method is the direct intravenous infusion of adenosine. The pharmacologic effect of adenosine is much more rapid than that of dipyridamole, but the degree of coronary dilatation is comparable, producing about three to five times baseline blood flow.

Patient Preparation. Contraindication to adenosine use and patient preparation are similar to those of dipyridamole. Caffeine should be avoided for 12 to 24 hours. Because dipyridamole potentiates the effects, and thus the side effects, of both endogenous and administered adenosine, its use should be withheld for 12 to 24 hours before adenosine infusion.

Adenosine Protocol. The usual dose is 0.14 mg/kg/min for 6 minutes, but doses may be titrated downward for unstable patients. The myocardial perfusion radiopharmaceutical is injected about halfway into the adenosine infusion (at 3 minutes), when maximal vasodilatation and myocardial hyperemia occur. No complementary exercise is usually used.

Side effects with adenosine are more common than those with dipyridamole and occur in 75% of patients. The three most common side effects are flushing, shortness of breath, and chest pain. These are usually transient and require no action or treatment. An uncommon but more serious side effect is atrioventricular block, which usually occurs in the first few minutes of infusion and is also transient. First-and second-degree block are more common. Because the biologic half-life of adenosine is extremely short (<10 seconds), its effects may be reversed by simply stopping infusion and beginning any specific treatments, if necessary.

Regadenoson Stress Imaging

As an alternative to adenosine stress, the selective A_{2A} receptor agonist, regadenoson, may be used for vasodilator cardiac stress. Side effects are similar to adenosine (flushing, headache, and dyspnea and chest discomfort) but may be less severe or less frequent. If persistent or severe, they may be reversed using IV aminophylline.

Regadenoson is administered as a rapid bolus of a fixed patient dose of 400 μg with the radiopharmaceutical injection immediately following. It provides results comparable to adenosine for detecting reversible, stress-induced myocardial defects.

Patient Preparation. As with adenosine stress, patients should avoid methylxanthines, including caffeine (coffee, tea, chocolate, and theophylline) for 1 to 2 days before administration, and therapeutic dipyridamole should be held 2 days in advance. Regadenoson can depress SA and AV nodal function, potentially leading to AV block or sinus bradycardia requiring intervention. It may also induce generalized arterial vasodilation and hypotension. Patients with hypotension, decompensated airway disease, or heart block should forego regadenoson stress.

Regadenoson Protocol. Instead of a dose by weight as with other pharmacologic stress agents, a fixed dose of 0.4 mg of regadenoson is given to all patients regardless of weight over 10 seconds by hand-administered IV push. The imaging radiopharmaceutical can be administered after 30 seconds. This reduces a 6-minute adenosine stress administration procedure to approximately 1 minute.

Dobutamine Stress Imaging

The mechanism of action of dobutamine pharmacologic stress is different from the direct coronary vasodilatation produced by dipyridamole or adenosine. Dobutamine is a β_1-agonist that acts in a manner similar to exercise by increasing myocardial oxygen demand through increases in both heart rate and myocardial contractility and, at higher doses, through increases in systolic blood pressure. In response, normal coronary arteries dilate to increase blood flow and satisfy increased oxygen demand. Stenotic arteries cannot dilate as much as normal vessels can, so a relative perfusion defect is produced in the myocardium supplied by the stenotic vessel. The increased blood flow of three times the baseline levels is somewhat less than that produced by the vasodilators dipyridamole or adenosine. Further, the success of dobutamine stress is limited in patients on β-blocker medications. Dobutamine is best reserved for those patients in whom dipyridamole or adenosine stress is contraindicated, such as in patients with asthma or chronic obstructive pulmonary disease, in those who have had caffeine or methylxanthine medications within 12 hours of the study, and in those taking oral dipyridamole therapeutically before adenosine stress

Dobutamine Protocol. The administration protocol consists of a gradually increasing intravenous infusion, beginning with 5 to 10 mcg/kg/min for 3 minutes, with the dose increasing every 3 minutes until a maximum dose of 40 mcg/kg/min is reached. The maximum dose administered may be titrated downward if significant symptoms, heart rate or blood pressure effects, or ECG evidence of ischemia occurs. The myocardial perfusion radiopharmaceutical is injected 1 minute after beginning the highest tolerated dose of dobutamine, and the infusion is maintained for an additional 2 minutes while the radiopharmaceutical localizes in the myocardium. Imaging is started at a time appropriate to the radiopharmaceutical used.

About 75% of patients undergoing dobutamine infusion experience side effects. The most common are transient and similar to those of adenosine infusion, including palpitation, chest pain, flushing, headache, and dyspnea. More worrisome is the common occurrence of premature ventricular contractions and, less commonly, unsustained ventricular tachycardia and atrial fibrillation. Patients with baseline atrial tachycardia should be infused with caution. Because the biologic half-life of dobutamine (≈2 minutes) is longer than that of adenosine, the occasional use of a rapidly acting β-blocker may be needed to reverse its effects when a rare, persistent, adverse reaction occurs. Contraindications to dobutamine stress include significant ventricular arrhythmias, hypotension, marked hypertension, and LV outflow obstruction.

Clinical Applications
Coronary Artery Disease
Diagnosis of Coronary Artery Disease.

SPECT Imaging Data. Stress and rest or redistribution myocardial perfusion is well recognized as an examination of high sensitivity and specificity for the detection of CAD. Its sensitivity for the detection of coronary artery stenosis increases directly with the severity of the stenoses and the extent of the disease (number of vessels involved). The overall sensitivity in the detection of stress-induced ischemia is about 80% to 90%, with a normalcy rate (percentage of normal patients with normal scans) of 85%. This represents a significant increase in sensitivity over exercise electrocardiography (60% to 70% sensitivity), with comparable or slightly increased specificity. This greater sensitivity is in large part attributable to the considerable number of patients with nondiagnostic exercise ECG tests because of baseline electrocardiographic abnormalities or inadequate stress.

Diagnostic stress myocardial perfusion imaging is most useful when it is applied to two broad groups of patients with suspected CAD: those in whom a routine exercise ECG test is nondiagnostic and those with an intermediate probability of disease. The latter group includes patients with high clinical suspicion of CAD based on symptoms and/or risk factors but with negative exercise ECGs, and those with a low pretest likelihood of CAD but with suggestive or positive ECGs at stress. Patients with underlying ECG abnormalities caused by left bundle-branch block, pacemakers, LV hypertrophy, baseline ST changes, or digoxin effect are also suitable candidates for myocardial perfusion imaging.

Although stress myocardial perfusion imaging is sensitive and specific for the diagnosis of CAD, it is less sensitive in determining the extent of disease. The presence of perfusion defects in more than one vessel distribution strongly indicates the presence of two- or three-vessel disease. However, a perfusion defect present in the distribution of only one vessel cannot be used to exclude the involvement of other vessels. False-negative studies may be caused by the phenomenon of balanced, symmetric, three-vessel CAD producing apparently normal, but uniformly reduced, flow through each artery. In this setting, transient LV dilatation or increased thallium lung activity may provide clues to the presence of underlying three-vessel CAD. Failure to reach adequate stress (>85% of maximum predicted heart rate during exercise stress) may also result in false-negative studies, especially in patients with moderate coronary stenoses.

GSPECT Functional Data. Assessing the severity of CAD can be enhanced by using the functional data derived from GSPECT. In most patients, any stress-induced ischemic segmental wall motion abnormalities quickly resolve after cessation of exercise. However, in approximately 30%, these areas of regional ischemic dysfunction persist as long as 1 hour after stress and are documented as focal wall motion abnormalities (stress-induced stunning)

and/or LVEF reductions on GSPECT imaging. Such regional stress-induced hypokinesia in myocardial segments exhibiting reversible perfusion defects predicts high-grade stenosis and increased severity of disease.

Because a common cause of a false-positive SPECT myocardial perfusion scan is soft-tissue attenuation artifact, especially in women, the ability to differentiate between a true fixed perfusion defect (characterized by diminished or absent wall motion and/or thickening) and artifact (demonstrating normal wall motion and thickening) is important in improving the specificity of the study. GSPECT wall motion displays may demonstrate the presence of wall motion in an apparent fixed perfusion defect, thus establishing the spurious nature of the abnormality consistent with an attenuation artifact. Conversely, the presence of a wall motion abnormality is compatible with scar or viable but hibernating myocardium. It should be noted, however, that wall motion in the region of some true fixed defects, especially small ones, may occasionally be observed because of recruitment by normally contracting adjacent myocardium or to the nontransmural nature of the injury. Normal post-stress wall motion in the region of a reversible defect neither confirms nor excludes an attenuation artifact.

In patients with three-vessel CAD, perfusion defects may not be seen in any or every coronary distribution, giving the false impression of absent or limited disease. The functional information obtained by GSPECT improves the detection of multivessel CAD, especially in cases of "balanced" global hypoperfusion, which may hinder the detection of segmental disease based on nongated perfusion data alone. In these patients, the ability to image post-stress ischemic wall motion/thickening abnormalities significantly increases the sensitivity of myocardial perfusion imaging for the identifying multivessel and left main CAD. A reduction in post-stress LVEF may also increase the sensitivity for multivessel disease and be the only indication of CAD in patients with "balanced" disease.

As a tool of differential diagnosis, GSPECT accurately distinguishes between patients with ischemic and nonischemic cardiomyopathy. Patients with nonischemic cardiomyopathy commonly present with diffuse wall motion abnormalities and globally abnormal LVEFs without the discrete perfusion defects usually noted with ischemic etiology. This differentiation has significant therapeutic implications.

Prognosis and Risk Stratification in CAD.

SPECT Imaging Data. In recent years, rather than simply identifying patients with CAD, the emphasis of myocardial perfusion imaging has shifted to identifying patients with CAD who are also at risk for cardiac death and thus are in most need of revascularization. Stress myocardial perfusion imaging has been shown to be effective for assessing risk of future cardiac events in patients with known CAD. Findings on abnormal stress myocardial perfusion imaging that have been found to represent potent prognosticators of future adverse cardiac events include the following: (1) the number of reversible defects (an indicator of multivessel disease), (2) the size and severity of the reversible defects (amount of myocardium at risk), (3) the extent of fixed defects (amount of infarcted myocardium), (4) reversible defects in the left main coronary artery distribution, (5) abnormal lung accumulation of ^{201}Tl, and (6) transient left ventricular dilatation at exercise (Table 5-3).

It should be remembered that the most severe or extensive reversible defect does not necessarily indicate the region most at risk for myocardial infarction. This correlates with the observation that mild plaques or stenosis ("vulnerable plaques") may be more subject to instability and to acute myocardial infarctions than more severe, established plaque/stenosis. Thus the myocardial perfusion findings indicate the overall risk of adverse cardiac events for the patient, not for a particular lesion.

Ideally, to adequately express the extent and severity of perfusion abnormality present in a given patient and thus to provide maximal prognostic information, quantitative or semiquantitative assessment is optimum, such as calculating summed perfusion scores as described earlier. The risk of both cardiac death and myocardial infarction both worsens as summed stress scores (SSS) as a measure of perfusion abnormality increases. The summed difference score (SDS) as a measure of ischemic myocardium at risk is a strong predictor of future myocardial infarction. This approach also facilitates comparison of serial follow-up perfusion studies.

In terms of favorable prognoses, patients with known CAD and an unequivocally normal stress myocardial perfusion study with adequate stress have a very good prognosis, with a

TABLE 5-3	Gated-SPECT Myocardial Perfusion Imaging: High Risk Findings
HIGH RISK FINDING	**DESCRIPTION**
Multivessel CAD-perfusion	Multiple perfusion abnormalities in more than one coronary artery distribution
Multivessel CAD-wall motion	Multiple regional wall motion or wall thickening abnormalities with or without perfusion defects
Large ischemic defect	Reversible myocardial defect >20% of LV
LAD ischemia	Reversible myocardial defects in LAD distribution
Diminished LVEF	LVEF <40% on gated-SPECT images
Lung activity	Increased lung/heart count ratio (>50%) with Tl-201 imaging
Transient ischemic dilatation (TID)	Apparent dilatation of LV cavity post stress (either exercise and pharmacologic) compared to resting cavity size. Likely caused by severe subendocardial ischemia, not actual cavity volume changes

CAD, Coronary artery disease; *LAD,* left anterior descending artery; *LV,* left ventricle; *LVEF,* left ventricular ejection fraction.

yearly rate of myocardial infarction or death of less than 1% to 2%.

GSPECT Functional Data. Assessment of risk in patients with CAD is enhanced by the addition of LV functional data to myocardial perfusion information. In patients with known CAD, a post-stress LVEF less than 45% or an end-systolic volume (ESV) greater than 70 mL confers a high mortality rate (≈8% to 9% per year), even in the presence of mild to moderate perfusion abnormalities. An LVEF greater than 45% or ESV less than 70 mL renders a low cardiac death rate (≈1% per year), even in the presence of severe perfusion abnormalities. When prediction of future nonfatal myocardial infarction is considered, the amount of ischemia present on the SPECT perfusion images appears to be a more accurate indicator than LVEF.

Hemodynamic Significance of Coronary Stenosis.

SPECT Imaging Data. Experimental evidence indicates that coronary artery diameter narrowing greater than 50% as determined by arteriography is likely to be hemodynamically significant. In many instances, however, the exact percentage of narrowing is difficult to ascertain on routine arteriography, and stress myocardial imaging can be useful in determining the hemodynamic significance of an angiographically demonstrated stenosis. Stress-induced ischemia of the myocardium supplied by a stenotic vessel may be interpreted as strong evidence of physiologic significance of the stenosis. Because myocardial perfusion imaging is not 100% sensitive, however, a normal stress perfusion study in a particular arterial distribution is less definitive in predicting the absence of significant narrowing.

Because coronary arteriography and myocardial perfusion imaging measure different parameters (anatomy and hemodynamics, respectively), discrepancies between the two tests are not unusual. The accuracy of the estimated degree of stenosis at angiography is highly dependent on the technical aspects of the study and the method of measurement used. In addition, the significance of an angiographically determined stenosis may be increased by the presence of superimposed spasm or small-vessel disease (such as in diabetic patients) or may be mitigated by the presence of adequately functioning collateral vessels. A lesion thought to be subcritical by diameter measurement may still be hemodynamically significant if it is a long stenosis, or if it occurs in a vessel of already small diameter or in a vessel with multiple low-grade stenoses. The assessment of hemodynamic significance on stress myocardial perfusion imaging may be further complicated in patients with multivessel stenoses, in whom exercise performance may be limited by the more severe lesions, so that an exercise level sufficient to induce ischemia in the distribution of a less severe but significant stenosis may not be reached.

These caveats aside, patients with angiographic stenoses, even left main or multivessel disease, have a relatively low risk for adverse cardiac events when no ischemia is identified on myocardial perfusion imaging.

GSPECT Functional Data. GSPECT performed within an hour or so after the completion of stress may reflect the post-stress status of LV function. The induction of post-stress wall motion/thickening abnormality in the region of a reversible stress-induced perfusion defect in the segment of myocardium distal to a stenosis provides independent highly specific evidence of stenosis severity. Reversible, stress-induced wall motion abnormalities confer high specificity for coronary stenoses greater than 70%.

Adequacy of Collateral Coronary Vessels. The functional significance of collateral vessels identified at coronary arteriography may be evaluated in a manner similar to that for coronary stenoses. Evidence suggests that in some patients, collaterals may maintain adequate rest perfusion to the myocardium distal to a stenosis but may not be able to meet the oxygen demands of this tissue during exercise. Therefore stress myocardial imaging may be able to give a clearer idea of the reserve perfusion potential of such collaterals by demonstrating the presence or absence of reversible stress-induced ischemia in the region of concern.

Evaluation of Myocardial Revascularization.

SPECT Imaging Data. Chest pain after coronary revascularization procedures may or may not have a cardiac origin, but the ability to distinguish between the two is significant. Recurrent pain from a cardiac cause may be related to occlusion of the bypass grafts or angioplasty vessel or to the progression of disease in indigenous vessels. In addition, about 25% of patients with restenosis may have no symptoms ("silent" ischemia). Postoperative exercise myocardial perfusion imaging gives information regarding the hemodynamic success of revascularization by comparing preoperative and postoperative stress images (Fig. 5-26).

After coronary artery bypass grafting, 10% to 20% of venous grafts occlude by 1 year, and up to 50% occlude by 10 years. Stress myocardial perfusion imaging is superior to both clinical findings and exercise ECG in predicting graft patency. The probability of graft occlusion increases significantly with worsening of defects that were present before surgery or with the appearance of new defects. Graft patency correlates with improved perfusion compared with presurgical scans. Reversible perfusion abnormalities not identified on the preoperative study suggest progression of disease in indigenous vessels, whereas new fixed defects may indicate perioperative myocardial injury.

Percutaneous transluminal coronary angioplasty (PTCA) is associated with a 30% to 40% restenosis rate by 6 months after the procedure. Although in general the addition of coronary stents to PTCA procedures has diminished postangioplasty restenosis compared with that

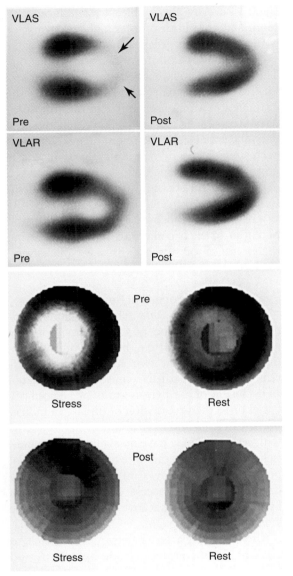

Figure 5-26. Preangioplasty and postangioplasty exercise SPECT myocardial perfusion imaging. Vertical long-axis stress (*VLAS*) and vertical long-axis rest (*VLAR*) images (*left side of upper rows*) obtained before angioplasty demonstrate a large apical reversible defect (*arrows*) consistent with stress-induced ischemia in the left anterior descending artery territory. Stress and rest vertical long-axis SPECT slices obtained 6 weeks after successful angioplasty (*right side of upper rows*) show that the apical defect has significantly improved. These results are also confirmed by the preangioplasty and postangioplasty stress and rest bull's eye plots (*lower rows*).

than 50% stenosis. Because of post-traumatic changes at the site of coronary arterial dilatation seen early after PTCA (including elastic recoil, spasm, intramural hemorrhage, and intraluminal debris), up to half of patients show a transient reduction in coronary flow reserve immediately after PTCA, which returns to normal in days to weeks. For this reason, false-positive myocardial perfusion scans may occur during the first few weeks after PTCA. When performed 4 to 8 weeks after PTCA, scans showing reversible perfusion defects are highly predictive for coronary restenosis and the recurrence of angina, whereas the absence of such defects correlates with vessel patency.

GSPECT Functional Data. In addition to myocardial perfusion assessment, the success of revascularization can be gauged by measuring any improvement in global LV function (LVEF) or regional wall motion after the procedure. A seemingly paradoxical circumstance may be observed in many patients who have undergone coronary artery bypass surgery. In these patients, apparent septal dyskinesia may be noted with preservation of systolic wall thickening. This finding is likely related to exaggerated translational cardiac motion after surgery and does not indicate underlying pathology.

Risk Stratification after Myocardial Infarction.

SPECT Imaging Data. In the post-myocardial infarction patient, myocardial perfusion imaging using submaximal exercise or pharmacologic stress provides important information regarding risk stratification. The primary strategy is to identify two distinctive groups of patients: (1) low-risk patients who require no further evaluation and may be discharged from the hospital, and (2) high-risk patients who are in need of further assessment and may benefit from revascularization therapy.

High-risk patients are identified by significant residual peri infarct ischemia (myocardium at risk) or ischemia remote from the acute injury (multivessel disease). If the walls of the LV appear to diverge from the base toward the apex, instead of converging toward the apex, an apical ventricular aneurysm complicating a myocardial infarct should be suspected (Fig. 5-27). Increased lung activity on thallium studies and transient ischemic dilatation are also high-risk indicators. Conversely, a normal study or a small, fixed

of PTCA alone by about one third, the range of in-stent restenosis still remains about 10% to 25% at 6 months. When properly timed, stress myocardial scintigraphy can document procedural success and can diagnose restenosis, defined angiographically as a return to more

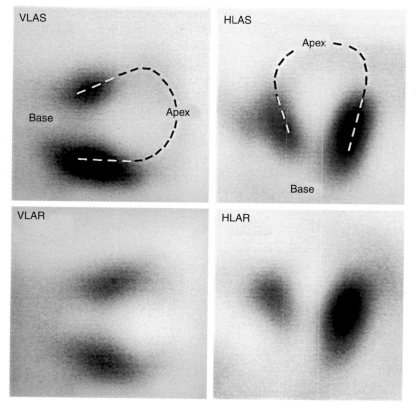

VLAS

Base

Apex

HLAS

Apex

Base

VLAR

HLAR

Figure 5-27. Left ventricular apical aneurysm. Vertical and horizontal long-axis SPECT sestamibi images at stress (*VLAS, HLAS*) and rest (*VLAR, HLAR*) demonstrate a fixed large apical defect compatible with a prior myocardial infarction with scarring. The walls of the left ventricle diverge as they go toward the apex and converge toward the base of the heart, indicating the presence of a left ventricular aneurysm at the apex.

defect in a single vascular territory allows low-risk classification, predicting about a 6% rate of cardiac events during the year after myocardial infarction.

GSPECT Functional Data. GSPECT can be used to determine residual LV function after myocardial infarction as a predictor of future adverse cardiac events. In post-myocardial infarction patients, the incidence of cardiac death or recurrent acute myocardial infarction with an LVEF less than 40% is about 40%, but the incidence is less than 10% in those with an LVEF greater than 40%.

Myocardial Viability Determination.

SPECT Imaging Data. In certain circumstances, it is important to distinguish fixed perfusion defects caused by myocardial scar from fixed defects representing viable but nonfunctional salvageable myocardium. This is especially true when revascularization procedures are under consideration as a means of restoring perfusion and thereby wall motion in the affected areas, thus improving overall LV function. Revascularization procedures provide no potential for improving cardiac function in areas of scarring and are associated with

significant morbidity. However, in fixed defects caused by viable but hibernating myocardium with accompanying regional wall motion abnormalities, myocardial contractile function may be restored by revascularization.

Hibernating myocardium is the result of severe coronary artery stenoses or partially reopened occlusions producing chronic hypoperfusion and ischemia. This leads to reduced cellular metabolism that is sufficient to sustain viability but inadequate to permit contractile function. Areas of hibernating myocardium usually present as segments of decreased perfusion and absent or diminished contractility, even when the patient is in a resting state. Because the myocardium is ischemic, but still viable, revascularization generally restores both perfusion and wall motion function.

Hibernating myocardium, a chronic process, should be distinguished from "stunned" myocardium, a more acute, temporary circumstance. Stunning is the result of ischemic and reperfusion injury secondary to an acute coronary artery occlusion that has reopened, either spontaneously or by thrombolytic therapy, before significant myocardial infarction can occur. Areas of stunned myocardium usually present with normal or near-normal perfusion but with absent or diminished contractility. Because the underlying myocardial cells are still viable, once blood flow has been restored, stunning generally spontaneously subsides over several weeks, with restoration of wall motion and improvement in LV function. Thus unlike hibernating myocardium, revascularization is not needed. However, if the reopened vessel does not sufficiently restore perfusion and there is residual ischemia, chronically hibernating myocardium may result. Recently a chronic form of so-called repetitive or cumulative stunning has been recognized in patients with CAD, which consists of multiple cycles of acute myocardial ischemia-reperfusion injury leading to chronic local contractile dysfunction. This may coexist with hibernation in ischemic heart disease to produce significant but potentially reversible LV dysfunction.

In the presence of fixed defects on routine myocardial perfusion imaging, additional effort over and above routine myocardial imaging must be made to establish the viability of a myocardial perfusion defect when it is crucial to patient management. In this setting, reinjection, delayed, or rest-redistribution thallium imaging techniques or ^{18}F-FDG PET, have demonstrated that a significant number of fixed defects (up to 50%) prove to be reversible, viable, but hibernating myocardium. Such evidence of viability is highly predictive of recovery of wall motion function in the involved segments after revascularization procedures, whereas lack of viability correlates with no recovery of myocardial function. ^{18}F-FDG PET for myocardial viability, the preferred technique in this setting, is discussed in the section of this chapter that addresses cardiac PET.

GSPECT Functional Data. Fixed or resting perfusion defects may be classified as viable if the presence of wall motion or thickening can be confirmed (Fig. 5-28). Detectable wall motion and/or wall thickening improves the likelihood of underlying viability and can predict regional recovery of function after revascularization compared with segments with no contractile function.

Administration of the inotropic drug dobutamine in low doses can be used to stimulate and measure myocardial contractile reserve, which enhances the accuracy of predicting recovery after coronary revascularization. Improved wall motion in a hypokinetic myocardial segment after dobutamine may increase the likelihood of postprocedural success. However, the technique appears less sensitive for predicting improvement in akinetic segments compared with that of quantitative perfusion imaging. In terms of global LV function, an increase in

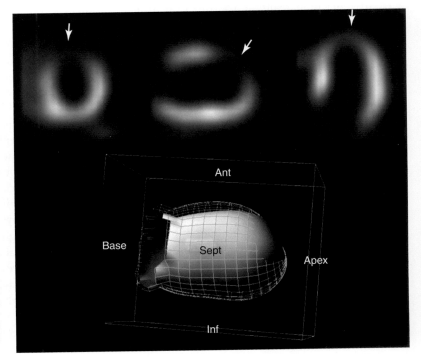

Figure 5-28. Anterior wall infarct. *Top,* Short-axis, horizontal long-axis, and vertical long-axis post-stress images from a GSPECT myocardial perfusion scan reveal a distal anterior wall defect *(arrows),* which was noted to partially reverse on rest images with a persistent fixed component. *Bottom,* Three-dimensional representation of the left ventricle at end systole shows marked regional hypokinesia with mild dyskinesia in the area of the perfusion abnormality. The lack of meaningful wall motion and focal dyskinesia are consistent with scarring, confirmed by lack of ^{18}F-FDG uptake. *FDG,* Fluorodeoxyglucose; *GSPECT,* gated single-photon emission computed tomography.

LVEF of more than 5% (5 ejection fraction units) after low-dose dobutamine may predict LVEF improvement after revascularization.

Evaluation of Acute Chest Pain. Patients with acute chest pain can be difficult to evaluate in the emergency setting because of the low sensitivity and specificity of clinical and ECG data available at the acute presentation. Because up to 10% of patients with acute chest pain discharged from the emergency room may develop a myocardial infarction within 48 hours, a conservative admissions policy is usually adopted, which may lead to a large number of inappropriate intensive care unit admissions. Under these circumstances, less than 30% of patients admitted to the coronary care unit have acute myocardial infarction. For these reasons, it has proved cost-effective in some acute care facilities to use resting myocardial perfusion imaging for the detection of defects associated with myocardial ischemia or infarct. Immediately on arrival in the emergency room, patients are injected at rest with 10 mCi (370 MBq) of ^{99m}Tc sestamibi or tetrofosmin and imaged after initial clinical evaluation and patient stabilization. Although sensitive in this setting, the rapid redistribution of thallium renders its use less practical.

Acute myocardial infarctions present as focal perfusion defects on the myocardial perfusion images. The detection of acute myocardial infarction by this technique is highly reliable in the first 24 hours after the insult. In fact, the sooner imaging is performed after the onset of symptoms, the more likely that the study will be positive. Almost all patients with myocardial infarction injected within 6 hours after onset of chest pain demonstrate perfusion defects. Sensitivity decreases thereafter with time, possibly related to the resolution of associated acute reversible ischemia in the region of infarction. However, a normal scan after this time likely confers a low risk but does not exclude acute coronary syndromes. The tracer may be injected regardless of whether the patient is experiencing chest pain at the time of injection, although the sensitivity of the study is lower if the patient's chest pain has resolved. By using this technique, patients may be triaged and treated expeditiously with significant cost-effectiveness. Because myocardial perfusion imaging does not distinguish between old and new myocardial infarctions, it may be most effective in patients without ECG or historical evidence of previous infarction or in patients with previous baseline imaging studies. The negative predictive value of a normal study approaches 100%.

Myocardial perfusion at rest has also been used to differentiate unstable angina pectoris from acute myocardial infarction. When the study is performed during an episode of pain, about half of patients with unstable angina demonstrate perfusion defects on initial resting images. Delayed images obtained after the pain has subsided (either by using thallium redistribution or ^{99m}Tc sestamibi reinjection techniques) demonstrate that these defects are usually reversible, as opposed to those associated with completed infarction. A normal study obtained during chest pain is a strong indicator that the pain is not related to myocardial ischemia.

Preoperative Risk Assessment for Noncardiac Surgery.

SPECT Imaging Data. Stress myocardial perfusion imaging can be used successfully to evaluate cardiac status before general surgical procedures. High risk for perioperative myocardial infarction is directly related to the number and extent of reversible myocardial perfusion defects. Normal studies or those disclosing only fixed defects confer a low risk of adverse cardiac events with a negative predictive value approaching 100%. Patients with significant reversible stress-induced ischemia should be considered for coronary arteriography (Fig. 5-29). Patients with lesser findings may proceed to surgery as necessary, with appropriate steps taken to lower surgical and anesthesia risks.

GSPECT Functional Data. There is incremental prognostic value in this setting with GSPECT compared with SPECT alone. The adverse perioperative cardiac event rate has been shown to increase with decreasing LVEF values (especially <35%) and with the number of hypokinetic LV wall segments.

Noncoronary Disease States

Valvular Lesions. Exercise-induced perfusion defects may be uncommonly identified in patients with mitral valve prolapse but without angiographic evidence of CAD. The cause and significance of such defects are uncertain, but when seen, ischemia as a cause must be excluded. A normal exercise myocardial perfusion study

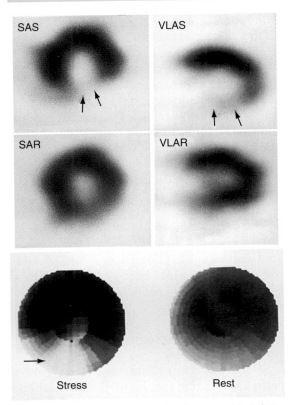

Figure 5-29. Inferior wall ischemia (reversible inferior wall defect). On these technetium-99m tetrofosmin SPECT images, the short-axis stress (*SAS*) and vertical long-axis stress (*VLAS*) images (*upper row*) show a defect in the inferior wall (*arrows*). There is much improved perfusion in these areas on the rest images (*middle row*) obtained earlier the same day with a smaller dose of ^{99m}Tc-tetrofosmin. Bull's eye plots (*lower row*) confirm the reversible stress-induced defect in the inferior wall (*arrow*). *SAR,* Short-axis rest; *VLAR,* vertical long-axis rest.

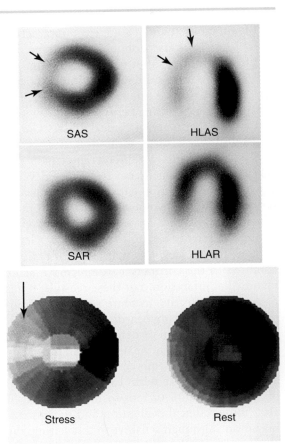

Figure 5-30. Left bundle-branch block (LBBB). On technetium-99m sestamibi SPECT short-axis stress (*SAS*) and horizontal long-axis stress (*HLAS*) images, there is a prominent perfusion defect in the septum (*arrows*). No discernible defect is seen on either short- or horizontal long-axis rest images (*middle row*). These findings are also seen on the bull's eye images (*lower row*). Coronary angiography was normal in this patient with LBBB. *HLAR,* Horizontal long-axis rest; *SAR,* short-axis rest.

in a patient with mitral valve prolapse, however, serves as evidence against superimposed CAD.

Patients with valvular aortic stenosis may present with angina-like symptoms in the absence of CAD. Forty percent to 50% of these patients may demonstrate reversible perfusion defects, which are thought to be related to a reduced perfusion gradient in the coronary arteries associated with tight aortic stenosis. Thus perfusion abnormalities after exercise in patients with aortic stenosis should be interpreted with caution. Patients with aortic regurgitation, but without CAD, may exhibit stress-induced reversible defects localized to the apex of the ventricle. With defects in other regions of the ventricle, CAD must be excluded.

Left Bundle-Branch Block. Because LBBB renders ECG stress testing nondiagnostic, a noninvasive diagnosis of CAD is often sought by using radionuclide myocardial perfusion

imaging. Patients with LBBB may demonstrate reversible septal or anteroseptal perfusion abnormalities during maximal exercise stress in the absence of demonstrable CAD (Fig. 5-30). Diminished septal perfusion at exercise resulting from asynchronous septal relaxation that is out of phase with diastolic coronary filling has been proposed as the mechanism for this phenomenon. Thus reversible perfusion defects at exercise in the septal region of patients with LBBB are an indeterminate finding. Reversible defects elsewhere in the LV myocardium, however, retain their specificity for the diagnosis of transient ischemia. Because the frequency of stress-induced septal defects in patients with LBBB is directly related to the heart rate achieved during exercise or dobutamine stress, pharmacologic stress with adenosine or dipyridamole (which

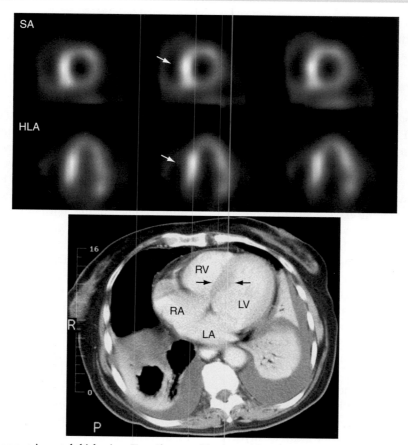

Figure 5-31. Asymmetric septal thickening. *Top,* Short- and horizontal long-axis rest slices from a technetium-99m tetrofosmin myocardial perfusion study show relatively decreased activity in the lateral wall of the left ventricle and normal or increased activity in the septum. This pattern persisted on the post-stress study, suggesting a lateral wall scar. *Bottom,* Post-contrast computed tomography scan shows an asymmetrically thickened interventricular septum (*arrows*) in a patient with hypertension. Coronary arteriography was normal. The findings on SPECT slices are due to relatively increased activity in the septum as a result of its hypertrophy with scaling of the images such that the normal activity in the lateral wall is suppressed, giving the false impression of a fixed perfusion abnormality.

produces no significant increase in heart rate) is a useful alternative to exercise stress or dobutamine, producing fewer false positive studies in this setting.

Hypertensive Myocardial Hypertrophy. Because hypertension is a major risk factor for CAD, hypertensive patients are often referred for myocardial perfusion scintigraphy. In patients with myocardial hypertrophy resulting from longstanding hypertension, myocardial perfusion imaging may demonstrate a relative increase in the septal wall activity on both stress and redistribution images. This increased septal count density may lead to an apparent relative decrease in activity in the lateral wall, especially on HLA SPECT images, causing a false impression of a fixed lateral wall defect (Fig. 5-31). Similar findings may occur in patients with idiopathic subaortic stenosis. Thus a history of

possible hypertension or idiopathic subaortic stenosis should be elicited in patients undergoing these studies.

PET CARDIAC IMAGING

Once a rarely used clinical tool, PET and PET/CT cardiac imaging has grown considerably in availability and application over the past decade. PET has inherent advantages that make it attractive for myocardial imaging. These include (1) better spatial resolution (2 to 3 mm) compared with that of SPECT (6 to 8 mm); (2) higher myocardial count rates, allowing better quality images; and (3) superior quantitative capabilities. As with gated-SPECT, gated-PET offers assessment of wall motion and LV function. Further, PET/CT has attenuation correction built into the technology, which considerably reduces the false-positive studies caused by attenuation artifacts.

In general, PET imaging provides assessment of myocardial perfusion or metabolism, depending on the radiopharmaceutical used.

PET Myocardial Perfusion Imaging

The physiologic principles and rationale involved in PET myocardial perfusion imaging in the setting of coronary artery disease are essentially the same as in SPECT imaging with ^{99m}Tc-labeled radiopharmaceuticals. Comparisons of PET with SPECT rest-stress myocardial perfusion imaging have generally shown a greater sensitivity (96% versus 85%) and specificity (80% versus 65%), and higher diagnostic accuracy (90% versus 80%) with PET for the diagnosis of coronary artery disease. Further, PET perfusion imaging with Rb-82 can be completed in a much shorter time than SPECT studies. In addition, lower patient absorbed doses are generally achievable with PET imaging agents, although occupational doses can be considerably higher.

Another potential benefit of assessing myocardial perfusion with PET agents is the ability to quantify absolute myocardial perfusion in millimeters per minute per gram of myocardium using dynamic imaging during the first pass of the radiopharmaceutical, especially with N-13 ammonia. This can be of great value in detecting balanced ischemia in patients with three-vessel coronary stenosis without visually detectable regional perfusion defects and thus, falsely normal-appearing images. However, at present, these studies are currently performed primarily for research purposes. Limitations of PET for myocardial perfusion imaging include higher costs and more complex procedures.

Radiopharmaceuticals

Several radiopharmaceuticals are available for PET imaging of myocardial perfusion either at rest or during pharmacologic stress. These include ^{13}N-ammonia chloride (^{13}NH$_3$), ^{15}O-water (H$_2$^{15}O), and rubidium-82 chloride (^{82}Rb). Because of their very short half-lives, the first two require an on-site cyclotron. ^{82}Rb is obtained from a ^{82}Sr/^{82}Rb generator that must be replaced every 4 weeks and requires a relatively high, consistent volume of patients because it is relatively expensive. With more favorable reimbursement and the decline in the cost of PET radiopharmaceuticals, especially

Rb-82 for rest-stress myocardial perfusion imaging, these studies have gained in usage.

H$_2$^{15}O is not used for routine clinical studies but is the gold standard for visual and quantitative assessment of myocardial perfusion. The half-life of O-15 is 123 seconds. It diffuses passively into and out of myocardial cells with high first-pass extraction, but with high blood pool background, which requires correction to produce diagnostic images of the myocardium. The overall patient radiation dose is low.

^{13}NH$_3$ initially diffuses passively across the capillary membrane with an extraction fraction approaching 100%, with rapid blood pool clearance. It may then enter the myocardial cells passively or by active transport. Approximately 80% is retained in the myocardial cells through incorporation of ^{13}N into the amino acid, ^{13}N glutamine. The remainder diffuses back into the blood pool.

Rubidium-82 is a potassium analog and behaves in vivo much as thallium-201 does. Its extraction fraction is about 50% to 60% at rest. It has a half-life of 76 seconds and more energetic positron emissions than F-18, rendering a less favorable image resolution. Because myocardial extraction of rubidium chloride is dependent on cell membrane transport in addition to blood flow, myocardial uptake may be affected by membrane function and cellular metabolism and can be diminished with systemic hypoxia and acidosis as well as myocardial ischemia.

Newer myocardial perfusion agents labeled with F-18 have shown promise and with a half-life of 110 minutes, allow for more flexibility in protocol selection and do not require an on-site cyclotron or generator.

Rb-82 CI Protocol

PET myocardial perfusion imaging with the potassium analog Rb-82 is well established. The Rb-82 is eluted from the generator by a computer-regulated elution pump and infused directly into patients using a commercially available IV infusion system. Because the Rb-82 supply is 90% replenished within 5 to 10 minutes of the last elution, serial studies can be performed in rapid succession maximizing patient throughput. Because of the short half-life of ^{82}Rb, pharmacologic stress is used instead of exercise.

Patient dosages are in the range of 20 to 60 mCi (0.74 to 2.22 GBq) and administered as a bolus lasting less than 30 seconds for each individual stress and resting acquisition, depending on the type of PET scanner, 2-D or 3-D acquisition, and imaging protocol used. To maximize accurate myocardial visualization, the start times of image acquisition post injection depends on the patient's LVEF: LVEF greater than 50% (70 to 90 sec); post injection, LVEF between 30% and 50% (90 to 110 sec); and LVEF less than 30% 110 to 130 sec). This delay allows for improved clearance of [82]Rb from the LV cavity blood pool activity, which can interfere with the detection and characterization of size and severity of adjacent myocardial perfusion defects. Image acquisition typically takes 5 to 6 minutes per image set. Imaging may be performed with or without ECG-gated technique for LV wall motion and functional data. Because of the short half-life of Rb-82 and the requirement of patient immobility during imaging, pharmacologic stress is used instead of physical exercise (Fig. 5-32). As the rest and stress images are performed in close succession, rest imaging should be performed before stress to avoid residual physiologic pharmacologic effects on the rest images. These images require significant smoothing to suppress noise.

When PET/CT is used, realignment of the transmission (CT) and emission (PET) is critical before reconstruction of the attenuation corrected PET myocardial images. It is also recommended that the rest and stress acquisitions should have their own dedicated transmission scan because of pharmacologic stress-induced changes in cardiac chamber and pulmonary volumes. The post-stress CT may be best obtained after the PET acquisition so that the effects of pharmacologic stress have subsided and less patient motion is likely. In some circumstances, a coronary CT angiogram may be obtained immediately following the PET/CT myocardial perfusion study.

N-13 Ammonia Imaging Protocol

N-13 ammonia PET imaging may be used for assessing both relative and absolute myocardial blood flow. However, its availability is limited; it requires an on-site cyclotron, and imaging protocols are complex. Thus this technique is not in wide clinical use.

To measure absolute myocardial perfusion (mL/min/g), the study must begin at the time of injection of the radiopharmaceutical with a dynamic acquisition to document its extraction and retention in the myocardial. For relative myocardial perfusion imaging, a typical

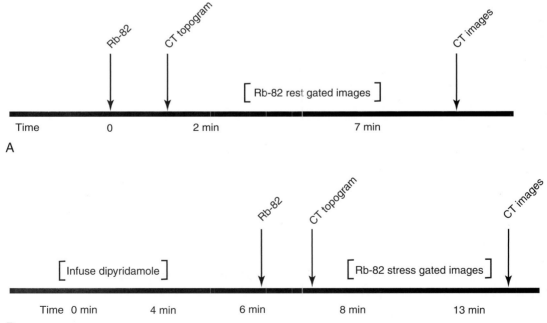

Figure 5-32. Rubidium-82 gated PET-CT dipyridamole myocardial perfusion protocol. Images are obtained at **A,** rest and with **B,** pharmacologic stress. In addition to dipyridamole, adenosine agents may be used as well but will vary the stress acquisition protocol slightly.

scanning doses of 10 to 15 mCi (370 to 555 MBq) for rest images and 30 mCi (1110 MBq) for stress images, depending on patient size, are administered as a bolus or 30-sec infusion. Although the physical half-life of approximately 10 minutes permits exercise stress to be used, pharmacologic stress is preferred and is more practical. Imaging is performed 3 to 5 minutes after injection, and each image series acquisition requires 10 to 15 minutes. Gated or nongated acquisition may be performed.

Interpretation

The images obtained in PET myocardial perfusion imaging may be analyzed using displays and methodologies similar to those used in SPECT imaging. Thus stress-induced reversible perfusion defects represent myocardial ischemia, and fixed defects are consistent with areas of scarring or hibernating myocardium. While attenuation artifacts common in SPECT imaging are largely corrected with PET, the effects of patient and respiratory motion artifacts on the images can be problematic and often are more difficult to detect. Image sets from a rotating SPECT camera allow assessment of patient motion by viewing cine of the individual images and determining on which images the patient moved. With a fixed ring of PET detectors, however, patient motion affects all of the simultaneously acquired projections. Thus careful observation and monitoring of patients during acquisition is important in assessing the degree of patient motion and in minimizing artifacts, which can blur the images. Because attenuation correction is critical in PET imaging, patient motion may induce artifacts from misregistration of the emission perfusion images with the transmission attenuation maps. Misalignments of just 1-2 cm can produce a 30% change in the apparent regional myocardial radioactivity producing artifactual perfusion defects. The position of these defects on the attenuation-corrected images depends on the direction and extent of misalignment. Most PET/CT scanners have software to correct transmission-emission misregistrations before image reconstruction and processing.

In addition to voluntary patient motion, changes in the cardiac situs between transmission-emission image acquisitions from altered breathing patterns and lung volumes associated with pharmacologic stress may produce areas of apparently increased activity in the inferior LV wall (over correction) and apparent perfusion defects in the anterior/anterolateral wall (undercorrection). Careful inspection of the co-registered transmission-emission images is necessary to determine whether misregistration has occurred. These artifacts may be corrected with the proper realignment of image set displacements in the appropriate planes. CT-related image reconstruction artifacts such as beam hardening from bone—"arms down"—or metallic objects (especially implantable cardioconverter defibrillator leads) in the field of interest are similar to those seen in PET/CT body imaging.

Also of note are differences in physiologic distribution of some PET radiopharmaceuticals in the normal myocardium, which must be recognized. For example, when imaging with N-13 ammonia, normal activity in the posterolateral wall of the LV is lower than elsewhere in the myocardium and may produce an apparent defect which may be misinterpreted as a perfusion abnormality. Further, occasional intense N-13 activity in the liver may hamper evaluation of the inferior wall.

As mentioned, the presence of significant cardiac blood pool activity caused by LV or RV dysfunction and prolonged circulation times may interfere with assessment of the size and severity of myocardial perfusion deficits.

Gated-PET images are presented for interpretation in many of the familiar formats used in SPECT imaging. Because gated-PET imaging assesses LV function during peak pharmacologic stress (rather than post stress with gated-SPECT), differences between LVEF at rest and peak stress can be used to predict the presence or absence of high risk CAD. Patients without significant CAD or single vessel diseases show an increase in LVEF from resting levels at peak vasodilator stress. Patients with multivessel CAD or left main CAD may show a decrease in LVEF even in the absence of perfusion defects. A rise in LVEF from rest to peak stress of 5% or more has an NPV of 97% for 3-vessel or left main CAD.

PET Myocardial Viability Imaging

Under normal fasting conditions, the normally perfused and oxygenated myocardium prefers long-chain fatty-acids as its primary metabolic substrate (70%) with 20% of energy demands fulfilled by glucose metabolism. However, under conditions of ischemia, the ability of the myocardium to metabolize fatty acids becomes markedly curtailed and is compensated for by a switch to greater anaerobic metabolism of glucose use to maintain myocardial energy needs. Exploitation of these adaptive changes in regional myocardial metabolism forms the basis of identification of chronically ischemic, but viable myocardium through PET imaging.

^{18}F-FDG is considered by many to be the gold standard for assessment of myocardial viability. As with other viable cells, F-18 FDG, as a glucose analog, enters the myocardial cells to become phosphorylated, and further metabolism essentially ceases. Being trapped in the myocardium for a considerable period allows imaging of viable myocardium. It is superior to delayed, reinjection, or rest thallium SPECT imaging strategies that may underestimate the amount of viable tissue.

A fixed defect on PET or SPECT myocardial perfusion studies may represent an area of prior infarction (scar) or hibernating myocardium. Both scars and hibernating myocardium present as wall motion dysfunction. However, while scars represent irretrievable, dead myocardium, hibernating myocardium represents a chronically ischemic but viable segment of myocardium that is salvageable by revascularization procedures. This oxygen-deprived tissue cannot effectively use oxidative metabolism of the preferred myocardial substrate (fatty acids) because of lack of oxygen. Consequently, as an adaptive mechanism, a hibernating segment switches to anaerobic metabolism of glucose and thus can be detected as metabolically viable by uptake of ^{18}F-FDG. This differentiates it from a fixed, metabolically inactive, perfusion defect caused by a postinfarction scar, which does not take up[18]F-FDG.

^{18}F-FDG Imaging Protocol

Typically, myocardial viability assessment entails combined resting perfusion and ^{18}F-FDG imaging protocols. The resting perfusion images using PET or SPECT define the perfusion deficit in the area of suspected hibernating myocardium, whereas the ^{18}F-FDG images determine the presence of any viable myocardium.

After a fasting period of 6-8 hours, oral glucose loading (25-100 g) of patients 1 to 2 hours before IV administration of 10-15 mCi (370-555 MBq) of ^{18}F-FDG is commonly used to increase endogenous insulin output, encouraging glucose uptake and metabolism by the myocardium. This optimizes FDG uptake in both normally perfused and ischemic, but viable myocardium. Imaging is performed approximately 1 hour after F-18 FDG injection and typically takes 10-30 minutes. In order to reduce absorbed dose to the bladder, frequent urination should be encouraged for several hours after the procedure.

Glucose loading can be challenging in diabetic patients as it is often not effective because of the limited ability to produce insulin. Exogenous insulin administration with blood glucose monitoring or imaging delayed by 2-3 hours post F-18 FDG administration may be successful alternatives.

Interpretation

Hibernating myocardium presents as a classic perfusion-metabolism mismatch defined by a fixed perfusion defect in an area that exhibits preserved or increased FDG uptake (Fig. 5-33).

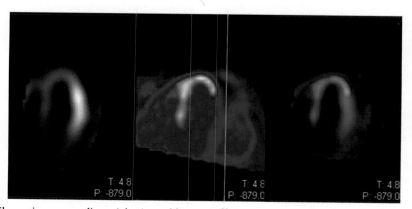

Figure 5-33. Hibernating myocardium. A horizontal long-axis ^{99m}Tc-sestamibi perfusion image (*left*) shows reduced perfusion to the septum and apex. The PET ^{18}F-FDG metabolism image (*middle*) has an inverse pattern indicating viable but hypoperfused myocardium in the septum and apex. The fused image is shown on the right.

This pattern correlates with improvement in myocardial perfusion and function (regional wall motion) after revascularization and restoration of perfusion to the area. Nonviable, unsalvageable myocardium related to myocardial scarring shows no evidence of perfusion or FDG uptake (Fig. 5-34). Thus viability imaging can be important in determining patient management and in avoiding unnecessary revascularization procedures in patients with scars.

Stunned myocardium may occur transiently after an acute episode of ischemia or after acute myocardial infarction with reperfusion therapy. Like hibernating myocardium, a stunned segment demonstrates diminished wall motion, but with normal or near normal perfusion (Fig. 5-35). Stunning may also occur in patients with severe chronic coronary artery

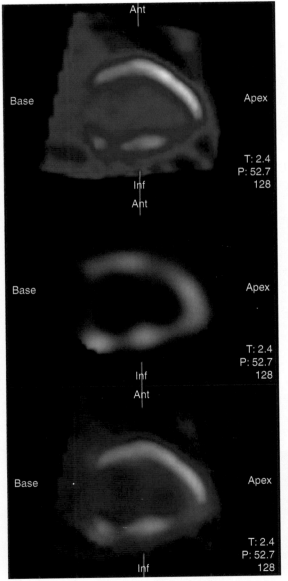

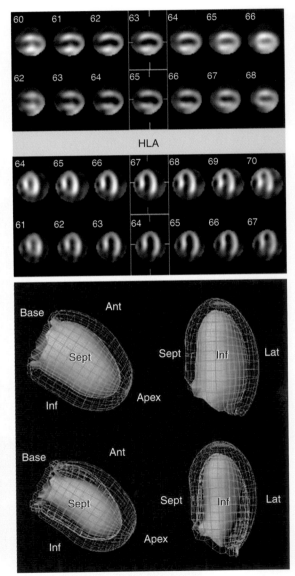

Figure 5-34. Hibernating LV anterior wall myocardium with inferior wall scar. The *HLA* ^{18}F-FDG image (*top*) shows a viable anterior wall with avid FDG uptake and a defect in the distal inferoapical wall consistent with a nonviable myocardial segment. The ^{99m}Tc-sestamibi perfusion scan (*middle*) demonstrates diminished perfusion to both. The fused images (*bottom*) confirm hibernating myocardium and a scar in the same patient.

Figure 5-35. Stunned myocardium. The top two stress/rest Tc-99m sestamibi image sets show normal to minimally decreased perfusion in the LV apex at rest and stress. However, the gated-SPECT sestamibi images show absent wall motion in the same region. The findings demonstrate an area of stunned myocardium with preserved perfusion but compromised function. *LV,* Left ventricle; *Tc,* technetium.

disease who experience repeated episodes of severe regional myocardial ischemia. Repetitive stunning may lead to a hibernating state as ischemia becomes more severe. Myocardial imaging in these patients typically demonstrates an area of normal perfusion at rest and normal metabolism, indicating viable myocardium, which is expected to improve functionally after revascularization. It is important to remember that a study demonstrating normal perfusion and metabolism at rest does not exclude the presence of coronary artery disease, and rest-stress perfusion imaging is necessary to do so.

Chronic myocardial ischemia may also be imaged on PET or SPECT as diminished uptake of labeled fatty acids, the primary metabolic substrate under normal aerobic conditions. A focal myocardial defect using 11C palmitate, I-123 labeled BMIPP, or other fatty acids, combined with increased ^{18}F-FDG uptake in the same area, substantiates the shift of metabolism from fatty acids to glucose indicative of ischemic but viable myocardium.

PET/CT in Aortic Dissection

Recent studies have indicated that ^{18}F-FDG PET/CT has the potential to distinguish between acute and chronic aortic dissections which can alter the course of patient treatment. Increased activity in the aortic wall compared to the adjacent aortic lumen blood pool activity correlates with acute injury and early reactive processes. Further, the more intense the activity in acute dissections, the more likely is the associated risk of rupture or progression of the dissection. While the mechanism of increased FDG accumulation remains unelucidated, it is hypothesized to be related to the accumulation of active cells such as macrophages and myofibrocytes in the vessel wall in acute dissections, as opposed to less active cells such as fibroblasts seen in tissue undergoing scar formation. In clinically unclear cases, FDG imaging may aid in determining the age of a dissection, the degree of risk for complication or progression, and the need for interventional therapy. FDG has been shown to accumulate in the macrophages of atheromas (vulnerable plaque) assumedly as a result of inflammation. The prevalance of FDG uptake in large arteries has been shown to increase with age.

RADIONUCLIDE IMAGING OF CARDIAC FUNCTION

Examinations that provide information about ventricular function play a decisive role in the detection and diagnosis of a variety of cardiac problems and in the management of patients with known heart disease. In this respect, radionuclide methods provide a noninvasive means to assess both right ventricle and LV pump performance at rest and during exercise and allow valuable insight into intracardiac and cardiopulmonary dynamics. Although these tests still have a place in clinical nuclear medicine practice, as general tools for evaluation of cardiac function, they have largely been supplanted for primary cardiac function evaluation by the widespread availability of echocardiography and the routine use of GSPECT for myocardial perfusion imaging.

Radionuclide tests of ventricular function are generally accomplished by four discrete methods:

- *GSPECT* using myocardial perfusion agents, as described earlier in the chapter, is the most frequently performed isotopic evaluation of cardiac function in clinical practice.
- *First-pass or first-transit radionuclide angiography (FP-RNA)* is the method in which imaging is undertaken during the initial rapid transit of an intravenously administered radioactive bolus through the heart, lungs, and great vessels.
- *Equilibrium radionuclide angiography (E-RNA),* in which images of the cardiac blood pool are obtained after a radiopharmaceutical has equilibrated within the intravascular space, is also known as gated blood pool ventriculography and multigated acquisition (MUGA) study.
- SPECT *equilibrium radionuclide angiography (SPECT-E-RNA)* is the method in which gated-SPECT imaging is performed instead of planar imaging.

Although first-pass and equilibrium methods require different procedural approaches, they provide essentially identical information for qualitative and quantitative assessment of LV function. Both techniques are accurate and reproducible compared with cardiac catheterization results. Therefore, although there are specific advantages and limitations to each, either method may be used for the evaluation of ventricular function at rest or during exercise.

Whichever technique is used, complete familiarity with and confidence in the procedure used provide the best approach for successful application.

Computer Methods

Among routine nuclear medicine procedures, those measuring cardiac function are perhaps the most dependent on computer methodology for the collection and processing of scintigraphic data. A basic knowledge of some specific computer methods is crucial to an understanding of these techniques.

Data can be acquired by a computer in *list mode* or *frame mode*. Basically, list mode involves digitizing and filing data in the time sequence in which it occurs, permitting later retrieval and manipulation of the data. In this manner, decisions concerning the sorting and formatting of the filed information and the discarding of unwanted information may be made at any time after the information is acquired. This flexibility allows the computer operator to format the data in varying time sequences, as may be dictated by the specific goals in mind. For instance, the data of a first-pass study may be formatted such that frames of several seconds' duration are generated and visual inspection of cardiac anatomy is possible. Alternatively, the data may be reformatted in frames of a fraction of a second's duration so that ventricular time-activity curves may be derived, allowing for quantification of ventricular function indices. Such flexibility necessarily has a price—the need for significant computer memory.

Frame mode acquisition requires formatting decisions to be made before the beginning of the study. After the information is collected, it cannot be reformatted to allow manipulation in varying time sequences. A major advantage is that frame mode requires substantially less computer memory.

Qualitative Data Display

When a computer system coupled with a gamma camera is used to acquire, analyze, and display the data obtained from nuclear cardiac studies, two types of information result:

■ Qualitative data, displayed as images
■ Quantitative data, expressed as numbers or curves

Computer-generated images of ventricular function can be processed by using computer software for edge or contrast enhancement, background subtraction, smoothing, filtering, or other manipulations to produce images of high quality. After images have been processed, they may be displayed as static images or more typically in an endless-loop cine format that allows visual inspection of the ventricular walls during cardiac contraction and thus permits qualitative assessment of ventricular segmental wall motion.

Quantitative Data Display

Computer manipulation of the statistical information contained within digitized equilibrium or first-pass images permits the quantitation of various indices of cardiac performance. These indices are derived from changes in activity (counts) in the ventricles during the cardiac cycle and as such are free from the errors inherent in the geometric methods used in contrast ventriculography. When meticulously performed, the results, including the LVEF, are very accurate and reproducible.

The basic principle underlying this count-volume (or time-activity) approach is the assumed proportionality between measured activity and the volume of blood in which it is contained. That is, as the radioactive bolus passes through the cardiac chambers, or after the administered radioactive agent has thoroughly mixed with the blood in the cardiac chambers, any change in the count rate obtained from a region of interest defining a particular chamber reflects a proportional change in the volume of blood within that chamber.

Regions of interest over the LV and a periventricular area of background to allow for subtraction of counts from structures overlying the ventricular area of interest are defined throughout the cardiac cycle either semiautomatically or manually, depending on operator preference. From these, a time-activity curve is generated. This curve represents changes in ventricular activity and therefore in relative ventricular volume during the cardiac cycle. It allows the calculation of perhaps the most important ventricular functional parameter: the global ejection fraction. By determining the number of counts present at end-systole and end-diastole, the difference, expressed as a percentage of the counts at end-diastole, gives the ejection fraction:

$$\text{Ejection fraction (EF)} = \frac{\text{End-diastolic counts} - \text{end-systolic counts}}{\text{End-diastolic counts} - \text{background counts}}$$

Usually the ejection fraction or changes are expressed as a percentage, although occasionally changes are expressed as ejection fraction units to avoid confusion. This solves the problem of whether a 10% decrease in a patient who previously had a 50% ejection fraction actually has a 40% or 45% ejection fraction. By stating that there is a decrease of 10 ejection fraction units, it would be clear that the resulting ejection fraction is 40%.

In most laboratories, a normal resting LVEF is at least 50%, usually in a range of 50% to 70%. The LVEF usually increases with exercise. A normal right ventricular ejection fraction is typically lower than the LVEF (by 5% to 10% [5 to 10 units]) because of the somewhat larger EDV of the right ventricle, but a stroke volume equal to the LV. A normal right ventricular ejection fraction is typically greater than 40% in normal patients. By mathematically differentiating the time-activity curves, ventricular ejection rates and filling rates may also be calculated. In addition to a global LVEF, regional ejection fractions may be derived by dividing the ventricle into segments. These ejection fractions serve as a measure of segmental LV wall motion and help quantify wall motion abnormalities.

As with any time-activity analysis of digitized images, the accuracy of the calculations depends largely on the precise selection of the regions of interest. Because it is important to determine accurately the edges of the LV and to exclude any activity in great vessels, lungs, and adjacent chambers, data processing protocols with computer algorithms for the automated detection of the LV edges as they change throughout the cardiac cycle are commonly used. These edge detection programs are accurate in most patients. It is important, however, that the physician analyzing the visual data correlate the calculated ejection fraction based on the computer selection of LV edges with his or her qualitative impression of LV function. Inaccurate definition of the aortic or mitral valve planes, with resultant inclusion of portions of either the ascending aorta or the left atrium in the LV region of interest, leads to underestimation of the LVEF. An artificially elevated LVEF may occur when a portion of the LV is excluded from the LV region of interest at end-systole. In some cases, manual selection of LV edges must be performed to ensure accurate ejection fraction determination.

Selection of the background region of interest is also of considerable importance so that the ejection fraction is not underestimated or overestimated. Overestimation and thus oversubtraction of background artificially elevates ejection fraction, whereas underestimation erroneously reduces ejection fraction values. There are various standard areas for placement of background regions of interest (usually periventricular), which should be consistently used for all such determinations to ensure the validity of technique.

Functional Images. By using various computer algorithms, functional or parametric images may also be generated. Rather than emphasizing spatial resolution, these images display global or regional changes in radioactivity, reflecting ventricular function. Although a number of functional images may be derived, those in common use include stroke volume, ejection fraction, phase, paradox, and amplitude images.

Stroke Volume Image. The *stroke volume* image may be obtained by subtracting the end-systolic frame of the ventriculogram from the end-diastolic frame and displaying the resultant distribution of activity in a gray-scale or color format (Fig. 5-36). This image presents the distribution of relative regional volume changes in each ventricle, reflecting the amount of blood ejected from each region of the ventricle during systole.

Ejection Fraction Image. The *ejection fraction image* is obtained through computer manipulation of the end-systolic and end-diastolic images to provide a static representation of the ejection fraction equation, that is, the stroke volume image divided by the end-diastolic image.

Typically, the ejection fraction and the stroke volume images obtained in the 45-degree left anterior oblique projection are similar. The images frequently resemble a horseshoe or incomplete doughnut because most of the volume and ejection fraction changes occur at the apex, posterior wall, and distal septal walls in this projection. Defects in the horseshoe or doughnut distribution of the "ejection shell" indicate areas of diminished stroke volume or ejection fraction, as may be found in regional hypokinesis or akinesis. Dyskinetic segments are not evaluated in these images because negative changes are given a zero value by the functional image program.

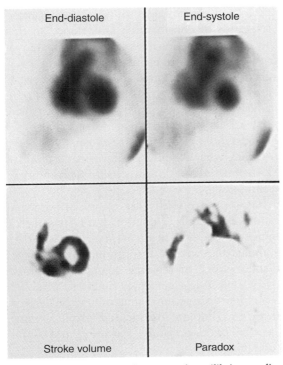

End-diastole   End-systole

Stroke volume   Paradox

Figure 5-36. Normal planar gated equilibrium radionuclide angiogram (E-RNA) with functional images. End-diastolic and end-systolic images of the heart in the 45-degree left anterior oblique projection are shown, with subsequent computer manipulation of the data to produce functional images. The *stroke volume image* demonstrates a darkened, circular shell, corresponding to left ventricular wall motion obtained by subtracting the end-systolic from the end-diastolic image. This shell corresponds to the amount of blood ejected from the left ventricle during systole (the stroke volume). The *paradox image* displays activity only in the regions of the atria that are contracting as the ventricles fill. No focal darkened area in the region of the left ventricular wall is seen to suggest the presence of localized dyskinesia (paradoxical wall motion).

Paradox Image. Dyskinetic segments, which may be associated with LV aneurysms, can be identified by using another type of functional image called the *paradox image*, in which the diastolic frame of the ventriculogram is subtracted from the systolic frame (Fig. 5-37). With normal LV contraction, no areas of focally increased activity should be identified in the region of the LV wall. Thus, in normal images, only the atria and the great vessels are seen. In the presence of regional dyskinesia, however, a focal area of increased activity appears in the image because the ESV in the region of paradoxical motion bulges beyond and thus exceeds the distribution of EDV. Thus subtraction of the two volume distributions leaves a focus of net increased activity at the site of dyskinesia.

Phase and Amplitude Analysis. These are examples of parametric functional images that display the sequence and degree of contraction of the cardiac chambers as well as individual wall segments of the left or right ventricle (Fig. 5-38). Such analysis permits sensitive evaluation of regional wall motion, as well as more precise differentiation between atrial and ventricular contraction. In this method, a summary of the characteristics of heart motion is derived through Fourier analysis of the digital data. The derived parameters of phase and amplitude are then displayed as functional images that allow the evaluation of the sequence of regional contraction and magnitude of segmental wall motion, respectively.

The phase image displays the time of contraction or motion of each myocardial segment independent of the degree or magnitude of movement. The amplitude image represents the extent of regional wall motion regardless of the time of occurrence within the cardiac cycle. In a normal phase analysis, the contraction pattern is expected to follow a standard sequence: atrial contraction fills the ventricular chambers, followed by contraction of the ventricles. Because the atria are filling when the ventricles are emptying and vice versa, they can be thought of as contracting with the phase difference of 180 degrees apart. Thus, the normal phase pattern, as seen in the functional image, shows the ventricles at one value of phase and the atria at 180-degree phase difference relative to the ventricles. A normal phase analysis is shown in Figure 5-39. Similarly, a dyskinetic, paradoxical myocardial segment would also be assigned a phase angle of about 180 degrees out of phase with the normal motion of the surrounding myocardium. Isolated regional phase abnormalities are commonly produced by scars, seen as areas of hypokinesia (Fig. 5-40), or by ventricular aneurysms producing focal areas of dyskinetic wall motion, which contract out of phase with the remainder of the ventricular wall (Fig. 5-41).

First-Pass Studies
Principle

In first-pass or first-transit radionuclide angiocardiography (FP-RNA), a bolus of radioactivity is injected into a large peripheral vein, and the initial rapid transit of the bolus through the heart, lungs, and great vessels is imaged in rapid

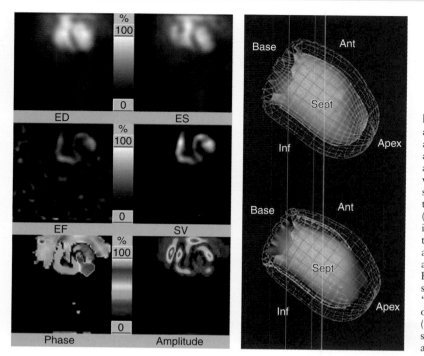

Figure 5-37. Left ventricular aneurysm. The end-diastolic (*ED*) and end-systolic (*ES*) frames from a gated equilibrium radionuclide angiogram (E-RNA) are displayed with the functional paradox and stroke volume images. The ejection fraction (*EF*) stroke volume (*SV*) images demonstrate a break in the stroke volume shell seen in the region of the left ventricular apex which could be interpreted as akinesia (absent wall motion). However, the phase image demonstrates apical wall motion which is "out of phase" with the remainder of the LV. This focal dyskinesia (paradoxical wall motion) is consistent with a left ventricular apical aneurysm.

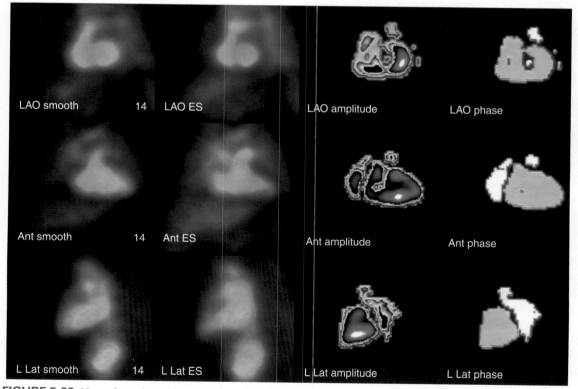

FIGURE 5-38. Normal gated equilibrium radionuclide angiography (E-RNA). Gated images of the cardiac blood pool are noted in the first two columns in static display of end-diastole and end-systole (*ES*) (from *left* to *right*). Left anterior oblique (*LAO*), anterior (*Ant*), and left lateral (*L Lat*) standard projections are presented. The amplitude and phase images give a static representation of the dynamic characteristics of the cardiac chambers, including sequence of contraction (*phase*) and degree of contraction (*amplitude*). The atria clearly show decreased contraction magnitude (less red) on the amplitude images compared with the ventricles. The phase images clearly separate the atria from the ventricles because of the normal alternating nature of their times of contraction (systole).

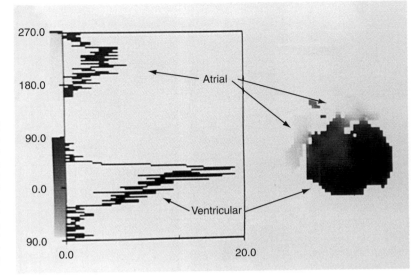

FIGURE 5-39. Phase analysis of a normal gated equilibrium radionuclide angiogram (E-RNA) in the left anterior oblique projection. The phase information is displayed as a histogram on the *left* and as a gray-scale image on the *right*. Clearly separated are the ventricular and atrial contraction peaks, with differentiation of the temporal sequence of atrial and ventricular contraction on the gray-scale image.

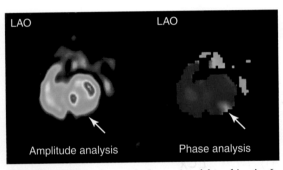

FIGURE 5-40. Left ventricular regional hypokinesia. In the phase and amplitude images, the arrows indicate an area of late (tardokinesia) or diminished (hypokinesia) contraction inferolaterally compatible with segmental myocardial scarring. The amplitude image demonstrates a defect compatible with severe hypokinesia or akinesia. The phase image indicates an abnormality in the timing of minimal wall motion, likely related to recruitment of the scarred area by adjacent viable myocardium.

sequence using a gamma camera. The data are processed by a computer, from which subsequent anatomic images can be obtained for visual interpretation, including ventricular wall motion. In addition, the quantitative analysis of the images can provide a number of hemodynamic indices, the most notable of which are left and right ventricular ejection fractions. The technique can be used in patients both at rest and during stress.

Radiopharmaceutical

Because the time for imaging of the first-pass study is necessarily limited, images of adequate statistical quality can be obtained only by administering a sufficient bolus of radioactivity, usually a minimum of 10 mCi (370 MBq). In addition, because each study requires a separate injection of radioisotope, a radiopharmaceutical that clears rapidly from the blood is necessary if multiple determinations are to be performed. Because of their rapid clearance by the liver and kidneys, respectively, ^{99m}Tc-labeled sulfur colloid and ^{99m}Tc-labeled diethylenetriamine pentaacetic acid (DTPA) are frequently used. Any ^{99m}Tc-labeled pharmaceutical may be used, however, if a repeat determination is not immediately contemplated. In fact, ^{99m}Tc blood pool agents may be used to obtain a first-pass study immediately before gated equilibrium imaging, so that both examinations are performed with only one radionuclide injection, allowing accurate determinations of both left and right ventricular ejection fractions.

Technique

The uniqueness of the first-pass examination is that the radioactive bolus progresses through the heart in such a manner that each chamber is visualized separately in temporal sequence, and problems with interfering activity in overlapping chambers, such as may be encountered with equilibrium imaging, are avoided (Fig. 5-42). A high sensitivity or general all-purpose collimator provides adequate statistical data collection. The examination may be performed in any view that places the cardiac ventricles reasonably near the camera face. The 30-degree RAO projection is most frequently used because

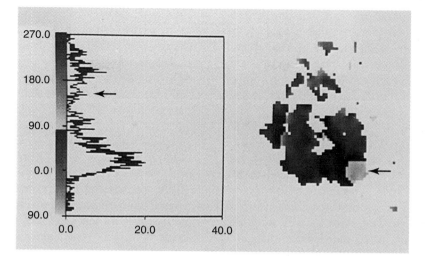

FIGURE 5-41. Phase analysis of a gated equilibrium radionuclide angiogram (E-RNA) demonstrating a left ventricular apical aneurysm. The phase information is displayed as a histogram on the *left* and as a gray-scale image on the *right*. On the histogram, a discrete peak for the ventricular contraction is seen, but there is significant broadening of the atrial peak compatible with a dyskinetic (out-of-phase) segment of left ventricular myocardium appearing during atrial contraction (*arrow*). The gray-scale image on the *right* clearly depicts the focal aneurysm (contracting paradoxically and "out of phase" with the remainder of the left ventricle) as a lighter shade of gray.

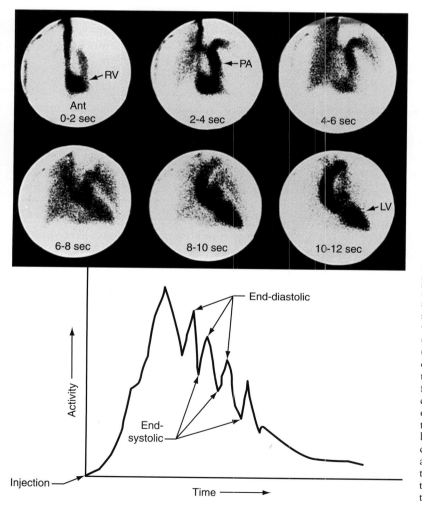

FIGURE 5-42. Normal first-pass radionuclide angiogram (FP-RNA). *Top,* Selected images from a normal FP-RNA demonstrate the sequential identification of right ventricle (*RV*), pulmonary artery (*PA*), lungs, and left ventricle (*LV*). Such temporal separation of chamber activity allows selective evaluation of both RV and LV function. *Bottom,* Time-activity curve obtained by using a region of interest over the RV displays the passage of the radionuclide bolus propelled by multiple cardiac cycles (usually 5 to 10), seen as peaks and valleys corresponding to sequential heart beats. RV ejection fraction can be derived from this curve.

it best allows separation of ventricular activity from atrial or aortic activity. Other projections may be used, depending on the particular aim of the study. Because only one projection can be obtained with each radionuclide bolus injection, multiple injections may be needed if several projections are required.

The collection of data in first-pass studies begins just before the injection of the radioactive bolus and is terminated after the activity traverses the left heart and is seen in the great arterial vessels. The entire study is normally completed in 30 to 60 seconds, over 5 to 10 cardiac cycles. Data are usually acquired by the computer in standard list mode as a sequence of images. Gated acquisition may also be used in synchrony with the patient's ECG, which allows better definition of the ventricular wall contours and evaluation of regional wall motion by the cine display of gated images. After the study has been acquired and processed, the data may be replayed and analyzed at the workstation.

Image Interpretation

First-pass radionuclide angiography is particularly well-suited to obtain the following functional information:

■ Measurement of right ventricle function (ejection fraction)
■ Assessment of ventricular function at peak exercise
■ Quantification of left-to-right intracardiac shunts

Because the first pass of the radioactive bolus through the heart and lungs takes place over multiple cardiac cycles, the data from several of these cycles can be analyzed or summed to form a single cycle of sufficient statistical nature for detailed visual and quantitative inspection. When viewed in endless-loop cine display, visual assessment of regional ventricular wall motion is possible. Although first-pass images of ventricular contraction are not of the statistical quality of equilibrium blood pool images and are usually limited to one projection only, the results are similar.

Cardiac Function. Quantitative assessment of the data presented in the digital images provides information regarding ventricular ejection fractions, ejection rates, cardiac output, and stroke volume as well as end-diastolic and end-systolic volumes. These parameters are usually acquired at rest. Uncommonly, the procedure may be performed at peak stress to assess ventricular contractile reserve and provides significant prognostic information in the setting of CAD. A significant fall in LVEF at peak exercise or an exercise LVEF of less than 40% confers a worse prognosis in patients with known CAD. Information concerning intracardiac and cardiopulmonary circulations can also be derived, including the calculation of pulmonary transit times.

Right Ventricular Function. Because of better separation of the right ventricle from the right atrium and left ventricle, first-pass determinations of right ventricular ejection fractions are in general more accurate than those obtained by using planar gated equilibrium technique, whereas LVEFs are comparable using the two techniques.

Intracardiac Shunts. In general, two-dimensional Doppler echocardiography is the initial procedure of choice in evaluating congenital heart disease and intracardiac shunts. However, in certain institutions offering expertise and experience in radionuclide techniques, FP-RNA can offer accurate assessment.

Left-to-Right Intracardiac Shunts. First-pass studies can provide information needed to diagnose and quantify left-to-right intracardiac shunts. This is made possible by analysis of time-activity curves obtained from a region of interest placed over a lung at a distance from the heart. A compact bolus of activity is essential to an accurate study. Early pulmonary recirculation of the radiopharmaceutical through a left-to-right shunt may be detected as an alteration in the normal curve, evidenced by a small second peak proportional to the size of the shunt. Various methods of analysis of FP-RNA data allow for shunt quantification, with accuracy equal to that of contrast arteriography. Although various mathematic approaches are available for the calculation of shunt size, the gamma variate function method provides the most accurate and reproducible technique. When using this method, pulmonary-to-systemic flow ratios of 1.2:1 or greater are considered evidence of left-to-right shunting.

Right-to-Left Intracardiac Shunts. Although right-to-left shunts may occasionally be defined on first-pass studies by early appearance of the radioactive bolus in the left heart or aorta through the intracardiac shunt before appearance of the bolus in the lungs, this method is not sensitive for the detection of such shunts, nor does it allow for accurate quantitation.

The magnitude of right-to-left shunts can be estimated by using an intravenous injection of the pulmonary perfusion radiopharmaceutical, ^{99m}Tc–macroaggregated albumin (MAA). In most patients, only about 4% to 6% of the injected ^{99m}Tc-MAA will bypass the lungs to localize in the capillaries of the systemic circulation. A whole-body scan, using regions of interest over the entire body and the lungs, allows an estimation of systemic activity, which is proportional to the size of the right-to-left shunt.

Equilibrium Radionuclide Angiography (Gated Blood Pool Ventriculography or MUGA Scans)
Principle
Equilibrium radionuclide angiography (E-RNA) or gated blood pool ventriculography consists of imaging the cardiac blood pool after the injected tracer has mixed thoroughly with the intravascular space. Images are typically obtained by synchronizing the gamma camera collection of data with the ECG signals from the patient at rest, but less commonly may be acquired during exercise or pharmacologic stress. Sophisticated, semi automated computer software is used to process the data, producing high quality cine images of the beating heart as well as a reproducible left ventricular volume curve from which ventricular functional parameters are derived. This output permits qualitative visual analysis of the size, configuration, and wall motion of the cardiac chambers and correlation with quantitative functional parameters of global and regional ventricular performance. Because the LV volume curve is based solely on LV blood pool count changes over the cardiac cycle, the LVEF derived is free of confounding geometric assumptions regarding LV shape and size and thus permits highly accurate, reproducible results.

Although E-RNA remains a valuable clinical technique, its use has significantly declined in recent years because of the widespread availability of echocardiography and the use of gated-SPECT myocardial perfusion imaging. However, when an accurate noninvasive determination of LVEF is desired, such as in patients in which echocardiography may be technically difficult, or when serial studies are needed to precisely monitor changes in LVEF, such as

during cardiotoxic chemotherapy, gated blood pool ventriculography can be quite useful.

Radiopharmaceutical
Basically, any radiopharmaceutical that is compartmentalized to the intravascular space for the time period required to obtain the study may be used. Technetium-99m labeled autologous red blood cells are the agent of choice.

Various methods of labeling autologous red blood cells with ^{99m}Tc have been described (see Appendix E-1), including in vivo, modified in vivo, and in vitro techniques. All methods use the initial introduction of stannous (tin) ion, which enters the red blood cells. The intracellular stannous ion then acts as a reducing agent, which permits the binding of subsequently introduced ^{99m}Tc-pertechnetate to the β-chain of the hemoglobin molecule. Superior labeling efficiency is obtained by using in vitro methods (such as the UltraTag method), in which the patient's blood sample is labeled externally and then reinjected, although, under most circumstances, adequate tagging of the red blood cells can be obtained by using in vivo methods.

The in vivo labeling procedure consists of intravenous injection of 0.5 to 1.0 mg of stannous ion, frequently as stannous pyrophosphate. After allowing the tin ion to equilibrate in the blood for 20 minutes, about 20 mCi (740 MBq) of ^{99m}Tc-pertechnetate is injected. With the tin acting as a complexing agent, a sufficient number of red blood cells are tagged in vivo to allow for labeling of the intravascular space. Although this technique provides sufficient tagging in most patients, a certain amount of injected ^{99m}Tc is rapidly lost from the intravascular space and does not participate in the labeling process. The percentage of injected technetium that remains intravascular and labels red blood cells is difficult to quantify but probably is about 75%. The percentage of radioisotope lost to the extravascular space contributes to longer imaging times as well as to background and thus to the degradation of images.

A modified in vivo technique provides for a combination of both in vivo and in vitro labeling procedures, giving a labeling efficiency of about 90%. This results in an increased intravascular concentration of ^{99m}Tc, with subsequent improvement in the quality of radionuclide images.

Because the technetium red blood cell bond lasts considerably longer than does the 6-hour half-life of ^{99m}Tc, the physical half-life of the radiopharmaceutical determines the length of time over which serial imaging is possible. With the use of 20 to 30 mCi (740 MBq to 1.11 GBq) of ^{99m}Tc-pertechnetate, delayed imaging is possible for up to 10 to 12 hours after injection.

Gated Planar Imaging Technique

Widespread use of cardiac ECG-gating was initially achieved in conjunction with equilibrium radionuclide angiography. The general principles involved have also been applied to gated-SPECT myocardial perfusion imaging as well.

After the cardiac blood pool has been labeled, gated images of the heart are obtained. Gating is performed by using a computer coupled with an R wave trigger or physiologic "gate" that signals the computer to begin recording data in the computer memory at the onset of the ECG R wave. This synchronizes the collection of data from the gamma camera with the onset of each cardiac cycle within the patient. The computer divides the R-R interval of each cardiac cycle into equal subdivisions, numbering from 16 to 32. Data collected from the scintillation camera are sorted during each cardiac contraction so that corresponding statistical information is filed temporally into one of the R-R interval segments, depending on its displacement in time from the initial R wave (Fig. 5-43). Such sorting of data over numerous cardiac cycles allows for the accumulation of enough statistical data in each interval subdivision to allow for creation of a series of single composite images, each representing one point of cardiac contraction.

When the sequence of individual images is subsequently played in cine format, an image of the blood in the chambers of the beating heart is produced, which represents a summation of the several hundred cardiac cycles needed to collect sufficient data. Images may be acquired for a certain number of counts ($\approx$3 to 6 million total counts) or, less frequently, for a set number of cardiac cycles. This gating process is the basis of all E-RNA and may be used in the collection of data from first-pass examinations as well.

Because of the inherent reliance of gated methodology on ECG input, the success of the technique is necessarily related to the consistency of cardiac rate and rhythm in a given patient. Ordinarily, because the length of systole does not change proportionally as the length of the cardiac cycle increases or

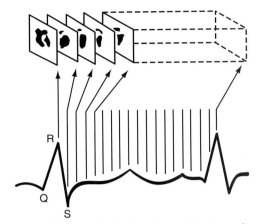

Figure 5-43. Gated technique for equilibrium radionuclide angiogram (E-RNA). Data collection is triggered by the R wave, with the cardiac cycle divided temporally into discrete frames. Counts arriving during any division are placed in the computer matrix relevant to that division. After several hundred cardiac cycles, there is enough information in each frame to form a useful image. These frames (images) can be sequentially viewed in a dynamic cine format as an endless loop of the same composite (summed) cardiac cycle replayed over and over.

decreases, minimal variations in heart rate during acquisition do not significantly affect the study. Severe disturbances in rhythm, however, cause distortion of the data obtained. Although a small number of aberrant cardiac cycles may be tolerated (<10%), as the number of such beats increases, there is a progressive degradation of the recorded data, which may give false information regarding such measurements as regional wall motion and LVEF. Computer software to access the quality of the data provides the operator with a histogram of distribution of the lengths of R-R intervals over the acquisition time of the study. In a patient with normal rhythm, the histogram demonstrates a single, well-defined peak. With aberrant beats, there are additional, smaller peaks (Fig. 5-44). These histograms allow for easy recognition of aberrant beats (Fig. 5-45).

In patients with occasional aberrant beats, the validity of the data may be preserved by *arrhythmia filtering* ("bad beat rejection"). This process allows for the rejection of cardiac cycles that do not conform to the average length of a cardiac cycle in a particular patient. However, because such arrhythmic information is excluded from the study, the time of acquisition for the examination increases. The most convenient method of arrhythmia filtering involves the use of

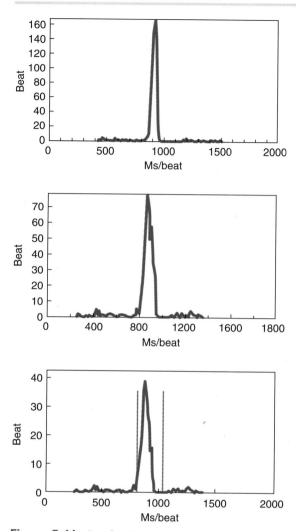

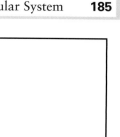

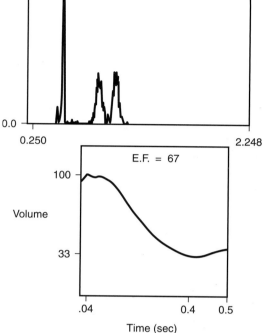

Figure 5-45. Cardiac arrhythmia. *Top,* The R-R histogram gives an indication of the number of normal and abnormal cardiac beats collected during gated equilibrium radionuclide angiography (E-RNA) based on variation of the lengths of their R-R intervals. The tall, thin peak is from the normal sinus rhythm. The lower, broader peaks correspond to aberrant beats with abnormally long R-R intervals. *Bottom,* A time-activity curve (left ventricular counts/volume curve) derived from these data is abnormal and does not return to baseline. This finding should raise the suspicion of a cardiac arrhythmia.

Figure 5-44. Gated technique, aberrant beat rejection. The histograms show the number of heart beats (cardiac cycles) collected during a gated acquisition which fall into different lengths (ms-milliseconds). At the *top* is a normal patient with no aberrant beats, so that all of the cardiac cycles are of the same length as noted by the sharp peak. In the *middle* is a patient with an arrhythmia, so that beats of longer and shorter length than normal can be seen on both sides of the normal peak. By selecting just the normal peak (*bottom*) between the two cut-off lines, the aberrant beats can be rejected from the data used to calculate LVEF and other functional parameters. *LVEF,* Left ventricular ejection fraction.

real-time list mode to hold the data briefly in a buffer while the R-R interval of a beat is measured. If the R-R interval is outside accepted limits (usually by ± 10% variation), the counts associated with the beat are rejected and thus do not contribute to the final image data set.

A high-resolution parallel-hole collimator may be used when performing planar E-RNA, provided that the count-rates are adequate.

This method provides the best spatial resolution for evaluation of regional wall motion. General low-energy, all-purpose, parallel-hole collimators may also be used at rest and provide a good compromise between sensitivity and resolution. General all-purpose and high-sensitivity collimators are often desirable for exercise studies because they provide increased sensitivity for the collection of images during the necessarily short intervals of exercise.

After the intravascular space has been labeled, resting studies usually require about 5 to 10 minutes per view, whereas exercise images are generally collected over several minutes. In resting studies, three views are normally obtained to allow for adequate visualization of the cardiac chambers and great vessels. These include (1) an anterior view, (2) a left anterior oblique ("best septal") view at about 45 degrees to visualize the septum and allow separation of the left and right ventricles (Fig. 5-46), and (3) a left lateral or 70-degree left anterior oblique view. A caudal tilt of the camera detector of about 10 degrees is recommended for acquisition of the 45-degree left anterior oblique view to maximize separation of the left ventricle from the left atrium. During exercise, usually only the 45-degree left anterior oblique view is imaged, to permit calculation of LVEF changes at various levels of stress.

Gated SPECT Imaging Technique

In addition to the routine planar imaging of the cardiac blood pool, gated-SPECT acquisition may be performed and the LV displayed as short- or long-axis tomographic slices or

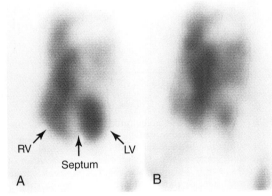

Figure 5-46. Normal gated equilibrium radionuclide angiogram (E-RNA). The views obtained in the left anterior oblique projection ("best septal view") depict **A,** end-diastole and **B,** end-systole. The right ventricle (*RV*), left ventricle (*LV*), and septum are easily identified.

three-dimensional volumetric images. Because of issues with overlapping cardiac chambers on planar images, imaging the cardiac blood pool using gated SPECT can be used to better isolate the structures of interest and allow more accurate assessment of motion in specific wall segments and calculation of individual chamber functional parameters (Fig. 5-47). Although not commonly used, it may be used to improve assessment of regional wall motion and to calculate absolute LV volumes as well as LVEF. In addition to more precise LVEFs obtained by excluding interfering left atrial activity, the method can also be used to measure RVEF without resorting to the more tedious first pass RNA methodology. It should be noted that the inherent differences between the planar and SPECT techniques can render significant discrepancy in the ejection fraction values obtained. LVEF is generally underestimated in planar mode, related to the persistent atrial activity in the systolic area of interest.

Elimination of such overlap using gated-SPECT often provides EF values greater than those using planar imaging. Thus a thorough understanding of the differences in normal values between SPECT and planar studies is necessary and should be considered in applying SPECT LVEF values in specific patient settings, such evaluating the effects of cardiotoxic chemotherapy

Image Interpretation

When E-RNA images are viewed cinematically in an endless-loop display, they present the image of the blood pool in a beating heart,

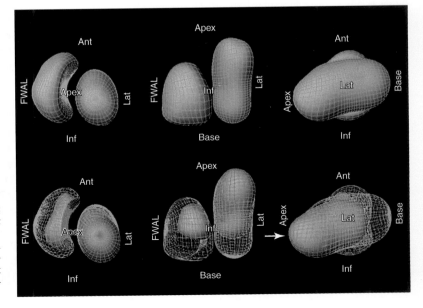

Figure 5-47. Gated SPECT E-RNA (blood pool ventriculogram). Gated SPECT of the cardiac blood pool can provide a better assessment of wall motion. These surface renderings of the cardiac blood pool show the right and left ventricles at end-diastole (*top row*) and end-systole (*bottom row*). In this patient, an area of focal dyskinesia at end-systole in the LV apex (*arrow*) is consistent with an aneurysm. *FWAL,* Free wall.

which can then be qualitatively and quantitatively analyzed by using various computer programs.

Qualitative Data. Cinematic computer display of gated images allows for the visual assessment of regional wall motion of both the left and right ventricles. In addition to ventricular wall excursion, relative sizes of the cardiac chambers, the size and position of the great vessels, the relative thicknesses of ventricular walls (particularly the septum) and the pericardial space, and any filling defects within the cardiac blood pool should be noted (Box 5-2).

Ventricular wall excursion is inferred by the impact of wall motion on the immediately adjacent portion of the blood-filled cavity. Once contraction begins, all ventricular wall segments should contract simultaneously, although some walls demonstrate greater absolute excursion than others. Generally, the anterior, posterior, and lateral walls appear to move to a greater degree than the septum, apex, and frequently the inferior wall.

Segmental wall motion abnormalities are usually described as *hypokinesis* (relatively diminished wall motion), *akinesis* (no wall motion), and *dyskinesis* (paradoxical wall motion). Areas of injured or scarred myocardium usually present as regions of hypokinesis or akinesis, whereas ventricular aneurysms appear as focal areas of dyskinesis. Lesions are localized as nearly as possible to particular segments of the LV wall by correlating the multiple views obtained. The evaluation of septal wall motion frequently presents a problem. Normally, the

---

Box 5-2   Gated Cardiac Equilibrium Blood Pool Imaging Visual Data Analysis

Quality of red blood cell labeling
Overall distribution of labeled red blood cells
Course and caliber of great vessels
Relative pulmonary blood pool activity
Thickness of pericardial–myocardial space
Shape and thickness of interventricular septum
Clot or mass within the cardiac chambers
Size of each chamber
Chamber wall motion
Sequence of chamber contraction

---

septum shortens or thickens and moves slightly toward the LV cavity during systole. Paradoxical septal motion (toward the right ventricle during systole) should be considered abnormal and is frequently associated with previous coronary artery bypass surgery or septal infarction.

Although wall motion abnormalities are almost always evident on visual inspection of cine images, the already described functional images generated by computer software may aid in the evaluation of regional wall motion.

Quantitative Data.

Systolic Function. By using a region of interest over the LV blood pool, a time activity curve is generated depicting the change in LV volume during the summed cardiac cycle. From this LV volume curve, LV functional parameters are derived. These include both systolic and diastolic indices, the most important of which is the LVEF.

In addition to LVEF and ejection rates, various other indices of LV function may be calculated as needed, including LV volumes and regional ejection fractions.

Because the LV is not temporally segregated from the other cardiac chambers, as in first-transit studies, a common problem for LVEF determination is the inclusion of a small amount of left atrium or left atrial appendage in the selected region of interest. Normally, the left atrium lies sufficiently posterior to the LV, so that counts within this chamber do not contribute significantly to LV activity. When the left atrium is enlarged, however, a portion of this structure may be included in the determination and falsely lower the ejection fraction. Differentiation of the LV from the atrium using gated SPECT E-RNA may give more precise results.

Unlike first-transit studies, right ventricular ejection fractions are often not reliably calculated from the equilibrium study because the right ventricle is not easily separated from the right atrium or an enlarged LV. If an accurate right ventricular ejection fraction is desired, it may be better obtained by performing a first-pass examination during the initial transit of the bolus at the beginning of the study. Furthermore, because data are obtained at equilibrium of the injected dose, shunt quantification is not possible with the gated blood pool technique.

Diastolic Function. Because diastolic dysfunction may precede abnormalities of systolic function (i.e., ejection fraction) in a variety of cardiac disease states, including CAD, quantitation of diastolic parameters may permit the early detection of LV functional impairment. The diastolic parameters available from the LV time-activity (volume) curve include ventricular filling and ejection rates. The most frequently derived LV diastolic parameter, peak filling rate (PFR), reflects the early, rapid-filling phase of diastole and is commonly seen as a measure of LV compliance. A normal PFR is usually greater than 2.5 end-diastolic volumes per second in young adults. Unlike LVEF, which remains relatively constant during aging, the PFR declines with age as compliance of the LV diminishes.

Diastolic dysfunction, as defined by parameters such as subnormal PFR, has been shown to occur in patients with CAD who have preserved systolic function (LVEF) and no evidence of active ischemia or previous infarction. Assessment of diastolic function parameters may also play an important role in the evaluation of congestive heart failure. About 40% of patients with a diagnosis of congestive heart failure demonstrate normal LV systolic function but impaired diastolic filling. Filling rate indices may be influenced by unrelated parameters, such as systolic ejection fraction and length of cardiac cycle, as well as by noncoronary diseases of the heart, including systemic hypertension, "normal" age-related decline in PFR, and anti-ischemic therapy.

Clinical Applications

Coronary Artery Disease. With the ascendancy of GSPECT myocardial perfusion imaging as the preferred radionuclide method for the diagnosis of suspected CAD and the risk stratification of patients with known CAD, the use of E-RNA in these settings has significantly declined, because LV perfusion and function are now available in a single test.

However, true resting LVEF in patients with known CAD obtained by either method remains a significant indicator of long-term prognosis in patients with stable CAD. Prognosis deteriorates as the LVEF at rest falls below 45% to 50%. Conversely, event rates are low in patients with normal resting LVEF.

Exercise or pharmacologic stress RNA is uncommonly used, using either first-pass or equilibrium technique, to obtain prognostic information in patients with known CAD. Most protocols involve an initial resting baseline determination of ventricular wall motion and ejection fraction, with subsequent serial images obtained over a period of stepwise increases in stress. Failure of the LVEF to rise by 5%, or a decrease during peak exercise, is considered abnormal. A decline in LVEF in response to stress or an abnormal peak exercise LVEF is an important indication of the severity of CAD and confers a worse prognosis. Further, a peak exercise LVEF of less that 30% indicates a high risk of future adverse cardiac events and reduced survival.

Myocardial Infarction. Prognosis after myocardial infarction is related to infarct size as reflected by global LVEF and extent and degree of wall motion abnormalities. Large infarcts may produce extensive wall motion abnormalities with significantly decreased LVEFs, whereas smaller injuries may produce only focal wall motion impairment with a normal or slightly decreased LVEF or no abnormality at all. Anterior infarcts generally lower LVEF to a greater degree than do inferior wall lesions.

The resting LVEF as determined by gated radionuclide ventriculography has proved to be a reliable measure of the impact of coronary occlusion on LV function in early myocardial infarction and, as such, has shown to be an important predictor of prognosis. In this setting, an ejection fraction of 0.30 during the first 24 hours after infarction appears to represent a watershed, with about 50% of the patients with values at or below this level succumbing to LV failure or death. This represents a nearly ninefold higher mortality rate than is seen in patients with a LVEF of greater than 30%. Conversely, only about 2% of patients with higher ejection fractions die acutely. During early recovery from the initial insult, a predischarge resting LVEF of 40% or less remains a potent predictor of future events and death, with the 1-year mortality rate increasing exponentially as the resting LVEF falls below 0.40.

Noncoronary Disease. Characteristic findings on gated blood pool imaging in patients with noncoronary heart disease are shown in Table 5-4. Radionuclide ventriculography may aid in the differential diagnosis of cardiopulmonary disease by helping distinguish dyspnea related to primary LV failure from that caused by chronic pulmonary disease, when differentiation on clinical grounds is not possible. Right ventricular dysfunction and cardiac chamber dilatation with a normal left ventricle are usually

TABLE 5-4	Characteristic Findings on Gated Blood Pool Imaging in Patients with Noncoronary Heart Disease
LESIONS	**FINDINGS**
Valvular	
Aortic regurgitation	Dilated LV cavity with hypertrophy; normal or decreased LVEF
Aortic stenosis	Normal LV cavity and LVEF; LV hypertrophy; dilated LA
Mitral regurgitation	Dilated LV cavity and normal or decreased LVEF; normal LV wall thickness; dilated LA
Tricuspid regurgitation	Dilated RV cavity and decreased RVEF; dilated RA
Hypertensive	
	LV concentric hypertrophy; normal or supranormal LVEF; diastolic dysfunction
Cardiomyopathy	
Dilated (congestive)	Dilatation of all four chambers; decreased LVEF and RVEF; decreased LV wall thickness
Ischemic	Normal or dilated LV cavity and decreased LVEF; decreased LV wall thickness; normal or dilated LA
Hypertrophic	Normal or small LV cavity; normal or supranormal LVEF; severe LV hypertrophy; normal or dilated LA
Restrictive	Normal LV cavity and normal or decreased LVEF; normal or increased RV cavity and normal or decreased RVEF
Septal defect	
Atrial	Dilated RV cavity and decreased RVEF; dilated RA with normal or dilated LA
Ventricular	Normal or increased LV cavity and normal or increased LVEF; dilated RV and normal or decreased RVEF; dilated LA

EF, Ejection fraction; *LA,* left atrium; *LV,* left ventricle; *RA,* right atrium; *RV,* right ventricle.

associated with chronic obstructive pulmonary disease, whereas pulmonary vascular congestion related to LV failure is accompanied by LV enlargement or functional abnormalities. In patients with known chronic obstructive pulmonary disease, a resting right ventricular ejection fraction of less than 0.35 is a relatively sensitive predictor of pulmonary artery hypertension.

Chemotherapeutic Cardiotoxicity. E-RNA is used in monitoring LV function in patients receiving cardiotoxic chemotherapy agents, principally because the technique is capable of detecting small serial reductions in LVEF with reproducible results.

The most common setting in this regard is the serial assessment of LVEFs to monitor the dose-related cardiotoxicity of anthracyclines, such as doxorubicin, during the course of treatment. The study is of use in selecting patients who may best tolerate the medication and in monitoring those who receive it to determine the onset of cardiac toxicity. Patients receiving doxorubicin usually do not have toxic cardiac responses below cumulative doses of about 400 mg/m2. With increasing dose, however, a largely irreversible dilated cardiomyopathy may result with diminished LV function, ultimately leading to congestive cardiac failure. Because administration of doxorubicin produces an acute transient reduction of LVEF, in addition to long-term toxicity, serial measurements should be taken about 2 weeks after the last dose to allow recovery to occur and to determine the new baseline value.

LVEF should be obtained in patients before doxorubicin therapy is begun to obtain a baseline value. This is especially important in patients with suspected or known cardiac dysfunction who are at greater risk of developing CHF. Doxorubicin therapy is initiated with special caution in patients with ejection fractions below the normal range. Parameters predictive of developing cardiotoxic CHF include a baseline LVEF less than 55%; a drop from baseline LVEF to 50% or less, and advancing age. A reduction from baseline LVEF of 10% or 5 ejection fraction units or to below 45% is usually considered significant. Frank congestive heart failure is preceded by a progressive fall in LVEF. Serial radionuclide studies permit the withdrawal of doxorubicin therapy in these patients, thereby preventing life-threatening cardiac complications.

Cardiomyopathy. Cardiomyopathies constitute a group of heterogeneous primary myocardial diseases usually classified as dilated, hypertrophic, or restrictive. Gated blood pool imaging has proved useful not only in detecting cardiomyopathies but also in evaluating the degree of systolic or diastolic functional impairment and assessing the effects of medical therapy. Hypertrophic cardiomyopathy typically presents with a normal or elevated LVEF and hyperdynamic systolic function, with evidence of ventricular wall thickening, especially in the basal interventricular septum, and a concomitantly small LV cavity. Eighty percent or more of these patients exhibit impaired diastolic function. Dilated cardiomyopathies typically present with LV chamber dilatation and diffuse hypokinesis, with a reduced LVEF of less than 40% (Fig. 5-48). Right ventricular dysfunction and dilatation may also be present. Generally, marked biventricular enlargement with global dysfunction is more likely to be of nonischemic origin, whereas the presence of focal left ventricular wall motion abnormalities and relatively preserved right ventricular function favor a diagnosis of ischemic cardiomyopathy.

Congestive Heart Failure. Although echocardiography is the initial procedure of choice in the evaluation of cardiac function in the setting of CHF, when E-RNA is performed, both LVEF and LV diastolic function should be assessed. Approximately 30% of patients presenting with congestive heart failure have isolated or predominant diastolic dysfunction, with hypertensive hypertrophic cardiomyopathy being the underlying cause in a large number. The E-RNA findings include a normal LV cavity, normal LVEF, and impaired LV filing as measured by a reduced PFR and exaggerated time to peak filling. Because the treatment for diastolic LV failure is different from primary systolic failure, this distinction has important therapeutic implications.

Cardiac Valvular Disease. In general, two-dimensional Doppler echocardiography is the procedure of choice in noninvasive evaluation of suspected valvular cardiac disease, although nuclear methods may be useful in some settings. In practice, E-RNA is not commonly used to evaluate valvular stenosis but may play a role in the assessment of valvular insufficiency. In patients with aortic or mitral regurgitation, as the resting LVEF declines below about 55%, patient prognosis worsens.

In patients with idiopathic hypertrophic subaortic stenosis, radionuclide findings include a markedly elevated LVEF and small LV cavity, with asymmetric thickening of the upper portion of the ventricular septum.

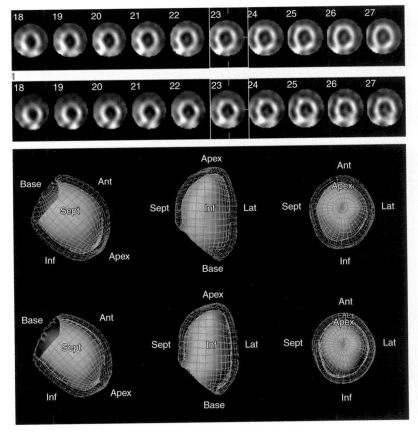

Figure 5-48. Dilated cardiomyopathy. This gated SPECT ^{99m}Tc sestamibi myocardial perfusion scan shows a persistently dilated left ventricle (LV) cavity with diffuse hypokinesia of the LV wall consistent with a dilated cardiomyopathy. No areas of myocardial ischemia are seen to indicate significant coronary artery disease.

PEARLS & PITFALLS

Myocardial Perfusion Studies

- The common indication for myocardial perfusion studies is to determine whether there is normal perfusion, ischemia, or infarction. The images obtained represent relative, not absolute blood flow.

- Technetium-99m sestamibi and tetrofosmin have a higher photon energy (140 keV) than do the mercury daughter x-rays (69 to 81 keV) from ^{201}Tl. As a result, there is less soft-tissue attenuation with ^{99m}Tc-labeled radiopharmaceuticals than with thallium.

- Myocardial uptake of ^{201}Tl-chloride and ^{99m}Tc-sestamibi or tetrofosmin is proportional to regional blood flow and requires cell viability.

- Thallium is actively taken up by the Na^+-K^+ pump in the cells, whereas ^{99m}Tc sestamibi and tetrofosmin passively diffuse across the membrane and localize primarily in cytoplasmic mitochondria.

- Thallium redistributes over time, so post-stress images must be obtained immediately after injection. Technetium-99m sestamibi and tetrofosmin do not redistribute, and the best images are made 30 to 90 minutes after injection to allow for clearance of interfering background activity from the liver but before the activity reaches the transverse colon.

- Infarcts and hibernating myocardium produce perfusion defects on the rest images.

- Stress images are needed to elucidate ischemia with lesser degrees of stenosis (50% to 90%). Stenoses less than 50% in diameter are not detected at rest and are variably diagnosed with exercise imaging.

- Stress may be physical or pharmacologic. Physical stress should be discontinued with patient exhaustion, claudication, severe angina or hypotension, arrhythmia or severe ECG changes, or attainment of more than 85% of maximal predicted heart rate (220 minus the patient's age in years).

- Dipyridamole, adenosine, and regadenoson are used instead of physical stress to dilate normal coronary arteries. Vessels in ischemic areas are already maximally dilated and do not dilate further.

- The adverse effects of dipyridamole are reversed with 100 to 200 mg of intravenous aminophylline. Dipyridamole and adenosine should not be used in patients with asthma or reactive airway diseases.

- Dobutamine is inotropic and chronotropic and is used as a form of pharmacologic stress. Adverse effects may be reversed by using short-acting β-blockers.

- The most common cause of false-negative examinations is submaximal stress. The most common cause of false-positive examinations is artifacts.

- The myocardium normally thins at the cardiac apex, in the membranous septum, and near the base of the inferior wall.

- A high degree of lung activity on exercise thallium images (greater than 50% of peak myocardial activity) is related to poor prognosis, more extensive disease, and LV dysfunction at exercise. On ^{99m}Tc sestamibi scans, lung activity is uncommon. When seen, its significance is unknown.

- Transient LV dilatation with exercise may be related primarily to subendocardial ischemia and less often to real LV dilatation. It is a sign of a multivessel CAD and poor prognosis.

- With adequate exercise, the sensitivity and specificity of myocardial SPECT are each about 85%.

- An occluded coronary artery with adequate collaterals or balanced three-vessel disease can produce an apparently normal scan.

- Real defects on myocardial perfusion images should be seen on at least two views (e.g., short and vertical or horizontal long axes).

- Defects seen at stress but not at rest are usually (but not always) ischemia. However, LBBB may produce reversible septal defects, mimicking ischemia. Patents with LBBB should be stressed with vasodilators, not by exercise or dobutamine, to avoid this artifact.

- A defect seen at the base of the heart is frequently artifactual unless it extends to the apex.

Continued

PEARLS & PITFALLS—cont'd

- Not all fixed defects (seen both at rest and post-stress) are infarcts or scars. They may also be soft-tissue attenuation artifacts, or hibernating or repetitively stunned myocardium.

- Hibernating myocardium is a chronically hypo-perfused myocardial segment that has reduced cellular metabolism and regionally decreased contractility. Revascularization is usually needed.

- Hibernating myocardium presents as a per-fusion-metabolism mismatch: a defect on myocardial perfusion imaging and F-18 FDG uptake on PET imaging, or as a perfusion defect with delayed Thallium-201 uptake on SPECT imaging.

- Stunned myocardium is due to an acute coronary occlusion with relatively rapid perfusion return. These myocardial segments have normal or near-normal perfusion and decreased contractility. Revascularization is not usually needed.

- Defects seen on rest (redistribution) images but not on post-stress images (reverse redistribution) are real but of uncertain cause and significance. They frequently are associated with prior myocardial injury or revascularization procedures.

- LV walls that diverge toward the apex should raise suspicion of a LV aneurysm.

- Diaphragmatic attenuation looks like an inferior wall defect. It often goes away on prone images.

- Diaphragmatic (cardiac) creep presents as a reversible inferior wall defect.

- Relatively intense gastrointestinal activity adjacent to the inferior wall can cause an apparent inferior myocardial defect on SPECT studies as a result of a reconstruction artifact.

- Breast attenuation usually causes an apparent defect in the anterior or lateral LV wall.

- Bull's eye plots underestimate apical defects and overestimate basal defects.

- GSPECT markers of high-risk CAD include the following: multiple perfusion defects indicative of multivessel disease; large, severe perfusion defects; transient LV dilatation; increased thallium lung/heart ratio; end-systolic volume (ESV) (greater than 70 mL); and a post-stress LVEF less than 40%.

- Compared to SPECT, PET myocardial perfusion imaging is more accurate, has a lower patient radiation dose, and can be completed in a shorter time period. Its costs are higher and the procedures more complex.

Equilibrium Radionuclide Angiography
- Gated equilibrium radionuclide angiograms (MUGA scans) are performed with ^{99m}Tc red blood cells. Common indications include assessment of LVEF and regional wall motion.

- The normal LVEF is 50% to 65%. The lower limit is 50% in older people. Ejection fractions higher than 70% may reflect hypertrophy, valvular regurgitation, or idiopathic hypertrophic subaortic stenosis (IHSS).

- The normal right ventricular ejection fraction is 40% to 50%.

- A time-activity (gated E-RNA LV volume) curve that does not come back to baseline may be due to a cardiac arrhythmia. Inspection of the R-R histogram reveals multiple peaks. More than 10% rejected beats will result in an inaccurate LVEF calculation.

- If the left anterior oblique view (best septal view) is not precise, overlap of the left ventricle with the left atrial appendage, right ventricle, or the great vessels may cause a falsely low LVEF. Oversubtraction of background will cause a falsely high LVEF.

- Regional wall motion abnormalities on a resting MUGA scan are usually due to myocardial infarction but may be seen in stunned or hibernating myocardium.

- A photopenic halo around the cardiac blood pool activity is usually due to a pericardial effusion.

SUGGESTED READINGS

Abraham A, Nichol G, Williams K, et al. ^{18}F-FDG PET imaging of myocardial viability in an experienced center with access to ^{18}F-FDG and integration with clinical management teams: the Ottawa-FIVE substudy of the PARR 2 trial. J Nucl Med 2010;51(4):567-74.

Baggish AL, Boucher CA. Radiopharmaceutical agents for myocardial perfusion imaging. Circulation 2008; 118(16):1668-74.

Bateman TM, Heller GV, McGhie AI, et al. Diagnostic accuracy of rest/stress ECG-gated Rb-82 myocardial perfusion PET: comparison with ECG gated Tc-99m sestamibi SPECT. J Nucl Cardiol 2006;13:24-33.

Botvinick EH. Current methods of pharmacologic stress testing and the potential advantages of new agents. J Nucl Med Technol 2009;37(1):14-25.

Einstein AJ, Moser KW, Thompson RC, et al. Radiation dose to patients from cardiac diagnostic imaging. Circulation 2007;116(11):1290-305.

Go V, Bhatt MR, Hendel RC. The diagnostic and prognostic value of ECG-Gated SPECT myocardial perfusion imaging. J Nucl Med 2004;45:912-21.

Hachamovitch R, Berman DS. The use of nuclear cardiology in clinical decision making. Semin Nucl Med 2005;35:62-72.

Machac J. Cardiac positron emission tomography imaging. Semin Nucl Med 2005;35(1):17-36.

Meine TJ, Hanson MW, Borges-Neto S. The additive value of combined assessment of myocardial perfusion and ventricular function studies. J Nucl Med 2004;45: 1721-4.

Nichols KJ, Van Tosh A, Wang Y, Palestro CJ, Reichek N. Validation of gated blood-pool SPECT regional left ventricular function measurements. J Nucl Med 2009;50(1): 53-60.

Paul AK, Nabi HA. Gated myocardial perfusion SPECT: basic principles, technical aspects, and clinical applications. J Nucl Med Technol 2004;32:179-87.

Salerno M, Beller G. Noninvasive assessment of myocardial perfusion. Circ Cardiovasc Imaging 2009;2(5):412-24.

Stabin MG. Proposed revision to the radiation dosimetry of [82]Rb. Health Phys 2010;99(6):811-3.

Travin MI, Bergmann SR. Assessment of myocardial viability. Semin Nucl Med 2005;35:2-16.

6 Respiratory System

Radionuclide lung imaging most commonly involves the demonstration of pulmonary perfusion using limited capillary blockade, as well as the assessment of ventilation using inspired inert gas, usually xenon, or technetium-99m (^{99m}Tc)-labeled aerosols. Although these studies are essentially qualitative, they have an advantage over most quantitative tests of global lung function in distinguishing between diffuse and regional pulmonary disease. Most significantly, the ability to display both regional airway and vascular integrity forms the basis for the noninvasive diagnosis of pulmonary emboli. Ventilation (V) and perfusion (Q) scans are often referred to as *V/Q scans*. Evaluation of lung cancer and staging are discussed in Chapter 11 on positron-emission tomography (PET) scanning. Some aspects of pulmonary infection and inflammation imaging are presented in Chapter 12.

ANATOMY AND PHYSIOLOGY

The trachea divides into the right and left mainstem bronchi, and these, in turn, divide to form lobar bronchi. The lobar divisions on the right are the upper-, middle-, and lower-lobe bronchi; on the left, there are just upper- and lower-lobe bronchi. The lobes are further divided into segments based on bronchopulmonary anatomy, which are shown in Figure 6-1. Knowledge of the anatomy of the lobes and segments of the lungs is essential for accurate interpretation of radionuclide pulmonary images.

Inspiration produces a negative intrapleural pressure, which is generated by action of the thoracic cage musculature and the diaphragm. Each terminal respiratory unit or alveolus is elastic, and this elasticity provides the major impetus for expiration. Adults have about 250 to 400 million alveoli, with an average diameter of 150 μm per alveolus. It is important to remember that the direct anatomic pathway is not the only means by which air can enter the alveoli. If a bronchiole is blocked, air may get into the distal alveoli through the pores of Kohn, which provide direct communication between neighboring alveoli. In addition, the canals of Lambert connect the respiratory bronchioles and alveolar ducts. Both of these indirect pathways allow collateral ventilation in the peripheral lung and often prevent collapse of an obstructed pulmonary segment or segments.

The main pulmonary arteries divide in each lung to follow the divisions of the bronchi and bronchioles to the level of the alveoli. Each alveolus is supplied by a terminal pulmonary arteriole, which, in turn, gives rise to capillaries. The capillaries that surround the alveoli are between 7 and 10 μm in diameter. The lungs also receive blood from the aorta via the bronchial arteries, which follow the bronchial tree as far as the respiratory bronchioles. The bronchial arteries anastomose at the capillary level with the pulmonary circulation, and most of the blood from

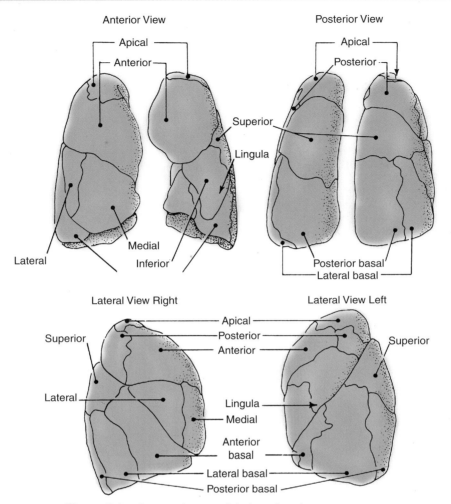

Figure 6-1. Schematic diagram of the bronchopulmonary segments.

the bronchial arteries returns to the left atrium via the pulmonary veins. The bronchial circulation supplies about 5% of the blood flow to the lung under normal circumstances.

Gravity and patient position have a significant impact on both ventilation and perfusion. However, the alteration of blood flow throughout the lungs with positional change is much more marked than accompanying changes in ventilation. In the upright position, intrapleural pressure is significantly more negative at the apices than at the lung bases. As a result of this negative pressure difference, the upper lung zone alveoli are held more open in expiration than are the lower lung alveoli, which are relatively collapsed. The increased potential volume in the lung bases provides a greater change in alveolus size during inspiration than at the apices, with the net effect

that ventilation (air exchange) is greater in the lower lungs. Normally, ventilation in the lower portion of the lung is about 150% of that in the apex.

Pulmonary perfusion is also unevenly distributed throughout the lungs. Maximal pulmonary blood flow normally occurs in the lung zone bracketing the junction of the lower third and upper two thirds of the lungs. In the upright position, the apex receives only about one third of the blood flow per unit volume as compared with the bases. In the supine position, however, perfusion is more uniform, although again there is relatively increased blood flow in the dependent portions of the lung. In patients who demonstrate more flow to the upper lobes, congestive failure with increased left atrial pressure or α_1-antitrypsin deficiency should be considered.

Thus in the normal, upright patient, both ventilation and perfusion increase progressively from the lung apex to the bases, although this gradient is more pronounced for perfusion. Because ventilation increases much less rapidly from apex to base, the ventilation/perfusion ratio changes in the reverse direction, increasing from base to apex. In the supine position, both ventilation and perfusion gradients are less pronounced, resulting in more even ventilation and perfusion throughout the lungs.

Uncommonly, acute changes in perfusion affect ventilation; local ischemia and hypoxia can cause reflex bronchoconstriction, with a resulting shift of ventilation away from the hypoperfused areas. However, this phenomenon appears to be transient and is uncommonly demonstrated in humans. Conversely, abnormalities of ventilation commonly cause redistribution of pulmonary perfusion; hypoventilation leads to regional hypoxia and reflex vasoconstriction with redistribution of perfusion away from the hypoventilated regions.

RADIOPHARMACEUTICALS
Perfusion Imaging Agents
Technetium-99m (^{99m}Tc) macroaggregated albumin (MAA) is the radiopharmaceutical used for pulmonary perfusion imaging. It localizes by the mechanism of capillary blockade. In general, fewer than 1 in 1000 (<0.1%) of the capillaries are blocked. In the absence of shunts, 95% of the particles are removed from the circulation on the first pass through the pulmonary capillary bed. About 5% of particles measure less than 5 μm in diameter and pass through the capillary system. For purposes of pulmonary perfusion imaging, it is important to use a sufficient number of particles to allow for good statistical distribution. In general, injection of a minimum of 100,000 particles and optimally between 200,000 and 600,000 particles is required.

The production of ^{99m}Tc-MAA entails aggregation of human serum albumin using heat and a reducing agent to form the particles. Visual inspection of the preparations through the use of a microscope and hemocytometer demonstrate whether the MAA particles are too large or have clumped. The particle size of ^{99m}Tc-MAA generally ranges from 5 to 100 μm, with most in the range of 10 to 30 μm. MAA has a biologic half-life in the lung of 2 to 4 hours, depending on the kit manufacturer and preparation. Some preparations begin to break down as early as 30 minutes after injection. The particle fragments enter the general circulation as smaller particles, which are usually removed from the circulation by the liver and spleen. The normal administered activity in adults is 3 to 5 mCi (111 to 185 MBq); in children 0.03 to 0.07 mCi (1.1 to 2.6 MBq)/kg. The lung is the critical organ. The absorbed dose to the lung is variable but is about 0.5 rad (5 mGy) for a 3-mCi (111-MBq) dose.

Technetium-99m MAA should be injected during quiet respiration, with the patient supine to minimize the normal perfusion gradient between the apex and lung base. Because the MAA particles tend to settle out in solution, the syringe should be gently agitated before injection to ensure even mixing. A peripheral vein is preferred, and administration through a Swan-Ganz catheter or any indwelling catheter port containing a filter generally should be avoided. To assist in homogeneous pulmonary distribution of the particles, injection should be made slowly, usually over three to five or more respiratory cycles, and the injected volume should be at least 1 to 2 mL. If blood is drawn into the syringe to confirm an intravascular needle location, it is important not to let the blood sit long in the syringe because this may allow the formation of small, clinically insignificant, labeled blood clots, which, when injected, result in focal hot spots on the perfusion scan (Fig. 6-2).

A relative contraindication to performing particulate perfusion lung scans is severe pulmonary hypertension because the blockade of additional lung capillaries may acutely exacerbate the condition and its cardiac complications. Care should also be taken in patients with known right-to-left shunts, although adverse effects on the coronary or cerebral circulations have rarely been observed. In these patients, however, as well as in infants and children, it is probably prudent to reduce the number of injected particles to 100,000 to 200,000. The presence of a right-to-left shunt can be easily recognized on posterior images by the immediate presence of renal activity, usually best seen on the posterior or lateral views, and can be confirmed by the demonstration of activity in the brain (Fig. 6-3). Sample imaging protocols and dosimetry are presented in Appendix E-1.

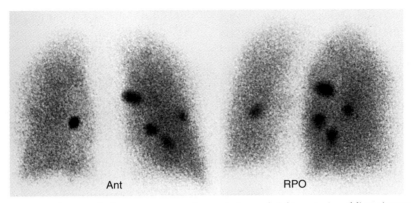

Figure 6-2. Hot spots on a lung perfusion scan seen on the posterior and right posterior oblique images. These represent labeled clots that formed when blood was inadvertently drawn into the syringe containing technetium-99m macroaggregated albumin (MAA) before injection. Note the relative decrease in activity in the remainder of the lungs, which could hamper detection of perfusion abnormalities.

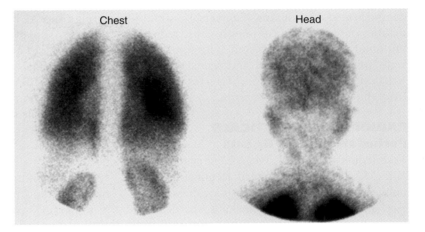

Figure 6-3. Right-to-left shunt. Two posterior images from a perfusion lung scan show ^{99m}Tc-macroaggregated albumin in the capillary bed of both the kidneys and the brain. No activity is seen in the thyroid or stomach, so this cannot be the result of free technetium pertechnetate (^{99m}TcO$_4$).

Ventilation Imaging Agents
Radiolabeled Aerosols

Technetium-labeled radioactive aerosols are commonly used to image ventilation. Unlike ventilation studies using radioactive gases, aerosol studies do not allow for dynamic single-breath or washout phase imaging but rather map the distribution of aerated lung volume. Once deposited in the lungs, the aerosol particles remain in place for sufficient time to permit imaging in multiple projections. Preparation of ^{99m}Tc-DTPA aerosol begins with the injection of about 30 mCi (1.1 GBq) of ^{99m}Tc–diethylene-triamine pentaacetic acid (DTPA) in a volume of 2 mL into the nebulizer of an aerosol delivery system. Oxygen tubing is then connected to the side port, and oxygen is supplied through a flow meter. Flow rates are in the range of 7 to 10 L/min. A mouthpiece with a nose clip is then used to administer the aerosol. If necessary, this can be connected to an endotracheal tube. The patient is usually in a supine position (which allows for an even distribution of aerosol) and breathes at tidal volume for 3 to 5 minutes.

The aerosols usually have a mean aerodynamic diameter of about 0.5 μm. The half-time clearance time from the lungs is 45 to 60 minutes in nonsmokers and 20 minutes in smokers. The larger the particle size, the more central its deposition in the bronchial tree. Central deposition is also common in patients with COPD, probably owing to turbulent flow in the central airways compared with that of normal people. The ^{99m}Tc-DTPA aerosol for ventilation imaging has several advantages, the most notable of which are the ready availability of ^{99m}Tc and its ideal imaging energy. Little patient cooperation is required. The aerosol can be delivered in a room separate from the camera room and can easily be delivered through mechanical ventilators or during normal tidal breathing. There is no need for special exhaust systems or traps, and, thus it can be used on a portable basis in intensive care units.

In most patients, DTPA aerosol particles cross the alveolar-capillary membrane with a half-time of about 1 hour, enter the pulmonary circulation, and from there are rapidly cleared by the kidneys. In smokers, clearance is significantly accelerated because of increased alveolar membrane permeability.

One of the major disadvantages in the use of ^{99m}Tc-DTPA aerosols is the small amount of activity actually delivered to the patient (2% to 10%) compared with that available in the aerosol generator. Usually about 30 mCi (1.11 GBq) is placed in the system nebulizer, with only 1 or 2 mCi (37 to 74 MBq) actually being delivered to the patient. Because both MAA and DTPA aerosols are labeled with ^{99m}Tc, sequential imaging of ventilation and perfusion requires the relative doses of each to be adjusted to prevent interference of one ^{99m}Tc-labeled agent with the other when imaging is performed.

Radioactive Gases

The use of radioactive inert gases to evaluate ventilation permits sequential imaging of both lung ventilation and perfusion in conjunction with ^{99m}Tc-MAA because of the rapid clearance of the gases from the lungs and the relative energy differences of the photon emissions.

Xenon-133 (^{133}Xe) is the primary isotope used for assessment of ventilation. It is relatively inexpensive and has a half-life of 5.3 days and a principal gamma ray energy of 81 keV. The low energy of these photons causes about half of them to be attenuated by 10 cm of inflated lung tissue. Thus overlying soft tissues, such as breasts, can produce substantial artifacts; these are usually avoided by performing xenon ventilation scans in the posterior position. The critical organ for ^{133}Xe is the trachea. Xenon-133 allows for the assessment of all phases of regional ventilation: initial single breath, wash-in, equilibrium, and washout. Single-breath images represent instant ventilation, wash-in and equilibrium images are proportional to aerated lung volume, and washout phases show regional clearance of activity from the lungs and delineate areas of air trapping. This complete characterization of ventilation renders ^{133}Xe imaging the most sensitive ventilation study for detection and assessment of airways disease.

Ventilation examinations are generally performed either to assess regional ventilation or to improve the specificity of a perfusion scan. Ventilation imaging using ^{133}Xe is limited in that images are usually obtained in only one projection and are performed before the perfusion study. The use of a single projection image ensures that some regional ventilation abnormalities will be missed because the lungs are not entirely imaged.

The ventilation study is usually performed before the perfusion scan using upright posterior views. The posterior view is selected because it is technically convenient and allows a ventilation survey of the greatest number of pulmonary segments with the least amount of overlying soft tissue. Although there are several common methods of performing ventilation imaging, the most complete involves three phases: (1) single wash-in or initial breath, (2) equilibrium, and (3) washout. Ventilation imaging with ^{133}Xe requires a considerable amount of patient cooperation because the patient must be able to tolerate breathing on a closed spirometer system for several minutes to reach equilibrium.

The single-breath phase involves having the patient exhale as deeply as possible and then inhale 10 to 20 mCi (370 to 740 MBq) of ^{133}Xe, holding his or her breath for about 15 seconds while a static image is taken. The equilibrium phase constitutes the rebreathing of the expired xenon diluted by about 2 L of oxygen contained in a closed system. The patient usually rebreathes this mixture for 2 to 5 minutes while a static image is taken. Thus, the ^{133}Xe image obtained at equilibrium essentially represents the distribution of aerated lung volume. After equilibrium is reached, fresh air is then breathed during the washout phase while serial 15-second images are obtained for 2 to 3 minutes as the xenon clears from the lungs. In patients with chronic obstructive pulmonary disease (COPD), the washout phase may be prolonged to 3 to 5 minutes, if necessary, to assess areas of regional airway trapping.

Xenon-133 is usually administered by using one of a number of commercially available delivery and rebreathing units. These generally allow the disposal of expired xenon by one of two methods. The simplest way is to exhaust the xenon to the atmosphere using a dedicated exhaust system. A more common method is to use an activated charcoal trap to accumulate the exhaled xenon gas until it has decayed to background. Although not required by specific regulation, ^{133}Xe imaging is optimally performed in a room with negative pressure in case of accidental leakage from the closed system, especially during administration to the patient. The exhaust vent should be placed near the floor because xenon is heavier than air.

Krypton-81m (^{81m}Kr) has also been advocated for use in ventilation imaging. Krypton-81m has a half-life of 13 seconds, with photon emissions between 176 and 192 keV. Krypton generators using the parent isotope rubidium-81 (^{81}Rb) are available, but they have a short shelf-life (half-life, 4.6 hours) and are therefore inconvenient. Unlike ^{133}Xe, ^{81m}Kr can be used in a continuous steady-state inhalation technique that is proportional to regional ventilatory rate rather than to lung volume; thus multiple images with good statistical information can be obtained. Because of its higher-energy photon emissions compared with ^{99m}Tc-MAA, ^{81m}Kr ventilation studies can be performed either before or after perfusion imaging, and the short half-life permits repeat studies to correlate with any specific perfusion views. The short half-life of ^{81m}Kr, however, precludes single-breath and washout images. In addition, ^{81m}Kr is expensive, limited in availability, and thus rarely used in clinical practice.

Another agent ^{99m}Tc-Technegas (Cyclomedica) consists of ultrafine carbon particles that behave physiologically like a gas at wash-in but lodge in alveoli. This agent is not currently available the United States.

TECHNIQUE

Sample technique protocols and dosimetry are presented in Appendix E-1.

Because most clinical situations dictate the performance of both ventilation and perfusion studies, the question may arise as to which study to perform first. When ^{99m}Tc-DTPA aerosol is used, the relative doses of ^{99m}Tc-MAA and the ^{99m}Tc-DTPA aerosol must be adjusted, with a reduction in the dose of the initial examination, depending on which is performed first. When ^{133}Xe gas is used, it is customary to begin with the ventilations because of the lower photon energy of xenon and its rapid clearance from the lungs. The disadvantage of this order is that the ventilation study may not have been performed in the projection that best

evaluates the region of a subsequently demonstrated perfusion defect. If the perfusion study is performed first and followed by the ventilation examination, it is helpful to decrease the dose of ^{99m}Tc-MAA and increase the dose of ^{133}Xe. This minimizes the effect of any Compton scatter from the ^{99m}Tc that may occur in the xenon window of the pulse height analyzer and degrade the ventilation images.

A number of authors have shown that the accuracy of lung scans can be improved somewhat by performing SPECT lung imaging (so called SPECT V/Q or V/P$_{SPECT}$). Xenon cannot be used for SPECT ventilation studies but ^{99m}Tc-DTPA aerosol and Technegas (in Europe) can be used. Other described techniques include SPECT V/Q combined with low-dose lung computed tomography (CT) and SPECT ^{99m}Tc-MAA perfusion images fused with CT. At the present time, there are a limited number of clinical comparison studies, and these more complicated techniques are not commonly available except during regular working hours.

NORMAL LUNG SCAN
Perfusion Scan

A normal perfusion scan is shown in Figure 6-4. In the posterior projection, there is some tapering of activity toward the bases as a result of the thinning of the lungs in the region of the posterior sulci. In the anterior view, the cardiac silhouette and the aortic knob are commonly identified. The left lateral view may show a substantial anterior defect because of the heart. A cardiac silhouette considerably larger than expected from the chest radiograph may occasionally be produced by hypermobility of the heart when lateral images are obtained, especially in the decubitus positions. In the lateral gamma camera views, about one third of the image statistics (or counts) come from the contralateral lung. This "shine through" frequently allows enough photons to be collected from the opposite lung to render a normal lateral image, even in the presence of a prominent defect seen in one lung on the anterior or posterior view. Oblique projections are often helpful but may be confusing to the uninitiated observer and frequently demonstrate prominent hilar defects. In general, defects suspected on the oblique projections should be confirmed on one of the four standard views.

Pleural disease may produce distinctive changes on an otherwise normal perfusion scan. Small

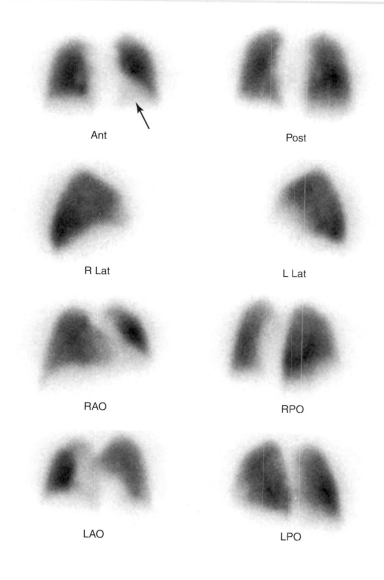

Ant

Post

R Lat

L Lat

RAO

RPO

LAO

LPO

Figure 6-4. Normal perfusion lung scan in the standard eight projections. The defect in the anterior left lower lung is caused by the heart.

pleural effusions may best be seen on the lateral or oblique views as posterior sulcus blunting or as a fissure sign, a linear defect caused by fluid in an interlobar fissure (Fig. 6-5). The fissure sign may also be produced by pleural scarring or thickening (even when not apparent on chest radiographs), by COPD, or, rarely, by multiple pulmonary microemboli. Moderate-sized pleural effusions may occasionally simulate segmental defects; if scanning is performed in the supine position in a patient with a pleural effusion, the fluid may collect in the superior part of the major fissure and mimic a superior-segment, lower-lobe defect. This defect, however, may disappear in the upright position. If an effusion is large, it may compress an entire lung and decrease the blood flow to that side generally or may surround the lung, producing the appearance of a small lung.

Perfusion defects may occur incidentally in asymptomatic people with normal chest radiographs and without a clinical history of pulmonary emboli. About 7% of young nonsmokers demonstrate small segmental defects, and 3% to 4% have lobular or segmental defects. If smokers are added to this population, as many as 10% may exhibit some type of perfusion defect.

Ventilation Scan

A normal ^{133}Xe ventilation study performed in the posterior projection is shown in Figure 6-6. After the initial breath, a relatively homogeneous distribution of activity should be seen

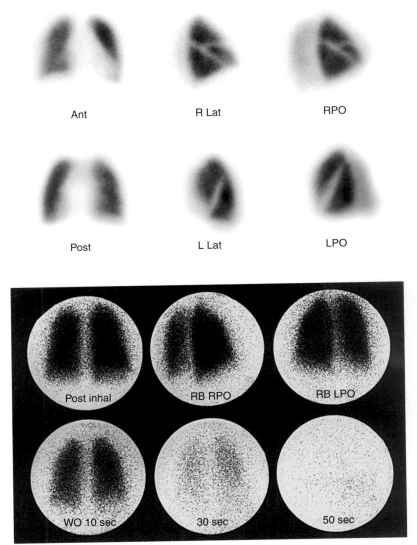

Figure 6-5. Fissure sign. There are linear defects in the region of the major and minor fissures. In this case, it is caused by fluid in the fissure in a patient with congestive heart failure.

Ant   R Lat   RPO

Post   L Lat   LPO

Post inhal   RB RPO   RB LPO

WO 10 sec   30 sec   50 sec

Figure 6-6. Normal xenon-133 ventilation scan. This shows an immediate posterior inhalation/inspiration (*Post inhal*) image and two oblique rebreathing (*RB RPO* and *RB LPO*) images followed by sequential posterior washout (*WO*) images.

throughout both lungs; the initial breath image reflects regional ventilatory rate if there is maximum inspiratory effort. The equilibrium-phase image indicates the aerated volume of lung and may be thought of as the "scintigraphic chest radiograph." Even in patients with abnormal single-breath and washout images, the equilibrium phase frequently is normal, particularly if rebreathing is performed for several minutes so that adequate collateral ventilation can occur. During the washout phase, activity clears from the lower portions of the lung at a faster rate than from the apices because the air exchange is greater. However, activity is frequently seen longer at the bases, owing to the relatively larger volume of lung present in that region. In most normal studies, the lungs are almost completely

clear of xenon within 2 or 3 minutes of beginning the washout phase because the normal half-time for xenon washout is about 30 to 45 seconds. Because washout is the most sensitive phase for the detection of trapping caused by airway obstruction, if xenon gas does not enter an area during equilibrium, washout cannot be evaluated. Thus, to a large extent, the sensitivity of the washout phase depends on performing sufficient rebreathing to obtain adequate equilibrium in as much of the lung volume as possible as well as on the length of the washout phase.

Because xenon is soluble in fat and partially soluble in blood, it may be deposited in the liver, resulting in increased activity in the right upper quadrant. This becomes apparent near the end of the xenon washout study and should not be

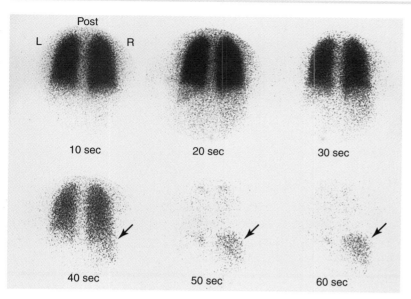

Figure 6-7. Fatty liver. Posterior sequential images of a xenon-133 ventilation scan show progressive accumulation of activity in the liver (*arrows*) as a result of fatty infiltration. This occurs because xenon-133 is soluble in fat.

mistaken for trapping of xenon in the right lower lung. The finding is particularly prominent in patients with disorders producing a fatty liver (Fig. 6-7). In children, activity may be seen in the left upper quadrant of the abdomen because of swallowing of the xenon gas during the study.

Normal DTPA aerosol ventilation images demonstrate homogeneous, symmetric aerosol deposition from apex to base. Areas in which there is no activity represent nonventilated regions. Normal aerosol scans resemble perfusion scans, except that the trachea and the bronchi are visualized. In addition, swallowed activity can sometimes be seen in the esophagus and stomach (Fig. 6-8).

CLINICAL APPLICATIONS

By far, the most important and frequent indication for a ventilation/perfusion lung scan is in the setting of suspected pulmonary emboli. Regardless of the reason for performing ventilation/perfusion pulmonary imaging, however, it cannot be overemphasized that a high-quality recent chest radiograph and pertinent clinical and laboratory findings should be fully used when interpreting lung scans. Use of poor-quality portable supine films can lead to mistakes in interpretation, although sometimes these are all that are available. Ideally, full-inspiration upright posteroanterior and lateral chest radiographs should be obtained as near as possible to the time the lung images are performed, certainly within 12 to 24 hours before performance of the scan or shortly thereafter.

Pulmonary Emboli

Pulmonary thromboembolism is a potentially fatal complication of deep vein thrombosis. Although anticoagulation and thrombolytic therapies are effective, they are not without potential morbidity. Thus, before the institution of treatment, determination of the reasonable likelihood of the presence or absence of pulmonary emboli is needed.

The clinical diagnosis of pulmonary embolism is often difficult. Less than one fourth of patients with pulmonary emboli show the classic signs or symptoms of the disease; hemoptysis is seldom observed, and blood enzyme and D-dimer determinations may be equivocal. Chest radiographic findings alone are nonspecific for the diagnosis of pulmonary embolism. However, an adequate chest radiograph is essential to diagnose conditions that can clinically mimic pulmonary emboli and is an important component of the interpretation of ventilation/perfusion lung scans. Clinical presentations are frequently vague and may be mimicked by a variety of thoracic and abdominal disorders, although the utilization of clinical pretest probability schemes, such as the modified Wells and simplified, revised Geneva scores has proved useful.

Although multislice spiral CT pulmonary angiography (CTPA) may be the initial test of choice to diagnose pulmonary embolism in many institutions, radionuclide ventilation/perfusion or perfusion only imaging, when properly performed and interpreted with a current chest

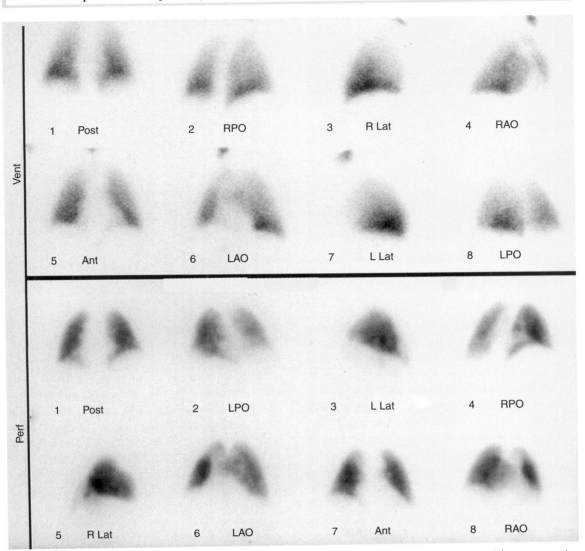

Figure 6-8. **DTPA aerosol and MAA scan.** Normal ^{99m}Tc-DTPA aerosol ventilation scan (*top*) with accompanying ^{99m}Tc-MAA perfusion scans (*bottom*).

radiograph, is an effective lower radiation dose procedure for the detection of pulmonary embolus. In addition, a normal perfusion scan essentially excludes the diagnosis, and the safety of relying on a normal V/Q scan for patient management has been reaffirmed by PIOPED I & II studies (discussed later). Even in the small percentage of patients in whom the studies are nondiagnostic, radionuclide imaging may be used to guide CT arteriography, thereby increasing the sensitivity of the examination. V/Q scans are often preferred over CT angiography for patients who have contrast allergies, are in renal failure, or who are too large for the CT-scanner table or gantry, as well as young patients (especially women) and those with clear lungs on chest radiographs.

Diagnostic Principle

The diagnosis of pulmonary thromboembolism by ventilation/perfusion imaging is based on the disassociation between ventilation and perfusion as a result of the obstruction of pulmonary segmental arterial blood flow by the embolus. With ^{99m}Tc-MAA imaging, the MAA particles are unable to enter the capillary bed distal to the arterial occlusion, so that the portion of lung supplied by the involved artery appears as a perfusion defect outlined by the normally perfused adjacent lung parenchyma. Because ventilation is generally unaffected, the xenon or aerosol images remain normal in the same distribution. Thus the most typical manifestation of the pulmonary emboli is as a wedge-shaped

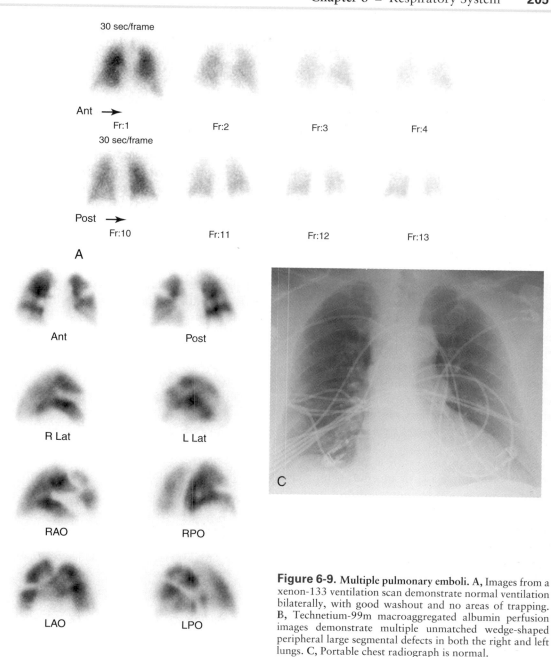

Figure 6-9. **Multiple pulmonary emboli. A,** Images from a xenon-133 ventilation scan demonstrate normal ventilation bilaterally, with good washout and no areas of trapping. **B,** Technetium-99m macroaggregated albumin perfusion images demonstrate multiple unmatched wedge-shaped peripheral large segmental defects in both the right and left lungs. **C,** Portable chest radiograph is normal.

perfusion defect with preserved ventilation: the segmental ventilation/perfusion mismatch (Fig. 6-9).

Although this principle is simple, its practical application in various clinical settings can present one of most difficult challenges confronting the nuclear imaging physician. For this reason, much effort has been directed toward defining the language used to describe the findings on ventilation/perfusion imaging as well as the criteria used to translate them into diagnostic conclusions. In this regard, a thorough

understanding of basic definitions and concepts is imperative.

Basic Concepts

A *normal pulmonary perfusion* scan has no perfusion defects or perfusion exactly outlines the shape of the lungs seen on the chest radiograph. It should be noted that a normal perfusion scan may demonstrate hilar and aortic impressions and the chest radiograph and/or ventilation study may be abnormal. A normal perfusion scan essentially excludes the presence of clinically significant pulmonary emboli, regardless of the ventilation scan findings.

A *perfusion defect* is a focus of absent or diminished pulmonary activity on perfusion images. Perfusion defects are nonspecific, and a list of differential diagnoses is given in Box 6-1. With a pulmonary embolism, perfusion does not have to be completely absent in the region of the defect because partially occluding pulmonary emboli are possible. Perfusion defects are classified as segmental or nonsegmental.

Segmental perfusion defects may involve all or part of a bronchopulmonary anatomic segment. Classically, these defects are pleural based and wedge shaped. They are best described by the particular bronchopulmonary segment that they occupy. Because segmental defects are the hallmark of pulmonary emboli and nonsegmental defects are not, the ability to distinguish between them is crucial to lung scan interpretation. This requires both careful characterization of defect configuration and an appreciation of the pulmonary segmental anatomy as it appears on perfusion lung images. Figure 6-10 shows the individual pulmonary segments in the projection that best visualizes each segment.

Historically, segmental defects have been characterized by size, with a large segmental defect occupying 75% or more of a lung segment, a moderate segmental defect occupying 25% to 75% of the segment, and a small segmental defect occupying less than 25% of the segment. Reproducibility of interpretation with such criteria has proven difficult. The significance of a defect with respect to the likelihood that it is caused by a pulmonary embolus is directly related to defect size and the number of defects present; larger segmental defects are more significant, and the probability of pulmonary emboli increases as the number of identifiable large defects increases. When assessing a pulmonary perfusion study for the number and size of defects, the PIOPED concept of segmental defect equivalence allows two moderate segmental defects to be summed so that they have the same diagnostic implication as one large segmental defect. Small defects, however, are not summed to form larger equivalents. Thus it is possible to assemble combinations of moderate and large segments to determine the total number of segments involved for assessment of the probability of the presence of pulmonary emboli.

An exception to the concept of defect size and significance is that solitary perfusion defects involving an entire lung (Box 6-2) or lobe of a lung represent uncommon presentations of pulmonary emboli. Both current and retrospective literature indicate that small segmental defects are uncommonly associated with pulmonary emboli.

Nonsegmental perfusion defects are those that do not correspond to bronchopulmonary anatomic segments and are generally not wedged shaped, but they may or may not be pleural based. In some instances, they are caused by nonpulmonary abnormalities, including hilar structures, alterations in diaphragmatic contour or position, cardiomegaly, or normal variants or pathology of hilar or mediastinal structures. Primary intrapulmonary abnormalities may also cause nonsegmental defects, including those produced by neoplasms, bullae, pneumonia, hemorrhage, edema, or other infiltrates. The significance of nonsegmental defects is that they are not associated with pulmonary emboli.

Perfusion segmental defects are further classified with respect to whether they exhibit ventilation. A *mismatch* refers to the circumstance in which a perfusion defect is seen to ventilate normally. Segmental mismatches are a hallmark of pulmonary emboli. Classically, a mismatch

---

Box 6-1 Causes of Defects on Perfusion Lung Scans

Pulmonary embolism (thrombotic, septic, marrow, or air)*
Bulla or cyst
Localized hypoxia caused by asthma, bronchitis, emphysema
Surgery (e.g., pneumonectomy)
Pleural effusion*
Tumor (including hilar or mediastinal)*
Metastases (hematogenous or lymphangitic)
Hilar adenopathy (lymphoma, sarcoidosis)
Pulmonary artery atresia or hypoplasia*
Fibrosing mediastinitis*
Radiation therapy*
Pneumonia
Pulmonary edema
Atelectasis
Fibrosis (postinflammatory, postradiation, pleural thickening)
Vasculitis*

*Entity may cause a ventilation/perfusion mismatch.

requires that the chest radiograph be normal in the same region. When a ventilation abnormality occurs in the same region as a perfusion defect, this constitutes a ventilation/perfusion *match*. Such ventilation abnormalities may occur as wash-in defects on aerosol or xenon studies, as washout abnormalities (focal trapping) on xenon images, or as both. Ventilation/perfusion matches may have significance in the diagnostic schema for the diagnosis of pulmonary emboli, depending on their size, number, and location in the lungs. The term *triple match* is often used to refer to a ventilation/perfusion match accompanied by a corresponding chest radiographic abnormality of the same size, usually, but not always, airspace opacity.

For purposes of regional localization of lung scan abnormalities, it is useful to divide the lungs into upper, middle, and lower zones of equal height, obtained by dividing the lungs into thirds from apex to base. The position of an abnormality, especially a single ventilation/perfusion match, with respect to these zones may add to its significance.

Analysis of Images

An orderly and consistent approach to lung scan analysis aids greatly in determining the findings to which interpretive criteria are to be applied. Analysis requires meticulous review and comparison of three separate sets of images: the perfusion images, the ventilation images,

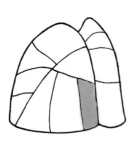
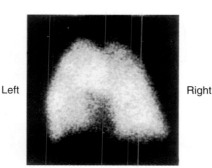

Left   Right

L. Posterior Oblique

A

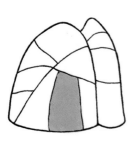
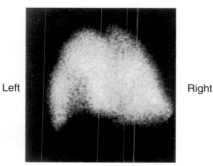

Left   Right

L. Posterior Oblique

B

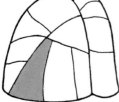
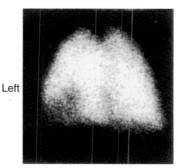

Left   Right

L. Posterior Oblique

C

Figure 6-10. **Segmental perfusion defects.** Each is shown diagrammatically and in the position that best demonstrates the defect on the perfusion scan. *Right, Left, Posterior,* and *Anterior* refer to the scintigrams. (From Mandell CH: Scintillation Camera Lung Imaging. New York: 1976, Grune & Stratton; pp 10-17, 20-27, 30-38, 42-51.) **A,** Left lower-lobe posterior basal segment. **B,** Left lower-lobe lateral basal segment. **C,** Left lower-lobe anterior medial basal segment.

Continued

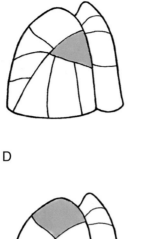

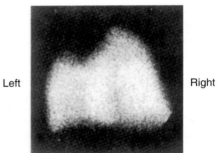

Left   Right

L. Posterior Oblique

D

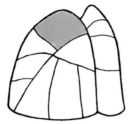

Left   Right

L. Posterior Oblique

E

Left   Right

L. Posterior Oblique

F

Figure 6-10, cont'd. D, Left lower-lobe superior segment. **E,** Left upper-lobe posterior apical segment. **F,** Left upper-lobe superior lingular segment. **G,** Left upper-lobe inferior lingular segment. The lingular segments are often difficult to identify because of the normal cardiac defect.

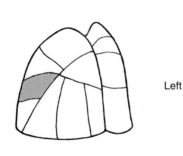

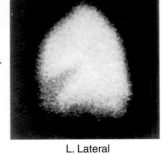

Anterior   Posterior

L. Lateral

G

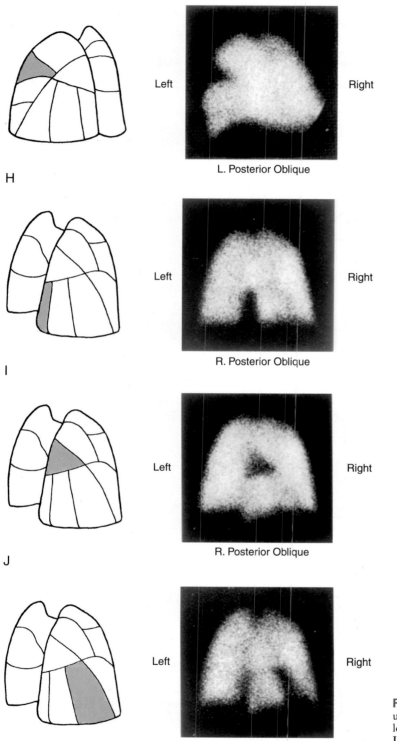

H

Left   Right

L. Posterior Oblique

I

Left   Right

R. Posterior Oblique

J

Left   Right

R. Posterior Oblique

K

Left   Right

R. Posterior Oblique

Figure 6-10, cont'd. H, Left upper-lobe anterior segment. **I,** Right lower-lobe posterior basal segment. **J,** Right lower-lobe superior segment. **K,** Right lower-lobe anterior basal segment.

Continued

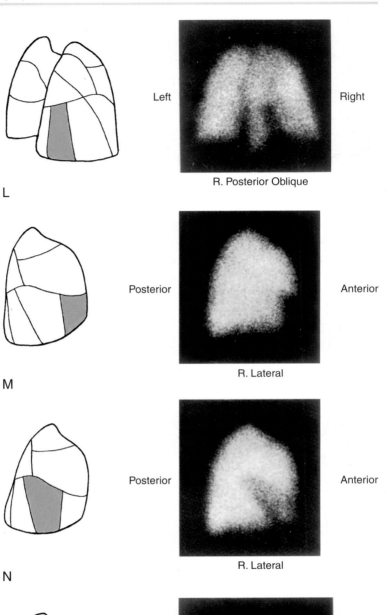

Left   Right

R. Posterior Oblique

L

Posterior   Anterior

R. Lateral

M

Posterior   Anterior

R. Lateral

N

Left   Right

R. Posterior Oblique

O

Figure 6-10, cont'd. L, Right lower-lobe lateral basal segment. M, Right middle-lobe medial segment. N, Right middle-lobe lateral segment. O, Right upper-lobe posterior segment.

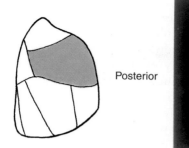

Posterior

Anterior

R. Lateral

P

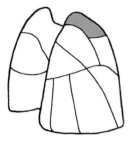

Left

Right

R. Posterior Oblique

Q

Figure 6-10, cont'd. P, Right upper-lobe anterior segment. Q, Right upper-lobe apical segment.

Box 6-2 Causes of Decreased Perfusion to One Lung

Pulmonary agenesis or stenosis
Swyer-James syndrome
Embolus
Pneumothorax
Massive effusion
Mediastinal fibrosis
Tumor

---

and the chest radiograph. Analysis of the perfusion scans first entails the identification and classification of any defects according to their appearance. Defects corresponding to anatomic divisions should be classified as lobar or segmental. Those defects that are not anatomic or do not respect segmental boundaries may be considered nonsegmental and unlikely to represent pulmonary emboli. Segmental defects, especially those of large or moderate size, should then be compared with the identical region on the ventilation scan to determine whether a corresponding ventilatory abnormality is present.

This allows characterization of the defect as matched or mismatched. Perfusion defects are then compared with findings on a recent chest radiograph to assess the presence of any correlative abnormalities, including infiltrates, pleural effusions, masses, or bullae. If available, any prior ventilation/perfusion lung scans should be reviewed as part of image analysis because persistent defects from previous pulmonary emboli are a common cause of false-positive findings for acute emboli.

Although lung scan interpretation is easiest in the presence of a clear chest radiograph, the presence of either a localized infiltrate or diffuse lung disease should not be seen as an insurmountable problem. Any approach that does not attempt to interpret pulmonary emboli in the presence of infiltrates or diffuse lung disease will result in a large number of scans being read as nondiagnostic and will unnecessarily subject a large number of patients to further studies. One of the most common situations involves the presence of one or more localized pulmonary infiltrates on the chest radiograph of a patient suspected of having pulmonary emboli. Certainly, the infiltrate or infiltrates could represent either inflammatory disease or pulmonary emboli with infarction. Because pulmonary emboli are generally multiple, however, and because only about 25% of such lesions progress to infarction, the likelihood is excellent that ventilation/perfusion mismatches suggesting pulmonary embolus may be found elsewhere, in areas of otherwise radiographically normal lung. In the absence of such findings, some diagnostic probability information can nevertheless be obtained by comparing the size of the radiographic infiltrate with the size of the corresponding perfusion deficit. When a perfusion defect is substantially smaller than the corresponding radiographic abnormality, the probability of pulmonary embolus is very low (Table 6-1). A perfusion defect that corresponds closely in size to an infiltrate is nondiagnostic. In this latter case, if clinical suspicion is high, CT angiography may be indicated.

Normal or near-normal perfusion lung scans may occur in a large percentage of patients with a diffusely abnormal chest radiograph, such as in the setting of pulmonary edema. Although the presence of perfusion abnormalities in such patients may cause difficulty in interpretation, the surprising number of normal or near-normal scans obtained indicates that pulmonary emboli can be effectively excluded in many patients with underlying lung diseases. As stated earlier, a normal ventilation/perfusion lung scan in any patient essentially excludes the possibility of recent significant pulmonary embolization.

With or without a normal chest radiograph, careful correlation of any perfusion abnormalities with the corresponding regions on the ventilation study should be undertaken to exclude airway disease as a cause for a perfusion defect. Multiple matched small ventilation/perfusion abnormalities with a clear chest radiograph demonstrate a low likelihood of pulmonary embolus.

Interpretive Criteria

The interpretation of ventilation/perfusion images in the setting of suspected pulmonary emboli involves the determination of the probability of pulmonary emboli, based on a set of specific interpretive criteria. These criteria have evolved over many years as experience with ventilation/perfusion lung imaging has increased. The sensitivity and specificity of different methods for imaging acute pulmonary emboli are shown in Table 6-2.

PIOPED: Prospective Investigation Of Pulmonary Embolism Diagnosis. A number of criteria have been defined by an extensive and ambitious project known as the Prospective Investigation Of Pulmonary Embolism Diagnosis (PIOPED). PIOPED and PIOPED II are multi-institutional studies involving tertiary care hospitals designed to evaluate the efficacy of various means of diagnosing acute pulmonary embolism. More specifically, the goal of PIOPED is to determine the sensitivity and specificity of V/Q lung scanning by using a specific set of diagnostic criteria to derive a probability (or likelihood ratio) for the presence of thromboemboli. The initial criteria were

TABLE 6-1	Angiographic Findings in Regions with Scintigraphic Perfusion Defects and Radiographic Abnormalities
SIZE OF PERFUSION DEFECT COMPARED WITH RADIOGRAPHIC ABNORMALITY	**PULMONARY EMBOLISM (%)**
Smaller	7
Equal	26
Larger	
V/Q mismatch	89
V/Q match	<5

Modified from Biello DR, Mattar AG, Osei-Wusu A, et al.: Interpretation of indeterminate lung scintigrams. Radiology 133: 189-194, 1979.
V/Q, Ventilation/perfusion ratio.

TABLE 6-2	Comparison of Interpretive Schema for Acute Pulmonary Emboli		
METHOD	**SENSITIVITY (%)**	**SPECIFICITY (%)**	**NONDIAGNOSTIC SCANS (%)**
Modified PIOPED II	85	93	27-27 (due to interpretation)
	77	98	(analysis after removal of nondiagnostic intermediate or low probability scans)
PISAPED	80-86	93-97	close to zero
Multidetector CT	83	96	6 (due to technical issues)

very complex and had significant variability in application among physicians as well as a high percentage of scans interpreted as indeterminate or nondiagnostic. Thus the data from the PIOPED studies have been refined with adjustments to simplify the original set of criteria. The current commonly used diagnostic schema is the *Modified PIOPED II Criteria*.

Modified PIOPED II Interpretive Criteria. The modified PIOPED II criteria are the most common criteria used in the United States. There are two versions of modified PIOPED criteria, a classic one which uses ventilation and perfusion scan with a chest radiograph and another that uses only a perfusion scan and chest radiograph. In both of these newer interpretive schemes, the classic PIOPED I categories of *high, moderate* (intermediate), and *low* probability of pulmonary emboli have been superseded by *high* (*PE-present*) and *very low* (*PE-absent*) categories, with an additional *nondiagnostic* classification for all other findings, including those criteria previously in the PIOPED *moderate* and *low* categories.

The modified PIOPED II criteria for combined ventilation/perfusion studies are compared with those of the modified PIOPED II criteria for perfusion scans only, in Table 6-3. A thorough familiarity with these criteria is crucial to the consistent and reliable interpretation of lung scans in the setting of suspected pulmonary embolism. The modified criteria can be used to classify V/Q scans as representing (1) a high probability of pulmonary emboli (PPV greater than 85%), (2) a very low probability (PPV less than 10%), or (3) a normal scan. All V/Q scans not falling into these categories are classified as nondiagnostic, which indicates the need for further patient evaluation. To maintain a high specificity for the patterns described, especially high probability, some sensitivity is unavoidably lost. It is the responsibility of the interpreting physician to communicate effectively the meaning of a reported probability to referring clinicians, so that patient management is optimized.

Ventilation/Perfusion (V/Q) Modified PIOPED II Criteria. There are several interpretation categories for the modified PIOPED II criteria when using both perfusion and ventilation scans in combination with a perfusion scan and a chest radiograph.

High Probability (V/Q): Using the modified PIOPED II criteria, there is only one criterion for a high probability scan: two or more large

(or summed equivalent) ventilation/perfusion mismatches are indicative of a high probability of pulmonary emboli (Figs. 6-11 and 6-12). This requirement seems reasonable because pulmonary emboli are multiple in 90% of cases and bilateral in 85%.

Very Low Probability (V/Q): Scans in this category have a positive predictive value (PPV) of less than 10% for the presence of pulmonary

TABLE 6-3	Ventilation, Perfusion, Radiographic (CXR) Interpretive Criteria
MODIFIED PIOPED II	**PERFUSION-ONLY MODIFIED PIOPED II**
High	**PE Present**
≥2 large mismatched V/Q segmental defects*	≥2 large mismatched (Q/CXR) segmental defects*
Nondiagnostic	**Nondiagnostic**
All other findings	All other findings
Very Low	**PE Absent**
Nonsegmental†	Nonsegmental†
Q defect < CXR lesion	Q defect < CXR lesion
Solitary matched V/Q/CXR defect (≤segment) in mid or upper lung	Solitary matched Q/CXR defect (≤1 segment) in mid or upper lung
1-3 small segmental defects*	1-3 small segmental defects*
≥2 matched (V:Q) defects, regionally normal CXR	
Stripe sign‡	Stripe sign‡
Solitary large pleural effusion§	Solitary large pleural effusion§
Normal	
No perfusion defects‖	

The modified PIOPED II criteria not using information from the ventilation images have been shown to perform equally to those using the ventilation images with fewer indeterminate studies.

Reprinted by permission of the Society of Nuclear Medicine; adapted from SNM Practice Guideline for Lung Scintigraphy v4.0. http://interactive.snm.org/Lung_Scintigraphy_V4_Final.pdf

CXR, Chest radiograph; *V/Q,* ventilation/perfusion.

*Or equivalent where a large defect (>75% of segment) equals 1 segmental equivalent, a moderate defect (25-75% of a segment) equals 0.5 segmental equivalents, and a small defect (<25% of segment) is not counted.

†For example, prominent hilum, cardiomegaly, elevated hemidiaphragm, costophrenic angle effusion, linear atelectasis with no other perfusion defect in either lung and no other radiographic lesions.

‡A stripe of perfused lung tissue between a perfusion defect and the adjacent pleural surface; best seen on a tangential view.

§One third or more of the pleural cavity with no other perfusion defect in either lung.

‖Perfusion exactly matches shape of chest-radiograph.

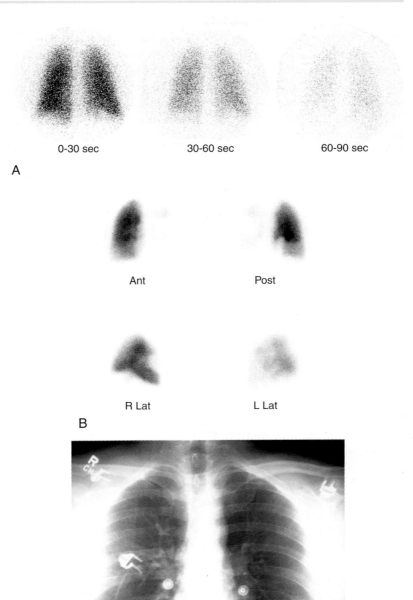

Figure 6-11. Large pulmonary embolism. A, Posterior xenon-133 ventilation scan is normal. **B,** ^{99m}Tc-MAA images show perfusion to the right lung only. **C,** Chest radiograph shows lucency from marked oligemia in the left lung (Westermark sign).

emboli. The criteria for very low probability scans are:
- Nonsegmental perfusion abnormalities
- Perfusion defect smaller than corresponding chest radiographic abnormality (regardless of ventilation findings)
- A perfusion defect with a stripe sign (see later section, Ancillary Signs)
- Solitary triple-matched (V:Q:CXR) defects in an upper or middle lung zone
- Matched V/Q abnormalities in two or more zones of a single lung, with regionally normal chest radiograph
- Pleural effusion equal to one third or more of the pleural cavity with no other perfusion defect in either lung

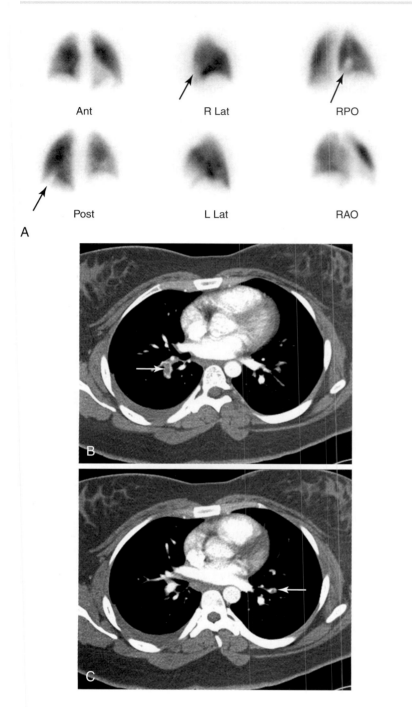

Figure 6-12. Small pulmonary emboli. In this patient with a normal ventilation scan and chest radiograph, on **A**, the perfusion scan, a single segmental defect is seen in the right posterior basal segment (*arrows*). The CT pulmonary angiogram, however, shows not only **B**, emboli on the right, but also **C**, small emboli on the left *(arrows)*. Using the modified PIOPED II criteria, this would be interpreted as nondiagnostic.

Normal: No perfusion defects. Clinically significant pulmonary emboli are excluded.

Nondiagnostic: All other findings than those listed previously are nondiagnostic. This category includes the findings listed in the moderate (intermediate) and low categories of the earlier PIOPED criteria.

Perfusion (Q) Only Modified PIOPED II Criteria. A set of modified PIOPED II criteria has also been developed that does not make use of ventilation findings, if any. These are referred to as the Perfusion-Only Modified PIOPED II Criteria. Using these criteria, lung perfusion scans are classified as *PE-present, PE-absent,* or *nondiagnostic.* These criteria have been shown to perform equally well to those that use ventilation scintigraphy with fewer nondiagnostic (indeterminate) studies.

PE Present (Q) Perfusion cans in this category have two or more large (or summed equivalent) segmental perfusion defects that are mismatched with regard to the chest radiograph (i.e., there is no segmental opacity exactly corresponding to the perfusion defect).

PE Absent (Q) Perfusion scans in this category are essentially the same as those defined as *very low probability* by the modified PIOPED criteria, with the exception that matched findings refer to perfusion scan-chest radiographic findings only(V/Q mismatch findings are excluded) because ventilation findings, if any, are not considered in this interpretive protocol. Normal perfusion scans are included in this category.

Nondiagnostic: All findings other than those listed previously are nondiagnostic.

PISAPED Interpretive Criteria. Another set of interpretive criteria has been derived from the Prospective Investigative Study of Acute Pulmonary Embolism (PISAPED) study. These criteria are primarily used in Europe.

PISAPED interpretive criteria do not use a ventilation scan but rely on only a perfusion scan and chest radiograph. The sensitivity and specificity are broadly comparable to the modified PIOPED II (V/Q) criteria but with fewer nondiagnostic (indeterminate) studies. These criteria are very similar to those used in the Perfusion-Only Modified PIOPED II interpretive schema.

PE Present: In contrast to the modified PIOPED II criteria (which requires two large segmental V/Q or Q/CXR mismatches), for a PE-present determination, the PISAPED criteria simply require the presence of one or more wedge-shaped perfusion defects.

PE Absent: Scans in this category include nonsegmental pulmonary perfusion defects, defects caused by the heart, mediastinum or diaphragm, or those with normal or near normal perfusion.

Nondiagnostic: All findings other than those listed previously are nondiagnostic.

Gestalt Interpretation. Gestalt, or overall pattern, interpretation of ventilation/perfusion scans by some physicians may add to the accuracy of lung scan assessment and is often used adjunctively in combination with specific criteria. This approach should be reserved for the very experienced interpreter because the basis for interpretation may be difficult to explain in a potential legal setting.

Optimizing Interpretation

Incorporation of Clinical Information. Interpretation of ventilation/perfusion images correlates well with the likelihood of finding pulmonary emboli with selective pulmonary angiography or pulmonary CT angiography. Even though the clinical presentation of pulmonary emboli is nonspecific, risk factors and clinical findings suggestive of pulmonary emboli may be used to formulate a clinical pretest likelihood of pulmonary emboli that may be combined with the ventilation/perfusion scan results to determine an overall likelihood of the presence of the disease.

The predictive value of lung scans is optimized when supported by clinical impressions suggesting either the presence or absence of emboli (Box 6-3 and Table 6-4). Such information can be especially useful when assessing the significance of low probability scans. Although patients with low or very low probability scans without significant risk factors have a

---

Box 6-3 Signs and Symptoms Associated with Probability of Predicting Acute Pulmonary Embolism

Tachycardia (>100 beats/min)
Sudden onset dyspnea
Hemoptysis
Malignancy
Older age
Hypocapnia (kPa Pa_{CO2} <5.1)
Hypoxemia (kPa Pa_{O2} <11.0)
Right ventricular overload
Signs or symptoms of deep venous
 thrombosis
PE more likely than alternative diagnosis
Immobilization or recent surgery
Previous DVT or PE
Chest radiograph findings of
 Oligemia
 Amputation of hilar artery
 Pleural-based consolidation
 Hemidiaphragm elevation
 Linear atelectasis

Generally, a patient with four or more of the above clinical signs or symptoms is at significantly increased probability of pulmonary embolism. Clinically unstable patients should have a CTPA rather than a lung scan because of the short time required for preparation and the procedure.
CTPA, Computed tomography pulmonary angiography; *DVT,* deep vein thrombosis; *PE,* pulmonary embolism.

combined prevalence of pulmonary embolism of only 4%, with one or more than one significant risk factors, the prevalence values are increased to 12% and 21%, respectively. Thus, in patients with low probability lung scans and important risk factors, further investigation, including lower extremity noninvasive venous studies and/or pulmonary CT angiography, may be warranted. Further, a low probability scan with a strong pretest clinical impression of the absence of pulmonary emboli makes the probability of pulmonary emboli remote. The presence of associated risk factors does not change the significance of a normal lung scan in essentially excluding a diagnosis of pulmonary embolism.

Ancillary Signs. The *stripe sign* consists of a thin line or stripe of activity representing perfused lung tissue between a perfusion defect and the adjacent pleural surface. Pulmonary emphysema is the most common cause of this sign. Perfusion defects presenting with a stripe sign are very unlikely to represent pulmonary emboli based on the assumption that non–pleural-based lesions are not emboli. These defects should be interpreted as having a very low probability of being pulmonary emboli in the absence of perfusion abnormalities elsewhere in the lungs (Fig. 6-13).

The *fissure sign* refers to linear perfusion deficits corresponding to the interlobar pulmonary fissures, both major and minor. This sign is commonly seen in the presence of pleural fluid in the fissures but may also be seen in the presence of fissural pleural thickening and is frequently observed in patients with COPD (see Fig. 6-5).

Special Situations

Pleural Effusions. Ipsilateral pleural effusions may occur in 30% to 40% of patients with pulmonary emboli. Such pleural effusions may produce perfusion defects by loculation or compression of lung parenchyma. There are conflicting reports regarding the significance of matched ventilation/perfusion defects corresponding to radiographic pleural effusions of similar size. Analysis of the PIOPED I and II data suggests that matched defects caused by small pleural effusions (those producing only costophrenic angle blunting) should be classified as *intermediate probability* (nondiagnostic), whereas defects caused by larger effusions (at least one third of the pleural cavity) should be classified as *low probability*. Still, some studies indicate that pulmonary emboli are associated with pleural effusions of all sizes, and thus all pleural effusion-related matched ventilation/perfusion abnormalities should be assigned an intermediate probability

TABLE 6-4	Pretest Probability for Pulmonary Embolism (Wells Criteria)	
Clinical signs and symptoms of deep venous thrombosis (minimum of leg swelling and pain with palpation of the deep veins)		3 points
Pulmonary embolism as or more likely than alternative diagnosis		3 points
Heart rate greater than 100/minute		1.5 points
Immobilization or surgery within the previous 4 weeks		1.5 points
Previous deep vein thrombosis or pulmonary embolism		1.5 points
Hemoptysis		1.0 point
Current or palliative treatment of malignancy within last 6 months		1.0 point

Score <2, low likeihood of PE (0.5-2.7%); score 2-6, moderate likelihood of PE (16%); and score >6, high likelihood of PE (41%). From Wells P, Anderson D, Rodger M, et.al. Excluding pulmonary embolism at the bedside without diagnostic imaging. Ann Int Med 2001;135(2):98-107.

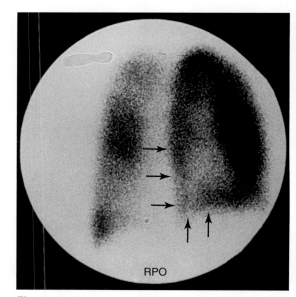

Figure 6-13. Stripe sign. Single view from a perfusion lung scan in a patient with chronic obstructive pulmonary disease shows a perfusion defect in the right lower lobe, but this does not extend all the way to the periphery of the lung. The rim of activity near the pleura (*arrows*) indicates a low probability of pulmonary embolus.

(nondiagnostic) of pulmonary emboli regardless of size. In general, pleural effusions that do not produce perfusion defects are irrelevant to the interpretation of a V/Q lung scan.

Diffuse Lung Disease. The overwhelming majority (75%) of patients with diffuse lung disease, such as relatively homogeneous infiltrates produced by pulmonary edema, have normal or near-normal perfusion lungs scans in the absence of pulmonary emboli (Fig. 6-14). Thus such diffuse abnormalities on chest radiographs should not discourage the use of

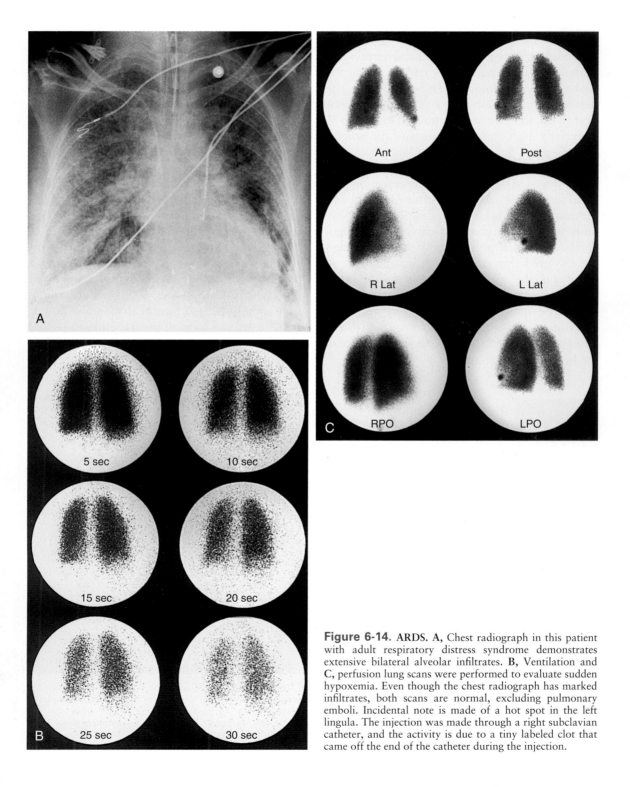

Figure 6-14. ARDS. A, Chest radiograph in this patient with adult respiratory distress syndrome demonstrates extensive bilateral alveolar infiltrates. **B,** Ventilation and **C,** perfusion lung scans were performed to evaluate sudden hypoxemia. Even though the chest radiograph has marked infiltrates, both scans are normal, excluding pulmonary emboli. Incidental note is made of a hot spot in the left lingula. The injection was made through a right subclavian catheter, and the activity is due to a tiny labeled clot that came off the end of the catheter during the injection.

ventilation/perfusion lung imaging because pulmonary emboli may be successfully excluded in the presence of a normal perfusion pattern.

Airway Disease (Chronic Obstructive Pulmonary Disease). Severe diffuse COPD may significantly lower the sensitivity and specificity of lung scans in diagnosing pulmonary embolism. In COPD, both nonsegmental and segmental perfusion defects may occur, making differentiation from superimposed pulmonary emboli impossible without an accompanying ventilation study. When COPD is severe and diffuse, even the combined ventilation/perfusion study may not provide an answer. CT angiography may be indicated if emboli are strongly suspected clinically. In the presence of severe COPD, however, even CT angiography may be fraught with interpretive error.

Location of Triple Matches. There is some evidence that pulmonary embolism is significantly more common in the presence of triple matches located in lower lung zones, where blood flow is greater, than with triple matches in the upper and middle lung zones. Thus matching ventilation/perfusion defects corresponding to chest radiographic opacities isolated to the upper and middle lung zones confer a very low probability of pulmonary emboli, whereas similar findings in the lower lung zones represent an intermediate (nondiagnostic) probability of pulmonary emboli. There appears to be no differences in the prevalence of pulmonary emboli among various sizes of triple matches.

Lobar or Whole-Lung Defects. Solitary lobar or solitary whole-lung perfusion defects are unusual presentations for pulmonary emboli. Other possibilities, including hilar masses, mediastinal fibrosis, and hypoplastic pulmonary artery (Fig. 6-15), should be considered.

Incorporation of Noninvasive Deep Venous Testing

Because pulmonary emboli are a complication of deep venous thrombosis, a noninvasive evaluation of the veins of the lower extremity, especially duplex ultrasound, has become an important diagnostic tool in patients with suspected pulmonary emboli. In patients with nondiagnostic lung scans and low clinical suspicion of pulmonary emboli, normal lower extremity noninvasive venous ultrasound may obviate further testing and allow conservative patient management. Positive noninvasive testing renders a patient a candidate for anticoagulation therapy. A combination of lower extremity ultrasound and plasma D-dimer assessment, a specific breakdown product of clot fibrinolysis, may provide even more information to direct patient management and may reduce the need for further imaging when both are negative.

Computed Tomography Pulmonary Arteriography (CTPA)

In many health care institutions, CT angiography is the preferred initial imaging study for suspected pulmonary embolus, and some recent clinical algorithms do not include radionuclide ventilation perfusion imaging. The advantages and disadvantages of CTPA and V/Q scanning are outlined in Box 6-4. To some extent, this may be the result of the high number of nondiagnostic scan interpretations and the generally perceived higher interobserver interpretive variance for V/Q imaging compared to spiral CT angiography. With current generation CT scanners, coverage of the entire chest in high resolution can be achieved in one short breath hold lasting a few seconds. Very high resolution axial images of the pulmonary arteries with three-dimensional reconstruction are possible. CT scanning is often definitive when nondiagnostic V/Q scan results are obtained (Fig. 6-16). The specificity for pulmonary emboli detection with multidetector CT is greater than that of V/Q and has greatly contributed to its use. Some difficulties with spiral CT protocols are the need for very precise timing of the contrast bolus to produce a diagnostic examination, and the clinical quandary presented by the detection of small peripheral emboli in normal persons or patients with minor symptoms. Incidental emboli are found in 1% to 5% of patients, and many of these patients have malignancies. Incidental emboli are even more common in very old patients. Findings from a number of studies suggest that while CT angiography may detect more pulmonary emboli, the detection of clinically relevant disease did not change. Thus the question of overdiagnosis of pulmonary emboli by CT angiography has been raised.

Despite the advantages of spiral CTPA, V/Q scans will likely continue to play a role in the evaluation of pulmonary emboli, right-to-left shunts, and regional pulmonary function. Selective pulmonary arteriography, which was the gold standard for diagnosis of pulmonary emboli, is now extremely rare.

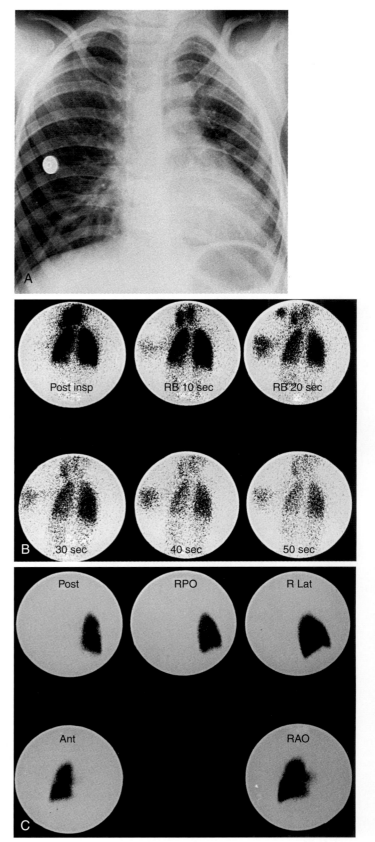

Figure 6-15. Hypoplastic or absent left pulmonary artery. A, Chest radiograph demonstrates the classic findings compatible with this entity, including volume loss and bronchial vascularity. **B,** Ventilation scan demonstrates good ventilation in both lungs, with slightly more rapid washout on the *left*. **C,** Perfusion scan demonstrates completely absent perfusion to the left lung. *Insp,* Inspiration; *RB,* rebreathing/equilibrium phase.

Lung Scan Follow-up of Pulmonary Emboli

Once the diagnosis of pulmonary embolism has been established, perfusion imaging may be used (and is often preferred over CTPA) to follow the course of the disease. Typically, there is some evidence of change in the pattern of perfusion defects in the first few days after the embolism. Defects may become smaller or disappear altogether, and new defects may appear. New defects may result from fragmentation of larger, centrally placed clots that pass to the lung periphery or from altered regional perfusion pressure in the lung, which may convert a

---

Box 6-4 Comparison of Lung Scanning and CT Pulmonary Angiography for Detection of Pulmonary Embolism

Lung Scan	Multidetector CT Pulmonary Angiography
Strengths	Strengths
High negative predictive value in low pretest probability	High accuracy
High positive predictive value in high pretest probability	More readily available
No contrast reactions	Rapid
Lower radiation dose (effective dose ~2 mSv)	Better for unstable patients
Weaknesses	Easier to interpret
Lower overall specificity	Can provide alternative diagnosis
Longer examination time	Weaknesses
	Higher radiation dose (effective dose ~15 mSv)
	Possible contrast allergies
	Incidental pulmonary emboli issue

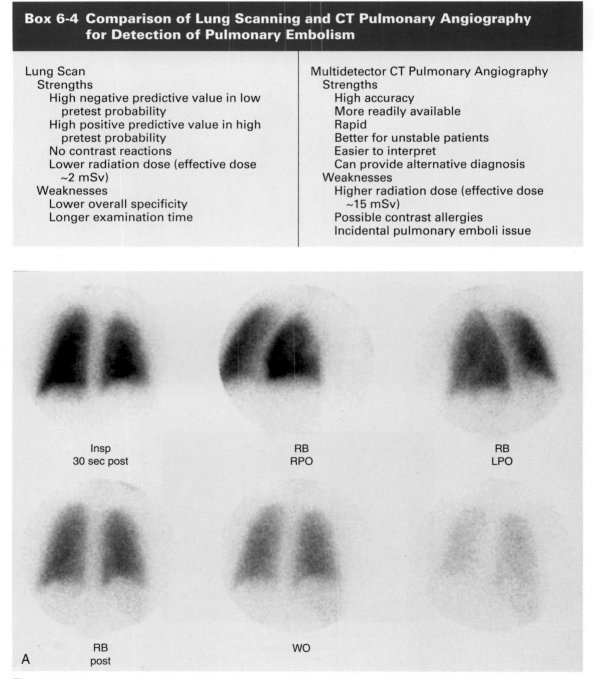

Insp
30 sec post

RB
RPO

RB
LPO

RB
post

WO

A

Figure 6-16. Large central partially occluding pulmonary embolism. **A,** Xenon ventilation images are normal. *RB,* rebreathing/equilibrium phase; *WO,* washout.

Continued

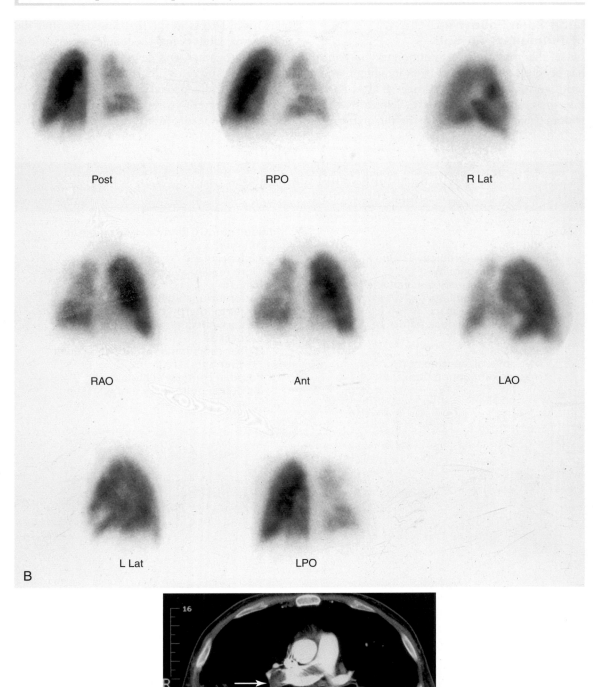

Post   RPO   R Lat

RAO   Ant   LAO

L Lat   LPO

B

C

Figure 6-16, cont'd. B, Perfusion images show substantially reduced blood flow to the right lung. **C,** Contrasted CT scan clearly shows a large filling defect (*arrow*) in the right main pulmonary artery.

partially obstructing clot to a complete obstruction. Of course, recurrent emboli also produce new defects, but the mere presence of new defects per se cannot be used to establish recurrent embolization during this period.

The ultimate fate of pulmonary emboli is variable and depends to some extent on the size of the emboli and the age of the patient. The larger the initial defect and the older the patient, the less likely is the pulmonary perfusion scan to return to normal. Emboli occurring in the presence of underlying diffuse diseases are also less likely to show complete resolution, as are those that produce actual infarction of lung. Because persistent defects may be mistaken for acute pulmonary emboli on subsequent ventilation/perfusion scans, it is strongly recommended that those patients with high probability scans or those with intermediate probability (nondiagnostic) scans who are treated for pulmonary emboli be followed with a 3-month baseline study for future reference if symptoms suggestive of new pulmonary emboli occur. Thromboembolic perfusion defects persisting at 3 months are likely to remain unresolved.

Pulmonary Hypertension

Pulmonary hypertension is defined as having a mean pulmonary arterial pressure greater than 25 mm Hg measured during right heart catheterization. The disease has multiple causes, including primary (idiopathic) pulmonary hypertension, chronic thromboemboli, left heart disease, and pulmonary parenchymal diseases. The differentiation among causes is important because management and prognosis depend on an accurate diagnosis. Untreated pulmonary hypertension (greater than 30 mm Hg) has a 5-year survival rate of about 30%. While less than 5% of cases of pulmonary hypertension are due to thromboembolic events, they can potentially be successfully treated with pulmonary endarterectomy. V/Q scanning has been reported to be more sensitive than CT pulmonary angiography in making the differentiation. A normal or low probability scan essentially excludes pulmonary hypertension caused by chronic pulmonary emboli. A high probability scan demonstrating segmental or subsegmental mismatches typical of pulmonary emboli has a sensitivity of over 96%, specificity of 95%, and accuracy of 95% as the cause of a patient's pulmonary hypertension. Importantly, inclusion of intermediate probability (nondiagnostic) scans

reduces these values only minimally and thus an intermediate probability (nondiagnostic) presentation is a useful finding in this setting. Primary pulmonary hypertension can have a normal V/Q scan or simply patchy perfusion. Parenchymal causes of pulmonary hypertension usually have matched defects. Because of accompanying perivascular fibrosis in patients with chronic pulmonary hypertension from various causes, the lung bases generally remain poorly perfused, regardless of the position in which the patient is injected. In addition, focal and segmental basilar perfusion defects may also be present.

Nonembolic Diseases
Chronic Obstructive Pulmonary Disease

Emphysema and chronic bronchitis are the most common forms of COPD. Both diseases are associated with patchy, uneven ventilation, reduced lung compliance, and increased peripheral resistance. In emphysema, there is parenchymal destruction distal to the terminal bronchioles, causing damage in the secondary pulmonary lobules; this includes damage to the alveoli as well as to the pulmonary capillaries. Extensive destruction may result in the formation of bullae. On ventilation/perfusion lung scans, these changes result in matched ventilation/perfusion abnormalities that typify airway disease.

Pulmonary ventilation imaging is most helpful in characterizing the regional distribution of airway abnormalities and, to a lesser extent, in delineating the clinical severity of the disease. It is not uncommon for a patient to have marked changes on the ventilation scan but a relatively normal chest radiograph because the typical radiographic changes are often late manifestations of emphysema.

In patients with early or mild COPD, the perfusion scan may be normal or near normal. As the destruction of lung parenchyma progresses, however, it characteristically produces multiple subsegmental or nonsegmental perfusion defects, which may be relatively focal and discrete or diffusely scattered throughout the lungs, giving a coarsely mottled pattern. Perfusion defects may also be caused by regional hypoxia, producing reflex vasoconstriction and by bullae themselves or their compression of adjacent lung. Large apical bullae may render strikingly reduced or absent perfusion to the upper lung zones.

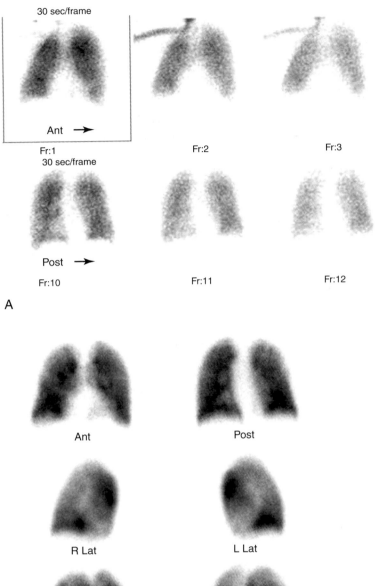

A

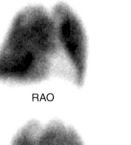

B

Figure 6-17. Chronic obstructive pulmonary disease. **A,** Xenon ventilation scan shows markedly delayed washout. **B,** Perfusion images show patchy distribution but no wedge-shaped segmental defects.

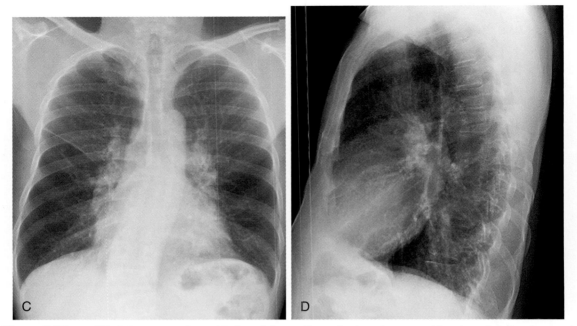

Figure 6-17, cont'd. C, Posteroanterior and **D,** lateral chest radiographs show the expected lung hyperinflation, increased anteroposterior chest diameter, and flattened hemidiaphragms.

In the presence of COPD, the perfusion scan is nonspecific unless accompanied by a ventilation study. Ventilation scans performed with ^{133}Xe characteristically reveal abnormalities in the involved areas on the single-breath images and less frequently on the equilibrium views. Washout images usually demonstrate areas of delayed clearance (trapping) that may correspond to the initial defects seen on the single-breath views. Ventilation abnormalities that correlate with defects seen on the perfusion scan constitute a ventilation/perfusion match, a hallmark of primary airway disease (Fig. 6-17). This finding may be of great value in distinguishing between COPD and superimposed pulmonary emboli when the latter are suspected. Many patients who present for ventilation/perfusion imaging for evaluation of pulmonary emboli have COPD. Thus it is important to correlate carefully the ventilation and perfusion scans. If all of the defects are small and subsegmental and have matched ventilation defects, emphysema is likely. Using the modified PIOPED II criteria, the diagnosis of pulmonary embolism is not made unless there are at least two superimposed mismatched large segmental defects.

The sensitivity of the ventilation scan for detection of chronic obstructive airway disease varies with the imaging phase of the examination. The ^{133}Xe single-breath image detects about 70%

of matched ventilation/perfusion abnormalities, whereas the equilibrium images detect only 20% of such defects. In fact, the equilibrium images may well be normal if rebreathing of xenon is sufficient to allow collateral pathway filling of postobstructive lung. The washout or clearance phase, however, is much more sensitive, detecting more than 90% of matched ventilation/perfusion lesions as regional trapping of xenon. Because the late phase is most sensitive, particular care should be given to this part of the examination. A ^{133}Xe washout study in patients with suspected COPD should continue for at least 3 to 5 minutes because single-breath and equilibrium images may be normal in these patients. When using ^{99m}Tc-DTPA aerosol ventilation imaging in patients with COPD, little or no peripheral activity may be seen in the lungs because increased turbulence in the large airways causes marked deposition in the trachea and bronchi (Fig. 6-18).

Ventilation/perfusion scintigraphy has also been used to investigate less common forms of COPD, such as α_1-antitrypsin deficiency and cystic fibrosis. α_1-Antitrypsin deficiency is a recessive inherited form of panlobular emphysema in which homozygotes demonstrate marked abnormalities of ventilation and perfusion predominating in the lower lungs, and even heterozygotes may show delayed clearance

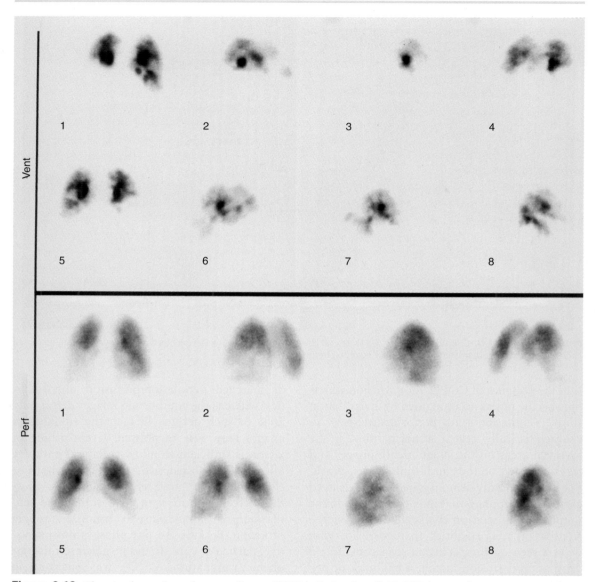

Figure 6-18. Chronic obstructive pulmonary disease (COPD). Technetium ^{99m}Tc-DTPA aerosol scan (*upper set*) shows marked central deposition of the aerosol caused by COPD, which limits interpretation for pulmonary embolism significantly. ^{99m}Tc-MAA perfusion images (*lower set*) are more normal but still inhomogeneous.

of xenon from these zones. Ventilation/perfusion studies performed in patients with cystic fibrosis demonstrate patchy segmental defects in perfusion and markedly disturbed ventilation, particularly in the washout phase.

Mucous Plugs

Mucous plugging of one or more airways is a common cause of hypoxia and may produce matched segmental ventilation/perfusion defects on lung scans. The ventilation scan demonstrates little or no activity in the involved lung segment on inspiration images and may demonstrate significant trapping on the washout images where there is collateral air drift (Fig. 6-19). Perfusion in the affected area is usually reduced, owing to reflex arteriolar constriction induced by local hypoxia. The chest radiograph may be normal or may show some volume loss associated with postobstructive atelectasis.

Asthma, Bronchiectasis, and Bronchitis

Asthma, bronchiectasis, and bronchitis all cause airway obstruction by different but often overlapping mechanisms. Asthma is primarily

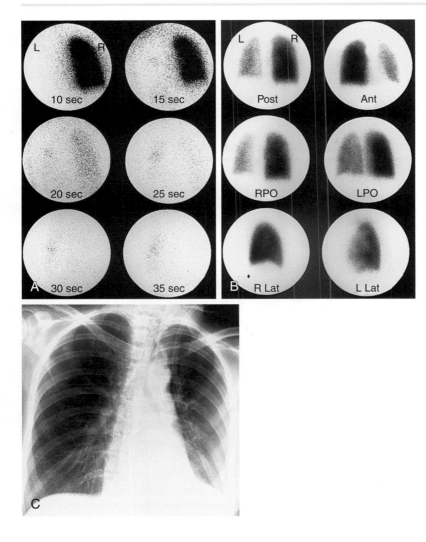

Figure 6-19. Mucous plug. **A,** Posterior xenon ventilation scan shows little or no activity in the left lung initially and a little trapping at 35 seconds. **B,** Perfusion scan shows a small left lung with generally diminished perfusion. **C,** Anteroposterior chest radiograph shows volume loss on the left as a result of postobstructive atelectasis. The findings were due to a mucous plug in the left mainstem bronchus.

related to acute spastic narrowing of the bronchi. Bronchiectasis destroys the elastic and muscular tissue in the bronchial walls, causing dilation and sometimes collapse, usually with associated infection. Bronchitis results in large amounts of viscous mucus in the bronchi. Often, all three disorders are present in the same patient (frequently a smoker) and may ultimately lead to emphysema. These diseases are characterized by acute episodic exacerbation, during which significant ventilation and accompanying perfusion abnormalities are found on pulmonary ventilation/perfusion scans. Despite the clinical symptoms, chest radiographs are often negative, and excluding the presence of superimposed diseases such as pulmonary emboli may be difficult.

Scattered matched segmental perfusion defects are generally present during an acute asthma attack, related to reflex vasoconstriction secondary to regional hypoxia. Corresponding ventilation defects are frequently noted during the single-breath xenon study but may become less apparent with rebreathing, and regional areas of delayed washout are also usually identified. The geographic location of these abnormalities within the lungs may characteristically change during the same or subsequent attacks, giving an altered pattern of ventilation/perfusion abnormalities on serial lung scans (Fig. 6-20). This provides a scintigraphic distinction from chronic emphysema, which results in a fixed location of the abnormalities. In asthmatic patients who do not have COPD, ventilation/perfusion scans frequently return to normal within 24 hours after treatment with bronchodilators. This may be used to distinguish between pulmonary emboli and asthma if they cannot be differentiated on the basis of initial clinical and scintigraphic assessment. The detection of

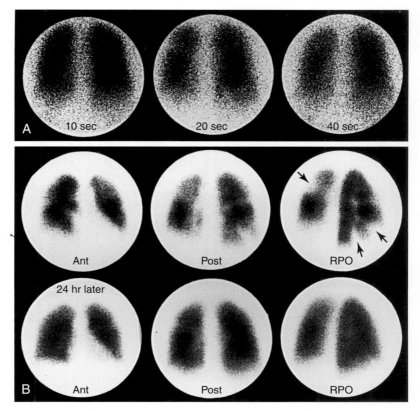

Figure 6-20. Asthma. A, Posterior images from the washout portion of a xenon ventilation scan show poor washout with little decrease in activity on the sequential 20-second images. **B,** Perfusion scan (*top*) shows multiple large and small segmental defects (*arrows*) that cleared within 24 hours after bronchodilator therapy (*bottom*).

wheezing or ascertainment of a prior history of asthma in a patient undergoing imaging for suspected pulmonary emboli may greatly aid in the interpretation of the images and in determining the need for repeat imaging after bronchodilator administration.

Unlike asthma, the perfusion defects produced by bronchiectasis are constant in location (generally restricted to the lung bases) and are in large part related to reflex vasoconstriction secondary to local hypoxia. Regional ventilation defects with or without associated trapping are the expected findings on the xenon study.

Lung Neoplasms

If large enough, any lung neoplasm, whether benign, malignant, or metastatic, may produce localized ventilation/perfusion defects corresponding to the lesion on a lung scan. If there is secondary pulmonary arterial or bronchial obstruction, then larger ventilation/perfusion abnormalities in the lung distal to the lesion may occur, with possible delayed washout of xenon. If the lesion is bronchial (such as an adenoma), there may be distal hypoxia with a reflex decrease in perfusion. With lesions

that cause arterial compression, the perfusion abnormality is generally more striking than is the ventilatory impairment (Fig. 6-21).

The use of ventilation/perfusion imaging in staging and evaluating the extent of local tumor invasion has been supplanted by CT. PET and PET/CT scanning are being used to stage and evaluate response to therapy of non–small-cell lung cancers and to evaluate solitary pulmonary nodules (Chapter 11). Preoperative radionuclide lung imaging, however, may still play a role in the assessment of regional lung function to predict expected residual function after surgical resection of a lobe or entire lung (Fig. 6-22). This is usually done in conjunction with standard spirometry. These evaluations are particularly important because coexistent chronic lung disease is common in these patients.

In patients with multiple tumor microemboli or lymphangitic carcinomatosis, there may be multiple small linear perfusion defects that outline the bronchopulmonary segments, a finding known as *contour mapping* (Fig. 6-23). Segmental contour mapping may be present even when the chest radiograph and ventilation scans are normal. The sign may be of value in differentiating these

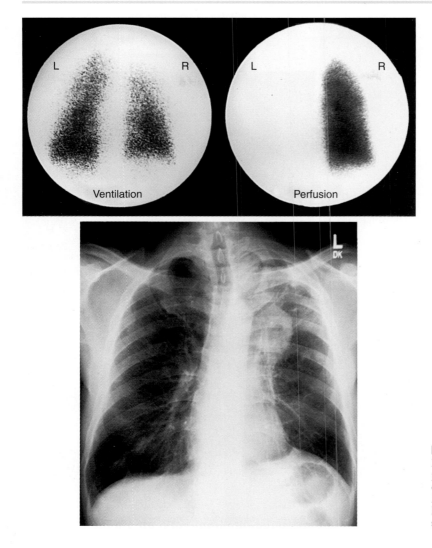

Figure 6-21. Lung cancer. *Top,* Posterior images from a ventilation/perfusion scan show ventilation of the left lung but no perfusion. *Bottom,* Chest radiograph shows a large left hilar mass that has constricted the left pulmonary artery.

conditions from suspected pulmonary embolism, in which the perfusion defects usually occupy all or parts of segments. This finding is usually seen incidental to imaging for other reasons because routine ventilation/perfusion lung scanning is of no real value in the detection or assessment of pulmonary metastases.

Inflammatory Disease

When a localized infiltrate is identified on the chest radiograph of a patient with thoracic symptoms, pneumonitis is the foremost consideration, although in certain patients other causes, such as pulmonary emboli, may need to be excluded. In the presence of any radiographic infiltrate, regardless of cause, both ventilation and perfusion are expected to be markedly decreased or absent in the involved area on lung imaging. The areas of infiltration usually

do not ventilate on the initial or rebreathing studies and do not retain xenon during the washout procedure unless there is associated obstruction. With pneumonic infiltrates, the ventilation defects are normally larger than are the perfusion defects (Fig. 6-24), and ventilation and perfusion abnormalities often persist for some time after an infiltrate has resolved on the chest radiograph. For this reason, if a perfusion defect appears significantly larger than is the corresponding radiographic infiltrate in a patient with presumed pneumonia, then a series of recent chest radiographs, if available, should be reviewed because a partially resolved pneumonia may be the cause of the discrepancy.

When the cause of an infiltrate is in doubt, the size of the perfusion defect in relation to that of the radiographic infiltrate may provide a clue to its etiology. In small or early pneumonias, there

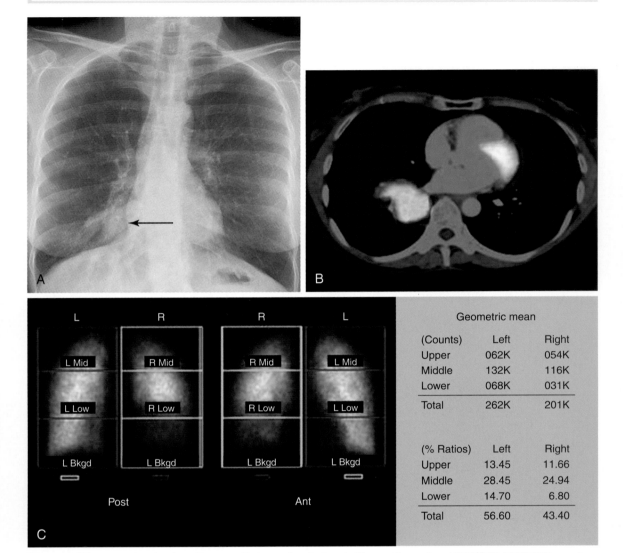

Figure 6-22. **Regional evaluation of lung ventilation and perfusion. A,** Chest radiograph and (**B**) ^{18}F-FDG PET/CT scan show a right lower lobe lung cancer. Quantitative split lung function can show (**C**) regional perfusion or ventilation for preoperative planning. Here the lungs are divided into thirds and the geometric mean of anterior and posterior images is calculated.

The Geometric mean table from panel C:

Geometric mean		
(Counts)	Left	Right
Upper	062K	054K
Middle	132K	116K
Lower	068K	031K
Total	262K	201K

(% Ratios)	Left	Right
Upper	13.45	11.66
Middle	28.45	24.94
Lower	14.70	6.80
Total	56.60	43.40

Figure 6-23. Lymphangitic tumor spread. The pattern seen on these anterior (*left*) and right posterior oblique (*right*) lung perfusion images is referred to as *contour mapping.* Thickening of the intersegmental interstitium at the periphery of the pulmonary segments has resulted in perfusion defects (*lines*) that outline the segments.

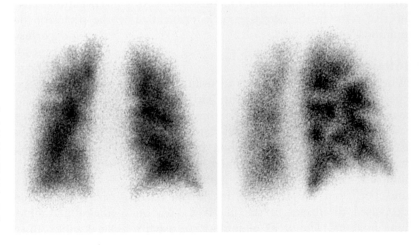

is almost always a perfusion defect that is smaller than or equal in size to the corresponding radiographic infiltrate. With large pneumonias (such as lobar pneumonia), the perfusion deficit is usually the same size as the radiographic infiltrate. Perfusion defects that appear significantly larger than the radiographic abnormality or that are

out of proportion to the ventilatory defect may raise a suspicion of pulmonary embolus in the appropriate clinical setting. Frequently, such a suspicion may be substantiated by the presence of segmental ventilation/perfusion mismatches in other areas of radiographically normal lung. In the absence of corroborating perfusion

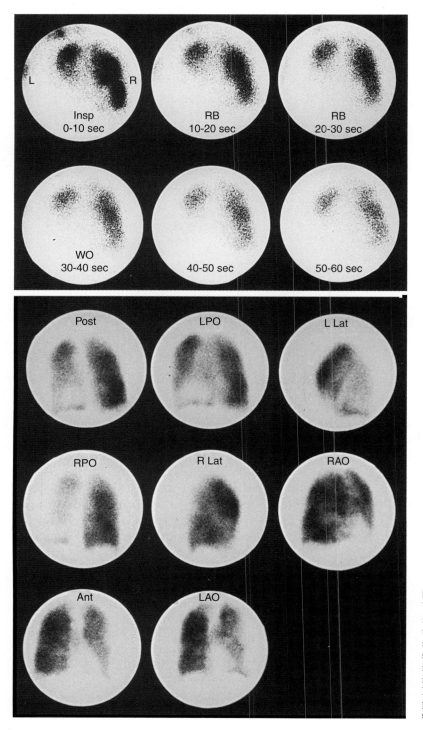

Figure 6-24. Pneumonia. *Top,* Ventilation scan demonstrates a marked area of nonventilation in the left lung base. *Bottom,* Perfusion scan shows a defect that is smaller than the ventilation defect, in the area where an infiltrate was identified on a chest radiograph. Note the presence of the stripe sign, particularly on the posterior perfusion image.

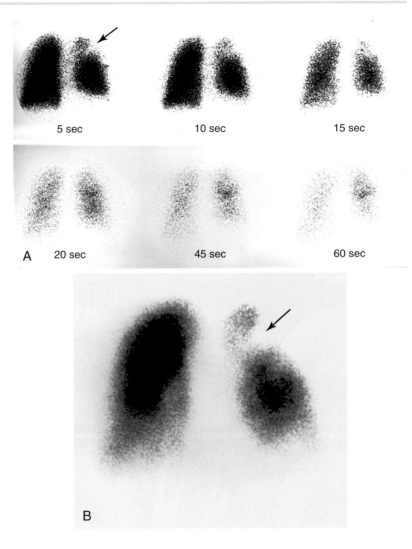

Figure 6-25. Tuberculosis. A, Posterior xenon ventilation scan shows an area of initially decreased ventilation (*arrow*), with trapping seen later in the same area. B, Posterior image from the perfusion lung scan shows decreased perfusion (*arrow*) in the same area (a matched defect).

defects elsewhere in the lungs, CTPA may be needed to exclude the diagnosis. Matched apical abnormalities may be seen with old tuberculosis (Fig. 6-25).

Cardiovascular Abnormalities

Normal cardiovascular structures commonly cause significant defects on the ventilation/perfusion images, which may be accentuated in disease. These defects are typically nonsegmental and usually conform to the radiographic appearance of the structures producing them. Thus it is important to examine the chest radiograph for cardiovascular abnormalities, particularly structural enlargement, abnormal contours, aneurysmal dilations, and changes caused by either congestive failure or pulmonary hypertension.

Uncomplicated congestive heart failure is typically characterized by nonsegmental perfusion defects, which are usually diffuse and scattered throughout both lungs but may occasionally be focal. Fissure signs may be present, as well as other abnormalities caused by pleural effusions, cardiac enlargement, redistribution of pulmonary blood flow to the upper lung zones, or pulmonary edema. Occasionally, superimposed pulmonary emboli may be suspected in patients with congestive heart failure, and differentiation of the two entities by scintigraphic techniques may be difficult, especially when congestive heart failure is manifested by pulmonary edema or pleural effusions. Diffuse interstitial edema is frequently not a problem because a relatively normal perfusion scan may be obtained in the absence of emboli. When patchy alveolar edema is present, however, focal perfusion defects may result, usually corresponding to localized alveolar densities seen on the chest radiographs.

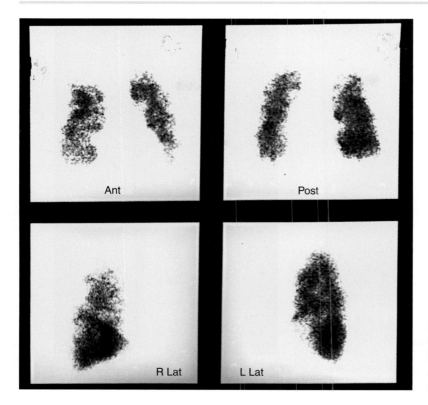

Ant   Post

R Lat   L Lat

Figure 6-26. Vasculitis. Perfusion scan images show bilateral patchy small segmental defects. This pattern could also be seen in a variety of abnormalities, including multiple small emboli.

In these cases, a high probability of superimposed pulmonary emboli may be assessed if segmental ventilation/perfusion mismatches are identified in areas of a relatively normal lung. If a distinction cannot be made, CT angiography may be necessary to establish the diagnosis.

Loculated pleural effusions accompanying congestive heart failure may cause peripheral defects in the lungs, but these are usually easily discernible on the chest radiograph and rarely appear segmental or multiple on upright views. To minimize the imaging problems, patients with pleural effusions are normally injected in the supine position and imaged in the upright position.

A multitude of other diseases related to the cardiovascular system can cause abnormalities on the ventilation/perfusion scans. However, these scan abnormalities can frequently be sorted out when reviewed with the benefit of clinical history and recent chest radiographs. Numerous bilateral, very small perfusion defects with normal ventilation should raise the possibility of either vasculitis (Fig. 6-26) or fat emboli (Fig. 6-27).

DEEP VENOUS IMAGING AND THROMBUS DETECTION

The introduction of radiolabeled monoclonal antibodies that recognize specific sites on activated components of clotted blood represents a new approach to the diagnosis of deep venous thrombosis; however, such techniques have not been clinically useful to date. One Food and Drug Administration-approved radiopharmaceutical is ^{99m}Tc-apcitide, a synthetic polypeptide, which binds to receptors on activated platelets and, to a lesser extent, to endothelial cells. There is normally activity present in the liver and kidneys and excretion via the urinary tract and biliary system. It is most sensitive for the detection of acute clots in the first 2 weeks after onset of clinical symptoms. Diagnosis is based upon significant asymmetry in activity between the two lower extremities. The agreement rate between this technique and the "gold standard" of contrast venography is only 50% to 75%, and thus is not a commonly used technique. It has low sensitivity for pulmonary emboli.

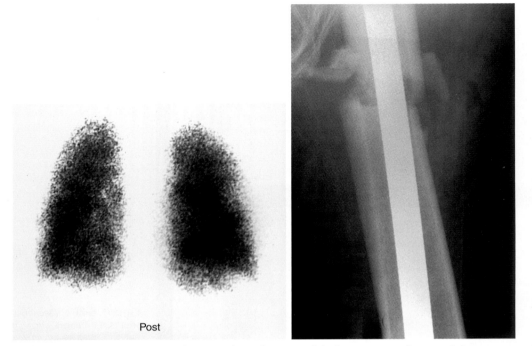

Figure 6-27. Fat emboli. Posterior image from a perfusion lung scan (*left*) demonstrates a fine, mottled pattern caused by fat emboli occurring after this patient had an intramedullary femoral rod (*right*) placed for a fracture.

PEARLS & PITFALLS

- While over 90% of pulmonary embolism studies are now performed by CT angiography, V/Q scans remain useful particularly in patients with renal failure, contrast allergies, or other situations in which CT is difficult, contraindicated or not available.

- Unless it is completely and absolutely normal, do not interpret a ventilation/perfusion scan without a recent chest radiograph. A radiograph within a day or two may be adequate for a stable patient but a radiograph within a few hours is needed in an unstable patient.

- A normal perfusion lung scan essentially excludes clinically significant pulmonary emboli. An abnormal ventilation scan or chest radiograph will not change this assessment.

- In addition to pulmonary thromboembolism, other causes of perfusion defects are COPD, pneumonia, asthma, tumor, mediastinitis, mucous plug, fat emboli, and vasculitis.

- Most perfusion defects caused by pulmonary emboli are segmental, wedge-shaped, and extend to the periphery. They are often bilateral and multiple. The defects can be areas of

- diminished activity because not all clots are completely occluding.

- Using the modified PIOPED II criteria, two or more large ventilation-perfusion mismatches are needed to make a determination of PE present. There are limited specific criteria (including a normal scan) used to make a determination of PE-absent. All other findings are nondiagnostic.

- In the interpretation of V/Q lung scans, an *unmatched or mismatched defect* refers to one that is seen on the perfusion scan without an accompanying ventilation abnormality. It does not refer to a defect on the ventilation scan when the perfusion scan is normal. Similarly, it does not refer to comparison of the perfusion scan to the chest radiograph (unless one is using the PIOPED perfusion-only criteria) or to comparison of the ventilation scan to the chest radiograph.

- Regardless of the ventilation scan findings, if there is a normal chest radiograph and the perfusion scan has one or more segmental defects, pulmonary embolism is likely present.

- Regardless of the ventilation scan findings, if there are only nonsegmental defects or defects

PEARLS & PITFALLS—cont'd

caused by the heart, diaphragm, mediastinum, bullae or large pleural effusion, pulmonary embolism is likely absent.

- Asthma, mucous plugs, and COPD can cause segmental perfusion defects, but they should not have normal ventilation scans.

- A stripe sign of peripheral activity around a perfusion defect is frequently seen with COPD and indicates a very low probability of pulmonary embolism.

- A fissure sign refers to identification of an intrapulmonary fissure as a corresponding linear defect on a perfusion scan. Common causes are pleural fluid or thickening and COPD.

- When there is an infiltrate on the chest radiograph and a smaller perfusion defect, pneumonia is a common cause. When there is a small infiltrate and a relatively larger perfusion defect, pulmonary emboli should be considered.

- If there is ventilation of one whole lung but no perfusion, the differential diagnosis includes congenital absence of the pulmonary artery, massive central pulmonary embolus, mediastinal fibrosis, or hilar neoplasm.

- A focal hot spot in the lung is due to an injected labeled clot that was either formed in the syringe or dislodged from the end of the central line through which ^{99m}Tc-MAA was injected.

- On an MAA perfusion scan, activity in the kidneys and brain indicates a right-to-left shunt. If a shunt is suspected before the perfusion scan, the number of particles should be reduced from about 400,000 to about 100,000.

- Pulmonary hypertension caused by chronic pulmonary emboli typically presents as a high or intermediate (nondiagnostic) probability scan with mismatched segmental or subsegmental defects and normal ventilation images. Other causes of pulmonary hypertension have normal scans or matched V/Q defects.

- Multiple tiny or small bilateral patchy defects on a perfusion scan should raise the possibility of fat emboli, tumor emboli, vasculitis, or an inadequate number of particles injected.

- On an aerosol ventilation scan, collection of activity in the central bronchi is an indication of COPD.

- Poor perfusion to the lung apices may be normal after lung transplantation.

- Extrapulmonary activity can be seen on a xenon scan as a result of a fatty liver, and this may be mistaken for air trapping at the right lung base. Esophageal activity can be seen on a DTPA aerosol scan as a result of swallowed activity, and activity in thyroid, salivary glands, and stomach is seen as the result of free technetium pertechnetate.

SUGGESTED READINGS

Anderson DR, Kahn SR, Rodger MA, et al. Computed tomography pulmonary angiography vs. ventilation-perfusion lung scanning in patients with suspected pulmonary embolism: A controlled randomized trial. JAMA 2007;298(23):2743-53.

Angelli G, Becattini C. Acute pulmonary embolism: Current concepts. N Engl J Med 2010;363:266-74.

Line BR. Scintigraphic studies of non-embolic lung disease. In: Sandler MP, Coleman RE, Patton JA, et al, editors. Diagnostic Nuclear Medicine. 4th ed. New York: Lippincott Williams & Wilkins; 2003, p. 377-412.

Reid JH, Coche EE, Inoue T, et al. Is the lung scan alive and well? Facts and controversies in defining the role of lung scintigraphy for the diagnosis of pulmonary embolism in the era of MDCT. Eur J Nucl Med Mol Imaging 2009;36:505-21.

Reinartz P. To PIOPED, or not to PIOPED. J Nucl Med 2008;49(11):1739-40.

Society of Nuclear Medicine. SNM practice guideline for lung scintigraphy 4.0, 2011, http://interactive.snm.org/docs/Lung_scintigraphy_V4_Final pdf. Accessed September 16, 2011.

Sostman HD, Miniati M, Gottschalk A, et al. Sensitivity and specificity of perfusion scintigraphy combined with chest radiography for acute pulmonary embolism. J Nucl Med 2008;49:1741-8.

Sostman HD, Stein PD, Gottschalk A, et al. Acute pulmonary embolism: Sensitivity and specificity of ventilation-perfusion scintigraphy in PIOPED II study. Radiology 2008;246(3):941-6.

Stein EG, Haramati LB, Chamarthy M, et al. Success of a safe and simple algorithm to reduce use of CT pulmonary angiography in the emergency department. AJR. Am J Roentgenol 2010;194:392-7.

Stein PD, Freeman LM, Sostman HD, et al. SPECT in acute pulmonary embolism. J Nucl Med 2009;50:1999-2007.

Tunariu N, Gibbs S, Win Z, et al. Ventilation-perfusion scintigraphy is more sensitive than multidetector CTPA in detecting chronic thromboembolic disease as a treatable cause of pulmonary hypertension. J Nucl Med 2007; 48(5):680-4.

7 Gastrointestinal Tract

LIVER–SPLEEN IMAGING
  Radiopharmaceuticals
  Planar Imaging and SPECT
  Normal Liver Scan
  Abnormal Liver Scan
HEPATIC BLOOD POOL IMAGING
SPLENIC IMAGING
  Normal Spleen Scan
  Abnormal Spleen Scan
GASTROINTESTINAL BLEEDING STUDIES
  Interpretation

MECKEL DIVERTICULUM IMAGING
HEPATOBILIARY IMAGING
  Radiopharmaceuticals
  Technique
  Normal Scan
  Clinical Settings
GASTROESOPHAGEAL FUNCTION STUDIES
  Esophageal Transit
  Gastroesophageal Reflux
  Gastric Emptying
ABDOMINAL SHUNT EVALUATION

LIVER–SPLEEN IMAGING

Computed tomography (CT) and ultrasound offer better anatomic display of liver and spleen architecture than does radionuclide liver–spleen imaging, which is seldom performed. However, there remain some indications for technetium colloid liver–spleen scanning, such as the confirmation or evaluation of suspected hepatocellular diseases, hepatomegaly or splenomegaly, and the confirmation of specific space-occupying lesions such as hepatic focal nodular hyperplasia. Although this section is primarily directed toward these applications, as with the interpretation of any examination, it is prudent to have an understanding of other important entities that may be present incidentally, as well as their scintigraphic appearance.

Radiopharmaceuticals

The liver and spleen are organs of widely differing functions, but radionuclide colloid imaging capitalizes on a function common to both: phagocytosis. The most commonly used agent is technetium-99m (^{99m}Tc) sulfur colloid, with an average particle size of 0.3 to 1.0 μm, which is larger than a true colloid. The uptake and distribution of ^{99m}Tc colloid in the liver reflect both the distribution of functioning reticuloendothelial cells and the distribution of hepatic perfusion. In normal patients, most particles are rapidly accumulated by the phagocytes of

the reticuloendothelial system of both the liver (Kupffer cells) and the spleen, allowing simultaneous imaging of both organs. Technetium colloid agents are cleared from the bloodstream with a half-time of 2 to 3 minutes. Under usual circumstances, 80% to 90% of the injected particles are sequestered by the liver, and 5% to 10% localize in the spleen. A small percentage of particles appears in other reticuloendothelial sites, particularly the bone marrow, but usually in amounts insufficient to permit imaging. In theory, there is some correlation between particle size and organ avidity for colloid: the larger particles are favored by the spleen, smaller particles go to the liver, and the smallest particles are sequestered by the bone marrow. As discussed later, visualization of uptake in the bone marrow on a technically satisfactory colloid liver–spleen scan is an abnormal finding. However, when amounts of ^{99m}Tc colloid significantly higher than the usual liver–spleen scanning dose are used, routine bone marrow imaging is possible.

Planar Imaging and SPECT

Sample imaging protocols for both planar and single-photon emission computed tomography (SPECT) imaging techniques as well as dosimetry are presented in Appendix E-1.

Imaging is performed using 4 to 6 mCi (148 to 222 MBq) of ^{99m}Tc sulfur colloid. Adequate accumulation of ^{99m}Tc sulfur colloid in the liver requires about 5 to 10 minutes in normal patients. This allows for an optimal target (liver–spleen)-to-background (blood pool) ratio. In patients with compromised hepatic function and/or portal hypertension, optimal liver concentration of the radiopharmaceutical may take considerably longer. In such patients, it is wise to wait 20 to 30 minutes before imaging.

Routine gamma camera images for liver–spleen scanning consist of anterior and posterior views as well as both lateral views. Each image is obtained for 500- to 1000-k counts by using a low-energy parallel-hole collimator. Various oblique images may be routinely obtained or performed as needed for further evaluation of a suspected abnormality in either organ. One anterior view with a lead marker identifying the right inferior costal margin is usually obtained as well. The marker should be of a known size so that hepatic and splenic measurements may be obtained. SPECT scanning of the liver occasionally adds additional information, although focal areas of decreased activity as a result of normal biliary and vascular structures often make interpretation difficult.

Tomographic imaging using ^{99m}Tc sulfur colloid requires a fundamental knowledge of cross-sectional anatomy of the liver and spleen as well as of surrounding unimaged structures. Transaxial images are displayed in the conventional CT format along with coronal and sagittal reconstructions. In general, defects thought to represent significant pathology should be seen in at least two orthogonal planes to be described with confidence. SPECT is most frequently used to evaluate known or suspected focal or multifocal space-occupying disease. In this setting, SPECT sensitivity and accuracy of localization have been shown to be superior to planar imaging. SPECT has proved especially useful in ^{99m}Tc red blood cell (RBC) blood pool imaging for suspected liver hemangiomas using the same technical parameters as for ^{99m}Tc sulfur colloid. Vascular structures appearing as characteristic defects on colloid SPECT images are usually identifiable as areas of increased activity on the labeled RBC images. Accuracy of interpretation may be improved by use of SPECT-CT fusion imaging.

Normal Liver Scan

In the normal liver, there is a homogeneous distribution of ^{99m}Tc sulfur colloid throughout the organ. The liver usually consists of a dominant right and a smaller left lobe (Fig. 7-1), which may occasionally be absent. Numerous variant liver shapes have been described, the most notable of which are a long, thin right lobe (Riedel lobe) and a prominent quadrate lobe. The porta hepatis is frequently identifiable as an area of decreased activity in the inferomedial aspect of the right lobe; this should not be mistaken for a lesion. Peripheral marginal indentations in the liver may normally be produced by the lateral rib margins, the xiphoid, the gallbladder, the right kidney, the suprahepatic veins, the heart, and intrathoracic abnormalities that affect the diaphragmatic configuration. A right lobe defect is commonly seen in many anterior views, owing to attenuation of the photons by overlying breast tissue. Activity seen in the bowel

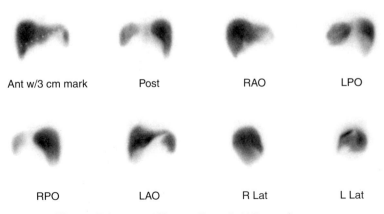

Figure 7-1. Normal ^{99m}Tc-sulfur colloid liver–spleen scan.

should raise the suspicion of a prior other type of nuclear medicine study (Fig. 7-2).

Normal length of the right lobe of the liver is generally 17 to 18 cm on the anterior view, measured from the highest point to the inferior tip of the right lobe. Evaluation of a liver–spleen scan should include (1) the size, shape, and position of the liver and spleen; (2) the homogeneity of activity within the organs; (3) the presence of any focal defects in activity; and (4) the relative distribution of colloid among the liver, spleen, and bone marrow.

Abnormal Liver Scan

Any localized space-occupying process in the liver may present as a focal area of decreased activity (commonly referred to as a *defect*) on a technetium colloid scan, provided that it is of sufficient size to be detected. Radionuclide imaging simply confirms the presence or anatomic location of focal lesions in the liver rather than providing a definitive histologic diagnosis. The size and location of a lesion are of paramount importance in determining whether it will be detected by gamma camera techniques. By using present technology, lesions as small as 8 mm may be identified. The nearer these lesions are to the surface of the organ, and therefore to the camera collimator surface, the more readily they may be detected.

Defects in the hepatic parenchyma are non-specific. Solitary intrahepatic defects may be produced by various lesions, any of which may also be multiple (Box 7-1 and Table 7-1). In any patient with several liver defects, however, metastatic disease must be a prime consideration, particularly when accompanied by hepatomegaly or a known primary lesion. In most instances, particularly in cases of equivocal liver scan findings, ultrasonography, CT, or MRI should be performed. A large area of decreased activity in the liver may be produced by the inclusion of part of that organ in a radiation therapy portal. This type of defect, however, is usually readily recognized by its sharp linear edges, which correspond to the sides of the treatment portal. In addition to primarily intrahepatic lesions, peripheral defects in the liver are frequently produced by adjacent extraparenchymal pathology, including subdiaphragmatic fluid accumulations or renal tumors, or by peripheral lesions of a primary hepatic origin, including subcapsular hematoma.

Increased radiocolloid concentration by the spleen and bone marrow compared with the liver (colloid shift) may be found in patients with diseases that cause derangement of hepatic function and/or portal hypertension. Among diffuse hepatocellular diseases, hepatic cirrhosis is the most common abnormality presenting in this fashion. Colloid shift accompanied

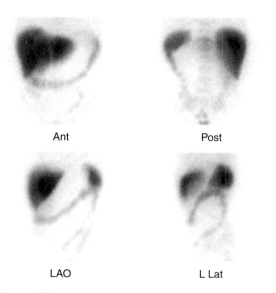

Ant   Post

LAO   L Lat

Figure 7-2. Normal ^{99m}Tc-sulfur colloid liver-spleen scan after a cardiac perfusion study on the previous day. Multiple planar images show colonic activity, which is the result of biliary excretion from a ^{99m}Tc-sestamibi study on the previous day.

Box 7-1   Differential of Focal Hepatic Lesions on Technetium-99m Colloid Scans

Decreased Uptake
Metastasis (especially colon)
Cyst
Hepatoma (especially in cirrhosis)
Adenoma
Hematoma
Hemangioma
Abscess
Pseudotumor (cirrhosis)

Increased Uptake
Focal nodular hyperplasia
Cirrhosis with regenerating nodule
Budd-Chiari syndrome (caudate lobe)
Superior vena caval obstruction (arm injection, quadrate lobe)

TABLE 7-1	Nuclear Imaging Appearances of Liver Lesions on ^{99m}Tc Colloid and Other Scans	
LESIONS	**APPEARANCE**	
Hepatic adenoma	Usually photopenic defect	
	Rarely normal activity	
	^{99m}Tc RBCs—normal	
	^{99m}Tc hepatobiliary: perfusion—normal, parenchymal—decreased, washout—delayed	
Focal nodular hyperplasia	30% photopenic defect	
	30% normal activity	
	40% increased activity	
	^{99m}Tc hepatobiliary: perfusion—increased, parenchymal—normal, washout—delayed	
Cavernous hemangioma	Photopenic defect	
	^{99m}Tc RBCs: perfusion—decreased, blood pool—increased	
Hepatocellular carcinoma	Photopenic defect	
	^{67}Ga—avidly increased	
	^{99m}Tc RBCs—rarely increased	
	^{99m}Tc hepatobiliary: perfusion—decreased, parenchymal—normal or decreased, washout—delayed	
Cholangiocarcinoma	Photopenic defect	
Metastases	Photopenic defect, early hyperperfusion	
Liver abscess	Photopenic defect	
	^{67}Ga—80% increased	
Focal fatty infiltration	Photopenic defect	
	^{133}Xe—increased	

^{67}Ga, Gallium-67; RBCs, red blood cells; ^{99m}Tc, technetium-99m; ^{133}Xe, xenon-133.

Box 7-2 Diffuse Pulmonary Uptake of Technetium-99m Sulfur Colloid

Hepatic cirrhosis
Chronic obstructive pulmonary disease with superimposed infection
Bacterial endotoxin
Estrogen therapy
Neoplasms (various primary tumors and metastases, including hepatoma)
Disseminated intravascular coagulopathy
Mucopolysaccharidosis type II (Hunter syndrome)
Histiocytosis X
Faulty colloid preparation (excess aluminum)
High serum aluminum level (antacids)
Children (normal minimal uptake)
Transplant recipients
Pulmonary trauma

---

by other typical scintigraphic findings is a hallmark of this disease. Even patients with diffuse hepatic metastases may show colloid shift. The distribution of colloid in the bone marrow should be carefully examined in such patients because localized defects in colloid activity indicating marrow involvement by tumor may be identified.

Other abnormal distributions of colloid include activity in renal transplants, diffuse lung activity, and focal hot spots in the liver (see Box 7-1). Diffuse pulmonary activity may be noted occasionally in cirrhosis, infection, and many other entities (Box 7-2). In the presence of superior vena cava or innominate venous obstruction, a bolus of activity injected into an ipsilateral arm vein can travel via the collaterals to a recanalized umbilical vessel, delivering a large amount of activity to the anterior mid-portion of the liver (quadrate lobe), which causes a focal hot spot. Other entities that may cause apparent focal areas of increased hepatic activity are Budd-Chiari syndrome (hepatic vein obstruction), focal nodular hyperplasia, and cirrhosis (regenerating nodules).

Hepatic Cirrhosis

A spectrum of technetium colloid scan findings is presented by hepatic cirrhosis. In its early phases, alcoholic hepatitis or fatty infiltration may present as a normal-sized or enlarged liver with diffusely diminished or inhomogeneous activity. As the disease progresses and parenchymal scarring becomes more prevalent, the liver may become smaller than normal. An oddity of this disease is that the right lobe is frequently more affected, giving a typical pattern of a small right lobe and a relatively enlarged left lobe. This probably occurs because the portal vein delivers more blood flow (and alcohol) to the right lobe of the liver.

Fatty infiltration of the liver may be focal or diffuse. Focal fatty infiltration is seen on CT as an area of low attenuation and can be confused with a neoplastic process. Usually, it can be differentiated from a true mass on CT

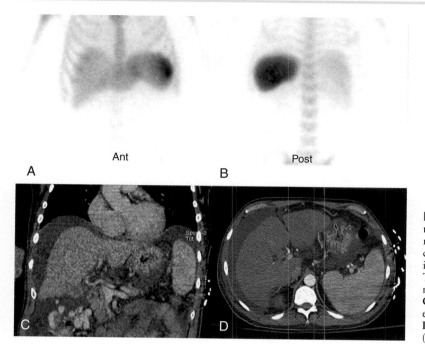

Ant   Post

A   B

C   D

Figure 7-3. Cirrhosis with ascites. **A,** ^{99m}Tc-sulfur colloid anterior and **B,** posterior images show colloid shift as increased activity in the bone marrow and spleen. The liver is small and displaced medially from the ribs by ascites. **C,** The ascites and small liver are easily appreciated on coronal and **D,** axial computed tomography (CT) scans.

by noting that there is no mass effect and that portal vessels run through the low-density area. If a technetium colloid scan is performed, the area typically shows normal reticuloendothelial activity. Fatty infiltration can also be noted as an incidental finding on a xenon ventilation lung scan by noting xenon retention in the liver, either focally or diffusely.

As the process of injury, scarring, and regeneration continues, activity within the organ becomes less homogeneous and is sometimes so coarsely mottled as to be confused with space-occupying lesions. In cirrhotic patients with this mottled pattern or with a large dominant defect, especially those who have demonstrated sudden unexplained clinical decompensation, superimposed hepatoma must be considered.

Colloid shift to the spleen and bone marrow is another prominent feature of all phases of hepatic cirrhosis. When hepatocyte function is severely depressed, persistence of technetium colloid in the blood pool may also be identified on static images, especially in the cardiac area. In the advanced stages of disease, the spleen is frequently enlarged, a finding that may correlate with portal hypertension. In some patients, ascites may be imaged on the anterior view as medial displacement of the right lobe of the liver from the ribs and lateral abdominal wall (Fig. 7-3).

Box 7-3   Causes of Hepatomegaly with Slightly Decreased Activity on Technetium-99m Sulfur Colloid Scans

Normal variant (i.e., large patient with soft tissue attenuation)
Diffuse hepatocellular disease (e.g., hepatitis)
Metastases
Diabetes mellitus
Fatty infiltration
Hemochromatosis
Amyloidosis
Lymphoma
Leukemia
Sarcoidosis
Lipid storage disorders
Passive congestion

Diffuse and Infiltrative Disorders

Any disease that secondarily invades the liver may produce a pattern of hepatomegaly, with or without focal defects, and commonly with diffusely diminished activity. Disease entities that may produce this pattern are listed in Box 7-3. Hepatitis may present in this manner, reflecting diffuse parenchymal edema. If hepatic function is compromised, colloid shift may also be seen.

Metastatic Disease

CT or MRI scanning is the initial test of choice if a hepatic tumor or metastasis is suspected. Radionuclide liver-spleen scanning usually detects these as serendipitous findings when the examination is performed for some other reason. Applications of tumor-specific radiopharmaceuticals are discussed in Chapters 10 and 11.

The most characteristic presentation of liver metastasis on a technetium colloid scan is as multiple focal defects, although the lesions may present as coarsely inhomogeneous activity or simply as hepatomegaly. By using discrete hepatic defects as the diagnostic criterion for metastatic disease, the liver scan demonstrates a detection sensitivity of about 75% to 80% for all types of primary tumors, especially when scintigraphic data are integrated with available clinical information. Individual sensitivity varies with the particular primary lesion.

Primary Liver Neoplasms

Hepatoma. Hepatoma usually presents as a focal defect on sulfur colloid images (Fig. 7-4), although uncommon multifocal forms exist. The lesions frequently occur in association with preexisting diffuse hepatic diseases, most notably alcoholic or postnecrotic cirrhosis. The appearance of a prominent localized colloid deficit in a patient with one of these associations should alert the physician to the possibility of hepatoma. Hepatomas are also noted to be generally gallium-67 (^{67}Ga)–avid and with variable FDG activity. Therapy for hepatoma may involve direct infusion of chemotherapeutic or embolic agents into the hepatic artery. Evaluation of the catheter placement and distribution of blood flow can be done either with contrast angiography or by administration of 1 to 4 mCi (37 to 148 MBq) of ^{99m}Tc macroaggregated albumin (MAA) (not colloid). The MAA lodges in the capillaries served by the catheter.

Focal Nodular Hyperplasia. The benign neoplasm of focal nodular hyperplasia generally occurs as an asymptomatic mass or as a serendipitously discovered lesion found predominantly in women. The lesions are unique because they contain adequate numbers of Kupffer cells, so that they normally concentrate and occasionally hyperconcentrate radiocolloid. Thus in most cases, they appear indistinguishable from normal hepatic parenchyma (Fig. 7-5); infrequently, they present as regions of increased activity on liver scans. When lesions discovered by other imaging modalities are of sufficient size to be detected by liver scintigraphy but appear normal on the liver scan, the diagnosis of focal nodular hyperplasia may be presumed in the proper clinical setting. In a minority of cases, insufficient colloid is concentrated by the lesions, so that they are perceived as photopenic areas on the scan. When this occurs, the mass cannot be differentiated from other causes of parenchymal defects.

Hepatic Cell Adenomas. Hepatic cell adenomas are usually encountered in young women who have used birth control pills. Although the disease usually is asymptomatic, hemorrhage, often of massive degree, occasionally occurs. Because Kupffer cells are not a prominent feature of these lesions, adenomas present as focal defects on technetium colloid images. When birth control pills are withheld, these lesions may rapidly regress.

Miscellaneous Focal Lesions

Abscess. Abscess commonly presents as a nonspecific solitary focal defect on liver scans, although multiple lesions may occur. The diagnosis is frequently suggested by history.

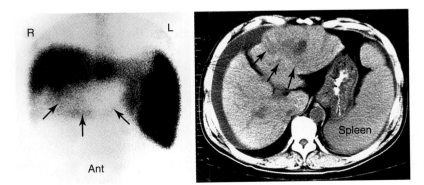

Figure 7-4. Hepatoma in a patient with cirrhosis. *Left,* The liver-spleen scan reveals a small liver and large spleen. There is a large cold defect (*arrows*) in the inferior aspect of the left lobe of the liver. *Right,* CT scan shows a bulging, poorly defined, low-density lesion in the left lobe (*arrows*), as well as ascites and splenomegaly.

Budd-Chiari Syndrome (Hepatic Vein Thrombosis). Hepatic vein thrombosis may occur secondary to tumor invasion or hypercoagulation syndromes, but frequently no underlying cause is identified. The disease usually presents as an enlarged, congested tender liver accompanied by ascites. With early or partial hepatic vein obstruction, technetium colloid activity in the liver becomes diffusely mottled. As thrombosis progresses, activity in both lobes steadily decreases. Typically, the caudate lobe simultaneously enlarges and shows relatively increased activity. This latter phenomenon has been explained by the presence of separate venous drainage directly into the vena cava for the caudate lobe, which is unaffected by thrombosis of the major hepatic veins.

HEPATIC BLOOD POOL IMAGING

Although hemangiomas and cysts are usually occult, asymptomatic lesions, ultrasound can reliably distinguish between cysts (which are hypoechoic) and hemangiomas (which are hyperechoic). CT with intravenous contrast is more specific, usually demonstrating characteristic progressive enhancement toward the center of a hemangioma. Cavernous hemangioma is highly likely when a defect seen with ^{99m}Tc sulfur colloid imaging shows increased activity after administration of a ^{99m}Tc blood pool agent, such as ^{99m}Tc red blood cells, owing to labeling of the blood pool in the lesion. To allow equilibration of the hemangioma blood pool with the labeled red blood cells, delayed imaging (sometimes over several hours) may be necessary when planar imaging is used. Dynamic or blood flow images frequently show normal or decreased perfusion of the lesions. Use of SPECT in the setting of suspected hepatic hemangioma increases the sensitivity of the study, especially when lesions are deep or less than 5 cm in diameter (Fig. 7-6). SPECT provides nearly 100% sensitivity for detection of hemangiomas larger than 1.5 cm in diameter; sensitivity is 50% or less for lesions smaller than 1.0 cm in diameter.

SPLENIC IMAGING
Normal Spleen Scan

On the posterior and anterior views of a technetium colloid scan, the normal spleen exhibits homogeneous activity equal to or less than that

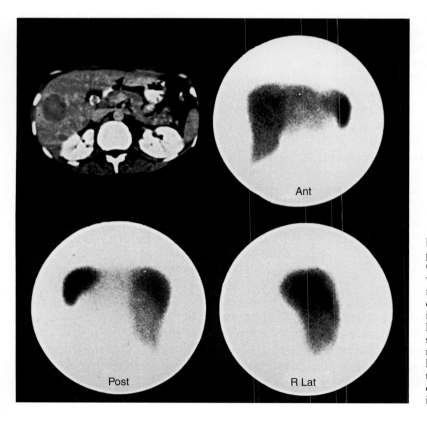

Figure 7-5. Focal nodular hyperplasia. A post-contrast abdominal CT scan of the liver in a young woman with right upper quadrant pain demonstrates a well-defined, focal, low-density lesion in the right lobe of the liver. A liver-spleen scan obtained in the same patient demonstrates a normal technetium-99m sulfur colloid distribution in the region of the lesion. When this discrepancy occurs, focal nodular hyperplasia is the prime consideration.

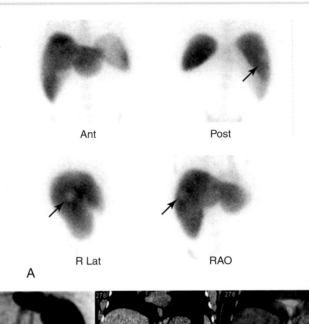

Ant

Post

R Lat

RAO

A

Figure 7-6. Hepatic hemangioma. **A,** Planar views of the abdomen on a technetium-99m sulfur colloid scan show a defect in the right lobe (*arrows*). **B,** Anterior ^{99m}Tc-RBC scan shows intense blood pool in the lesion, coronal CT shows an area of decreased attenuation in the right lobe, and the coronal SPECT/CT shows the area to be congruent.

B

of the liver. The organ is ovoid in configuration, with occasional thinning of the anterior aspect. The normal length of the spleen on a posterior scan is about 10 ± 1.5 cm and should not exceed 13 cm. When imaging the spleen with colloid, routine anterior, posterior, and lateral liver-spleen scan views are obtained. Left anterior oblique and left posterior oblique views at varying degrees of obliquity also may be useful. Occasionally a right posterior oblique view may be needed to separate the left lobe of the liver from the spleen. After surgery or trauma, there may be questions about splenic remnants or accessory spleens. Historically, these were imaged with heat-damaged red blood cells; however, for most purposes, use of ^{99m}Tc sulfur colloid is adequate (Fig. 7-7).

Abnormal Spleen Scan
Focal Lesions

Solitary or multiple splenic defects are nonspecific and may be produced by a number of abnormalities. Careful correlation with pertinent clinical history is necessary to distinguish among these. More common abnormalities that may present as defects within the organ are cysts, hematomas, abscesses, infarctions, and neoplasms. Peripheral wedge-shaped defects may often be correlated with infarcts, especially when a pertinent history, such as of hemoglobinopathy, is obtained.

Metastatic lesions to the spleen are uncommon, although tumors such as lymphoma, melanoma, chorioepithelioma, or soft-tissue sarcoma may present with splenic lesions. Primary splenic neoplasms are extremely rare. Focal areas of decreased activity in the spleen occur in less than 1% of liver-spleen scans. If trauma is excluded as a cause, one third of such defects are due to splenic infarcts, one third to lymphoma, and one third to metastatic disease. A history of immunosuppression or drug abuse increases the likelihood of abscess.

Splenomegaly

Liver-spleen scans may be ordered to confirm clinical suspicion of splenomegaly, although ultrasound is less expensive and does not use ionizing radiation. The causes of splenomegaly are numerous (Box 7-4), and unless focal space-occupying disease is identified, scans are generally unhelpful in determining the cause. Infiltrative disorders produce varying degrees of splenomegaly, with or without alterations in

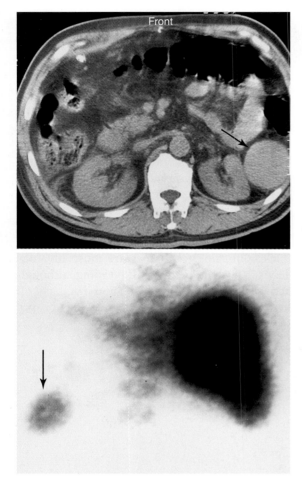

Figure 7-7. Accessory spleen. *Top,* In this patient who had a previous splenectomy, a CT scan revealed a soft-tissue mass (*arrow*) lateral to the left kidney. *Bottom,* A posterior image from a technetium-99m colloid scan in the same patient demonstrates functioning tissue (*arrow*), which represents an accessory spleen or splenic remnant.

splenic activity. The findings are largely nonspecific and are best interpreted in light of clinical observations. Perhaps the one exception to this is massive splenomegaly, which is most often caused by chronic lymphocytic leukemia.

Trauma

CT is the imaging method of choice for acute splenic trauma. The role of radiocolloid spleen imaging is usually very limited. After abdominal trauma, splenic tissue may seed to other locations (splenosis), such as the lung and peritoneal cavity. Such tissue fragments usually accumulate radiocolloid or heat damaged RBCs (Fig. 7-8) and, when identified on ultrasound or CT imaging, can be substantiated as splenic tissue.

Box 7-4	**Diseases Affecting Splenic Size and Activity**

Massive Enlargement
Chronic leukemia
Myelofibrosis
Glycogen storage diseases
Thalassemia major

Moderate Enlargement
Cirrhosis with portal hypertension
Hepatitis, acute or chronic
Hemolytic anemia
Mononucleosis
Lymphoma*

Minimal Enlargement
Congestive heart failure
Metastatic disease*
Collagen disease
Infections
Increased activity
Portal hypertension
Anemia
Leukemia
Lymphoma*
Sepsis
Melanoma*
Stress (recent surgery or chemotherapy)
Hepatocellular dysfunction (colloid shift)

*Depending on disease stage, these entities may also cause decreased activity.

Nonvisualization of the Spleen

In certain cases, the spleen may not be visualized on a ^{99m}Tc colloid scan even in the absence of a history of splenectomy (Box 7-5). Congenital asplenia may be associated with a number of cardiovascular, pulmonary, and abdominal anomalies. In sickle cell anemia, the spleen may not be seen because of atrophy related to repeated infarctions (autosplenectomy); in some of these patients, the spleen remains anatomically intact but with depressed or absent reticuloendothelial function, owing to reversible mechanical obstruction of blood flow by the abnormal configuration of the red blood cells (functional asplenia).

GASTROINTESTINAL BLEEDING STUDIES

Technetium-99m in-vitro labeled red blood cells are the radiopharmaceutical of choice in the investigation of GI hemorrhage, especially in cases of intermittent or slow bleeding, with a sensitivity for active bleeding of greater than 90%. Because the agent remains in the intravascular space, imaging may be performed over a period of 24 hours. Any free technetium that is not bound to red blood cells is excreted by the kidneys and gastric mucosa and passes into the bladder, small bowel, and colon. This latter problem is obviated somewhat by use of in vitro or modified in vivo labeling techniques, which allow for a higher degree of red blood cell tagging and therefore a lower percentage of free technetium. With red blood cells, most bleeding sites show an initial focus of activity, which increases and changes position and/or configuration with time. If the activity remains in the same location, static vascular abnormalities, such as an aneurysm or angiodysplasia, should be suspected. When delayed imaging is necessary to identify a bleeding site, there may be uncertainty with respect to the site of origin.

If the extravasated intraluminal agent is not identified shortly after its deposition, it may move to a more proximal or distal site during any prolonged intervals between images, especially with the increased peristalsis present in most patients with GI bleeding. However, establishing the mere presence of slow bleeding into the bowel remains possible, and, therefore, the study is undoubtedly of value in many patients. The sensitivity with both is significantly greater than with angiography for the detection of lower GI bleeding, with the added advantage of being noninvasive. Because of significant background activity in the upper abdomen and the diagnostic efficacy of endoscopy in the GI tract, nuclear imaging techniques are most advantageous in evaluating lower GI bleeding, although active small-bowel, duodenal, and distal gastric hemorrhage are routinely detected when proper

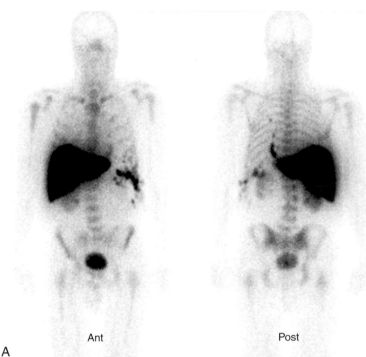

Ant   Post

A

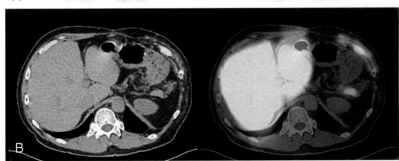

Figure 7-8. Splenosis. A, In this patient who had prior surgery for a shotgun wound of the spleen, a heat damaged ^{99m}Tc-red blood cell scan demonstrates scattered activity in the left upper quadrant and lower left lung. **B,** SPECT/CT scan shows splenic tissue in the left upper quadrant as small soft tissue masses as well as scattered in the anterior left abdominal wall and ribs.

timing and technique for imaging are used. The accuracy of endoscopy in making the diagnosis of upper GI bleeding exceeds 90%.

The common causes of lower GI bleeding in adults are diverticular disease, angiodysplasia, neoplasms, and inflammatory bowel disease. Preoperative localization of a bleeding site permits a more rational, tailored approach to angiography and surgical intervention. Because bleeding from these causes is frequently intermittent, chances of detecting the site of hemorrhage are enhanced by a radiopharmaceutical with a long intravascular half-life, such as labeled red blood cells. Angiography may be negative in patients with intermittent bleeding or bleeding

rates below 1.0 mL/minute. With radionuclide techniques, bleeding rates on the order of 0.2 mL/minute are reliably detected, and the sensitivity has been reported to be good even for bleeding rates as low as 0.04 mL/minute, although a total volume of 2 to 3 mL of blood is necessary. These techniques are best applied to patients who are bleeding acutely. Patients with chronic, low-volume blood loss presenting with guaiac-positive stools or chronic anemias seldom benefit from the examination. Details of the technique are presented in Appendix E-1.

If ^{99m}Tc-RBCs are unavailable or if time does not allow for the labeling procedure, ^{99m}Tc sulfur colloid may be used as a gastrointestinal (GI) hemorrhage imaging agent.

Interpretation

A positive scan shows a focal site of increased activity within the abdomen or pelvis, which progresses distally in the bowel (Figs. 7-9 and 7-10; Box 7-6). Once bleeding is identified, multiple sequential images aid greatly in establishing its origin by recording the pattern of progression of the radionuclide within the bowel. Optimally, the images are viewed in cine mode. Because blood is an irritant to the intestine, movement of activity is often rapid and can be bidirectional. This is often true in the small bowel where a rapid serpiginous course of the labeled red blood cells from the left upper abdomen to the right lower quadrant is characteristic. The earlier in a study that the bleeding is seen, the more accurate is the localization. Because the main purpose of the examination is to localize the site of bleeding, the study should be continued for a sufficient length of time to follow the progress of the labeled blood and permit mapping of bowel anatomy, which may

---

Box 7-5 Causes of Splenic Defects on Technetium-99m Colloid Scan

Focal Defects
Infarct
Lymphoma
Metastasis
Cyst
Abscess
Hematoma or splenic artery aneurysm
Anatomic variation
Artifact

Nonvisualization
Splenectomy
Sickle cell disease (functional or autosplenectomy)
Congenital absence of spleen (isolated or Ivemark syndrome)
Tumor replacement
Infarction
Traumatic avulsion or volvulus
Functional asplenia

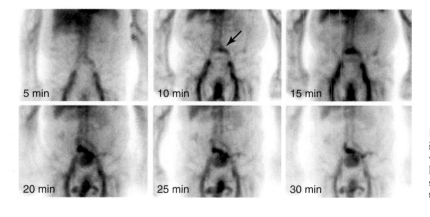

Figure 7-9. Small-bowel bleeding. This study was performed with technetium-99m in-vitro labeled red blood cells and demonstrates a focus of active bleeding in the mid small bowel (*arrow*).

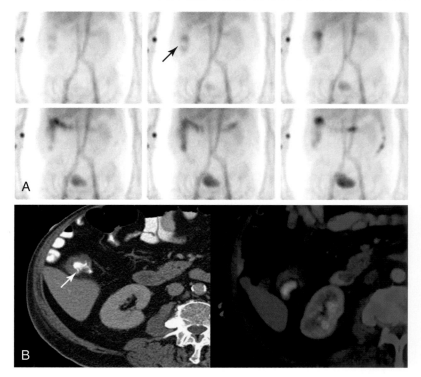

Figure 7-10. Lower gastrointestinal bleeding. **A,** Bleeding is seen as a focus of activity that initially appears in the right transverse colon (*arrow*) and then subsequently moves both antegrade and retrograde from the site of bleeding. **B,** Subsequent CT and ^{18}F-FDG scan show a colon cancer as the cause of the bleeding. *FDG,* Fluorodeoxyglucose.

Box 7-6   Interpretation of Labeled Red Blood Cell Scans for Gastrointestinal Bleeding

Criteria for Active Bleeding
Activity appears and conforms to bowel anatomy
Usually increase in activity with time
Must move antegrade and/or retrograde in bowel

False-Positive
Free technetium-99m pertechnetate
Urinary tract activity
Uterine or penile blush
Accessory spleen
Hemangioma (hepatic)
Varices

False-Negative
Bleeding rate too low
Intermittent bleeding

---

vary somewhat from patient to patient. An area of activity that remains fixed in location over time should raise the suspicion of causes other than intraluminal bleeding. Occasional confusion of bladder activity with a rectosigmoid bleed can usually be resolved on postvoid views or lateral pelvic images. Interfering genital activity is usually identified by its location on anterior oblique or lateral pelvic views. Carefully performed labeled red blood cell studies show a high degree of sensitivity (>90%), with a low false-negative results rate. In addition to providing evidence of active GI bleeding and its location, the examination may also be used as a guide for selective abdominal arteriography and to assess the results of interventional therapy.

MECKEL DIVERTICULUM IMAGING

Meckel diverticulum occurs in about 2% of the population and predominantly affects male patients. Although most (96%) of the lesions remain asymptomatic throughout life, complications (obstruction, hemorrhage, intussusception, and volvulus) occur in a small percentage of patients. The most common presentation in a child is painless rectal bleeding. In virtually all cases accompanied by bleeding, ectopic gastric mucosa with or without associated ulceration can be demonstrated in the diverticulum. The traditional method of radionuclide investigation of a patient with bleeding from suspected Meckel diverticulum is based on visualization of the ectopic mucosa with intravenously administered ^{99m}Tc-pertechnetate. Negative results are

Box 7-7   Interpretation of Meckel Scans

Positive
Usually mid abdomen or right lower
  quadrant and anterior
Appear and fade in same temporal pattern
  as stomach mucosa

False-Positive
Urinary tract activity
Other ectopic gastric mucosa
Hyperemic inflammatory lesions
Arteriovenous malformation, hemangioma,
  aneurysm
Neoplasms
Intussusception

False-Negative
Minimal amount of gastric mucosa
Rapid washout of pertechnetate
Meckel diverticulum with impaired blood
  supply
Sensitivity may be enhanced using
  pentagastrin, cimetidine, or glucagon
  (see text).

common in patients whose diverticula do not contain ectopic gastric tissue (Box 7-7).

The study consists of intravenous injection of 8 to 12 mCi (296 to 444 MBq) of ^{99m}Tc-pertechnetate in adults or about 200 to 300 µCi/kg (7.4 to 11.1 MBq/kg) in children. Sequential anterior abdominopelvic images are then obtained for 45 to 60 minutes. A typical positive scan consists of a focal area of increased activity in the right lower quadrant or mid-abdomen, which on lateral view is seen to be anterior and unrelated to any ureteral activity (Fig. 7-11). This finding generally appears in the first 30 minutes of the study but may take up to 1 hour to appear, depending on the amount of gastric mucosa present. False-positive results have been reported secondary to intussusception (possibly related to the associated hyperemia), urinary tract activity (often secondary to obstruction), various small-bowel lesions, inflammatory bowel disease, vascular lesions, and rarely, intestinal duplication cysts containing gastric mucosa. False-negative scans have been reported in patients with malrotation of the ileum, small amounts of ectopic mucosa, and localized bowel irritability, which causes rapid clearance of the pertechnetate from the

area. The overall specificity and sensitivity of the examination, however, are about 90%.

Several pharmacologic interventions have been proposed to increase the sensitivity of Meckel diverticulum imaging, with varying degrees of success. These include the use of H$_2$ blockers (cimetidine, famotidine, or ranitidine) to block release of pertechnetate from the ectopic mucosa, pentagastrin to enhance mucosal uptake of ^{99m}Tc-pertechnetate (^{99m}TcO$_4^-$), and glucagon to decrease small-bowel (diverticular) motility. Cimetidine is administered in an oral dose of 300 mg four times daily for adults or 20 mg/kg/day for children for 2 days before the study. Some laboratories use glucagon, given intravenously 10 minutes after the start of the study.

Actively hemorrhaging patients with suspected Meckel diverticulum may be initially investigated with radionuclide techniques intended to detect the bleeding site rather than the ectopic gastric mucosa.

HEPATOBILIARY IMAGING

The ^{99m}Tc-labeled hepatobiliary agents enable accurate and convenient imaging in acute and chronic biliary disease. Common indications are for acute (calculous or acalculous) cholecystitis, biliary patency, identification of biliary leaks, and, in neonates, differentiation of biliary atresia from neonatal hepatitis. Less common uses are for the evaluation of biliary dyskinesia and sphincter of Oddi dysfunction.

Radiopharmaceuticals

A number of ^{99m}Tc–iminodiacetic acid (IDA) analogs are available, providing excellent quality routine imaging of the biliary system. The IDA imaging agents have strong chelating properties and therefore bind readily to ^{99m}Tc, forming a stable complex. In general, increasing the length of the alkyl chain substituted on the benzene ring of IDA increases the biliary excretion of the radiopharmaceutical and reduces renal clearance. This added biliary excretion can be of great value in imaging patients with elevated bilirubin levels.

Perhaps the most widely used IDA compound is diisopropyl IDA (DISIDA; disofenin or Hepatolite), which with its longer substituted chain allows for increased biliary excretion and visualization of the hepatobiliary system at serum bilirubin levels approaching 20 mg/dL. Mebrofenin (trimethyl bromo IDA or Choletec) is also

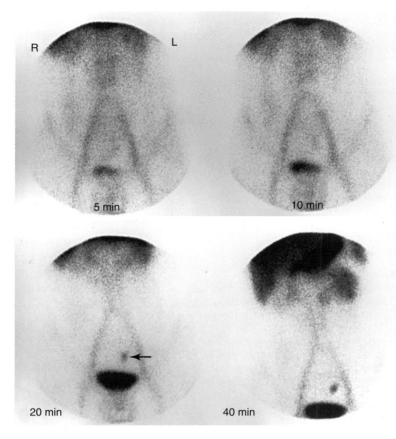

Figure 7-11. Meckel diverticulum. In this 2-year-old boy with rectal bleeding, sequential technetium-99m pertechnetate scans reveal a focus of activity (*arrow*) that appears at 20 minutes in the mid-abdomen. This did not move over time and was located anteriorly in the abdomen on a lateral view (not shown).

used and can demonstrate biliary visualization with bilirubin levels up to 30 to 40 mg/dL. Although biliary duct visualization with these agents can occur at high bilirubin levels, visualization of the gallbladder is not ensured. Persistent visualization of the cardiac blood pool after 5 to 10 minutes and renal excretion are signs of hepatic dysfunction. The radiopharmaceutical is normally rapidly removed from the circulation by active transport into the hepatocytes and secreted into the bile canaliculi and then into the biliary radicles, bile duct, gallbladder, and small intestine. In contrast to bilirubin, the IDA is excreted without being conjugated. Hepatic uptake is normally about 90% for disofenin and 98% for mebrofenin. The half-time of liver clearance for both agents is 15 to 20 minutes.

Technique

For elective studies, patients are given nothing by mouth beginning at midnight the night before the examination. In patients with acute disease, a minimum of 2 hours' fasting is suggested. Fortunately, in emergency patients with suspected acute cholecystitis, fasting has generally been self-imposed. In patients whose gallbladders are being stimulated by the presence of food in the upper GI tract, the intermittent contraction of the gallbladder interferes with biliary filling and therefore may render a false-positive study. In 65% of patients who have eaten 2 to 5 hours before the study, the gallbladder will not be visualized in the first 60 minutes of the study. In addition, prolonged fasting in some patients has been implicated as a source of false-positive examinations because a gallbladder distended with bile may not be able to accept IDA excreted by the liver in order to visualize the gallbladder.

Subsequent to the intravenous injection of 3 to 10 mCi (111 to 370 MBq) of ^{99m}Tc-labeled IDA, sequential anterior gamma camera images of the abdomen are obtained with the patient in the supine position. Images of 500- to 1000-k counts are obtained at 5-minute intervals for the first half-hour of the study. Similar images are then obtained at 10-minute intervals. Continuous, dynamic imaging may also be used. Normally, the gallbladder is visualized within

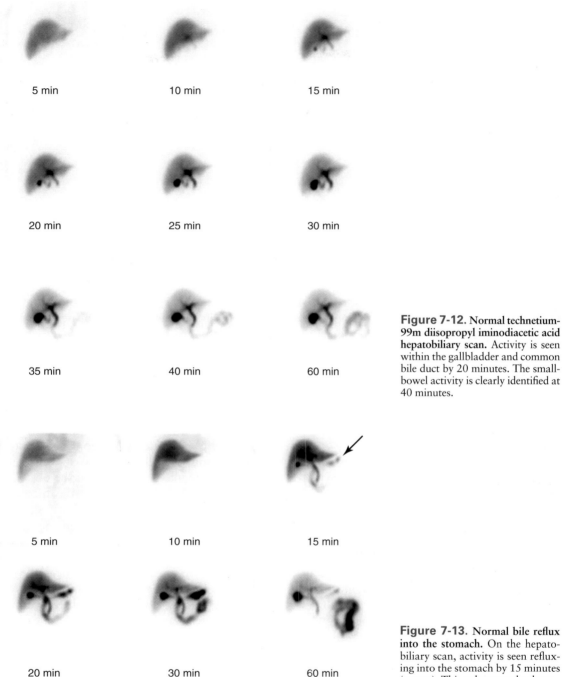

5 min

10 min

15 min

20 min

25 min

30 min

35 min

40 min

60 min

Figure 7-12. Normal technetium-99m diisopropyl iminodiacetic acid hepatobiliary scan. Activity is seen within the gallbladder and common bile duct by 20 minutes. The small-bowel activity is clearly identified at 40 minutes.

5 min

10 min

15 min

20 min

30 min

60 min

Figure 7-13. Normal bile reflux into the stomach. On the hepato-biliary scan, activity is seen refluxing into the stomach by 15 minutes (*arrow*). This subsequently clears.

the first half-hour of the study, as are the common bile duct and duodenum (Fig. 7-12). If these structures are not identified at 1 hour, delayed images should be obtained hourly for up to 4 hours after injection, or as discussed later, intravenous morphine may be used to shorten the examination. Some bile reflux into the stomach can be a normal finding (Fig. 7-13).

In jaundiced patients with increased renal excretion of the radiopharmaceutical, a right extrarenal pelvis may be confused with gallbladder activity (Fig. 7-14). This activity may be differentiated from gallbladder activity by obtaining a right lateral image, on which the characteristic anterior abdominal location of the gallbladder can be identified. At times, the

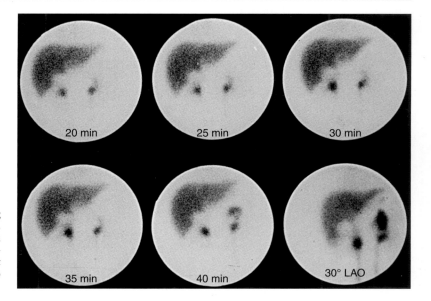

Figure 7-14. Long-standing common bile duct obstruction. This scan was performed with technetium-99m diisopropyl iminodiacetic acid. A significant amount of renal excretion but no hepatic excretion is noted.

gallbladder activity may be obscured by activity collecting in the adjacent duodenal loop, or on delayed images, in the transverse colon. In the case of duodenal activity, an additional view in the left anterior oblique or right lateral position can be used to distinguish the two structures. If this fails to provide the answer, the patient may drink water to clear the duodenum of activity.

Normal Scan

In the normal patient, sufficient ^{99m}Tc-IDA is present in the liver in 5 minutes to allow good visualization of that organ. If for any reason additional views of the liver are sought, they should be obtained in the first 10 or 15 minutes of the examination. After this time, there is progressive clearance of the radiopharmaceutical from the liver, and it becomes less apparent. As the radiopharmaceutical is excreted into the biliary tree, the major hepatic ducts and common duct are visualized first. Next, the gallbladder is filled as labeled bile flows through the cystic duct. About two thirds of biliary flow bypass the gallbladder and enter the duodenum, and about one third enters the gallbladder. The amount and timing of entry into the gallbladder depend on a number of factors, including the nutritional state of the patient, administration of various drugs, and the tone in the sphincter of Oddi. In the presence of a patent common duct, activity flows promptly into the duodenal sweep and proximal small bowel. Normally, visualization of these structures is complete by 1 hour. Occasionally, a small amount of bile reflux into the

stomach can be seen as a normal variant, but it should not be a large amount or persistent.

Clinical Settings
Acute Cholecystitis

Hepatobiliary imaging has proved to be of greatest value in the diagnosis of acute cholecystitis. More than 95% of patients with acute cholecystitis have cystic duct obstruction. In this group of patients, radiopharmaceuticals excreted into the bile by the liver cannot enter an inflamed gallbladder through the obstructed cystic duct. This fact provides the theoretical basis for using ^{99m}Tc hepatobiliary agents to diagnose the disease.

In the proper clinical setting, the diagnosis of acute (calculous or acalculous) cholecystitis in a fasting patient may be reliably made in the presence of normal hepatic uptake and excretion of the radiopharmaceutical through the common duct, but without visualization of the gallbladder over a period of 4 hours after injection (Fig. 7-15). In several large series, accuracy of cholescintigraphy for diagnosis of acute calculous cholecystitis has been greater than 95%, and the accuracy for acute acalculous cholecystitis is only slightly less. In addition, this imaging modality is usually unaffected by modest levels of jaundice. The accuracy of ultrasound for the detection of acute cholecystitis is only about 80% to 85%, even if liberal criteria are used. A normal hepatobiliary scan with gallbladder visualization almost always excludes a diagnosis of acute cholecystitis.

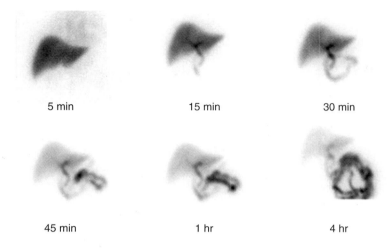

5 min   15 min   30 min

45 min   1 hr   4 hr

Figure 7-15. Acute cholecystitis. There is activity in the small bowel and common duct at 30 minutes on this technetium-99m hepatobiliary scan. This study was continued for 4 hours, with no visualization of the gallbladder.

Box 7-8   Interpretive Difficulties in Diagnosis of Acute Cholecystitis by Hepatobiliary Scan

False-Positive
Recent meal within 4 hr of imaging
Total parenteral nutrition
Alcoholism
Pancreatitis (some cases)
Chronic cholecystitis
Hepatocellular dysfunction
Cholangiocarcinoma of cystic duct
Prolonged fasting for 24 hr or
   hyperalimentation
Severe intercurrent illness

False-Negative
Acalculous cholecystitis
Duodenal diverticulum simulating
   gallbladder
Accessory cystic duct
Biliary duplication cyst

Occasionally the gallbladder may not be seen in a patient with chronic cholecystitis, but this is uncommon. Usually the gallbladder is visualized within 4 hours after injection. Visualization of the gallbladder during this period effectively excludes the diagnosis of acute gallbladder disease. Thus it is essential that this delayed sequence of images be a routine part of IDA imaging for acute cholecystitis. As discussed later, morphine may be used to shorten the study. Box 7-8 lists some sources of error in IDA scan interpretation when a diagnosis of acute cholecystitis is being considered.

The *rim sign* has been described in patients with acute cholecystitis. This has also been called *pericholecystic hepatic activity sign,* and it refers to a curvilinear band of increased activity along the right inferior hepatic edge above the gallbladder fossa (Fig. 7-16). This sign is seen in about 20% of patients whose gallbladders are not visualized on hepatobiliary scans. The rim sign is important because about 40% of such patients have either a perforated or a gangrenous gallbladder, and 70% to 85% have acute cholecystitis. The mechanism involved in the production of the rim sign is uncertain. It may be the result of inflammation causing regional hepatic hyperemia, with more radiopharmaceutical being delivered to this area of hepatic parenchyma; or it may be caused by edema causing localized delayed biliary excretion; or both.

The *cystic duct sign* has also been described in acute cholecystitis (Fig. 7-17). This is seen as a small nubbin of activity in the cystic duct proximal to the site of obstruction. It is usually seen between the common hepatic duct and the gallbladder fossa.

Various pharmacologic adjuncts have been suggested to increase the sensitivity of hepatobiliary imaging in the evaluation of patients for acute cholecystitis (Box 7-9). The sensitivity of the hepatobiliary scan may be increased by emptying the gallbladder before the administration of the radiopharmaceutical; this, theoretically, reduces the false-positive rate of the test in patients with chronic cholecystitis, viscous bile, parenteral nutrition, or prolonged fasting. Initially, fatty meals were used, but these proved variable in their ability to produce gallbladder contraction. Consequently, a synthetic

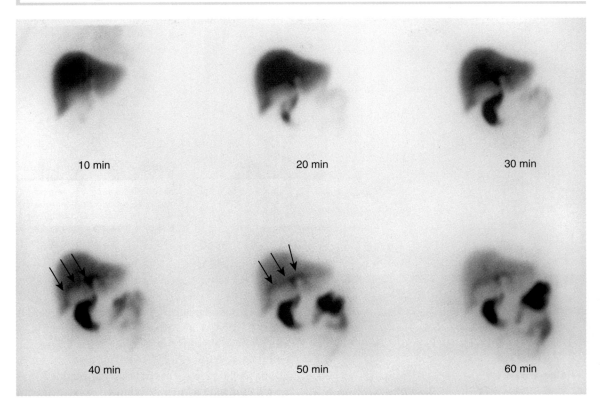

Figure 7-16. Rim sign of acute cholecystitis. On anterior planar images a rim of increased activity outlining the gallbladder fossa is seen at the inferior edge of the right lobe of the liver (*arrows*).

octapeptide of cholecystokinin (CCK-8 or sincalide, Kinevac) can be used. This causes gallbladder contraction, relaxation of the sphincter of Oddi, and increased bile secretion and bowel motility. In normal patients, there is prompt gallbladder contraction, reaching a maximum effect at 5 to 15 minutes after slow (over 5 to 10 minutes) intravenous administration of sincalide, although slow infusions over 15 to 60 minutes are usually performed. The standard dose is 0.02 mcg/kg in 10 mL of saline, although larger volumes for slower infusions may be used. Intravenous bolus administration should be avoided because it produces abdominal discomfort and less complete gallbladder emptying because of inducement of gallbladder neck spasm.

Although these maneuvers may reduce the false-positive rate, such premedication may potentially obscure the diagnosis of chronic cholecystitis by speeding up the visualization of the gallbladder in patients who would otherwise present with delayed visualization. Further, delayed biliary to bowel transit occurs in half the patients given sincalide before cholescintigraphy, which raises a question of partial common duct obstruction. These problems may

be obviated by reserving the administration of CCK or sincalide until the failure to visualize the gallbladder at 30 to 60 minutes is demonstrated. At this time, intravenous CCK can be administered, followed 15 to 30 minutes later by reinjection of the IDA radiopharmaceutical.

Intravenous morphine is commonly used to improve the diagnostic accuracy of hepatobiliary scanning. Morphine causes increased tone in smooth muscle and decreases peristalsis. Because morphine causes constriction of the sphincter of Oddi, there is a rise in intraductal pressure in the common duct by 60%, producing increased flow of the radiopharmaceutical into the gallbladder. Thus if after the passage of the radiopharmaceutical into the common duct and small bowel there is no gallbladder visualization, intravenous morphine can be administered. The typical dose is 0.04 mg/kg diluted in 10 mL of saline and administered over 3 minutes. This is usually well tolerated by patients, without significant aggravation of symptoms. If there is enough residual radiopharmaceutical in the liver and if the cystic duct is patent, the gallbladder usually fills in 5 to 10 minutes (Fig. 7-18). Peak effect is in about 5 minutes. If there is not enough activity

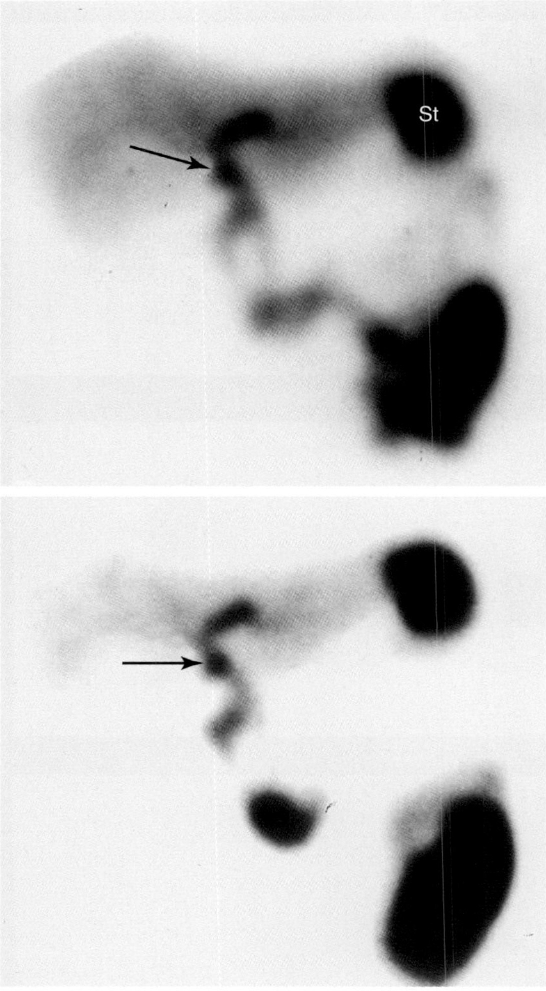

Figure 7-17. Cystic duct sign. In this patient with right upper quadrant pain, 30- and 60-minute images (*top* and *bottom*) from a technetium-99m hepatobiliary scan show activity in the liver, hepatic ducts, and common bile duct. The gallbladder is not seen, but there is a small focus of activity adjacent to the common duct (*arrow*), which represents activity in the portion of the cystic duct proximal to the obstruction. Incidental note is made of a large amount of bile reflux into the stomach (*St*).

> ### Box 7-9   Use of Pharmacologic Intervention with Hepatobiliary Imaging
>
> **Cholecystokinin (sincalide)**
> Administer 0.02 mcg/kg slow IV infusion.
> Empty the gallbladder in a patient fasting >24 hr before DISIDA scan.
> Evaluate sphincter of Oddi dyskinesia.
> Differentiate functional from anatomic duct obstruction.
> Calculate gallbladder ejection fraction.
>
> **Morphine**
> 0.04 mg/kg IV
> Use to shorten the imaging time when gallbladder is not visualized at 1 hr and sufficient activity is still in hepatobiliary tree
> Use advisedly in patients with cystic duct sign
>
> **Phenobarbital**
> 5 mg/kg/day orally for 5-7 days before examination
> Use to prime hepatic enzymes to increase IDA excretion in distinguishing between biliary atresia and neonatal hepatitis

DISIDA, Diisopropyl iminodiacetic acid; IDA, iminodiacetic acid.

remaining in the liver and common duct, it is best to first reinject the patient with more hepatobiliary agent and then to administer morphine 15 to 20 minutes later. Nonvisualization of the gallbladder 30 minutes after morphine administration has the same implication as lack of visualization on 4-hour images and indicates acute cholecystitis. Morphine should be used advisedly if a cystic duct sign is present because the back pressure may force activity past the cystic duct obstruction into the gallbladder. This nonphysiologic maneuver may convert a true-positive result into a false-negative result. Further, after morphine administration, CCK should not be used because it induces gallbladder contraction against a contracted sphincter of Oddi, increasing patient discomfort.

Chronic Cholecystitis

Although delayed gallbladder visualization correlates well with chronic gallbladder disease, it also occurs in a small number of patients with acute cholecystitis. Thus although late visualization strongly suggests chronic cholecystitis, acute acalculous disease with partial cystic duct obstruction cannot be completely excluded. In those patients in whom the gallbladder is visualized after 1 hour and in whom acute disease is strongly suspected on clinical grounds, the contractile response of the gallbladder to administered CCK may provide a clue to the true nature of the disease. A gallbladder that fails to contract on stimulation with CCK should be held in suspicion for acute gallbladder disease until excluded by other modalities, such as ultrasonography. However, an abnormal response does not definitively distinguish between acute and chronic disease. If the

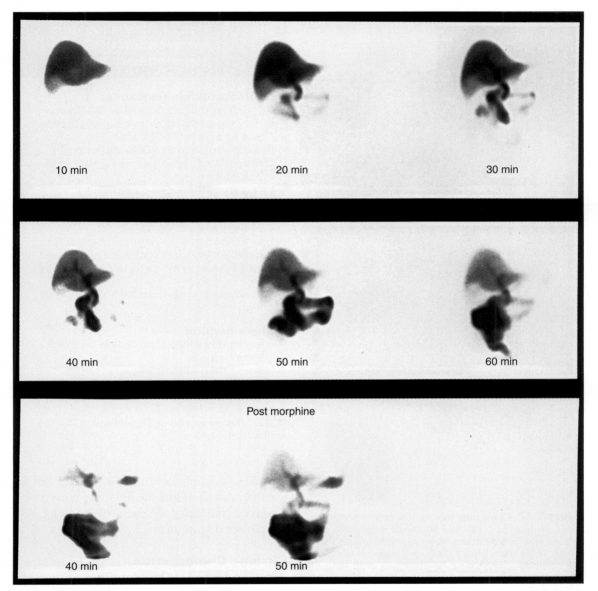

Figure 7-18. Morphine augmentation. On these anterior technetium-99m hepatobiliary scan images, the gallbladder is not visualized by 60 minutes, indicating either acute or chronic cholecystitis. Rather than wait 4 hours for a delayed image, morphine was given in hope of increasing back pressure and filling the gallbladder. Even 50 minutes after morphine administration, the gallbladder was not seen, indicating acute cholecystitis.

gallbladder does respond, continued investigation of presumed chronic cholecystitis is indicated.

Computer acquisition of a CCK gallbladder stimulation study allows the calculation of a gallbladder ejection fraction, the percentage of radiolabeled bile ejected from the gallbladder after CCK administration. This is a measure of gallbladder contractility and thus function. (Fig. 7-19). Generally, an ejection fraction of less than 35% is considered abnormal (Fig. 7-20). Unequivocally normal ejection fractions are greater than 50%. The normal mean is 75% with a standard deviation of about 20%. The normal emptying rate is about 6% per minute. CCK is administered slowly intravenously with various recommended infusion times from 15 to 60 minutes. The slower the infusion the less likely the patient is to experience abdominal pain and the less variability in ejection values obtained in normal patients. If CCK is not available, a fatty meal can be used to induce gallbladder emptying, but the mean ejection fraction is lower ($\approx$50% with a standard deviation of 20%), and the emptying rate is slower

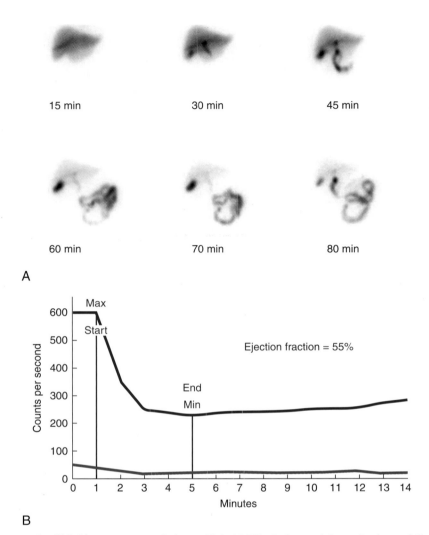

Figure 7-19. Normal gallbladder response to cholecystokinin (CCK). A, Sequential anterior hepatobiliary images show normal gallbladder and small bowel activity at 60 minutes after injection of ^{99m}Tc-DISIDA. **B,** After subsequent administration of 1.6 mcg of CCK, the gallbladder contracts well within 5 minutes as the time activity ejection fraction curve shows.

($\approx 2\%$ per minute). An abnormal ejection fraction can be used, along with clinical information, to suggest the presence of gallbladder dysfunction. A reduced ejection fraction is suggestive, but not specific for chronic cholecystitis or biliary dyskinesia. Other causes of a reduced ejection fraction include sphincter of Oddi spasm, cystic duct syndrome, chronic acalculous cholecystitis, and medications (morphine, atropine, calcium channel blockers, octreotide, progesterone, indomethacin, theophylline, benzodiazepines, and histamine-2 receptor antagonists).

Aside from delayed gallbladder visualization, several other scintigraphic patterns demonstrate correlation with the diagnosis of chronic cholecystitis. Delayed biliary-to-bowel transit time in the presence of normal gallbladder and common duct visualization is suggestive of chronic gallbladder disease but it can be a normal variant in up to 20% of individuals. The longer that intestinal visualization is delayed, the more likely is a diagnosis of chronic cholecystitis; however, this finding alone is by no means diagnostic.

Finally, poor but definite visualization of the gallbladder, filling defects within the gallbladder or common duct, and a less-than-optimal contractile response to CCK stimulation have all been reported in patients subsequently proved to have chronic cholecystitis. Identification of cholelithiasis is extremely poor unless

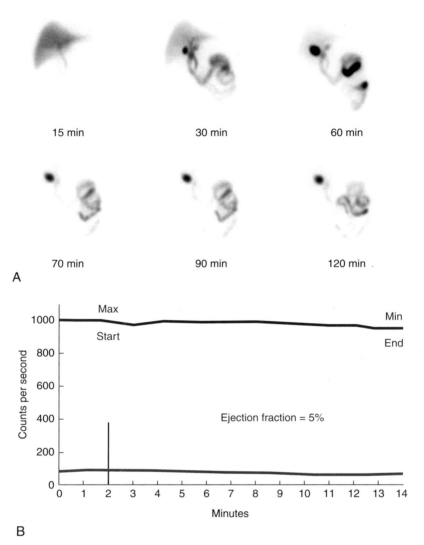

Figure 7-20. **Abnormal gallbladder response to cholecystokinin (CCK). A,** Multiple images from a technetium-99m hepatobiliary scan show normal activity in the gallbladder by 60 minutes. **B,** After subsequent infusion of CCK, the images and ejection fraction curve show that gallbladder does not contract. This suggests a functional abnormality, which may be the result of a number of causes, including gallbladder dyskinesia, chronic acalculous cholecystitis, sphincter of Oddi spasm, and multiple medications.

the stones are large. None of these findings, however, correlates as well with the disease as does delayed gallbladder visualization.

Biliary Obstruction

Suspected biliary obstruction is usually first imaged using ultrasound, CT or magnetic resonance cholangiopancreatography (MRCP), which provide excellent detailed anatomic and diagnostic information when required. However, it is still important to understand the appearance of biliary obstruction on hepatobiliary scans because a significant number of patients being evaluated for acute cholecystitis

have stones in the common duct that cause some degree of obstruction.

Lack of visualization of the biliary tree with good visualization of the liver (the so-called *liver scan sign*) is typical with acute complete obstruction of the common bile duct (Fig. 7-21). Obstruction may be mechanical, owing to calculi or neoplasm, or functional, as seen in some cases of ascending cholangitis. Intrahepatic cholestasis, such as that produced by obstruction of the canaliculi by certain drugs, or hepatitis may also yield a pattern indistinguishable from complete common duct obstruction. With partial bile duct obstruction, the biliary tree is visualized to the

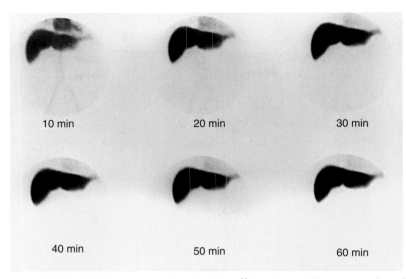

Figure 7-21. Liver scan sign. Anterior sequential technetium-99m (^{99m}Tc) hepatobiliary images show the liver but no biliary system or bowel activity. There is constantly increasing activity in the liver throughout the study. Also note that there is activity seen above the liver in the heart for at least 30 minutes. This blood pool activity normally should be cleared by 5 to 10 minutes. This is called the *liver scan sign* because it looks like a ^{99m}Tc colloid liver-spleen scan without the spleen. Acute high-grade common duct obstruction is the prime consideration in such cases.

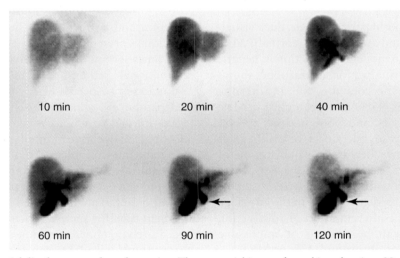

Figure 7-22. Partial distal common duct obstruction. The sequential images from this technetium-99m hepatobiliary scan show that the liver accumulates activity slower than normal but that there is some hepatic clearance by 120 minutes. The gallbladder and common duct are clearly seen up to the point of obstruction (*arrow*). The obstruction could have been caused by a common duct stone, tumor, or sphincter of Oddi dyskinesia, but, in this case, it was purely functional and iatrogenic. The referring physician had given the patient morphine for pain relief before performing the study, constricting the sphincter of Oddi and producing a false-positive scan.

level of obstruction (Fig. 7-22), and occasionally a filling defect is identified at that point.

All of these patterns depend on good hepatocyte function (Fig. 7-23). In the past, severe hepatocellular disease or dysfunction precluded a diagnostic study because insufficient excretion of the radiopharmaceutical into the major biliary ducts rendered it impossible to distinguish between nonvisualization of the ducts secondary to primary liver disease and high-grade obstruction of the common duct. The use of longer-chain IDA analogs that allow good hepatic concentration and excretion, even in the presence of marked jaundice, has made this diagnostic problem considerably less frequent.

The sequence of events occurring after acute complete distal biliary obstruction is as follows: 0 to 24 hours, hepatocyte function is normal

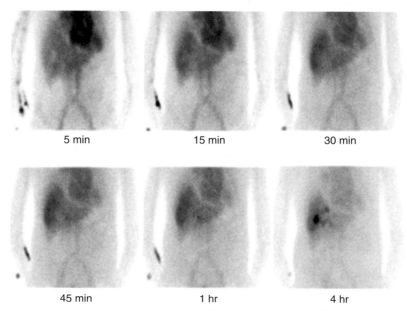

Figure 7-23. Hepatocellular dysfunction. Anterior sequential images from a hepatobiliary scan in this patient with hepatic failure show markedly delayed clearance of the tracer from the blood pool and soft tissues. The cardiac blood pool is normally not visualized after 30 minutes even in cases of severe biliary obstruction.

and there is good hepatic and bile duct visualization (ultrasound at this time is normal); 24 to 96 hours, mild to moderate reduction in hepatic and bile duct visualization (ultrasound shows enlargement of the common bile and hepatic ducts); and after 96 hours, prolonged cardiac blood pool activity and poor hepatic uptake, with no activity in bile ducts or gallbladder (ultrasound shows beginning of dilatation of intrahepatic ducts). In all of these events, there is no visualization of intestinal activity unless there is partial obstruction only. In the late stage (after 96 hours), differentiation of obstruction from hepatitis can be difficult or impossible without the use of ultrasound, CT, or MRI.

Partial duct obstruction is suggested by persistent visualization of the common duct or delayed clearance of activity from the duct. Delayed appearance (>60 minutes) of activity in the duodenum and small bowel is nonspecific and can occur in 20% to 25% of normal people. Partial obstruction can be caused by a common duct stone, benign or malignant stricture, or sphincter of Oddi dysfunction with elevated sphincter pressure.

Post-Traumatic and Postsurgical Biliary Scans

The confirmation and localization of biliary leaks after abdominal surgery or trauma using ^{99m}Tc-IDA agents may lead to the early detection and correction of the problem. This technique presents several advantages and overcomes several of the disadvantages of using conventional radiographic methods for the evaluation of suspected biliary fistula.

Hepatobiliary scintigraphy has also proved useful in the postcholecystectomy patient by allowing the identification of persistent cystic duct remnants and biliary leaks (Figs. 7-24 and 7-25) and the assessment of biliary patency. In attempting to detect a remnant of the cystic duct, it is important to obtain delayed images to permit sufficient time for such a structure to be visualized. Rarely, retained common duct stones may be identified on the IDA scan as photon-deficient areas in the visualized common duct. This finding should be followed by ultrasonography, although stones may be missed in the presence of a normal-caliber common bile duct. Finally, the functional significance of a dilated common duct on ultrasound after gallbladder surgery may be clarified with cholescintigraphy by determining the patency or obstruction of the duct.

When imaging for a possible bile leak, it is important to image the right paracolic gutter and to obtain pelvic images to look for subtle leaks, which may accumulate in the pelvis. Often, postsurgical bile leaks may cause the accumulation of labeled bile in the gallbladder fossa, producing a biloma that may mimic

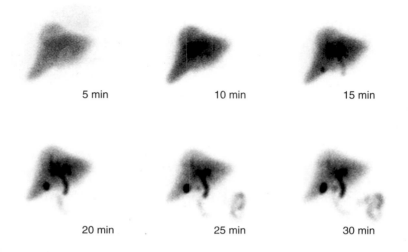

5 min   10 min   15 min

20 min   25 min   30 min

Figure 7-24. Bile leak post-cholecystectomy. The anterior sequential images show activity being excreted into the common duct and what appears to be the gallbladder. Without the history of recent cholecystectomy, the diagnosis may have been missed. The leaking bile can pool in the porta hepatis and mimic a gallbladder.

gallbladder visualization. Labeled bile may also track superiorly in the perihepatic spaces, coating the liver surface. When this occurs, it may give the appearance of paradoxically increasing activity in the liver after the liver has largely emptied activity, producing the *reappearing liver sign.* It may also give the appearance of an alteration of liver shape compared to initial images.

On occasion, cholescintigraphy may be used to investigate surgically altered biliary and GI anatomy or stent patency evaluation by providing appropriate functional information. As with all postsurgical studies, it is important to obtain a precise understanding of the type of surgical procedure performed and the postsurgical anatomy before proceeding with the examination.

Biliary Atresia and Neonatal Hepatitis

Radionuclide techniques have traditionally been used to differentiate between biliary atresia and neonatal hepatitis in the jaundiced infant. Because the successful surgical treatment of biliary atresia depends greatly on early intervention, prompt diagnosis is essential. Frequently, the diagnosis cannot be made on clinical, laboratory, or even needle biopsy grounds, and cholescintigraphy may provide the only clue to the proper diagnosis.

Imaging with ^{99m}Tc-IDA analogs has been used to exclude a diagnosis of biliary atresia

by demonstrating patent extrahepatic biliary systems in jaundiced neonates (Fig. 7-26). In the absence of visualization of the biliary tree, however, atresia may not be successfully differentiated from severe hepatocellular disease produced by neonatal hepatitis (Fig. 7-27). Thus every effort should be made to permit visualization of the biliary tree, including delayed imaging at 24 hours. The relatively short physical half-life of ^{99m}Tc is disadvantageous in that imaging beyond 24 hours is not practical, and, therefore, biliary flow into the small bowel more than 24 hours after injection may not be detected. There is some evidence that the examination using ^{99m}Tc-IDA analogs is more diagnostic when the liver is primed first with 5 to 7 days of phenobarbital therapy, 2.5 mg/kg orally twice a day, which stimulates better hepatic excretion of the radiopharmaceutical and therefore earlier identification of a patent biliary tree. In addition to biliary atresia, other anomalies of the biliary tract, such as choledochal cysts and Caroli disease, have been identified successfully by using ^{99m}Tc-IDA imaging.

GASTROESOPHAGEAL FUNCTION STUDIES

Radionuclide techniques provide a convenient, noninvasive, and direct method to assess GI motility. By using imaging and computer-assisted quantitation, numerous physiologic parameters of upper GI function may be evaluated. These

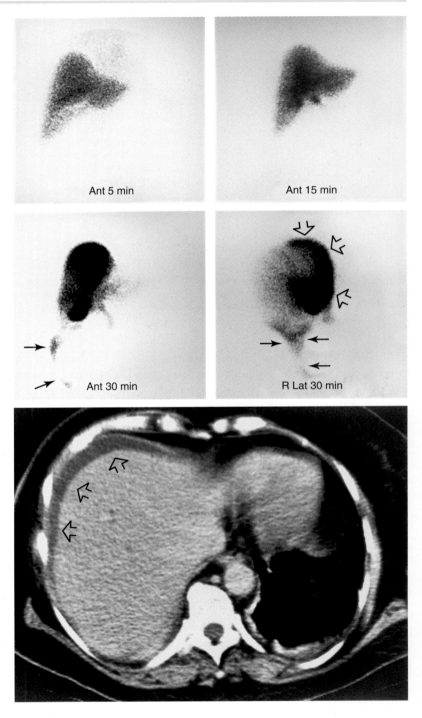

Figure 7-25. Bile leak. *Top,* Sequential images from a hepatobiliary scan show increasing perihepatic activity by 30 minutes that no longer conforms to the shape of the liver that was seen at 5 or 15 minutes. Also, activity has tracked inferiorly in the right pericolic gutter (*small arrows*). Most of the activity on the 30-minute images are along the anterior surface of the liver (*open arrows*). *Bottom,* Fluid (*arrows*) is also seen anterior and lateral to the liver on the CT scan.

include (1) esophageal transit, (2) the detection and quantitation of gastroesophageal and enterogastric reflux, and (3) gastric emptying rates.

Esophageal Transit

Scintigraphic methods are useful to quantitate esophageal transit. Several methods are used, and most of these use an orally administered liquid bolus and measure the time to esophageal clearance. Although the scintigraphic study is useful as a quantitative measure, it has limited anatomic resolution and, therefore, is not a replacement for a barium esophagram. The initial evaluation of a patient with esophageal symptoms should include a barium study. A number of radiopharmaceuticals can be used with success; however, ^{99m}Tc-sulfur colloid is used most often. It has the advantages of being readily available,

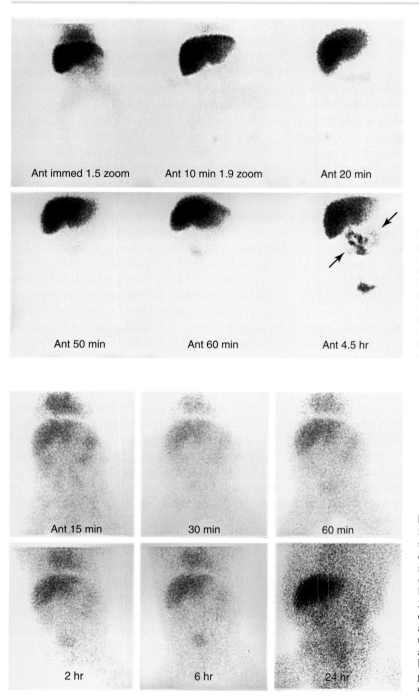

Ant immed 1.5 zoom   Ant 10 min 1.9 zoom   Ant 20 min

Ant 50 min   Ant 60 min   Ant 4.5 hr

Figure 7-26. Neonatal hepatitis. Sequential images from a technetium-99m hepatobiliary scan in this 2-week-old, jaundiced infant show only liver activity on the initial images; however, on the 4.5-hour image, activity is seen in the bowel of the central abdomen (*arrows*), indicating a patent biliary system. This finding excludes a diagnosis of biliary atresia.

Ant 15 min   30 min   60 min

2 hr   6 hr   24 hr

Figure 7-27. Biliary atresia. Sequential technetium-99m hepatobiliary images show markedly delayed clearance of radiopharmaceutical from the blood pool (heart) and poor concentration by the liver, even at 6 hours. The 24-hour image shows a great deal of residual liver and soft-tissue activity, with some excretion by the kidneys but no evidence of biliary or bowel activity. The resultant bladder activity must be distinguished from bowel activity, and catheterization may be helpful.

nonabsorbable, and inexpensive. The radiation absorbed dose from this procedure is about 20 mrad (0.2 mGy), compared with several rads (a few tens of mGy) for a barium esophagram.

The patient should fast for at least 6 hours before the procedure. The patient is placed supine under a gamma camera with the field of view, including the entire esophagus and proximal stomach. The supine view negates the effects of gravity. An upright view may be better to assess results of therapy in abnormalities such as achalasia and scleroderma. The patient is instructed to swallow 300 µCi (11.1 MBq) of ^{99m}Tc-sulfur or albumin colloid in 10 mL of water at the same time that acquisition by the camera and computer is begun. The patient then "dry" swallows every 15 seconds for 5 minutes. Because there may be variability between swallows, many laboratories repeat the procedure up to five times. After the acquisition is complete, regions of interest are outlined on the computer image to generate time-activity curves. A global esophageal region is used with optional divisions of the esophagus into thirds, with each as an additional region of interest. The global esophageal emptying time measures the time from the appearance of the radionuclide bolus in the proximal esophagus to the clearance of more than 90% from the entire esophagus. The esophageal transit time consists of the time interval between peak activity in the time activity curve from the proximal third of the esophagus and the peak in the distal third of the esophagus.

In normal persons, esophageal transit time for water is 5 to 11 seconds, and at least 90% of the activity should have traversed the esophagus globally by the end of 15 seconds. In patients with scleroderma and achalasia, transit may be reduced to levels as low as 20% to 40%. Patients with various other motor disorders of the esophagus usually have intermediate values.

Gastroesophageal Reflux

In patients with symptoms of heartburn, regurgitation, or bilious vomiting, computer-assisted scintigraphic studies provide a sensitive and useful method for reflux determination and quantitation. Alternative methods are limited in usefulness. Fluoroscopic barium studies are not sensitive and depend on the expertise and persistence of the fluoroscopist. Acid-reflux testing is the standard that is used for comparison but requires intubation. Esophageal manometry is sometimes used, but it also requires intubation to measure the decreased resistance of the lower esophageal sphincter in cases of reflux.

Technetium-99m colloids are the radiopharmaceuticals of choice. The procedure calls for the oral administration of 300 μCi (11.1 MBq) of ^{99m}Tc sulfur colloid in 150 mL of orange juice combined with 150 mL of 0.1 normal hydrochloric acid. The patient should fast overnight or for at least 2 hours after a liquid meal. An abdominal binder is placed around the upper abdomen. While in a sitting position, the patient drinks the 300 mL of solution, and, after 30 seconds, a single image is obtained to see that all of the liquid is in the stomach. An additional 30 mL of water is then given to rinse residual activity from the esophagus. The patient is placed under the gamma camera in the supine position with a field of view that includes

the esophagus and stomach. Serial 30-second images are then obtained with the abdominal binder at 0, 20, 40, 60, 80, and 100 mm Hg. In this method, position, pressure, and the presence of acid are all used to aggravate reflux. In addition to visual interpretation, regions of interest drawn over the stomach and the esophagus are used to calculate the percentage of gastric radiopharmaceutical refluxing into the esophagus.

A variation of this scintigraphic method using ^{99m}Tc colloid mixed with milk or infant formula may be used to study gastroesophageal reflux and pulmonary aspiration of gastric contents in infants; it is often referred to as a *milk scan*. In this case, an abdominal binder is not used, and imaging for reflux is performed in the left anterior oblique position rather than supine. If aspiration is suspected, anterior delayed images are obtained 2 to 4 hours later to look for activity in the lungs. In older children, ^{99m}Tc sulfur colloid or, preferably, indium-111 (^{111}In)–diethylenetriamine pentaacetic acid (DTPA) can be administered as a liquid meal at bedtime with imaging performed over the lungs during the following morning. The detection of aspiration occurring during esophageal reflux studies is reported to be 0% to 25%.

By this technique, esophageal reflux is expressed as the percentage of the gastric counts obtained at the beginning of the study (before reflux) that subsequently reflux into the esophagus. The upper limit for gastroesophageal reflux in normal people is 3%. Between 3% and 4% is considered indeterminate, and more than 4% reflux is abnormal (Fig. 7-28). The sensitivity of this study is about 90%; however, if acidified liquid, abdominal binder, and supine position are not used, the sensitivity of the study decreases. The study can be used in the initial diagnosis of reflux as well as in the evaluation of various therapeutic modalities.

Gastric Emptying

Scintigraphic studies of gastric emptying are the gold standard for measuring gastric emptying. Gastric emptying evaluation is complicated because liquid and solid contents empty from the stomach at different rates, and a host of factors regulates this process. Liquids empty from the stomach in an exponential fashion, whereas solid foods empty in a more linear manner. Osmolality, pH, volume, caloric content, amount of protein, carbohydrate, fat, weight, time of day, position, drugs, and sex of the patient all

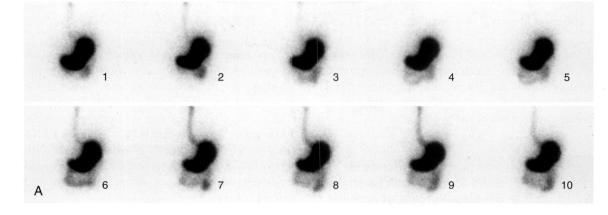

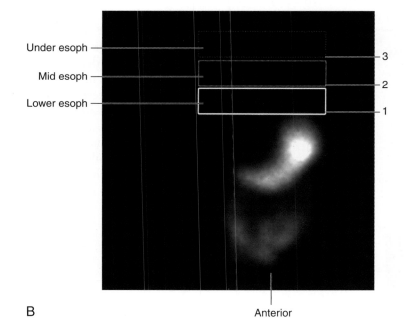

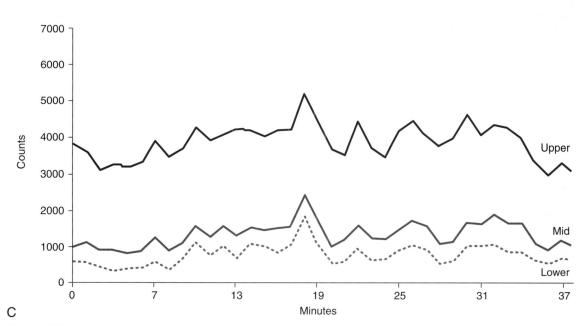

Figure 7-28. Gastroesophageal reflux. A, Anterior 1-minute images of the chest and upper abdomen shows activity within the stomach; however, sequential views show intermittent activity in the esophagus. **B,** Three regions of interest over the proximal, mid, and distal esophagus allow **C,** time activity curves to be generated. These show the spikes of refluxed activity in the esophagus.

affect emptying rate. For example, distention of the stomach accelerates gastric emptying, whereas lipids are potent inhibitors. In general, the emptying of solid foods is more relevant to postprandial abdominal symptoms.

TABLE 7-2	Interpretation Criteria for Solid Meal Gastric Emptying Studies (Percent of Activity in the Stomach at Specified Times)	
TIME (MIN)	**RAPID EMPTYING (%)**	**DELAYED EMPTYING (%)**
30	<70	
60	<30	>90
120		>60
180		>30
240*		>10

*The emptying value at 240 minutes is the most sensitive for delayed gastric emptying.

Two main classes of radiopharmaceuticals are used for the evaluation of gastric emptying: (1) those for the solid phase and (2) those for the liquid phase. The solid phase study may use ^{99m}Tc colloid eggs or egg whites. Perhaps the most widely used method is to mix 0.5 to 1 mCi (18.5 to 37 MBq) of ^{99m}Tc sulfur colloid with scrambled egg whites served as a white bread sandwich with 30 g of strawberry jam and 120 mL of water.

The patient should consume the radiolabeled solid meal within 10 minutes along with about 120 mL of water. The patient is then imaged in the upright position immediately after consuming the meal with additional images obtained every 60 minutes up to 4 hours. Recent evidence suggests that determining the degree of gastric emptying at 4 hours is more sensitive for gastroparesis than a 1- or 2-hour measure. In children, imaging may be stopped after 2 hours. The patient should sit up between the images and must not consume solids or liquids for the 4-hour imaging period. Vomiting during this

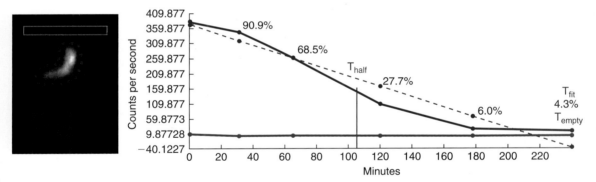

Figure 7-29. **Normal gastric emptying.** Anterior and posterior sequential images are used with a computer region of interest around to generate a time activity curve. Delayed gastric emptying occurs if there is >90% present in the stomach at 1 hour, >60% at 2 hours, >30% at 3 hours, or >10% at 4 hours. The 4-hour value is the best criteria.

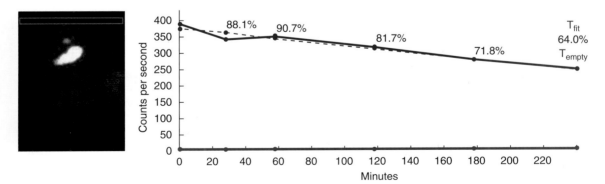

Figure 7-30. **Delayed gastric emptying.** Anterior and posterior images taken after the patient ingested technetium-99m colloid solid meal were used to generate a time-activity curve. It shows that more than half of the activity has remained in the stomach at 4 hours.

period renders the results invalid. Computer acquisition is mandatory, and regions of interest are selected over the stomach and appropriate background areas. If a dual-head camera is available, simultaneous anterior and posterior images acquisition with the geometric mean values for calculations is the most accurate methodology, although a left anterior oblique view acquisition with a single-headed camera is often satisfactory.

In most facilities, only a solid-phase study is performed using the technique described in Appendix E-1. The criteria for rapid and delayed emptying are shown in Table 7-2. A computer time-activity curve is obtained from a region of interest drawn over the stomach (Figs. 7-29 and 7-30). Emptying curves for solid meals typically display a flat initial portion (lag phase) and then

---

Box 7-10   Causes of Abnormal Gastric Emptying

Delayed
Hyperglycemia
Acidosis
Connective tissue diseases
Ileus
Diabetes mellitus
Gastroesophageal reflux
Vagotomy
Proximal partial gastrectomy
Chronic gastritis
Gastric ulcer disease
Malignancies
Psychiatric disorders
Drugs
　Opiates
　Antacids
　Anticholinergic agents
　Tricyclic antidepressants
　Cholecystokinin
　Gastrin
　Progesterone
　Calcium-channel blockers
　Levodopa

Rapid
Zollinger-Ellison syndrome
Duodenal ulcer disease
Sprue
Pancreatic insufficiency
Distal partial gastrectomy with vagotomy
Drugs
　Metoclopramide
　Domperidone
　Cisapride
　Erythromycin
　Motilin

---

a linear portion. In normal patients, retention of activity in the stomach is 30% to 60% at 2 hours and 0% to 10% at 4 hours. Patient radiation absorbed doses for solid-phase-only studies are quite low.

If a liquid phase alone is desired for infants, ^{99m}Tc sulfur colloid can be given in milk or formula. Under these circumstances, 2.5 to 5.0 µCi (0.09 to 0.18 MBq) are added per milliliter of liquid. Rarely, a simultaneous liquid-phase study is desired while performing a solid-phase gastric emptying study. This can be accomplished by using another radionuclide, such as ^{111}In-DTPA (125 µCi [4.6 MBq] in 300 mL of water) and performing a computer analysis of different photopeaks. Because dual-phase studies add cost and radiation dose, and, because the solid phase is more sensitive than is the liquid phase for detection of delayed gastric emptying, usually a solid-phase study is all that is needed. The half-time for emptying of the liquid phase is 40 (12 to 65) minutes. The normal half-time reported for infants given milk or formula varies widely in the literature from 25 to 48 minutes with breast milk, to 60 to 90 minutes with formula and bovine milk.

Major uses of gastric emptying studies are to confirm gastroparesis as a cause for persistent nausea and vomiting and to monitor the effects of therapy in patients with abnormal gastric motility (Box 7-10), such as diabetic patients. As is the case with esophageal transit studies, the initial workup of a patient with symptoms of gastric outlet obstruction should include an anatomic imaging examination to exclude structural disease.

ABDOMINAL SHUNT EVALUATION

Various shunt procedures have been developed that involve the peritoneal cavity. Evaluation of ventriculoperitoneal shunts for relief of hydrocephalus is discussed in Chapter 3. LeVeen shunts are sometimes placed for relief of intractable ascites. They drain the peritoneal cavity through a one-way pressure valve into the superior vena cava. In the event of suspected shunt failure, a pulmonary perfusion agent, such as ^{99m}Tc-MAA, can be introduced into the ascites by paracenteses. Subsequent activity in the lung indicates a patent shunt (Fig. 7-31). ^{99m}Tc-sulfur colloid also can be used with delayed activity in the liver, indicating patency.

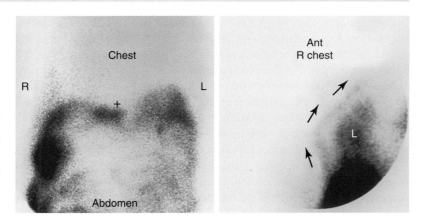

Figure 7-31. Patent LeVeen shunt. In this patient with intractable ascites, intraperitoneal injection of technetium-99m macroaggregated albumin allows an evaluation of the shunt. *Left,* An initial anterior image of the abdomen shows the activity throughout the peritoneal cavity outlining viscera and bowel. *Right,* An anterior image of the right chest shows the tracer progressing through the shunt (*arrows*) and localizing in the lungs (*L*).

PEARLS & PITFALLS

Colloid Liver–Spleen Imaging

- Common indications are for evaluation of hepatocellular disease (cirrhosis), hepatomegaly, splenomegaly, and focal abnormalities in the liver or spleen seen on ultrasound or CT.

- These studies are performed with ^{99m}Tc sulfur colloid. On the posterior view, the spleen should be equal to or less intense than the liver. With colloid shift, usually indicative of hepatocellular disease, the bone marrow is easily visualized, and increased splenic activity relative to the liver is seen.

- If there is a colloid shift, look for ascites (a space between the ribs and the lateral right lobe of the liver) and for a photopenic liver lesion that may represent a hepatoma.

- Photopenic lesions in the liver can be the result of anything that does not have reticuloendothelial activity (cyst, hematoma, abscess, hepatic adenoma, hepatoma, metastasis). Cold splenic lesions are usually infarct, tumor, or cyst.

- If there is a photopenic lesion, make sure that it triangulates in the same place in the organ on all images; otherwise, it may be the result of an artifact (such as barium in the colon or a bad photomultiplier tube).

- Focal nodular hyperplasia can accumulate ^{99m}Tc sulfur colloid, but hepatic adenomas and other tumors do not.

- Focal hot lesions in the liver are often the result of focal nodular hyperplasia, regenerating nodule in cirrhosis, or flow abnormalities. Collateral flow can deliver radiopharmaceutical to a specific portion of the liver. A hot area in porta hepatis region (quadrate lobe) suggests superior vena caval obstruction, and a hot caudate lobe suggests Budd-Chiari syndrome.

Blood Pool Imaging of the Liver

- This study is commonly performed to differentiate cavernous hemangioma from other focal liver lesions seen on ultrasound or CT.

- Hemangiomas are not seen to be hypervascular on early arterial images. On late blood pool images, a hemangioma usually shows activity that is more intense than the normal liver.

- Hypovascular tumors are photopenic on early and late images, and hypervascular tumors are usually increased in activity on early images but may be hot or cold on delayed images.

Gastrointestinal Bleeding Studies

- These are best performed with in-vitro ^{99m}Tc-labeled red blood cells. Salivary and thyroid activity indicate poor labeling.

- A focus of bleeding should change shape and location on sequential images. If the activity does not move, it may represent a vascular abnormality, such as an aneurysm, or an intussusception.

- On static images, the best way to pinpoint the bleeding site is to find an image in which there is a definite abnormality and then to look at the earlier images and find the first image in which the activity can be seen. This is necessary because activity seen as a result of bleeding can

PEARLS & PITFALLS—cont'd

go both antegrade and retrograde in the bowel. Review of dynamic (cine) images in addition to any static image series is optimum.

- Minimum bleeding detection rates are 1 mL/min for contrast angiography and 0.1 mL/min for the radionuclide study.

- Bladder activity from free ^{99m}Tc-pertechnetate can be confusing, and sometimes it is necessary for the patient to void or be catheterized.

Meckel Diverticulum Imaging

- These scans are performed with ^{99m}Tc-pertechnetate, which concentrates in normal and ectopic gastric mucosa.

- Most (about 70%) of Meckel diverticula do not contain ectopic gastric mucosa, but the ones that bleed almost always do.

- Look for a focus of activity in the mid-abdomen or right lower quadrant. It should increase in activity similar to the stomach mucosa and should remain in a fixed spot.

- A Meckel diverticulum should be seen anteriorly on lateral or oblique views.

- Cimetidine can be used to fix the radiopharmaceutical, and pentagastrin can increase the uptake in the gastric mucosa, thus increasing the sensitivity of the study.

- Bladder activity from the ^{99m}Tc-pertechnetate is normal. The patient may need to void or be catheterized if there is a suspicious lesion nearby.

Hepatobiliary

- The most common indications for a hepatobiliary study are to differentiate between acute or chronic cholecystitis, to look for suspected bile leaks or biliary obstruction, and, in the setting of neonatal jaundice, to differentiate neonatal hepatitis from biliary atresia.

- Technetium-99m hepatobiliary (IDA) agents are cleared and excreted by the hepatocytes but not conjugated. It then follows biliary excretion into the bowel.

- Cardiac blood pool activity should clear by 5 to 10 minutes. Lack of clearance indicates poorly functioning hepatocytes. Renal and bladder activity may be seen if the liver cannot efficiently excrete the radiopharmaceutical.

- If there is persistent cardiac blood pool activity, poor liver activity, and no biliary excretion, the differential diagnosis includes hepatocellular diseases (hepatitis) and severe biliary obstruction.

- If there appears to be only liver activity on sequential images and no cardiac, biliary, or bowel activity, this may be the *liver scan sign* of complete biliary obstruction, although this sign is not specific.

- Bowel activity should be seen by 1 hour. Delayed biliary-to-bowel transit can be the result of a number of entities, including common duct calculus, tumor, stricture, morphine, sphincter dyskinesia, or chronic cholecystitis.

- For hepatobiliary scans performed to differentiate biliary atresia from neonatal hepatitis, delayed 24-hour images to look for evidence of excretion into the bowel are often necessary. If bowel activity is present, biliary atresia is excluded. If no bowel activity is seen, the child may have either severe hepatitis or biliary atresia.

- The normal gallbladder with a patent cystic duct is usually seen by 30 minutes and should almost always be seen by 1 hour.

- A small amount of bile reflux from the duodenum into the stomach can be normal.

- Gallbladder activity can be confused with duodenal activity. To differentiate between these, either have the patient drink water and repeat the image or use a right lateral view and a left anterior oblique view (the gallbladder is anterior).

- Nonvisualization of the gallbladder is most likely the result of acute or, less often, chronic cholecystitis. Always determine whether the patient has had a cholecystectomy before interpreting the study.

- Nonvisualization of the gallbladder at 4 hours or after administration of morphine at 1 hour is most likely caused by acute cholecystitis.

Continued

PEARLS & PITFALLS—cont'd

- Morphine contracts the sphincter of Oddi and can help fill the gallbladder, but it will delay transit of activity into the small bowel.

- Nonvisualization of the gallbladder at 1 hour but visualization at 4 hours or after morphine administration is most likely caused by chronic cholecystitis.

- Look for either the rim sign (increased activity along the inferior edge of the right lobe of the liver) or cystic duct sign of acute cholecystitis if the gallbladder is not seen by 1 hour. A rim sign increases the likelihood of complicated cholecystitis (gangrene, abscess, or rupture).

- Bile leaks often pool in the region of the porta hepatitis, along the right lateral aspect of the liver, in the right pericolic gutter, and in the lower pelvis. If the gallbladder was recently removed, the bile may pool in the gallbladder fossa and mimic a gallbladder.

- Subtle bile leaks are often identified by comparing the shape and intensity of the liver on the first image to its apparent shape on the delayed views. When the liver appears to change shape or grow more intense owing to perihepatic accumulation of radiolabeled bile, a bile leak is likely.

- CCK can be used to initially empty the gallbladder in a fasting patient, to differentiate common duct obstruction from functional causes, and assess for a low ejection fraction in a patient with acute or chronic cholecystitis. CCK should be infused over 15 to 60 minutes. There is less abdominal pain and less variability of gallbladder ejection fraction values in normal patients with longer infusions.

- Generally, a CCK-stimulated gallbladder ejection fraction below 35% is considered abnormal. An unequivocally normal gallbladder ejection fraction after CCK is more than 50%.

Gastric Emptying Studies

- These studies usually are performed to assess the rate of emptying of solids from the stomach; they are most commonly performed with ^{99m}Tc colloid mixed into liquid egg whites before they are scrambled. It is served as a white bread sandwich with 30 g of strawberry jam and 120 mL of water.

- 1-minute standing anterior and posterior images are obtained at 1, 2, 3, and 4 hours, and the geometric mean is used to generate a time-activity curve.

- Delayed gastric emptying occurs if there is more than 90% present in the stomach at 1 hour, more than 60% at 2 hours, more than 30% at 3 hours, or more than 10% at 4 hours. The 4-hour value is the best criteria.

- Solids leave the stomach in a linear fashion, liquids exponentially.

- Portions of the stomach have different functions and may have different emptying rates. The proximal portion of the stomach relaxes to accommodate food and for liquid emptying, while the antrum is more associated with mechanical grinding and solid emptying.

SUGGESTED READINGS

Donohoe KJ, Maurer AH, Zeissman HA, et al. Procedure guideline for adult solid meal gastric emptying study 3.0. http://www.snm.org/guidelines. Accessed June 29, 2011.

Mariani G, Pauwels EK, AlSharif A, et al. Radionuclide evaluation of the lower gastrointestinal tract. J Nucl Med 2008;49(5):776-87.

Society of Nuclear Medicine Procedure guideline for hepatobiliary scintigraphy, Version 4.0, approved 2010. http://www.snm.org. Accessed June 29, 2011.

Urbain JC, Vekemans MM, Malmud LS. Esophageal transit, gastroesophageal reflux and gastric emptying. In Sandler MP, Coleman RE, Patton JA, et al. Diagnostic Nuclear Medicine, 4th ed. New York: Lippincott Williams & Wilkins; 2003. p. 487-502.

Ziessman HA: Acute cholecystitis, biliary obstruction and biliary leakage. Semin Nucl Med 2003;33:279-96.

Zuckier LS: Acute gastrointestinal bleeding. Semin Nucl Med 2003;33:297-311.

8 Skeletal System

The availability of stable technetium-labeled bone-seeking pharmaceuticals with good soft-tissue clearance has led to sensitive, high-resolution images, which accounts for the widespread use of these agents in bone scanning. Bone imaging with these technetium agents will probably remain clinically useful for a long time, despite the rapid advances in other technologies, such as positron emission tomography combined with computed tomography (PET/CT) and magnetic resonance imaging (MRI). The bone scan often provides an earlier diagnosis and demonstrates more lesions than are found by radiographic procedures. Although the presence of a lesion on a bone scan is nonspecific, its monostotic or polyostotic status and anatomic distribution can usually be determined, and these findings often provide important clues to the differential diagnosis. For optimal performance of bone scans, both the physician and the technologist need to understand the limitations and uses of skeletal imaging procedures.

ANATOMY AND PHYSIOLOGY

The basic structure of bone is a crystalline lattice composed of calcium, phosphate, and hydroxyl ions, which form the inorganic mineral hydroxyapatite. The other major constituents of bone include collagen, ground substance, and other minerals. Anatomically, the skeleton is composed of two parts: the axial and the appendicular portions. The axial skeleton includes the skull, spine, and thoracic girdle. The appendicular skeleton includes the upper extremities, pelvis, and lower extremities. This is a relatively important distinction because some diseases favor either the appendicular or the axial skeleton.

RADIOPHARMACEUTICALS

Bone-seeking radiopharmaceuticals are analogs of calcium, hydroxyl groups, or phosphates. By far, the most widely used radiopharmaceuticals for skeletal imaging are technetium-labeled diphosphonates, most often methylene diphosphonate.

Diphosphonates contain organic P–C–P bonds, which are more stable in vivo than are inorganic P–O–P bonds (pyrophosphates), primarily because of their resistance to enzymatic hydrolysis. Because the diphosphonates have rapid renal excretion, they provide a high target-to-nontarget ratio in 2 to 3 hours after injection, with 50% to 60% of the activity localizing in bone and the remainder being cleared by the kidneys. Factors that impair renal function result in increased soft-tissue activity, which reduces the quality of the bone scan. With most diphosphonates, maximal skeletal uptake occurs at about 5 hours. The biologic half-life is about 24 hours.

Care should be taken to avoid the injection of air into the mixing vial during preparation of phosphate radiopharmaceuticals because the resultant oxidation of technetium causes poor tagging of the phosphates. Bone radiopharmaceuticals should be routinely checked with chromatography before injection; a 95% tag is acceptable. If the radiopharmaceutical is administered more than 4 hours after preparation,

---

Box 8-1 Possible Mechanisms of Increased Activity on Bone Scans

Increased osteoid formation
Increased blood flow
Increased mineralization of osteoid
Interrupted sympathetic nerve supply

Box 8-2 Causes of Increased Activity on Bone Scan

Localized
Primary bone tumor
Metastatic disease
Osteomyelitis
Trauma
Stress or frank fractures
Battering
Postsurgical osseous changes
Loose prosthesis
Degenerative changes
Osteoid osteoma
Paget disease, melorheostosis, fibrous
  dysplasia
Arthritis
Locally increased blood flow
Hyperemia
Decreased sympathetic control
Decreased overlying soft tissue (e.g.,
  postmastectomy)
Soft-tissue activity (see Box 8-5)

Generalized (Superscan)
Primary hyperparathyroidism
Secondary hyperparathyroidism
Renal osteodystrophy
Diffuse metastases
Prostate
Lung
Breast
Hematologic disorders

---

gastric and thyroid visualization on bone scans may be seen as the result of free pertechnetate.

The initial accumulation of technetium-labeled radiopharmaceuticals in bone is primarily related to blood supply; however, roles are also played by capillary permeability, the local acid–base relation, fluid pressure within bone, hormones, vitamins, the quantity of mineralized bone, and bone turnover. Increased radionuclide activity in bone may result from accentuation of any one of these factors. Factors that may be responsible for greater than usual activity are listed in Boxes 8-1 and 8-2. For example, regionally increased blood flow causes increased delivery of the radiopharmaceutical to the bone, with resultant increased regional deposition of the agent. The converse is also true: interference with any of these factors may cause decreased skeletal activity. For instance, in cases of decreased cardiac output, bone scans may be of poor quality, owing to inadequate delivery of radiopharmaceutical to the bone. The relation between blood flow and radionuclide bone activity, however, is not linear; a fourfold increase in blood flow increases bone uptake by only 30% to 40%.

Initial deposition is thought to be attributable to *chemisorption* on the bone surface. In some patients, this accumulation can be affected by administered drugs. Technetium-99m (^{99m}Tc) diphosphonates concentrate not in osteoclasts or osteoid but rather in the mineral phase of bone, which is two thirds crystalline hydroxyapatite and one third amorphous, noncrystalline calcium phosphate.

^{18}F sodium-fluoride (^{18}F NaF) is an analog for the hydroxyl ion in the bone matrix. The fluoride ion exchanges with the hydroxyl ion in the hydroxyapatite crystal for localization with high initial extraction efficiency. ^{18}F NaF PET scanning has been recognized as an excellent technique for imaging areas of altered osteogenic activity in bone. ^{18}F NaF has desirable characteristics for this use, including rapid bone uptake, very rapid blood clearance (resulting in a favorable bone-to-background tissue ratio within 1 hour after ^{18}F NaF intravenous administration), and a reasonable decay half-life (110 minutes). ^{18}F NaF was initially approved for bone scanning by the U.S. Food and Drug Administration (FDA) in 1972, but until recently it was not reimbursed. With the advent of fast PET/CT scanners and local cyclotron production of ^{18}F, the methodology has become practical. The quality of the PET/CT ^{18}F NaF bone scans is better than ^{99m}Tc- methylene diphosphonate (MDP) in terms of spatial and anatomic resolution. There are a number of articles in the literature quoting greater sensitivity and specificity of ^{18}F NaF scanning over ^{99m}Tc- MDP. While ^{18}F-NaF scanning may be more sensitive, it is not yet clear whether it also has less specificity because small benign appearing sclerotic lesions and small degenerative changes can actively accumulate the radiopharmaceutical and be mistaken for metastatic disease. Further, ^{18}F NaF PET/CT scanning is significantly more expensive and has a radiation dose about seven times higher than that of ^{99m}Tc-MDP scans.

TECHNIQUE

Technical aspects, sample protocols, and dosimetry for planar and single-photon emission computed tomography (SPECT) and PET/CT skeletal imaging are presented in Appendix E-1.

For routine planar scans, the patient is normally injected intravenously with 10 to 20 mCi (370 to 740 MBq) of the technetium diphosphonate radiopharmaceutical and imaged 2 to 4 hours later. The site of injection should be distant from any suspected osseous pathology and should be recorded. Often, even a slight extravasation of isotope at the injection site causes a focus of markedly increased soft-tissue activity. In patients suspected of having either osteomyelitis or cellulitis, a radionuclide angiogram and initial blood pool image are performed after injection, and routine images are obtained at about 2 to 3 hours. This is termed a *three-phase study*. Sometimes, additional images are performed 18 to 24 hours after injection (*four-phase study*). A four-phase study is rarely needed but can be useful in patients in renal failure who have poor soft-tissue clearance.

Gamma camera imaging usually employs a moving table which results in whole-body images. If multiple spot films are obtained, the entire skeleton should be imaged. The patient is normally scanned in both the anterior and posterior projections. Detailed spot views of particular regions may be obtained as dictated by patient history or symptoms. In addition, selective pinhole or high-resolution collimator views allow for enhanced resolution in any areas of interest. These are especially useful when imaging small bones and pediatric patients.

The rapid urinary excretion of phosphate radiopharmaceuticals causes large amounts of activity to accumulate within the bladder, which may obscure pelvic lesions; therefore voiding before imaging should be routine. Voiding, however, particularly in incontinent patients, may result in radioactive contamination of skin or clothing; this may obscure underlying pathology or mimic a lesion. Removal of contaminated clothing and cleansing of skin may be necessary to obtain accurate results. After injection and

before scanning, patients should be hydrated. The resultant more frequent voiding decreases the bladder and pelvic radiation dose.

SPECT imaging may significantly improve skeletal lesion detection in patients with specific regional complaints and may establish or better localize an abnormality suspected on routine planar images. SPECT is most valuable in complex bony structures, such as large joints, the spine, and the pelvis.

The technique for ^{18}F NaF PET/CT scans includes intravenously administered activity of about 20 mCi (740 MBq). Whole body scanning is done 1 hour post injection, and the CT scan is done without the use of IV or gastrointestinal contrast. Limited body scanning is sometimes done for suspected focal entities, such as osteomyelitis. Scans are typically reviewed and interpreted on a workstation, which allows viewing rotating images and also provides automatic fusion of the PET and CT data.

NORMAL SCAN

The normal scan (Fig. 8-1) varies significantly in appearance between children and adults. In children, areas of growth in the region of the epiphyses show intense radionuclide accumulation (Fig. 8-2). In adults, the quality of the bone scan can be related to age; in general, the older the patient, the higher the proportion of poor-quality scans. There usually is good visualization of the skull, with relatively increased accumulation of activity in the region of the nasopharynx, which may be secondary to the high proportional blood flow in this region. Activity in the skull is often patchy, even in normal patients, so care must be taken in assessing skull lesions without an accompanying radiograph. Often, there is focal maxillary or mandibular alveolar ridge activity in adults, owing to dental disease. There is activity throughout the spine, and it is common to see focal areas of increased activity in the lower cervical spine even on anterior images, usually representing degenerative changes or simply a result of the lordosis of the cervical spine rather than activity in the thyroid cartilage or the thyroid itself. Areas of tendon insertion, chronic stress, and osseous remodeling caused by any reason also demonstrate increased activity. On the anterior view, there is prominent visualization of the sternum, sternoclavicular joints, acromioclavicular joints, shoulders, iliac crests, and hips. Increased

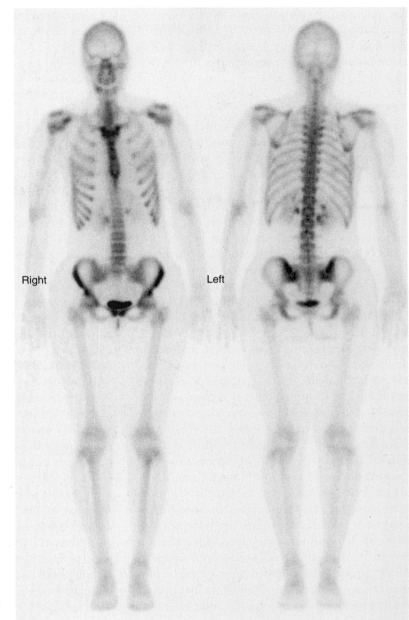

Right   Left

Figure 8-1. Normal adult bone scan. Anterior (left) and posterior images.

activity in the knees in older patients is relatively common because of the propensity for arthritic changes. On the posterior view, the thoracic spine is well seen, as are the tips of the scapulae. The spine often demonstrates increased activity in areas of hypertrophic degenerative change, and the sacroiliac joints are usually pronounced.

Because the human skeleton is symmetric, any asymmetric osseous activity should be viewed with suspicion. In addition, it is important on the posterior view to examine the scan for the presence and location of renal activity; on the anterior view, for bladder activity. The kidneys and bladder should be routinely scrutinized for focal space-occupying lesions producing photopenic defects in the renal cortex or displacement of the kidneys or bladder. Asymmetric renal activity is not uncommon. Because the scans are usually obtained in the supine position, activity may accumulate in extrarenal pelves. If urinary tract obstruction is suspected, kidney views should be repeated after the patient has ambulated to distinguish obstruction from position-related collecting system activity (Fig. 8-3).

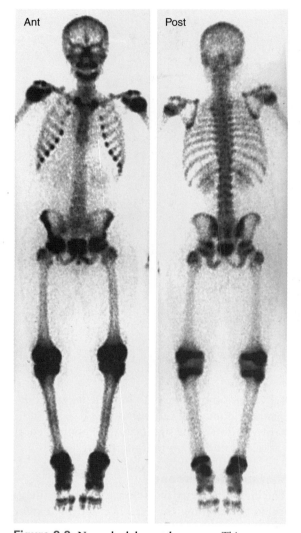

Ant   Post

Figure 8-2. Normal adolescent bone scan. This scan was performed on a 15-year-old boy. Anterior (*left*) and posterior (*right*) images demonstrate markedly increased activity around the epiphyseal plates. This is usually best seen around the knees, ankles, shoulders, and wrists.

If there is extravasation of the radiopharmaceutical at the site of injection, the radiopharmaceutical will be slowly resorbed. In such cases, lymphatic drainage may also occur, resulting in the visualization of one or more lymph nodes, not infrequently seen in the axilla or supraclavicular region on the side of an upper extremity injection. (Fig. 8-4).

Localized areas of increased soft-tissue or skeletal activity in an extremity distal to the site of injection (the *glove phenomenon*) may be a result of inadvertent arterial injection of the radionuclide. Regional blood flow changes may also be reflected in the scan (either relative ischemia if the activity is decreased, such

as with atherosclerotic disease or gangrene, or hyperemia if the activity is locally increased, such as with cellulitis or other inflammation). When pathology is suspected in the hands, wrists, or forearms, and a three-phase study is being performed, it is important to release the venous tourniquet and wait for about 1 minute before injecting the radiopharmaceutical. If this is not done, there can be confusion of actual pathology, with transient hyperemia resulting from vasodilatation caused by the tourniquet (Fig. 8-5). Differential blood flow also may be secondary to neurologically or autonomically mediated abnormalities (sympathectomy or neuropathy), or even to altered stress.

Recognition of the details of normal imaging anatomy becomes even more important when SPECT images of specific skeletal regions are obtained. Reviewing the images in three orthogonal planes generally aids interpreter orientation and thus allows more accurate localization of pathology. The specific reconstructions of greatest value depend on the area being evaluated. The complexity of the spine makes it particularly amenable to SPECT imaging to localize an abnormality in the vertebral body, disk space, or posterior elements. Transverse images of the spine resemble those of CT sections, whereas coronal and sagittal SPECT images are analogous to anteroposterior and lateral radiographic tomograms, respectively. The curvature of the thoracolumbar spine results in sequential rather than simultaneous visualization of the anatomic parts of adjacent vertebrae. With a careful view of the sequential images on a computer monitor display, proper orientation generally is not difficult.

CLINICAL APPLICATIONS

The following are some common indications for bone scanning:

- Detection and follow-up of metastatic disease
- Differentiation between osteomyelitis and cellulitis
- Determination of bone viability: infarction or avascular necrosis
- Evaluation of fractures difficult to assess on radiographs (stress fractures, fractures of complex structures, and possible fractures in battered children)
- Evaluation of prosthetic joints for infection or loosening
- Determination of biopsy site

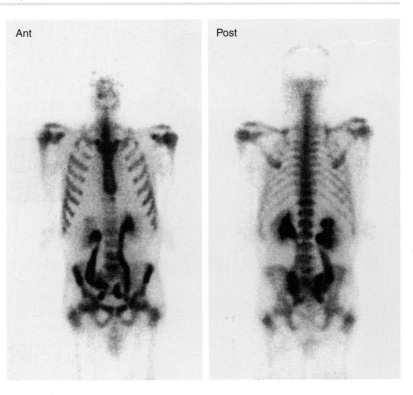

Figure 8-3. Hydronephrosis. This 50-year-old woman with cervical cancer had a bone scan because of back pain and suspected metastatic disease. Anterior (*left*) and posterior (*right*) images show markedly increased activity in both kidneys and ureters 3 hours after injection.

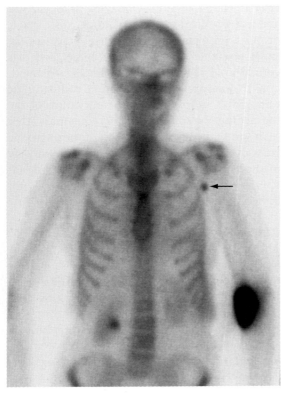

Figure 8-4. Activity in axillary lymph node (*arrow*) after extravasation of injection into left antecubital fossa.

■ Evaluation of bone pain in patients with normal or equivocal radiographs

■ Evaluation of the significance of an incidental skeletal finding on radiographs

Metastatic Disease

The high sensitivity of radionuclide bone imaging in determining the presence and the extent of metastatic disease makes it an extremely important tool in decision making, particularly because survival rates in patients with multiple distant osseous metastases from many tumors are worse than for those patients with localized disease. Although the prognostic value of bone scanning for some tumors is disputed, the answer probably depends on the natural history of each tumor type and adequate actuarial analysis. Finding metastases is frequently important to clinical decisions affecting quality of life. Serial bone scanning in patients with known metastases is thought to be valuable in therapeutic decision making (Fig. 8-6), particularly if it is used in combination with other clinical information. This may prove of particular value in the detection of lesions in critical weight-bearing areas, such as the femur.

For a lytic lesion to be visualized by radiography, localized demineralization of about 30% to 50% must occur, and there is little question

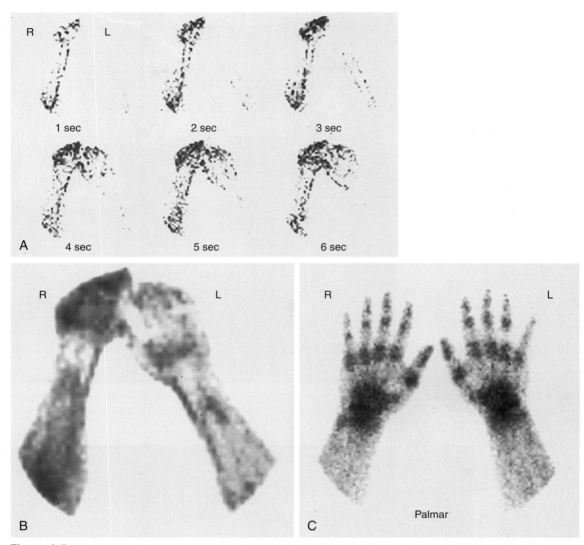

Figure 8-5. Tourniquet phenomenon in a normal patient. A tourniquet applied to the arm before intravenous administration of radiopharmaceutical causes distal ischemia and physiologic vasodilatation. **A,** When the tourniquet is released and the injection made within 30 to 60 seconds, there is increased blood flow and **B,** blood pooling in the forearm and hand. In this patient, the tourniquet was applied to the right arm, and the injection was made quickly because the patient was uncooperative and moving. **C,** Note that the delayed 3-hour images of the hands are normal.

that bone scans usually demonstrate metastatic lesions much earlier than radiography does. The false-negative rate of radiographic skeletal surveys may be as high as 50% with certain tumors, whereas the overall false-negative rate of bone scanning for the most common neoplasms may be as low as 2%. Some tumors are more likely than are others to produce a false-negative bone scan. These include highly aggressive anaplastic tumors, reticulum cell sarcoma, renal cell carcinoma (Fig. 8-7), thyroid carcinoma, histiocytosis, neuroblastoma, and especially multiple myeloma. When multiple myeloma is seen on a bone scan, it is often secondary to a

pathologic fracture or impending fracture. For patients in whom some lesions cannot be identified easily by bone scanning, the radiographic skeletal survey or MRI remain the procedures of choice.

About 80% of patients with known neoplasms and bone pain have metastases documented by the bone scan. Because 30% to 50% of patients with metastases do not have bone pain, a good case may be made for scanning patients with asymptomatic tumors that have a propensity to metastasize to bone (e.g., breast, lung, and prostate); but for tumors with low rates of osseous metastases (e.g., colon, cervix,

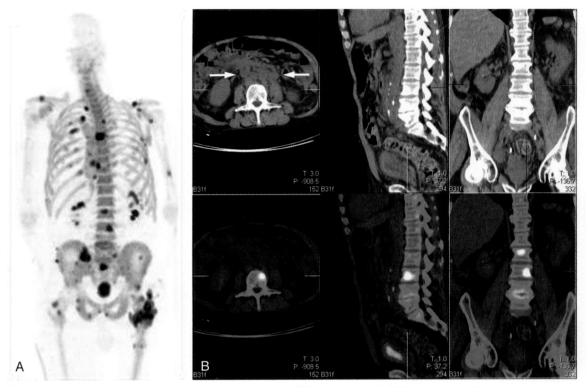

Figure 8-6. Metastatic prostate cancer. **A,** Anterior view of ¹⁸F-sodium fluoride PET scan shows the metastatic deposits as areas of increased activity. **B,** PET/CT scan shows the osseous metastases. Note, however, that the lymphadenopathy (*arrows*) is seen on only the CT portion of the study.

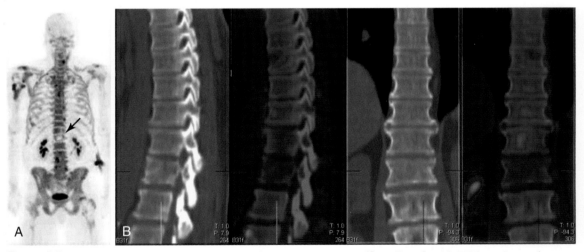

Figure 8-7. Cold defects caused by metastases. **A,** In this patient, an anterior ¹⁸F-sodium fluoride PET scan image shows an area in the spine that has no bony activity (*arrow*). **B,** PET/CT sagittal and coronal images of the thoracolumbar spine show multiple areas of decreased activity in areas where the CT scan shows minimal changes.

uterus, head, and neck), the procedure may not be cost-effective.

Even though most metastases are multiple and relatively obvious, there are times when the interpretation may be difficult. If a single lesion is identified, the false-positive rate for attributing the finding to a metastasis is high. Only about 15% to 20% of patients with proven metastases have a single lesion (most commonly in the spine). A single focus of increased activity elsewhere is often secondary to benign disease, especially in a rib where this is attributable to metastasis in only about 10% of cases. A notable exception to this is a single sternal lesion in a

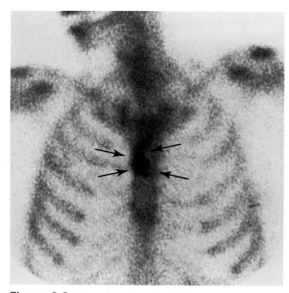

Figure 8-8. Sternal metastasis. This young woman was treated for breast cancer 1 year earlier. The follow-up bone scan reveals only one focus of increased activity, which is in the sternum. Round or eccentric sternal lesions in breast cancer patients have about an 80% chance of being a metastasis.

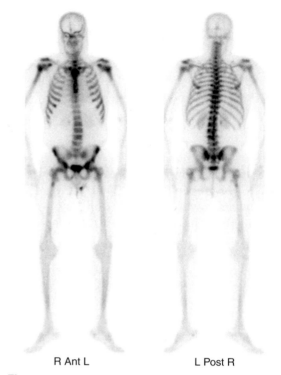

R Ant L   L Post R

Figure 8-9. Superscan. Diffuse osteoblastic metastases from carcinoma of the prostate. There is involvement of the entire axial and proximal appendicular skeleton. There is minimal renal or bladder activity identified because the metastases have accumulated most of the radionuclide.

patient with breast cancer (Fig. 8-8), which can be a result of metastasis in almost 80% of cases. If two consecutive ribs are involved by adjacent discrete foci of increased activity, the lesions are almost always secondary to trauma. In a patient with a known malignancy and a solitary abnormality on bone scan without an obvious benign explanation on radiographs, additional imaging is often warranted to exclude the possibility of metastases.

When multifocal areas of increased activity are seen in noncontiguous ribs, especially if in a linear configuration along the rib, however, the likelihood of metastatic disease is high. In multifocal metastatic disease, the regional distribution of lesions for common bone-seeking primary tumors is as follows: thorax and ribs, 37%; spine, 26%; pelvis, 16%; limbs, 15%; and skull, 6%. The reason for this distribution is that most bone metastases are caused by hematogenous spread to the red marrow, with subsequent erosion of the surrounding bone.

Follow-up bone scans in patients undergoing treatment for advanced breast and prostate cancer should be interpreted with caution. Within the first 3 months of chemotherapy, a favorable clinical response by focal bone metastases may result in healing that causes increased uptake at involved sites, which is usually a good

prognostic sign. If not clinically correlated, this *flare phenomenon* can give the false impression of new lesions or the extension of existing metastatic sites. Bone lesions that appear 6 months or later after treatment almost always indicate disease progression.

Diffuse involvement of the skeleton by metastases can be deceptive; it may initially appear as though there has been remarkably good, relatively uniform uptake in all of the bones. This has been referred to as a *superscan* (Fig. 8-9). A hallmark of the superscan caused by metastases is significantly decreased renal activity with diffusely increased activity noted throughout the axial skeleton. A superscan is most commonly a result of prostatic carcinoma, although diffuse metastases from other tumors, such as breast cancer and lymphoma, may also cause this appearance. In the absence of neoplasm, a superscan involving bones throughout the entire skeleton (both axial and peripheral) should raise suspicion of metabolic conditions, such as primary or secondary hyperparathyroidism. Increased activity primarily in the peripheral skeleton may be seen in hematologic disorders. For example, a patient with chronic anemia, such as occurs in sickle cell disease or thalassemia, may show increased activity in the skull and around the knees and ankles as a result of expanded marrow and an accompanying increase in blood flow to these regions.

In some patients who have metastatic disease, chemotherapy results in immunosuppression, and treatment may involve the use of granulocyte-macrophage colony-stimulating factor. This treatment causes marrow hyperplasia and increased marrow blood flow, resulting in bone scans with symmetrically increased activity around the major joints (particularly the knees).

Detection of bone metastases from prostate cancer is best assessed using a bone scan. Prostate-specific antigen (PSA) has been shown to be a marker for both primary and metastatic prostatic cancer. In asymptomatic patients presenting with well or moderately differentiated prostate cancer and PSA levels of less than 10 ng/mL, the likelihood of bone metastases is very low (less than 2%). Unless these patients have focal bone pain, a bone scan is likely not indicated. In patients who are not receiving adjuvant hormonal therapy, it is relatively rare (2%-10%) to see a positive bone scan if the serum PSA does not exceed 20 ng/mL. Contrarily, PSA levels can be normal in patients with osseous metastases receiving hormonal therapy. There are rare prostate cancers that do not produce detectable levels of PSA.

In searching for metastatic disease, it is important not only to delineate the areas of increased activity (see Box 8-2), but also to look for cold lesions (Box 8-3), which are usually much more difficult to identify. In cancer patients, focal photon-deficient lesions are attributable to metastatic disease in more than 80% of cases. They may occur if the tumor is extremely aggressive, if there is disruption of the blood supply to the bone, or if there is significant marrow involvement, particularly in a vertebral body. When multiple adjacent bones have a decreased radionuclide accumulation, other causes, such as radiation therapy, should be considered (Fig. 8-10). Other causes of cold lesions include infarction (particularly in patients with sickle cell anemia) and avascular necrosis. Both infarction and aseptic necrosis in the healing phase can show increased activity.

Box 8-3 Causes of Cold Lesions on Bone Scan

Localized
Overlying attenuation artifact caused by pacemaker, barium, etc.
Instrumentation artifact
Radiation therapy
Local vascular compromise
Infarction
Intrinsic vascular lesion
Early aseptic necrosis
Marrow involvement by tumor
Early osteomyelitis
Osseous metastases from:
Neuroblastoma
Renal cell carcinoma
Thyroid carcinoma
Anaplastic tumors (e.g., reticulum cell sarcoma)
Cyst

Generalized
Older age
Inadequate amount of radiopharmaceutical
Chemotherapy

Malignant Bone Tumors

The bone scan appearance of *osteogenic sarcoma* varies widely, depending on the vascularity and aggressiveness of the tumor and on the amount of neoplastic and reactive bone production (Fig. 8-11). Increased activity in these lesions is usually intense and often patchy with photopenic areas. Only about 2% of these patients present with osseous metastases from the primary site. Exact assessment of tumor extent by bone scanning is often complicated by reactive hyperemia in the affected limb, which may produce increased activity in the entire extremity. In this setting, MRI may provide more exact information regarding tumor extent, particularly in soft tissues. Evaluation of various bone tumors with ^{18}F-fluorodeoxyglucose (FDG) PET/CT is discussed in Chapter 11.

In the past, follow-up bone scans were not thought to be worthwhile in patients with osteosarcoma because pulmonary metastases almost always developed before osseous metastases. Aggressive chemotherapy, however, has altered the natural history of osteosarcoma, and now about 20% of patients develop osseous metastases before pulmonary disease. Thus follow-up bone scans are now recommended.

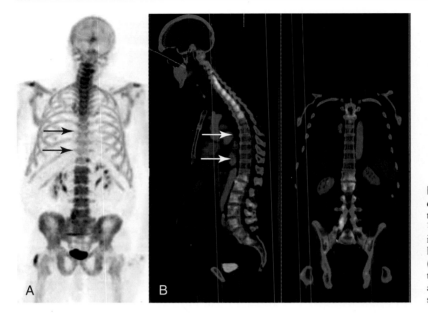

Figure 8-10. Radiation therapy defect. This patient had radiation therapy to the spine. **A,** Anterior ^{18}F-sodium fluoride PET scan image. Multiple contiguous vertebral bodies with decreased activity (*arrows*) are the result of radiotherapy, not metastases. **B,** Sagittal and coronal PET/CT scans of the spine show the same defects.

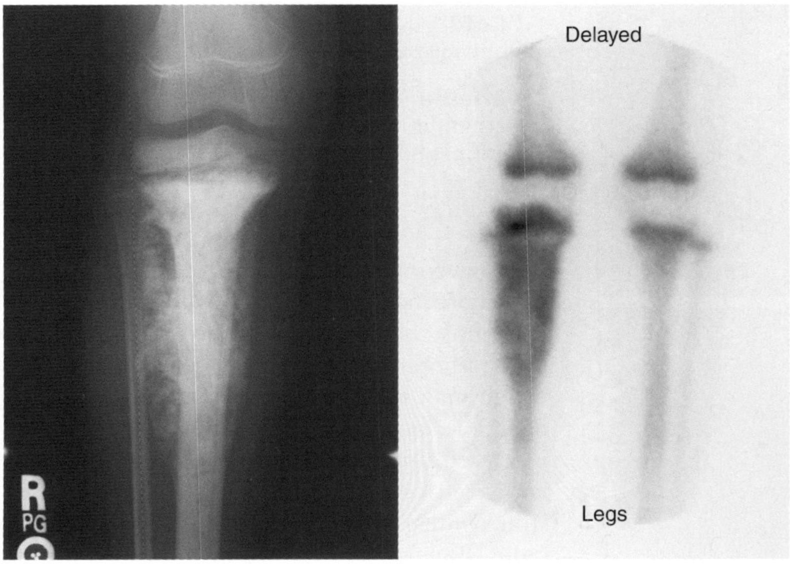

Delayed

Legs

Figure 8-11. Osteogenic sarcoma. Radiograph (*left*) reveals mottled sclerosis and periosteal reaction in the proximal tibia of a teenager. *Right,* Increased activity is seen on the bone scan as well. There is normal physiologic activity seen at the epiphyseal plates.

In interpreting follow-up scans, care must be taken not to mistake postamputation reactive changes at the amputation site for tumor recurrence. Because osteosarcomas are bone-forming lesions, soft-tissue metastases may be seen as foci of extraskeletal increased activity, especially in the liver and lung.

Ewing sarcoma is a relatively common primary bone tumor, frequently occurring in the pelvis or femur. Activity is often intense and homogeneous. The tumor is very vascular and may mimic osteomyelitis on three-phase bone imaging. Up to 11% of patients present with osseous metastases (Fig. 8-12). About 40% to 50% of patients with either Ewing sarcoma or osteosarcoma develop osseous metastases within 2 years of presentation, and follow-up bone scans are recommended. Reactive hyperemia producing increased activity in the adjacent uninvolved bone is not usually seen with Ewing sarcoma.

Benign Osseous Neoplasms

Benign osseous neoplasms have variable appearances on bone scan (Box 8-4). Angiographic and blood pool images obtained shortly

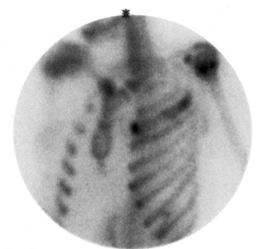

A   LAO

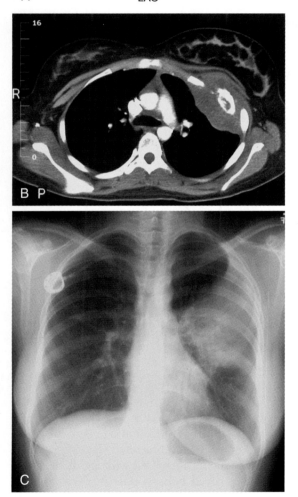

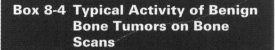

Box 8-4 Typical Activity of Benign Bone Tumors on Bone Scans

Intense
Fibrous dysplasia
Giant cell tumor
Aneurysmal bone cyst
Osteoblastoma
Osteoid osteoma

Moderate
Adamantinoma
Chondroblastoma
Enchondroma

Mild or Isointense
Fibrous cortical defect
Bone island
Cortical desmoid
Nonossifying fibroma
Osteoma

"Cold"
Bone cyst without fracture

Variable
Hemangioma
Multiple hereditary exostosis

Figure 8-12. Ewing sarcoma of the left third rib. **A,** On the bone scan, an oblique view of the ribs shows abnormal uptake in the anterior-lateral left third rib. **B,** Computed tomography scan shows the soft-tissue mass associated with rib destruction. **C,** Chest radiograph shows increased density as a result of a soft-tissue mass arising from the anterior left third rib.

after injection of bone scanning agents indicate that most malignant lesions are hyperemic and that most benign lesions initially accumulate little radiopharmaceutical. An early blood pool image may therefore be helpful in identifying benign lesions because it may show little or no increased uptake. The major exception to this is osteoid osteoma (Fig. 8-13), which demonstrates intense activity at the site of the vascular nidus. Bone scans are often of value in detecting these lesions when they occur in sites that are difficult to evaluate on a radiograph, such as the spine. On delayed images, benign lesions may show a wide range of activity. Osteoblastomas, osteoid osteomas, chondroblastomas, and giant-cell tumors usually have intense activity on delayed images. Enchondromas can be warm or hot (Fig. 8-14), chondroblastomas are usually of intermediate activity (Fig. 8-15), and fibrous cortical defects and nonossifying fibromas are of normal intensity or warm. Bone islands, hemangiomas, and cortical desmoid tumors rarely show increased activity and usually cannot be distinguished from normal bone. Bone cysts are usually cold centrally but may have a

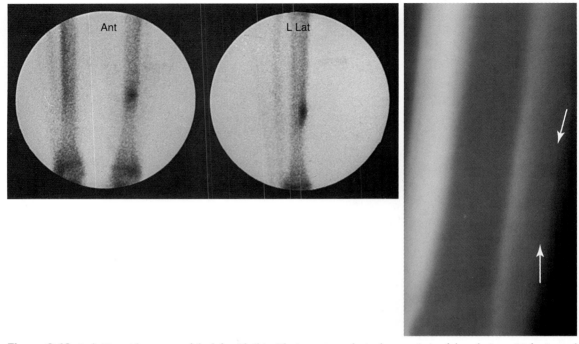

Figure 8-13. *Left,* **Osteoid osteoma of the left mid-tibia.** The intense uptake is characteristic of these lesions. *Right,* Lateral radiographic tomogram demonstrates the lesion (*arrows*) with a central nidus.

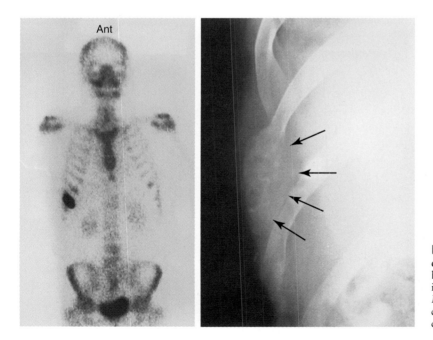

Figure 8-14. **Multiple enchondromas.** *Left,* On the anterior bone scan, areas of increased activity are noted, including in the ribs. *Right,* Rib radiograph shows a characteristic expansile lesion with central matrix (*arrows*).

warm rim caused by increased bone remodeling, or even a hot area caused by a pathologic fracture. *Fibrous dysplasia* is another benign disease of bone that may present as single (Fig. 8-16) or multiple areas of increased activity.

Both polyostotic fibrous dysplasia and Paget disease are sometimes confused with multifocal metastatic disease, although the distribution and radiographic presentation of lesions are frequently characteristic. Both osteochondromas

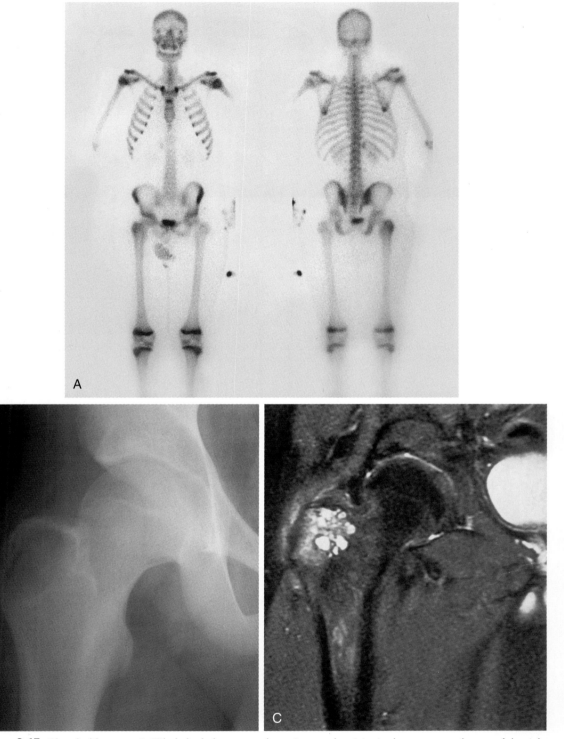

Figure 8-15. Chondroblastoma. **A,** Whole-body bone scan shows increased activity in the greater trochanter of the right hip. **B,** Radiograph shows a lytic lesion in the same region. **C,** Magnetic resonance imaging scan demonstrates the chondroid matrix.

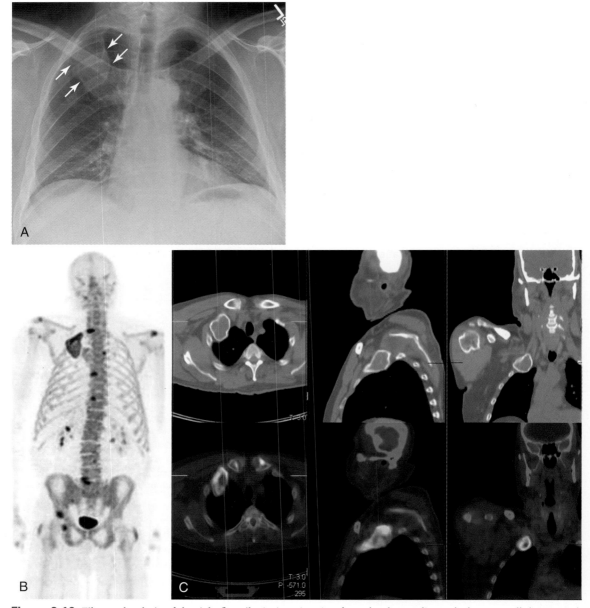

Figure 8-16. Fibrous dysplasia of the right first rib. A, Anterior view from the chest radiograph shows a well-demarcated, expansile, lucent lesion of the right first rib (*arrows*). **B,** Anterior image from a ^{18}F-sodium fluoride PET scan shows markedly increased activity in this area as do **C,** PET/CT images. Note that a number of other focal areas of increased activity in **B** can easily be mistaken for metastatic disease. In reality, these represent degenerative changes that are much more obvious on an ^{18}F-sodium fluoride PET scan than on a typical ^{99m}Tc-MDP scan.

and enchondromas are frequently seen as areas of increased activity.

Soft-Tissue Uptake

Activity may be seen in soft-tissue structures on the bone scan, and many possibilities can be considered when this occurs (Box 8-5). Soft-tissue activity may be secondary to any process that evokes soft-tissue calcification or infarction. The first and most obvious item to be excluded is surface contaminations by urine or by the radionuclide during injection.

Soft-tissue neoplasms or their metastases (especially in the liver) may calcify, resulting in soft-tissue activity. These tumors are often mucin-producing tumors from breast (Fig. 8-17), gastrointestinal (Fig. 8-18), and ovarian primaries (Fig. 8-19); lung cancer, lymphoma,

Box 8-5 Causes of Extraosseous Activity on Bone Scans

Generalized
Poor radiopharmaceutical preparation
Renal failure

Localized
Injection sites
Kidney (normal)
Obstructed kidney or ureter
Urine contamination
Hepatic necrosis
Tissue infarction (brain, muscle, heart, spleen)
Myositis ossificans
Polymyositis
Pulmonary or stomach calcification (hyperparathyroidism)
Vascular calcification
Hematoma
Steroids (breast uptake)
Sites of intramuscular iron injection or calcium injection extravasation
Chemotherapy (kidneys)
Radiotherapy treatment portals
Tumoral calcinosis, dystrophic, and metastatic calcification
Calcific tendinitis
Free pertechnetate (stomach, thyroid)
Amyloidosis
Soft tissue (tumors)
Breast
Ovary (especially mucinous)
Gastrointestinal (especially colon)
Neuroblastoma
Endometrial carcinoma
Uterine fibroids (leiomyoma)
Gastrointestinal lymphoma
Hepatic metastases
Meningioma
Lung carcinoma
Malignant ascites or effusions

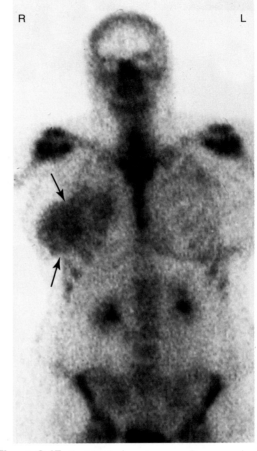

Figure 8-17. Activity in breast cancer. Bone scan in this patient with a right breast tumor shows marked asymmetric increased activity in the tumor (*arrows*).

osteogenic sarcoma (Fig. 8-20); and neuroblastoma (Fig. 8-21). Malignant pleural effusions or malignant ascites may also be demonstrated on bone scans as diffusely increased activity in the chest or abdomen (Figs. 8-22 and 8-23). Other causes of soft-tissue activity include dystrophic calcification such as occurs around joints in paraplegics, dermatomyositis (Fig. 8-24), calcific tendinitis, and other enthesopathies, postoperative scars, inflammation, amyloidosis, and uterine fibroids.

Areas of recent infarction in skeletal muscle (rhabdomyolysis) (Fig. 8-25), brain, heart, and spleen (Fig. 8-26) may often be demonstrated on the bone scan. Renal failure evoking secondary hyperparathyroidism (renal osteodystrophy) may cause localized activity within the walls of the gastrointestinal tract (particularly in the stomach), lungs, and kidneys, owing to excessive parathyroid hormone production and subsequent calcium deposition (Fig. 8-27). Infiltration of skeletal and cardiac muscle, liver, stomach, and skin by amyloid can likewise cause soft-tissue activity. Calcification in regions of trauma, secondary to calcifying hematomas or myositis ossificans, has also been reported as a cause of soft-tissue accumulation of bone-imaging radiopharmaceuticals. Some surgeons use bone scans as a measure of inflammatory activity in myositis ossificans and delay possible surgery until the activity in the soft tissue is similar to activity in normal bone (Fig. 8-28), so that recurrence is minimized. Dystrophic calcification around joints as a result of

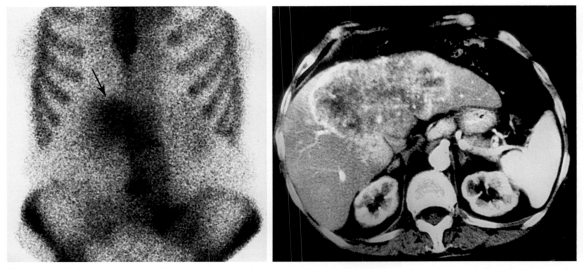

Figure 8-18. **Liver metastases.** This patient with a known mucinous colon carcinoma was thought to have hepatomegaly. *Left,* Bone scan done as part of the workup shows soft-tissue activity in the right upper quadrant (*arrow*). *Right,* Subsequent computed tomography scan clearly demonstrates a large hypervascular metastasis in the left lobe of the liver.

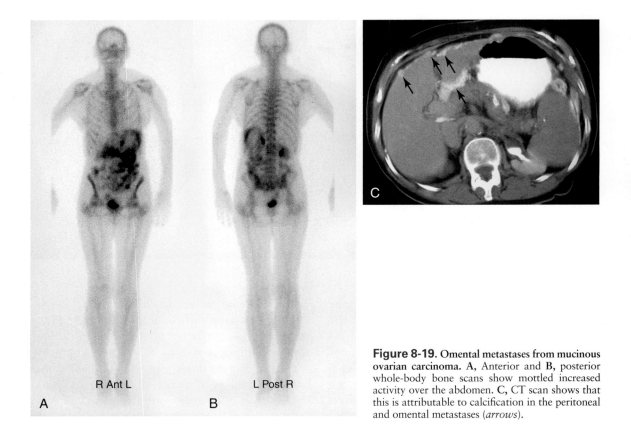

R Ant L

L Post R

A

B

C

Figure 8-19. Omental metastases from mucinous ovarian carcinoma. **A,** Anterior and **B,** posterior whole-body bone scans show mottled increased activity over the abdomen. **C,** CT scan shows that this is attributable to calcification in the peritoneal and omental metastases (*arrows*).

trauma (Fig. 8-29) or tumoral calcinosis also shows increased activity.

Breast activity may be increased in menstruating women, breast carcinoma, mastitis, trauma, and other benign conditions. Soft-tissue changes can be noted on bone scans after mastectomy. The ribs are usually more clearly seen on the mastectomy side, because there is less overlying soft tissue. Radiation therapy may produce increased chest wall activity in the early weeks

Post   RPO

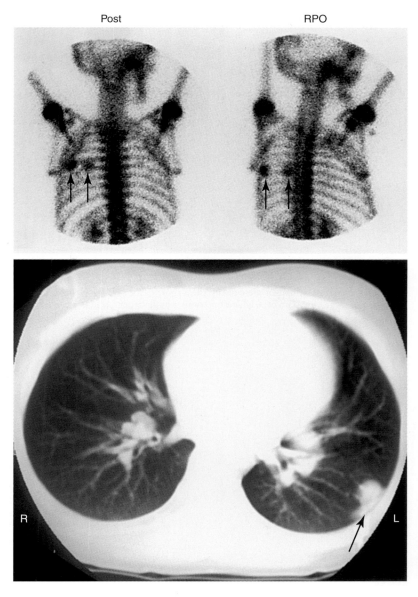

Figure 8-20. Osteosarcoma metastasis. This child had a right knee tumor that was resected 1 year earlier. *Top,* Follow-up bone scan showed foci of increased activity (*arrows*) projecting between posterior left ribs (and therefore probably in the lung). *Bottom,* Computed tomography scan confirmed the presence of lung metastases (*arrow*).

after treatment and several months later may produce relatively decreased activity at the treatment site.

A generalized increase in soft-tissue or blood pool activity is seen in some patients receiving chemotherapy or who have chronic iron overload. Soft-tissue injection of iron dextran may produce focal areas of increased activity. Renal failure commonly produces delayed clearance of the radiopharmaceutical and generalized increased activity throughout the soft tissues caused by diminished excretion of the radiopharmaceutical. Unilaterally increased activity in one kidney may be attributable to a number of causes, most commonly

an extrarenal pelvis or obstruction. Persistently increased diffuse activity in the kidney parenchyma can be attributable to radiotherapy, chemotherapy (Fig. 8-30), hyperparathyroidism, amyloidosis, or sarcoidosis. Some reported causes of increased hepatic and renal activity on bone scans are given in Boxes 8-6 and 8-7.

Trauma

Fractures not apparent on routine radiographs may be readily detected with CT, MRI, or radionuclide bone scanning (Fig. 8-31). MRI can detect the disruption of the cortex as well as edema in the marrow. MRI is most useful

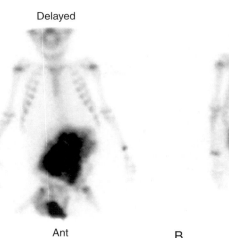

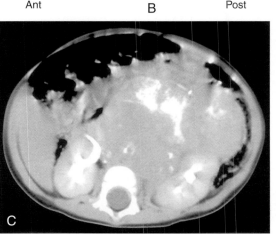

Figure 8-21. **Neuroblastoma.** A 2-year-old child with a left retroperitoneal mass was referred for a bone scan. There is increased activity in the region of the mass seen on anterior (**A**) and posterior (**B**) images. The activity is too large and too intense to be normal renal excretion and is the result of calcification in the tumor, which is easily seen on the CT scan (**C**).

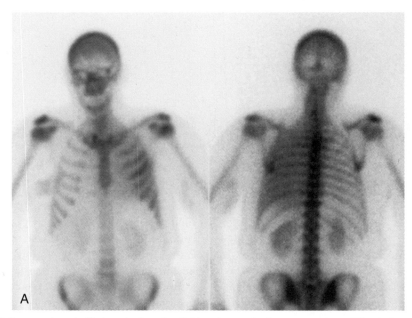

Figure 8-22. **Malignant pleural effusion. A,** Anterior (left) and posterior bone scans show diffusely increased activity over the left hemithorax. Nonmalignant effusions uncommonly accumulate activity.

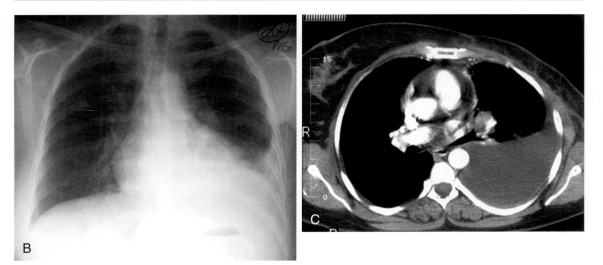

Figure 8-22, cont'd. B, Chest radiograph and **C,** CT scan demonstrate the effusion.

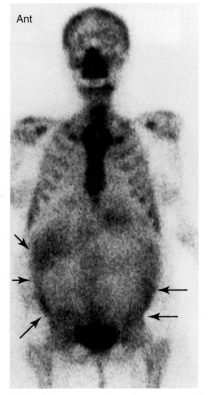

Figure 8-23. Malignant ascites. This 45-year-old woman has known ovarian carcinoma. Three-hour images from the bone scan show diffusely increased activity (*arrows*) over the entire peritoneal cavity.

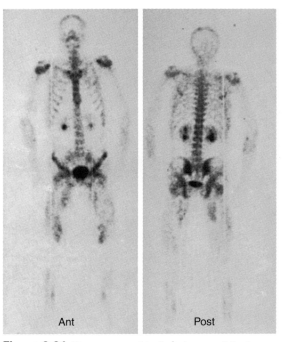

Figure 8-24. Dermatomyositis. Soft-tissue activity is seen on the bone scan in the large muscle groups of both lower extremities of a patient with dermatomyositis.

for occult hip and knee fractures or in cases in which the site of pain is well localized. When multifocal trauma (such as child abuse) is suspected, bone scanning may be more effective.

Bone scan appearance after fracture may be divided into acute, subacute, and healing phases. The acute phase usually lasts from 3 to 4 weeks and demonstrates a generalized diffuse increase in radionuclide activity around the fracture site. The subacute phase follows and lasts 2 to 3 months, with the activity more localized and intense. The healing phase may occur over a much longer period and is accompanied by a gradual decline in intensity of radiotracer activity. The time after fracture at which the bone scan becomes abnormal is shown in Table 8-1.

The percentage of fractures returning to normal at various times is shown in Table 8-2.

Most fractures show early increase in activity as a result of hyperemia and inflammation. Repair begins within a few hours and reaches a maximum in 2 to 3 weeks. The location of the fracture determines the time of appearance of increased activity on the bone scan. In the first 3 days, only 30% of pelvic and spine fractures show increased activity. Virtually all recent fractures in the axial skeleton and long bones can be seen by 14 days. Skull fractures

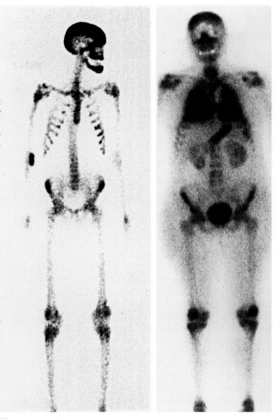

Figure 8-27. Hyperparathyroidism. Anterior bone scans in two different patients with hyperparathyroidism. *Left,* The first case demonstrates a typical superscan with lack of significant renal or bladder activity and with diffusely increased activity throughout the skeleton. Of note is the particularly increased activity in the calvarium, facial bones, mandible, and large joints that has been described in patients with hyperparathyroidism. *Right,* Bone scan of a second patient with hyperparathyroidism demonstrates increased activity around the major joints and significantly increased activity in the lungs, stomach, renal parenchyma, and thyroid, compatible with so-called metastatic calcification, which may be found in certain soft-tissue organs in severe cases of this disease.

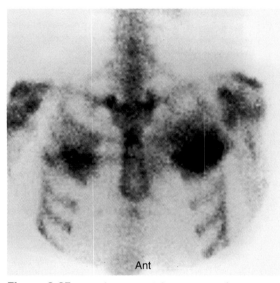

Figure 8-25. Muscle trauma. This young air force recruit experienced anterior chest wall pain after weight-lifting. The bone scan demonstrates increased activity in both pectoral muscles as a result of the trauma (rhabdomyolysis). Increased activity is also commonly seen for several weeks in various muscle groups after marathons or Ironman competitions.

Figure 8-26. Splenic infarction. Selected images from a diphosphonate bone scan demonstrate increased activity in the spleen in a patient with sickle cell disease. This activity has been attributed to ongoing splenic infarction.

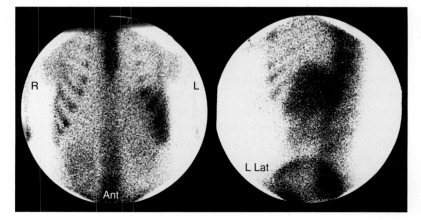

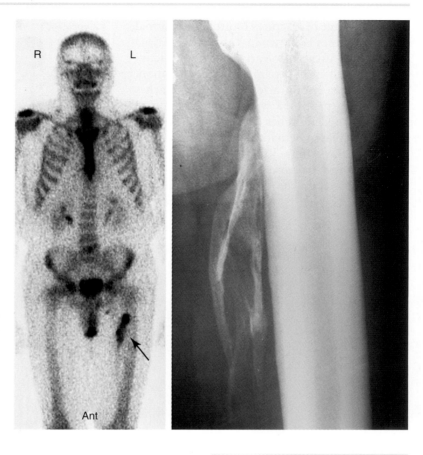

Figure 8-28. Myositis ossificans. This college football player had a history of trauma to the inner left thigh with residual firm swelling and limitation of motion. *Left,* Bone scan shows soft-tissue activity that is greater than the nearby bone, indicating that the process is not mature and should not yet be removed. *Right,* Radiograph shows the well-defined soft-tissue calcification.

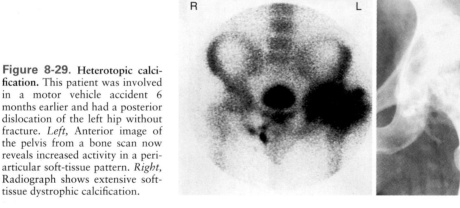

Figure 8-29. Heterotopic calcification. This patient was involved in a motor vehicle accident 6 months earlier and had a posterior dislocation of the left hip without fracture. *Left,* Anterior image of the pelvis from a bone scan now reveals increased activity in a periarticular soft-tissue pattern. *Right,* Radiograph shows extensive soft-tissue dystrophic calcification.

constitute a major exception and may not show any increase in activity on bone scan. Rib fractures almost always show intense activity and can often be recognized by their location in consecutive ribs (Fig. 8-32). Single rib fractures are often difficult to distinguish from a metastasis, but eliciting a trauma history from the patient is often helpful. In addition, rib fractures present as punctate foci of increased activity, whereas neoplastic lesions frequently have a more linear distribution following the long axis of the ribs.

Age of the patient was initially thought to be relevant to time of appearance of fractures on a bone scan, but subsequent work has shown this to be a minor variable. However, about 3 days are needed to reliably detect an occult hip fracture in an elderly patient on bone scan. Thus many clinicians prefer to order an MRI

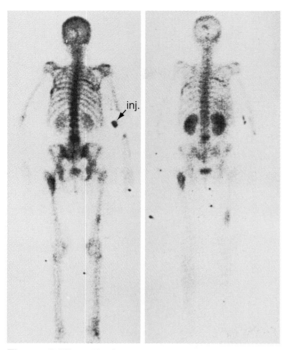

Figure 8-30. Diffusely increased renal activity. Posterior bone scans in the same patient obtained for osseous metastases. *Left*, Initial scan demonstrates the osseous metastases. *Right*, Follow up scan 2 months later after vincristine chemotherapy shows markedly decreased bone activity and relatively increased activity in the parenchyma of both kidneys. *Inj.*, Extravasation at injection site.

Box 8-6 Hepatic Uptake of Technetium-99m Phosphate Compounds

Common
Artifactual—after technetium-99m sulfur colloid study (diffuse activity)
Apparent—attributable to abdominal wall or rib uptake (focal activity)
Metastatic carcinoma (focal)
Colon
Breast
Ovary
Squamous cell carcinoma of esophagus
Oat cell carcinoma of lung
Malignant melanoma

Uncommon
Diffuse hepatic necrosis (diffuse activity)
Elevated serum Al^{3+} (diffuse activity)

Rare
Cholangiocarcinoma (focal activity)
Improper preparation of radiopharmaceutical causing microcolloid formation (diffuse activity)
Amyloidosis (diffuse activity)
Hepatoma

Box 8-7 Increased Uptake of Technetium-99–Labeled Bone Imaging Agents in the Kidneys

Focal

Common
Urinary tract obstruction

Uncommon
Calcifying metastases (breast cancer, poorly differentiated lymphocytic lymphoma)
Radiation therapy to the kidney

Rare
Renal carcinoma
Renal metastasis from carcinoma of the lung

Diffuse

Common
Urinary tract obstruction
Idiopathic

Uncommon
Metastatic calcification
Malignant (transitional cell carcinoma of bladder, malignant melanoma)
Hyperparathyroidism
Chemotherapy with cyclophosphamide, vincristine, and doxorubicin
Thalassemia major

Rare
Multiple myeloma
Crossed renal ectopia
Renal vein thrombosis
Iron overload
Administration of sodium diatrizoate after the injection of technetium-99m phosphate compound
Paroxysmal nocturnal hemoglobinuria
Acute pyelonephritis

---

scan and do prompt surgery, rather than leave an elderly person in bed and wait to do a bone scan.

Return of the bone scan appearance to normal after fracture or surgical trauma is variable. Fractures and even craniotomy defects in older patients may be visible on bone scans for several years. Few fractures of weight-bearing bones return to a normal scan appearance within 5 months, whereas about 90% are normal within 2 years. More intense and prolonged uptake has been demonstrated in fractures in

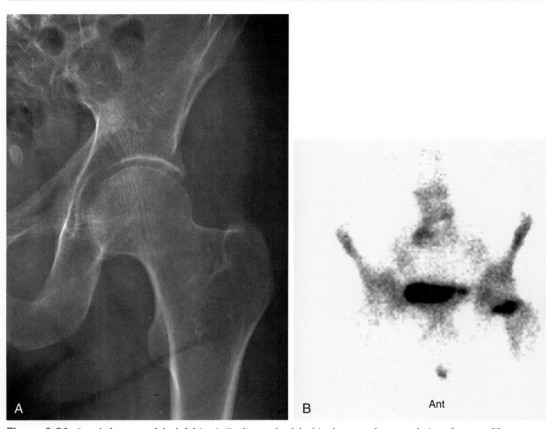

Figure 8-31. Occult fracture of the left hip. A, Radiograph of the hip does not show an obvious fracture. However, anterior bone scan of the pelvis (**B**) shows increased activity in the femoral neck fracture.

TABLE 8-1	Time after Fracture at which Bone Scan Becomes Abnormal	
TIME AFTER FRACTURE	**PERCENTAGE ABNORMAL**	
	Patients <65 yr	**All Patients**
1 day	95	80
3 day	100	95
1 wk	100	98

which open reduction was performed or a fixation device applied.

Subtle trauma, such as that from *stress fractures,* is often difficult to visualize on a plain radiograph. Often, these fractures are not visualized for 7 to 10 days, by which time interval decalcification becomes apparent radiographically around the fracture site. On the other hand, radionuclide bone scans are frequently positive at the time of clinical presentation and offer a means of early diagnosis and treatment.

Bone scans are an excellent way to diagnose either fatigue or insufficiency stress injuries.

In patients with *shin splints* (*medial tibial stress syndrome*), normal blood flow and normal blood pool are seen on a three-phase bone scan (Fig. 8-33). On delayed images, there is typically linear increased activity along at least one third the length of the posteromedial tibial cortex at the insertion of the soleus muscle. Stress fractures tend to be more focal or fusiform on delayed images (Figs. 8-34 and 8-35) and show increased activity on blood flow and blood pool phases of a three-phase bone scan. Insufficiency-type stress fractures usually occur in the pelvis or around the knees as a result of bone weakened by osteoporosis (Fig. 8-36).

Because fractures may be identified by bone scans as early as 24 hours after occurrence, bone imaging has been useful in the assessment of suspected battered children. In infants and small children, characteristic rib and thoracic spine fractures are a strong indication of physical abuse. Failure to find areas of increased

TABLE 8-2	Time after Fracture at which Bone Scan Returns to Normal			
FRACTURE SITE	**PERCENTAGE NORMAL**			**MINIMUM TIME TO RETURN TO NORMAL (mo)**
	1 yr	**2 yr**	**3 yr**	
Vertebrae	59	90	97	7
Long bones	64	91	97	6
Ribs	79	93	100	5

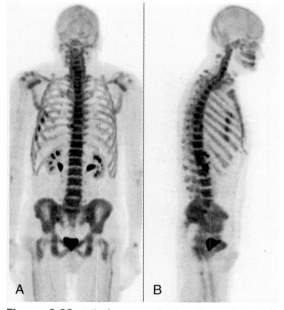

Figure 8-32. Rib fractures. A, Anterior and **B,** right lateral images show rib fractures in this patient who was in an auto accident. These can be confidently diagnosed because there are consecutive right rib abnormalities, and they have relatively rounded (not elliptical) foci of increased activity.

activity is useful in excluding the diagnosis of child battering. Detection of trauma at the ends of long bones may be complicated by the often intense activity in the physes of children. In most cases, a combination of bone scan and radiographs is the best approach to evaluation.

In elderly patients, the bone scan may not show the fracture for several days. A negative bone scan obtained a week after trauma, however, effectively excludes an occult fracture. SPECT scans may occasionally be useful for the demonstration of occult fractures, particularly in the spine (Fig. 8-37). SPECT imaging of the spine may also be helpful for the detection of pseudoarthrosis. Pronounced increase in uptake more than 1 year after fusion is highly indicative of motion in a failed spinal fusion.

Another use of bone scans in trauma is in the *assessment of hip prostheses.* In the initial postsurgical period, activity is noted around cemented prostheses, although this usually rapidly decreases and returns to normal within 12 months. With a porous coated prosthesis, generalized increased activity may be seen even at 2 years because fixation depends on bony ingrowth. Persistent activity at the trochanter and at the tip of the prosthesis may be taken as an indication of loosening (77% specific and 100% sensitive) (Fig. 8-38). For hip and knee prostheses, loosening may also be assessed by injecting the joint with 99mTc sulfur colloid (nuclear medicine arthrogram) to determine whether activity accumulates around the stem of the prosthesis, an indication of loosening. Postsurgical heterotopic bone formation may be visualized around a hip joint on bone scans, but this usually is easily recognized by its position predominantly lateral to the acetabulum.

Generalized increase in activity around a hip prosthesis, especially the shank (stem), may be indicative of osteomyelitis (Fig. 8-39). Historically, a gallium scan was often used because a normal scan effectively excludes osteomyelitis as the cause of symptoms. If gallium and 99mTc diphosphonate distributions are spatially incongruent, or if they are spatially congruent but gallium activity exceeds the technetium activity, osteomyelitis should be considered. If the gallium and technetium images are partially congruent and equal in intensity, the study is considered equivocal. An infected joint replacement is more specifically diagnosed by comparing an [111]In- or ^{99m}Tc-labeled leukocyte image with a technetium colloid marrow scan. When there is periprosthetic leukocyte accumulation without corresponding marrow activity on the colloid images, the study is positive for infection. Use of ^{18}F-FDG scanning has been reported to have sensitivity, specificity, and

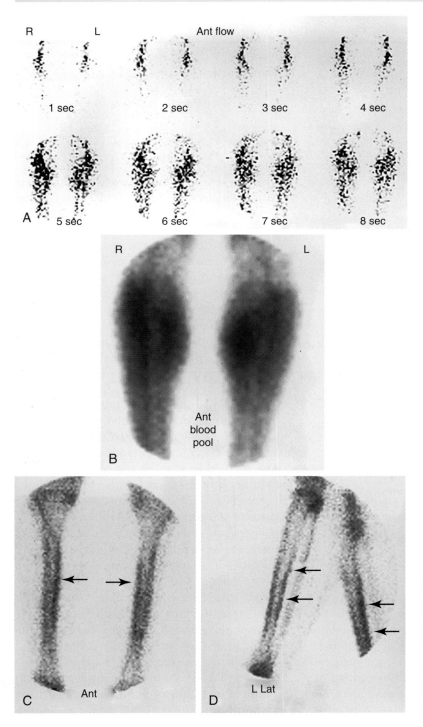

Figure 8-33. **Shin splints.** This athlete had bilateral lower leg pain. **A,** Three-phase bone scan shows normal and symmetric blood flow on the angiographic images. **B,** Blood pool image is also normal. (There is normally a lot of blood flow to the calf muscles.) **C** and **D,** On delayed 3-hour images, there is increased activity (*arrows*) in a long linear distribution of the postero-medial tibial shafts.

accuracy of 85% to 90% for infected hip and knee prostheses.

Osteomyelitis, Cellulitis, and Septic Arthritis

Early involvement of bone by an inflammatory disease process is often difficult to detect on radiographs. A number of imaging modalities can be used to evaluate osteomyelitis. MRI is highly effective and has excellent spatial resolution, but it is expensive and its use is limited in patients who have an infected metallic prosthesis. The earliest radiographic signs of osteomyelitis are nonspecific and include demineralization and loss of the soft-tissue fascial margins. At this stage, scanning with

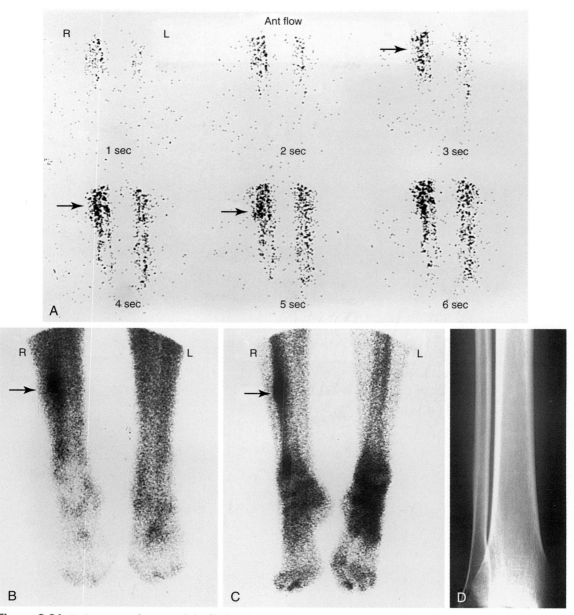

Figure 8-34. Fatigue stress fracture of the fibula. This jogger had pain in the lower right leg. **A,** Three-phase bone scan shows asymmetric increased activity on the angiographic phase. Note that between the blood pool image (**B**) and the 3-hour delayed image (**C**), the activity (*arrows*) becomes more intense and focal. **D,** Radiograph of the area is normal. Most tibial stress fractures occur in the proximal or middle tibia, and most fibular stress fractures occur distally.

radionuclides often demonstrates strikingly increased activity, both in the soft tissues and in the underlying bony structures. However, if soft-tissue inflammation is a prominent feature, it occasionally may be difficult to distinguish primary bone involvement from bone activity secondary to the hyperemia that accompanies simple cellulitis.

A number of radiopharmaceuticals are available to evaluate osteomyelitis. These include ^{99m}Tc-diphosphonate, indium-111- (^{111}In-) or

^{99m}Tc-labeled leukocytes, ^{18}F-FDG, and, much less commonly, gallium-67 citrate.

To differentiate osteomyelitis from cellulitis on a ^{99m}Tc diphosphonate bone scan, a radionuclide angiogram and an immediate blood pool image should be obtained after injection, and routine images should be taken at 2 to 3 hours. Such three-phase scintigraphy has been widely advocated to improve bone scan specificity in this setting. *Cellulitis* presents as increased blood flow (perfusion) and diffusely

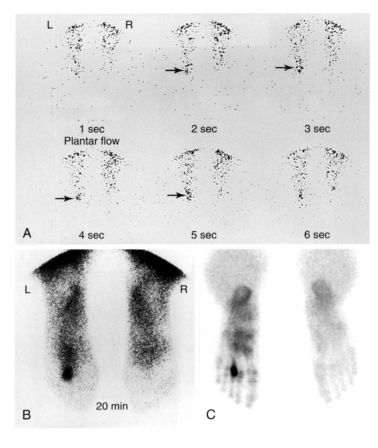

Figure 8-35. Fatigue stress fracture of the foot. This college soccer player had persistent foot pain. **A,** Plantar views on this three-phase bone scan reveal an abnormality of the left third distal metatarsal with increased blood flow (*arrows*), **B,** increased blood pooling, and **C,** a more intense and focal increase in activity on 3-hour delayed views.

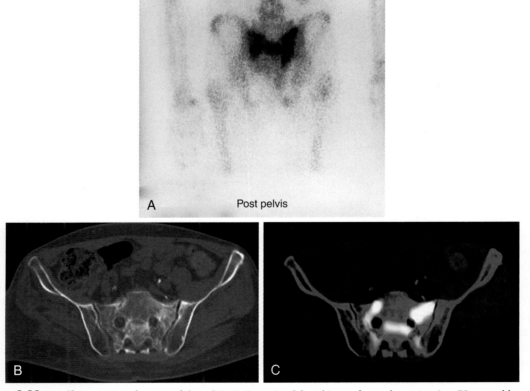

Figure 8-36. Insufficiency stress fracture of the pelvis. A, Posterior delayed image from a bone scan in a 70-year-old woman with pelvic pain shows an H-shaped area of increased activity in the sacrum (Honda sign). **B** and **C,** Axial images from an 18F-sodium fluoride PET/CT scan show the abnormality in better detail.

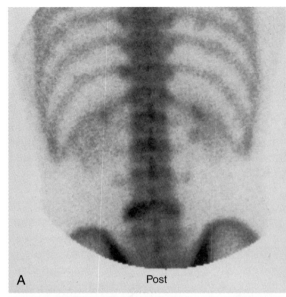

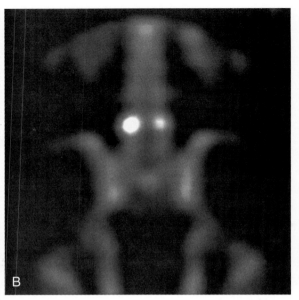

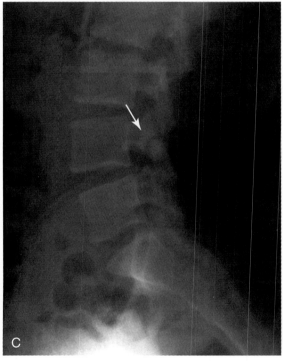

Figure 8-37. Pars defect. A teenager with back pain was referred for a bone scan. **A,** Planar and **B,** single-photon emission computed tomography images show increased activity at the pedicles of L4. **C,** Lateral lumbar spine shows the pars defect (arrow) as well.

increased soft tissue on early images, with decreasing activity on later scans (Fig. 8-40). No significant foci of increased bony activity should be seen on the delayed images in the area of concern. *Osteomyelitis,* on the other hand, demonstrates increased blood flow and blood pool activity with accumulation of bone activity that becomes more focal and intense on delayed scans (Fig. 8-41). The absence of increased perfusion and blood pool activity casts serious doubt on a diagnosis of osteomyelitis as a

cause for a focus of increased activity in bone on delayed images. Although scintigraphy is extremely sensitive, some false-negative scans have been reported early in the disease, perhaps secondary to disruption of the blood supply to the bone. Subperiosteal collections of pus may even produce focal photopenic defects (especially in young children).

Use of planar ^{99m}Tc-MDP for osteomyelitis has a sensitivity of greater than 80% and a limited specificity of about 50%. The specificity

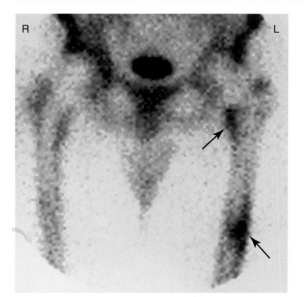

Figure 8-38. **Loose hip prosthesis.** This patient had bilateral cemented hip replacements 3 years ago. The prostheses account for the cold defects seen in the proximal femurs on this ^{99m}Tc-MDP image. The left prosthesis is loose, causing increased activity near the lesser trochanter and the distal tip of the prosthesis (*arrows*). The activity at the lesser trochanter is the fulcrum site, and the tip is the portion of the prosthesis with the greatest movement.

increases to above 80% with use of SPECT/CT. WBC scanning has sensitivity and specificity above 90% and ^{18}F-FDG/CT is reported to have sensitivity of about 95% and specificity of about 85%. The use of labeled leukocytes and ^{18}F-FDG PET/CT in the evaluation of complicated osteomyelitis is discussed in Chapter 12.

Septic arthritis is almost always seen as increased activity in all phases of a three-phase bone scan. Usually, it can be differentiated from osteomyelitis by the presence of diffusely increased bone activity on both sides of the joint (Fig. 8-42), as opposed to osteomyelitis in which the bony activity is typically focal and increased on only one side of the joint.

Diskitis is a condition of uncertain etiology that usually occurs in children. On bone scan, there is usually increased activity of two contiguous lumbar vertebral bodies, often just the adjacent end-plates, and radiographs may show a narrowed disk space (Fig. 8-43).

Benign Non-Neoplastic Disease
Paget Disease

Paget disease characteristically displays a marked increase in activity in large part attributable to the greatly increased regional blood

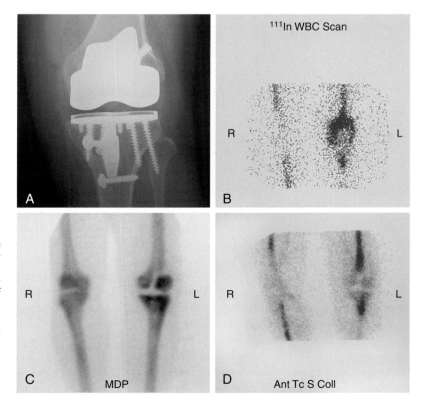

Figure 8-39. **Infected prosthesis. A,** Radiograph of the left knee shows a total knee arthroplasty that was painful. **B,** Indium-111 white blood cell scan shows activity about the proximal portion of the prosthesis and spatial nonconformity with **C,** minimal activity in distal femur on ^{99m}-Tc-MDP bone scan. **D,** Bone marrow scan done with technetium-99m sulfur colloid shows that the indium activity is not related to localized marrow hyperplasia.

flow. The increased activity usually conforms to the shape of all or part of the involved bone. There is often notable expansion or enlargement of the bone, and the increased activity characteristically extends to one end of the bone when a long bone is involved (Figs. 8-44 and 8-45). The disease is polyostotic in about 70% to 80% of cases. Although the osteolytic phase of the disease is often difficult to appreciate on radiographs, it is almost always represented by increased activity on bone scans. The dense sclerotic lesions seen late in the osteoblastic stage of the disease may demonstrate varying degrees of increased activity, and some "burned out" lesions may show only minimally increased or normal activity. At some institutions, serial quantitative bone scans using computer assessment of bone activity are performed to evaluate response of Paget disease to therapy. Sarcomatous degeneration occurs in approximately 1% of Paget disease patients (Fig. 8-46). This initially results in increasing activity in the area of involvement over time. Later, the

malignant area may appear photopenic, likely resulting from necrotic areas within the lesion.

Hypertrophic Pulmonary Osteoarthropathy

Hypertrophic pulmonary osteoarthropathy causes periosteal reaction, particularly in the long bones. It is most commonly seen in patients with lung cancer. The appearance on bone scan is that of distinctive parallel lines of activity along the cortex of the shafts and ends of the tibias, femurs, and radii (Fig. 8-47), especially around the knees, ankles, and wrists. This activity may decrease after treatment of the underlying disease.

Aseptic Arthritis

Bone scanning may be used as a method for documenting the early presence of various forms of arthritis as well as for assessing serial changes in the disease. Unfortunately, juxta-articular increased activity on a ^{99m}Tc diphosphonate bone scan is nonspecific and cannot

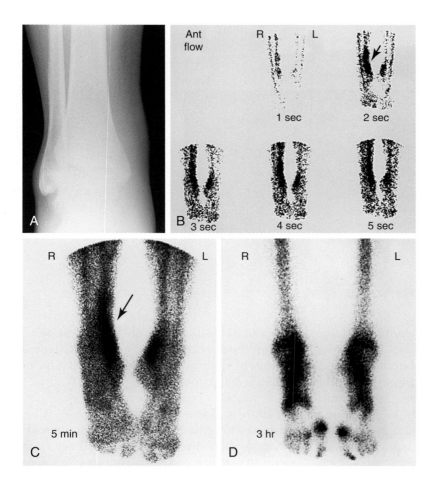

Figure 8-40. Cellulitis. This drug abuser had pain, redness, and swelling over the medial aspect of the right ankle. **A,** Soft-tissue swelling was evident on the anteroposterior radiograph of the ankle. **B,** On the bone scan, there is increased activity on the angiographic images and **C,** blood pool image at 5 minutes (*arrows*). **D,** By the 3-hour image, the asymmetric activity has faded, indicating no evidence of osteomyelitis.

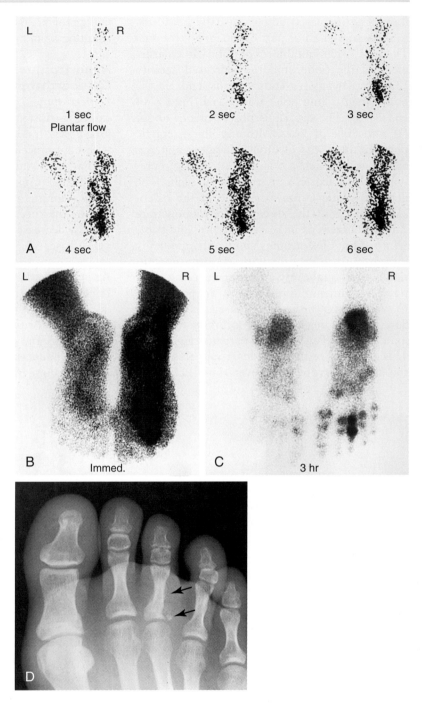

Figure 8-41. Osteomyelitis. **A,** Plantar images from a three-phase bone scan show increased flow, increased blood pooling in the whole foot (**B**), and increased intense focal activity on the delayed view in the region of the right third toe (**C**). The findings are compatible with osteomyelitis. **D,** Normal radiograph of the right foot at the time of the bone scan became frankly abnormal 2 weeks later (*arrows*).

reliably distinguish among synovitis, active arthritis, and old inactive disease. Both intravenously administered ^{99m}Tc pertechnetate and the diphosphonate bone imaging agents have been used for arthritis imaging. Technetium-99m pertechnetate is probably more specific for regions of synovial inflammation because it is able to diffuse across the synovial surface and into joint effusions, whereas phosphate compounds localize primarily in adjacent bone. Because bone scanning for arthritis is limited by lack of specificity, radiologic correlation of results is mandatory.

Metabolic Bone Disease

As discussed earlier, primary hyperparathyroidism and renal osteodystrophy resulting from secondary hyperparathyroidism may produce

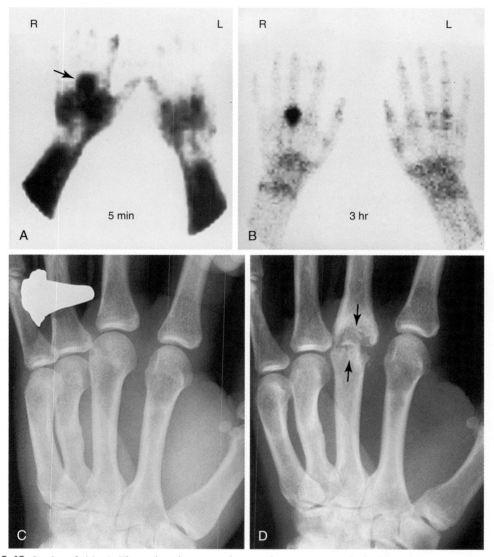

Figure 8-42. Septic arthritis. A, Three-phase bone scan done on this young man who had been bitten over the third metacarpal joint shows increased activity (*arrow*) on blood pool and **B,** delayed images. **C,** Normal radiograph at the time of the bone scan became positive 3 weeks later (**D**). Note bony destruction (*arrows*) involving both sides of the joint.

a *superscan* with diffusely increased activity throughout the skeleton, including the skull, mandible, and long bones, and relatively diminished or absent renal activity. This may be accompanied by increased activity in the thyroid, lungs, stomach, and kidneys caused by so-called *metastatic calcification* in these organs. When brown tumors are present, focal areas of increased activity in the skeleton may be seen.

Avascular Necrosis

Avascular necrosis is often a result of trauma, but it may have a variety of other causes, including steroid administration and vascular disease. Initially, there is generally decreased tracer activity in the affected area. This is followed by a hyperemic or repair phase, which is characterized by increased activity. Correlation with the radiographs is mandatory to diagnose avascular necrosis accurately. MRI is probably more accurate and thus more widely used for this diagnosis (Fig. 8-48). Some laboratories have used bone scans to demonstrate femoral head viability in patients with femoral neck fractures. Either diphosphonate or sulfur colloid imaging may be used. The usual procedure is to compare the normal side with the suspected abnormal side. Relatively decreased activity in the femoral head suggests avascularity. For these studies, a pinhole collimator should be used to

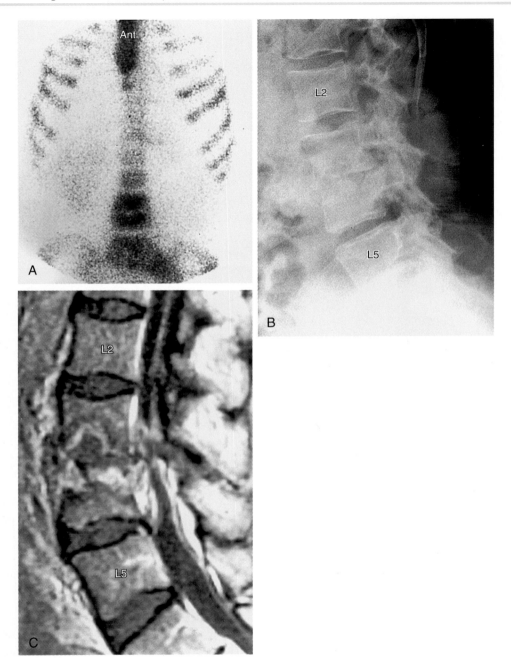

Figure 8-43. Diskitis. **A,** In this child with persistent back pain, the delayed bone scan image shows increased activity in two contiguous vertebral bodies. **B,** Lateral radiograph shows accompanying loss of L3-4 disk space. **C,** Magnetic resonance image shows involvement of the vertebral bodies. The cause of this entity remains obscure.

provide the high-quality detail needed for accurate diagnosis.

Spontaneous Osteonecrosis of the Knee

Spontaneous osteonecrosis of the knee usually presents as acute knee pain, especially medially, in elderly, often osteoporotic females. Intensely increased activity in the medial femoral condyle

essentially establishes or confirms the diagnosis in this setting. The disease may also occur in the medial tibial plateau or lateral femoral condyle.

Radiation Therapy

Radiation therapy constitutes a form of calculated iatrogenic trauma. Multiple factors determine the bone scan findings after radiation

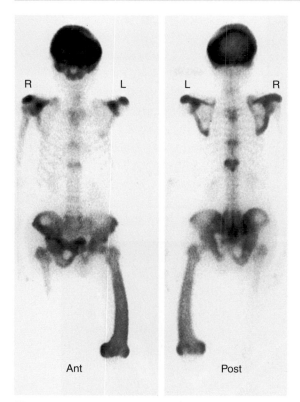

R   L   L   R

Ant   Post

Figure 8-44. Extensive Paget disease. In this deaf patient with the sclerotic form of Paget disease, there is markedly increased activity in the skull and left femur. The femur is bowed, owing to associated bone softening. The marked increase in activity seen on the bone scan is predominantly the result of increased blood flow.

treatment, including the cumulative amount of radiation, fractionation of doses, and length of time after therapy that the bone scan is performed. After fractionated radiation doses of 4000 to 5000 rad (40 to 50 Gy) to bone, there is a decrease in localized vascular patency in the area of treatment within the first month. The vascularity may return to near normal in about 6 months and then is reduced again, owing to endothelial proliferation and arteriolar narrowing. An abrupt geometric area of decreased osseous activity should raise the suspicion of skeletal trauma as a result of radiation therapy (see Fig. 8-10).

Complex Regional Pain Syndrome (Reflex Sympathetic Dystrophy)

Complex regional pain syndrome (CRPS), formerly known as *reflex sympathetic dystrophy (RSD) syndrome*, consists of pain, tenderness, swelling, and vasomotor instability in the affected limb. Its cause is obscure, but RSD is usually precipitated by trauma, myocardial infarction, or neurologic abnormality. The most common variants are *Sudeck atrophy* and *shoulder-hand syndrome*. Radiographically, there is usually patchy periarticular osteoporosis. Classically, three-phase bone scanning demonstrates increased blood flow to the affected limb with increased asymmetric periarticular radionuclide activity. Diffusely increased juxtaarticular activity around all joints of the hand or foot on delayed images may be the most sensitive indicator of RSD (Fig. 8-49). About one third of adult patients with documented RSD do not show increased perfusion and uptake. In children, decreased perfusion and uptake is a common manifestation.

BONE MARROW IMAGING

Bone marrow scans can be used to define marrow distribution. The most common agent is ^{99m}Tc sulfur colloid, which localizes in marrow because the particles are phagocytized by the resident reticuloendothelial cells in the marrow. The widespread availability and excellent anatomic resolution of MRI has reduced the need for most radionuclide marrow scans. On colloid marrow scans, intense liver and spleen activity may need to be shielded during imaging. In the adult, the marrow is usually restricted to the skull, ribs, sternum, vertebral bodies, pelvis, and proximal humeri and femurs. In children, the normal marrow extends more peripherally into the extremities.

BONE MINERAL MEASUREMENTS

The accurate measurement of bone mineral density using noninvasive methods can be of value in the detection and evaluation of primary and secondary causes of decreased bone mass. This includes primary osteoporosis and secondary disorders, such as hyperparathyroidism, osteomalacia, multiple myeloma, diffuse metastases, and glucocorticoid therapy or intrinsic excess.

By far, the largest patient population is that encompassed by primary osteoporosis. Osteoporosis is an age-related disorder characterized by decreased bone mass and increased susceptibility to fractures in the absence of other recognizable causes of bone loss. Primary osteoporosis is generally subdivided into type 1 (postmenopausal osteoporosis), which is related to estrogen deprivation, and type 2 (senile osteoporosis), which occurs secondary to aging.

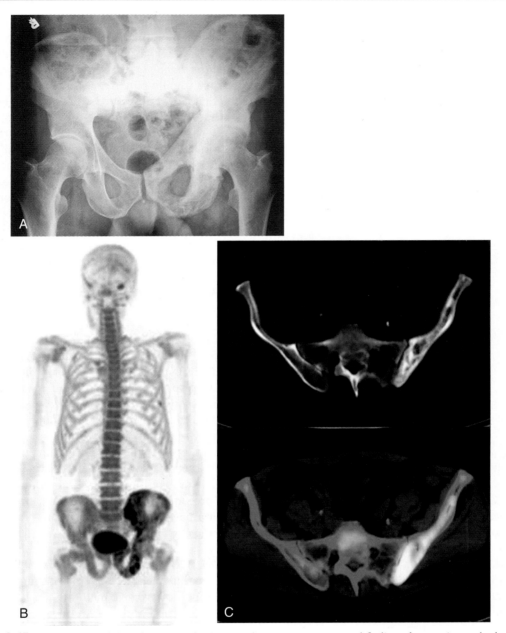

Figure 8-45. Paget disease of the pelvis. A, In this patient, there was an unexpected finding of expansion and sclerosis in the left hemipelvis on barium enema scout film. **B,** Anterior and **C,** axial images from an ^{18}F-sodium fluoride PET bone scan show intensely increased activity confined to the left side of the pelvis. This increase of activity in one hemipelvis is characteristic and is probably the most common presentation of Paget disease.

Primary osteoporosis is a common clinical disorder and a major public health problem because of the significant number of related bone fractures occurring annually. Because the risk of vertebral and femoral neck fractures rises dramatically as bone mineral density falls below 1 g/cm^2, fracture risk in individual patients may be estimated. Furthermore, in estrogen-deficient women, bone mineral density values may be used to make rational decisions about hormone replacement therapy, or other bone mineral therapies, and as follow-up in assessing the success of such treatment.

A number of methods have been devised to permit the accurate and reproducible determination of bone mineral content. The advent of radionuclide absorptiometry using dual-photon technique evoked a sustained interest in the

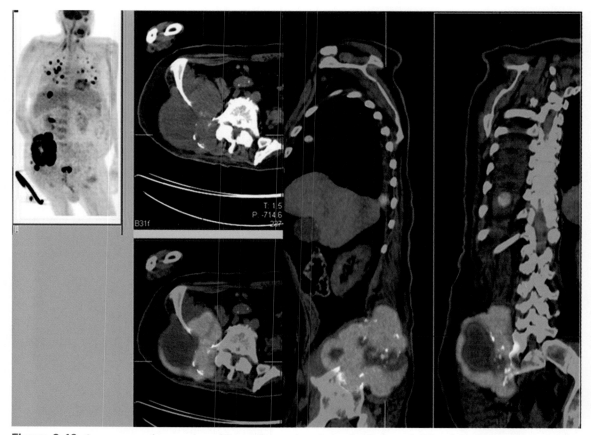

Figure 8-46. **Sarcomatous degeneration of Paget disease.** Anterior and reformatted CT and fluorodeoxyglucose (FDG) images from ¹⁸F-FDG PET/CT scan show intense activity in the right pelvis as a result of a large soft-tissue mass destroying bone as well as metastases to the lungs.

screening of patients for osteoporosis. However, dual x-ray absorptiometry (DEXA) has replaced the radionuclide method for determination of bone mineral. DEXA uses a highly collimated fan beam of x-rays that passes through the soft tissue and bony components of the body to be detected on the opposite side by a solid state detector. Because absorption by the body part examined (primarily by bone mineral) attenuates the photon x-ray beam, the intensity of the beam exiting the body part is indirectly proportional to the density of the bony structure being evaluated. The intensity of the exit beam is then compared with exit beam intensity from standard phantoms of known density, so that a bone mineral density can be determined. The results are expressed in grams per square centimeter.

The DPA and DEXA beams consist of photons or x-rays of two discrete energies, which obviate the need for assumptions about soft-tissue shape and attenuation. It also allows for evaluation of thicker body parts and bones involving complex geometry, such as the femoral neck and the spine. When the spine is examined, the hips are flexed to flatten the normal lumbar lordosis. When scans of the femoral neck are performed, the femur should be in slight internal rotation.

By using an x-ray tube rather than a radionuclide source, purchase of replacement radionuclide sources and recalibration are unnecessary. In addition, scan time is only 2 to 5 minutes for DEXA, compared with 20 to 40 minutes for DPA. Precision and image quality are also much better for DEXA than for DPA.

Falsely elevated bone mineral content when evaluating the spine may result from marked aortic calcification, scoliosis, hypertrophic degenerative disease, compression fractures, calcium or barium within the gastrointestinal tract, renal lithiasis, bone grafts, focal sclerotic bone lesions, or recent intake of aluminum-containing antacids. Falsely low bone mineral results may be obtained in patients who have had a laminectomy or lytic bone lesions. Most of the time,

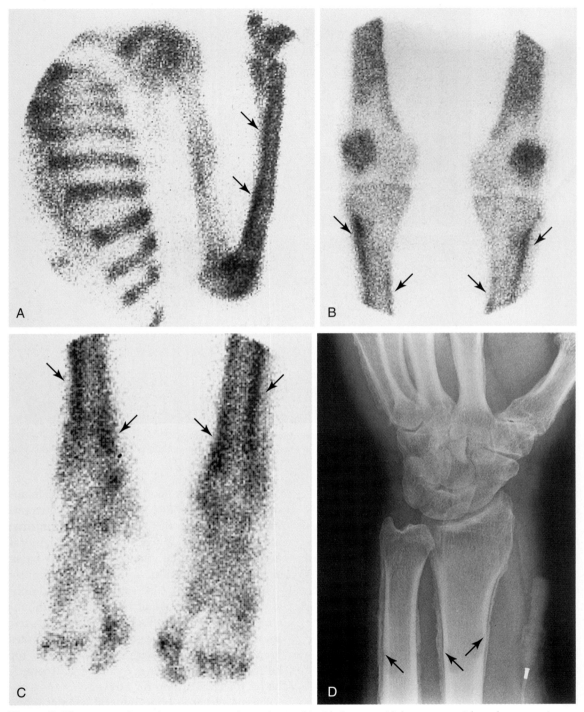

Figure 8-47. Hypertrophic pulmonary osteoarthropathy. In this elderly man with lung cancer, 3-hour bone scan images show increased activity (*arrows*) in the cortical regions of the shafts of the radius (**A**) and both tibias (**B** and **C**). **D,** Radiograph of the wrist shows marked periosteal reaction (*arrows*).

these problems can be identified from the plain radiograph if available before the test.

The use of bone mineral measurement has been controversial. Some of this controversy is because of the wide variation of measurements in the normal population. Also, the criteria for selecting the optimal skeletal site for evaluation have not been well defined because bone mineral loss does not progress at the same rate at different body sites. Measurement of the hip

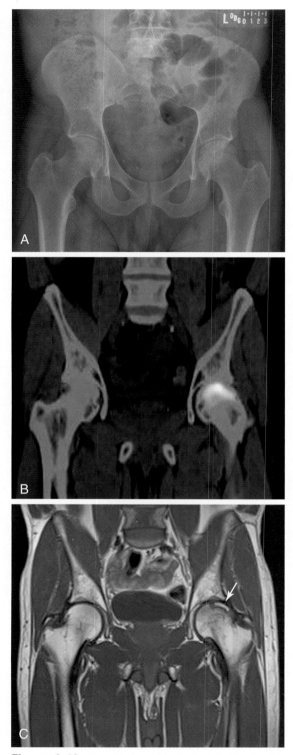

Figure 8-48. Aseptic necrosis of the left hip. In this 50-year-old male with left hip pain, the radiograph (**A**) is only minimally abnormal. **B,** Coronal image from an ^{18}F-sodium fluoride PET/CT scan shows increased activity in the same area as the defect (*arrow*) identified on the MRI scan. *MRI,* Magnetic resonance imaging (**C**).

bone mineral density is done to evaluate the risk for hip fracture, whereas vertebral bodies are regarded as the optimal site for monitoring response to treatment. Care must be taken to look at the images to ensure that extensive degenerative changes or surgical defects are not causing erroneous values (Fig. 8-50).

Most manufacturers express results that compare the patient's bone mineral density either to age-matched controls (Z score) or to a young normal population (T score) felt to be representative of peak bone mass. These comparisons may be expressed as percentiles or as standard deviations from the normal range. As determined by the World Health Organization (WHO), a T score of greater (less negative) than −1.0 (less than 1 standard deviation below young normal controls) is considered normal. Between −1.0 and −2.5 is considered to be evidence of osteopenia. Less (more negative) than −2.5 is consistent with osteoporosis. Thus the method can be used to determine the presence of osteopenia or osteoporosis and to evaluate effectiveness of a therapeutic maneuver by using serial scans in which the patient acts as his or her own control. A normal result, or a bone mineral content in the upper end of the normal range, identifies a patient in whom therapy may not be needed.

PALLIATIVE THERAPY OF PAINFUL OSSEOUS METASTASES

A large number of patients have extensive and diffuse painful blastic osseous metastases from various primary lesions that are not amenable to external beam radiotherapy or that are unresponsive to chemotherapy. Many of these patients are men with prostate cancer. Therapies with intravenously administered radionuclides are directed at palliation of pain (not at cure), decreased need for opiates, and improved quality of life. With most of the methods, the patient may have a transient increase in pain beginning 2 to 3 days after treatment and lasting for several days as a result of transient swelling of the treated lesions. Palliative symptomatic improvement usually begins 7 to 20 days after treatment and often lasts 3 to 6 months. Pain will not be relieved if it is caused by a pathologic fracture or is of nonosseous origin (such as epidural metastases with pressure on the spinal cord or soft-tissue masses pressing on nerves). A routine bone scan should be performed before this type of therapy to ensure that there will be

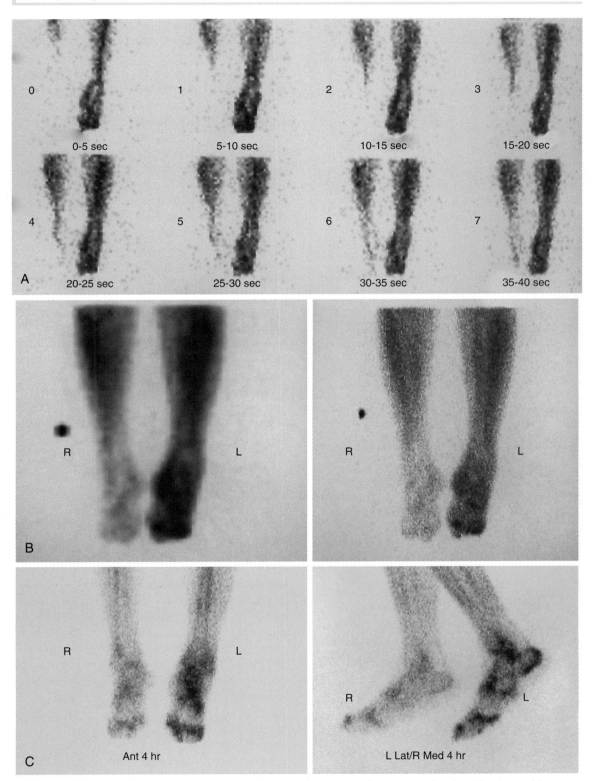

Figure 8-49. Complex regional pain syndrome (reflex sympathetic dystrophy). A young female with minor ankle trauma had continuing pain. **A,** Angiographic and **B,** blood pool images show diffusely increased activity to the entire lower extremity. **C,** Delayed images show increased activity in a periarticular distribution.

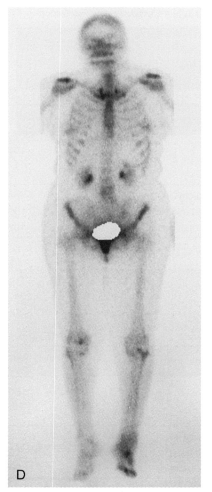

D

Figure 8-49. cont'd

uptake of the therapeutic radiopharmaceutical. A normal bone scan would suggest another source of pain. External beam teletherapy is recommended if there are only one or two lesions causing the patient's pain or if there is impending spinal cord compression.

The most commonly used radionuclide is strontium-89 (^{89}Sr) chloride (Metastron). The radionuclide decays by beta emission with a physical half-life of 50.5 days. The average and maximum range of the beta emission in tissue is 2.4 and 8 mm, respectively. After intravenous administration, localization in bone occurs in areas of active osteogenesis. Metastases with a blastic response have significantly more concentration and longer retention than does normal bone. Excretion is primarily urinary and to a lesser extent fecal. For the first week, medical staff handling these items should wear gloves and follow local disposal regulations.

Strontium-89 chloride therapy depresses the bone marrow and should not be used if the leukocyte count is below 2400/μL or if the platelets are below 60,000/μL. The typical dose is 40 to 60 μCi/kg (1.5 to 2.2 MBq/kg) up to 4 mCi (148 MBq) given by slow (1 to 2 minutes) intravenous injection using syringe shielding (especially plastic) appropriate for a beta-emitting radionuclide. After administration, peripheral leukocyte counts are usually obtained every 2 weeks until marrow recovery occurs. Repeated doses are usually not given at intervals of less than 3 to 4 months, and it is unusual to give more than three doses without being cautious about bone marrow reserve. Because excretion is primarily urinary, ^{89}Sr therapy should be used advisedly in patients with decreased renal function. Pain relief typically takes 1 to 3 weeks to become apparent, and, generally, this therapy should not be used in patients with a life expectancy of less than 3 months. In addition, issues relative to handling of a deceased patient recently treated with ^{89}Sr need to be addressed. Many states have regulations prohibiting cremation in this setting, and some have allowed only certain funeral homes to service these patients.

Other radiopharmaceuticals have been developed and used with success. These are rhenium-186 (^{186}Re) hydroxyethylene diphosphonate (HEDP or etidronate) and samarium-153 (^{153}Sm) ethylenediaminetetra methylene phosphonic (EDTMP) acid, also known as ^{153}Sm lexidronam (Quadramet). These agents have been used in patients with more metabolically active metastases from prostate and breast cancer, as well as in those from osteogenic sarcoma. Rhenium is in the same chemical family as technetium, and much of the same chemistry can be used. The physical half-life is 90 hours, which allows a large radiation dose to be delivered in a relatively short time. In addition to beta emissions, there is gamma emission (187 keV), which allows imaging. Unfortunately, the dose to normal bone is high. This has not been approved for use in the United States but is widely used in Europe. Another radiopharmaceutical for metastatic prostate cancer which is not yet approved in the United States is radium-223 chloride (Alpharadin).

Samarium-153 (lexidronam or Quadramet) EDTMP has a beta particle with an average soft tissue range of 0.6 mm and many of the

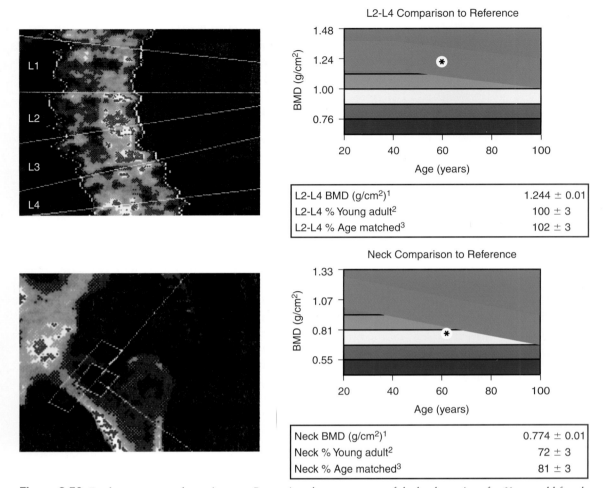

L2-L4 Comparison to Reference

L2-L4 BMD (g/cm²)[1]	1.244 ± 0.01
L2-L4 % Young adult[2]	100 ± 3
L2-L4 % Age matched[3]	102 ± 3

Neck Comparison to Reference

Neck BMD (g/cm²)[1]	0.774 ± 0.01
Neck % Young adult[2]	72 ± 3
Neck % Age matched[3]	81 ± 3

Figure 8-50. **Dual energy x-ray absorptiometry.** Bone mineral measurements of the lumbar spine of a 61-year-old female with lumbar scoliosis (*upper row*) suggest that the bone mineral measurements are normal. This is actually an artifact attributable to extensive osteophytes. When the region of interest is taken over the femoral neck (*lower row*), it can be seen that the patient has low bone mineral density. *BMD,* Bone mineral density.

advantages of rhenium, including a short half-life (46 hours) and, in addition to beta rays, a gamma photon (103 keV, 29% abundance) that can be imaged. Imaging is usually done at 6 hours after administration. There may be an initial increase in bone pain within 72 hours, which usually responds to analgesics. Pain relief may begin at about 1 week and reaches a maximum in about 3 weeks. About 70% of patients report pain relief, and about 35% report to be "much better" or "completely improved." No additional advantage is obtained by dose escalation. There can be bone marrow suppression, and about 95% of patients will have a nadir of white blood cell counts and platelets to about 40% to 50% of baseline at 3 to 5 weeks. As a result, it should not be given concurrently with radiation therapy or chemotherapy unless marrow status has been adequately evaluated. The recommended dose of ^{153}Sm lexidronam is 1.0 mCi/kg (37 MBq/kg) administered intravenously over a period of 1 minute followed with a saline flush. Hydration following injection is recommended to reduce bladder dose because about one third of the administered activity is eliminated in the urine in the first 6 hours. Precautions should be in place for 12 hours by using a toilet instead of urinal and flushing several times. Blood counts should be monitored weekly for at least 8 weeks. No other radiation protection precautions are necessary relative to family members and the public.

PEARLS & PITFALLS

Musculoskeletal

- Common indications for bone scans include evaluation of primary osseous or metastatic neoplasms, avascular necrosis of the hips or shoulders, trauma, infection, and, less commonly, arthritis or RSD in the peripheral skeleton.

- When bone scans are performed with ^{99m}Tc diphosphonate agents, normal skeletal activity should be reasonably symmetric on the left and right sides. About 50% of injected activity is localized in the skeleton at 2 to 4 hours.

- PET/CT bone scans can be performed with ^{18}F-sodium-fluoride. They have excellent resolution and sensitivity but they are more expensive and have about a sevenfold higher radiation dose.

- Look at kidney activity for potential abnormalities. A large amount of diffuse soft-tissue activity remaining at 4 hours is frequently a result of renal insufficiency.

- The vast majority of focal activity in the lower cervical region is a result of benign causes such as degenerative arthritis.

- A lesion that is hot on all three phases of a bone scan can be osteomyelitis but also may be an acute fracture, hypervascular tumor, neuropathic joint, or RSD.

- Most osseous metastases begin in the red marrow, and therefore about 80% are in the axial skeleton (skull, ribs, spine, pelvis, and proximal extremities). Metastases at distant appendicular sites are most commonly from lung cancer.

- In a patient with known metastases, an increasing apparent number and intensity of lesions compared with prior bone scans can indicate more disease or may indicate the flare phenomenon from recent treatment. A flare phenomenon is most likely seen within 1 to 3 months of therapy completion.

- Not all multifocal hot lesions are metastases; also consider fractures, multifocal osteomyelitis, multiple enchondromas, polyostotic fibrous dysplasia, or Paget disease.

- Paget disease is commonly seen as intense activity in the skull, femur, vertebral body, or half of the pelvis. It is usually polyostotic (80%), but it may be monostotic and may cause bowing of a femur.

- Excellent visualization of the bones and not of the kidneys may indicate a superscan attributable to diffuse metastases or hyperparathyroidism. If the skull is hot and the distal extremities are well seen or if there is stomach and/or lung activity, it is probably hyperparathyroidism.

- Focal hot lesions in multiple adjacent ribs are essentially always a result of fractures. Elliptical lesions with the long axis running along the length of a rib are not usually fractures.

- Cold lesions can be a result of poor perfusion of an area of bone, lack of bony matrix (aggressive tumor), overlying attenuating material, or gamma camera dysfunction, such as a bad photomultiplier tube.

- Multiple sequential cold vertebral bodies are almost always a result of radiation therapy.

- Tumors that commonly cause cold (photopenic) metastatic lesions include kidney, lung, thyroid, and breast tumors.

- Stress fractures usually occur in the pelvis and below the knees. They can be seen as focal or fusiform, primarily cortical activity. Shin splints have normal angiographic and blood pool images but are hot on delayed views in the posteromedial aspects of the tibias (insertion of the soleus muscle).

- Bilaterally increased activity along the cortex of the tibias may be a result of shin splints, hypertrophic osteoarthropathy, or periosteal reaction of other causes.

- A loose hip prosthesis is suggested by activity at the tip and near the lesser trochanter. An infected prosthesis usually has activity all along the length of the shaft. Postoperative activity around a cemented prosthesis can normally persist for 6 months to 1 year, and activity around a noncemented prosthesis can normally persist for 2 to 3 years.

- Focal soft-tissue activity can be a result of a process that makes bone (osteosarcoma metastases), calcifies (cancer of the colon, ovary, breast,

Continued

PEARLS & PITFALLS—cont'd

neuroblastoma), or causes dystrophic calcification (infarction, myositis ossificans, tumoral
calcinosis, dermatomyositis, and polymyositis).

- Diffuse liver activity on a bone scan is probably
a result of hepatic necrosis or a radiopharmaceutical problem. Focal liver activity is often a
result of metastases from colon, breast, ovary,
or lung. Diffuse splenic activity is probably
attributable to splenic infarction (e.g., sickle cell
disease). Diffuse renal parenchymal activity is
probably attributable to chemotherapy, especially if bone metastases are present.

- Increased activity in two adjacent vertebral bodies in the absence of compression fractures suggests diskitis, especially in a child.

- Osteomyelitis, acute fractures, vascular tumors,
such as Ewing sarcoma, and RSD are hot on
angiographic, blood pool, and delayed bone
scan images. Cellulitis is hot on the first two
phases but fades on delayed images. Osteomyelitis usually does not cross joints. Increased
activity seen on both sides of a joint is more
likely the result of septic arthritis.

SUGGESTED READINGS

Bridges RL, Wiley CR, Christian JC, et al. An introduction to Na^{18}F bone scintigraphy: Basic principles, advanced imaging concepts, and case examples. J Nucl Med Technol 2007;35(2):64-76.

Charron M, Brown ML. Primary and metastatic bone disease. In: Sandler MP, Coleman RE, Patton JA, editors. Diagnostic Nuclear Medicine. 4th ed. New York: Lippincott Williams & Wilkins; 2003. p. 413-28.

Chengazi VU, O'Mara RE. Benign bone disease. In: Sandler MP, Coleman RE, Patton JA, editors. Diagnostic Nuclear Medicine. 4th ed. New York: Lippincott Williams & Wilkins; 2003. p. 429-62.

Dotan ZA, Bianco Jr FJ, Rabbani F, et al. Pattern of prostate-specific antigen (PSA) failure dictates the probability of a positive bone scan in patients with an increasing PSA after radical prostatectomy. J Clin Oncol 2005;23(9):1962-8.

Even-Sapir E, Metser U, Mishani E, et al. The detection of bone metastases in patients with high risk prostate cancer: ^{99m}Tc-MDP planar bone scintigraphy, single and multi-field-of-view SPECT, ^{18}F-fluoride PET and ^{18}F-fluoride PET/CT. J Nucl Med 2006;47(2):287-97.

Fogelman I, Blake GM. Different approaches to bone densitometry, continuing education. J Nucl Med 2000; 41:2015-25.

Gomez P, Manoharan M, Kim SS, et al. Radionuclide bone scintigraphy in patients with biochemical recurrence after radical prostatectomy: When is it indicated? BJU Int 2004;94(3):299-302.

Grant FD, Fahey FH, Packard AB, et al. Skeletal PET with ^{18}F-fluoride: Applying new technology to an old tracer. J Nucl Med 2007;49(1):68-78.

Love C, Tomas M, Marwin S, et al. Role of nuclear medicine in diagnosis of the infected joint replacement. Radio-Graphics 2001;21:1229-38.

Segall G, Delbeke D, Stabin M, et al. Society of Nuclear Medicine practice guideline for sodium ^{18}F-fluoride PET/CT bone scans. Version 1.0 approved 2010. http://www.snm.org. Accessed September 21, 2011.

Silberstein EB, Buscombe JR, McEwan A, et al. Society of Nuclear Medicine Procedure guidelines for palliative treatment of painful bone metastases. Version 3.0 approved 2003. http://www.snm.org. Accessed September 21, 2011.

9 Genitourinary System and Adrenal Glands

Radionuclide evaluation of the genitourinary system includes quantitative estimates of renal perfusion and function. With the widespread use of ultrasound and computed tomography (CT), the evaluation of renal anatomy by nuclear techniques has diminished, and the role of nuclear renal imaging has become more confined to functional analysis. Indications for renal scanning include sensitivity to radiographic contrast material, assessment of renal blood flow, and differential or quantitative functional assessment of both native and transplanted kidneys. Nuclear techniques have also proved of value in evaluating ureteral or renal pelvic obstruction, vesicoureteral reflux, and suspected renovascular hypertension, with pharmacologic interventions used when indicated. Imaging of genitourinary cancers with positron emission tomography (PET) scanning is discussed in Chapter 11. Osseous metastases from prostate cancer are discussed in Chapter 8.

PHYSIOLOGY

The excretory function of the kidneys consists of two primary mechanisms: passive filtration through the glomerulus and active secretion by the tubules. These processes are tempered by the varying reabsorption of certain substances by the tubules. Twenty percent of renal plasma flow is cleared by glomerular filtration and 80% by tubular secretion. The glomerulus acts as a semipermeable membrane, allowing only those compounds of a relatively small molecular size to pass through. Larger materials, such as proteins, do not pass through the glomerulus but may reach the urine by tubular secretion.

RADIOPHARMACEUTICALS

Radiopharmaceuticals commonly used for evaluating renal function and anatomy fall into three main categories:

- Those excreted by tubular secretion
- Those excreted by glomerular filtration
- Those bound in the renal tubules for a sufficiently long time to permit cortical anatomic imaging

A thorough knowledge of the biodynamics of these classes of radiopharmaceuticals is essential for choosing the best radiopharmaceutical for a particular clinical setting. Sample imaging protocols and radiation dosimetry are presented in Appendix E-1.

Glomerular Filtration Agents

Technetium-99m diethylenetriamine pentaacetic acid (DTPA) is the radiopharmaceutical used for the evaluation of glomerular filtration function.

As the DTPA complex is cleared by the renal glomeruli, serial images may be obtained that demonstrate sequential visualization of the kidneys and collecting systems, ureters, and bladder. Measurement of its excretion can also provide an accurate estimate of the glomerular filtration rate (GFR). The normal GFR is 125 mL/min. Because a small amount (≈5% to 10%) of injected DTPA is bound to plasma proteins, it tends to underestimate the GFR slightly. For routine clinical applications, however, this is generally not significant. About 20% of ^{99m}Tc-DTPA is extracted from the blood with each pass through the kidney (extraction fraction), so that about 90% of DTPA is filtered by simple exchange or diffusion into the urine within 4 hours. This makes it an inexpensive agent for renal imaging and as a substitute for contrasted CT in patients who are allergic to radiographic contrast and if ultrasound or MRI are not available. Because the nephrogram phase of the examination is brief, however, it is not an ideal agent for demonstrating intraparenchymal renal lesions. In addition, it may not be the agent of choice in patients with obstruction or impaired renal function in whom tubular agents with higher extraction efficiencies allow for increased excretion and better renal visualization. Technetium-99m DTPA is normally administered in activities of 10 to 20 mCi (370 to 740 MBq).

Tubular Secretion Agents

Technetium-99m-labeled agent mercaptoacetyltriglycine (mertiatide or MAG3) is protein bound and is cleared predominantly by the proximal tubules (95%) with minimal filtration (less than 5%), and it behaves much as radioiodinated orthoiodohippurate does. Its ^{99m}Tc label produces much better images. In addition, with an extraction fraction of 40% to 50% (more than twice that of ^{99m}Tc-DTPA), it provides more satisfactory images than does ^{99m}Tc-DTPA, especially in patients with obstruction or impaired renal function. The clearance of MAG3 by the kidneys, when used with a correction factor, can be used to measure effective renal plasma flow (ERPF). Activities administered are 10 to 20 mCi (370 to 740 MBq) in adults.

Renal Cortical Agents

The two radiopharmaceuticals commonly used for visualization of the renal parenchyma are ^{99m}Tc-dimercaptosuccinic acid (DMSA) and ^{99m}Tc-glucoheptonate. Both of these agents bind sufficiently to the renal tubules to permit renal cortical imaging.

Technetium-99m DMSA is an excellent cortical imaging agent, with about 40% of the injected dose concentrated in the renal cortex at 6 hours and the remainder being slowly excreted. DMSA is of particular value when high-resolution images of the renal cortex are needed and when there is no need to identify abnormalities in the ureters or bladder because these structures are not effectively imaged. DMSA localizes by binding to the sulfhydryl groups in the proximal renal tubules. Only 10% of the radiopharmaceutical is excreted in the urine during the first several hours. The radiopharmaceutical activity normally used is 1 to 5 mCi (37 to 185 MBq). The radiation dose to the kidneys with DMSA is high because there is a long, effective half-life of the radiopharmaceutical in the kidneys. Another disadvantage of ^{99m}Tc-DMSA is its short shelf-life after preparation. In addition, because of its slow clearance rate, delayed images 1 to 3 hours after injection are frequently necessary in patients with poor renal function to allow for improved kidney-to-background ratios.

Technetium-99m glucoheptonate is a radiolabeled carbohydrate cleared by the kidneys both by glomerular filtration and by the renal tubules. Thus early images permit the assessment of renal perfusion as well as evaluation of the renal collecting systems and ureters. Early camera images demonstrate the renal cortex and the collecting system, although the renal cortex remains well visualized 2 to 4 hours after administration. Ten percent to 15% of the injected dose remains bound to the renal tubules, and 40% is cleared through the urine at 1 hour. Thus 1- to 2-hour images permit excellent visualization of the renal cortex. Technetium-99m glucoheptonate is stable and may be used for up to 5 hours after preparation. The usual administered activity is 10 to 20 mCi (370 to 740 MBq).

RADIONUCLIDE RENAL EVALUATION

Evaluation of the kidneys with radiopharmaceuticals may be performed by using a variety of methods, each providing a slightly different approach to the assessment of renal function or anatomy. These methods include the following:

■ Functional imaging (visual assessment of perfusion and function)
■ Renography (time-activity curves representative of function)
■ Quantification of renal function (GFR and ERPF determinations)
■ Anatomic imaging (visual assessment of the renal cortex)

Functional Renal Imaging

Radionuclide imaging with ^{99m}Tc-labeled agents provides anatomic, functional, and collecting system patency information. Imaging may be adequately performed in most patients by using either ^{99m}Tc-MAG3 or ^{99m}Tc-DPTA.

Functional imaging of the kidneys may be divided into assessment of blood flow, parenchyma, and excretion. Normally, both kidneys can easily be imaged on a standard or large-field-of-view gamma camera with a parallel-hole collimator. Image information is usually collected in digital dynamic mode or on an interfaced computer and reformatted in temporal sequences that reflect both initial renal perfusion and subsequent function.

Renal Perfusion Imaging

Evaluation of renal blood flow and function of native kidneys is performed from the posterior projection, whereas the evaluation of transplant blood flow and function is performed from the anterior projection. Normally, a small bolus of high-activity (10 to 20 mCi [370 to 740 MBq]), ^{99m}Tc-labeled radiopharmaceutical (^{99m}Tc-DTPA or ^{99m}Tc-MAG3) is injected intravenously, preferably into a large antecubital vein. Imaging renal perfusion is usually begun as the bolus is visualized in the proximal abdominal aorta, with subsequent serial images made every 1 to 5 seconds, depending on the instrumentation available and the preferences of the interpreter. A typical renal blood flow study is seen in Figure 9-1. The activity reaches the kidneys about 1 second after the bolus in the abdominal aorta passes the renal arteries. Time-activity curves reflecting renal perfusion during the first minute may be generated by drawing regions of interest over the aorta and each kidney. Each of the renal curves may then be compared with the time-activity curve of the abdominal aorta to assess relative renal perfusion. Occasionally, the spleen overlies the left kidney, giving a false impression of asymmetrically increased left renal perfusion or of a "phantom kidney" in patients with prior left nephrectomy.

Renal Function Imaging

At the end of the renal perfusion sequence, imaging for renal function begins. Dynamic or sequential static, 3- to 5-minute ^{99m}Tc-DTPA or ^{99m}Tc-MAG3 (Fig. 9-2) images are then obtained over 20 to 30 minutes. Evaluation of the images includes attention to renal anatomy and position, symmetry and adequacy

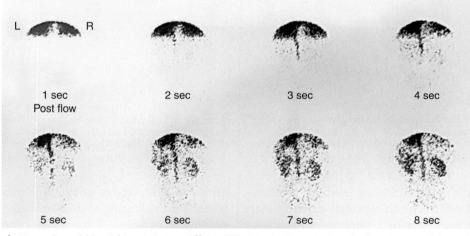

Figure 9-1. **Normal renal blood flow.** A bolus of ^{99m}Tc-DTPA in the lungs is visualized at the top of the serial images at 1 second. By 3 seconds, the aorta is fully visualized. By 5 to 6 seconds, both kidneys are clearly seen. The flow is symmetric to both kidneys. Note that in normal perfusion, the activity seen in the kidneys is about equal to that seen in the aorta just above the aortic bifurcation. Maximal activity in the kidneys usually is reached later, between 30 and 60 seconds. *DTPA*, Diethylenetriamine pentaacetic acid.

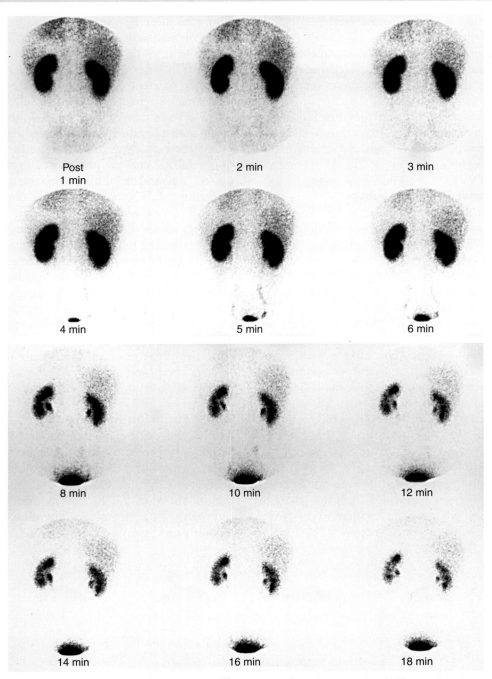

Figure 9-2. Normal renogram. After administration of ^{99m}Tc-mertiatide (MAG3), maximal kidney activity is seen at about 3 to 5 minutes, and, by 4 to 5 minutes, the bladder can be identified at the bottom of the images. By about 8 to 12 minutes, most of the activity has cleared the parenchyma and is seen in the collecting systems, making the kidneys appear slightly smaller than on the early images.

of function, and collecting system patency. With ^{99m}Tc-MAG3, the maximal parenchymal activity is seen at 3 to 5 minutes, with activity usually appearing in the collecting system and bladder by about 4 to 8 minutes. Some laboratories routinely use furosemide to clear activity from the renal collecting systems.

However, post-void or post-ambulation images to enhance collecting system drainage may be obtained as needed. Time-activity (renogram) curves for each kidney, reflective of relative renal function, are also usually created from regions of interest over the renal parenchyma, as discussed below.

Renography

A renogram is simply a time-activity curve that provides a graphic representation of the uptake and excretion of a radiopharmaceutical by the kidneys. Information is displayed from the time of injection to about 20 to 30 minutes after injection. The classic renogram curve is obtained by using agents that are eliminated by tubular secretion (e.g., ^{99m}Tc-MAG3). Renogram curves are generated by placing a region of interest around each kidney, usually the entire kidney, but occasionally just around the renal cortex if a considerable amount of collecting system activity is present. Background subtraction regions of interest are selected just inferior to each kidney (Fig. 9-3). An aortic region of interest may be used to assess the discreteness and adequacy of the injected bolus as well as relative renal perfusion.

The normal computer-generated renogram curve using a tubular radiopharmaceutical consists of three phases (Fig. 9-4). Initial renal perfusion, or the *vascular transit phase*, lasts about 30 to 60 seconds and represents the initial arrival of the radiopharmaceutical in each kidney. Reconstruction of the first 30 to 60 seconds of the curve by using different axes may be performed to assess more carefully the renal perfusion phase. Generally, renal peak activity during the perfusion phase equals or exceeds that of the aorta and should be reasonably symmetric between the two kidneys. The second phase is the *cortical* or *tubular concentration phase* of initial parenchymal transit. This phase occurs during minutes 1 through 5 and contains the peak of the curve. The initial uptake slope closely correlates with ERPF values. The third phase is the *clearance* or *excretion phase*, which represents the down slope of the curve and is produced by excretion of the radiopharmaceutical from the kidney and clearance from the collecting system.

Patients should be well hydrated when renography is performed because in the presence of dehydration, an abnormal renogram curve demonstrating delayed peak activity, delayed radiopharmaceutical clearance, or an elevation of the excretion slope may result.

Overall, the renogram curves for each kidney should be reasonably symmetric, although slight asymmetries are not unusual. The shapes of curves should also be inspected individually

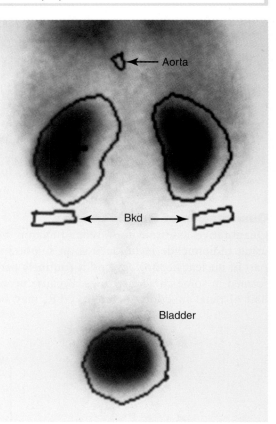

Figure 9-3. Typical regions of interest for computer analysis. Outlined regions of interest are drawn over the aorta, the kidneys, and the bladder. Areas of background activity (*Bkd*) are also drawn. Time-activity curves are then generated for each of these after appropriate background subtraction has been made.

for alterations in the normal configuration. Semiquantitative indices derived from the curves may be helpful in this respect. Data commonly derived from ^{99m}Tc-MAG3 renograms include the following:

- *Time to peak activity.* Normal is about 3 to 5 minutes.
- *Relative renal uptake ratios at 2 to 3 minutes.* This is an index of relative renal function between the two kidneys. Activity in each kidney should be equal, ideally 50%. A value of 40% or less in one kidney should be considered abnormal.
- *Half-time excretion* is the time for half of the peak activity to be cleared from the kidney. Normal is about 8 to 12 minutes.
- *Differential cortical retention at 15 minutes.* The percentage of retained activity about 15 minutes after injection in each kidney should be relatively equal. Differences of 20% or more should be considered abnormal.

■ *The 20 minute-to-peak count ratio.* This is the activity measured in each kidney at 20 minutes and expressed as a percentage of peak curve activity. As renal function deteriorates, delayed transit of the radiopharmaceutical in the kidney results in an abnormal renogram curve, which can be quantitated by using this index. In the absence of pelvic calyceal retention, or if only a cortical region of interest is used, a normal 20-minute maximal cortical ratio for ^{99m}Tc-MAG3 is less than 0.3 (or 30%).

Quantitation of Renal Function

Quantitative assessment of renal function by using radionuclide techniques is an important part of nuclear nephrology and is routinely performed in some clinical settings. Because up to half of renal function, including GFR, may be lost before serum creatinine levels become abnormal, direct measurement of GFR and ERPF by using radiopharmaceuticals plays an important role in the assessment of renal function.

The classic measures of renal function involve the ability of the kidneys to clear certain substances from the plasma. These so-called clearances are expressed as volume of plasma cleared of a particular substance per minute (mL/min) as the plasma passes through the kidneys. The significance of the clearance depends on the substance used. The clearance of inulin, which is entirely filtered, defines the GFR; and the clearance of para-aminohippurate (PAH), which is both filtered and secreted by the tubules, defines renal plasma flow. The radiopharmaceutical analogs for calculation of these clearances are the totally filtered radiopharmaceutical ^{99m}Tc-DTPA

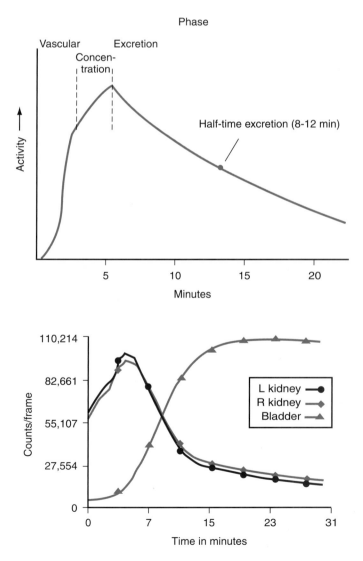

Figure 9-4. Typical renogram curves. *Top,* Schematic drawing demonstrates the conceptual portions of the time-activity curve within the kidney. *Bottom,* Actual renogram shows symmetric activity between right and left kidneys, rapid drop-off after the peak, and a long tail extending to the right. The curve also shows increasing activity within the bladder after about 4 minutes.

for inulin clearance and GFR estimation, and
^{99m}Tc-MAG3, which is primarily secreted by the
tubules, for PAH clearance and ERPF. The latter
index is termed *effective* because the radiopharmaceuticals used closely estimate, but do not
equal, the PAH clearance.

Two dominant radionuclide methods of determining GFR and ERPF are used: (1) plasma
sample-based clearances, which are more tedious
but more accurate, and (2) camera-based clearances, which do not require sampling of plasma
or urine.

Plasma Sample-Based Clearances

These measurements are generally obtained by
determining the plasma levels of the injected
radiopharmaceutical at a specified time,
although some techniques require urine collection as well. For tubular agents such as
^{99m}Tc-MAG3, ERPF can be estimated by a
single, timed blood sample obtained about
45 minutes after injection. Because the glomerular agent ^{99m}Tc-DTPA is cleared more
slowly than are tubular agents, plasma samples are obtained 60 and 180 minutes after
injection. The amount of activity remaining in
the blood at these times is a measurement of
activity not yet cleared by the renal mechanism
and therefore is indirectly a measure of activity already cleared. These techniques require
meticulous attention to detail and personnel
expertly trained in in-vitro techniques. When
performed correctly, GFR and ERPF measurements are theoretically more accurate than are
those based on camera measurements.

Camera-Based Clearances

State-of-the-art gamma cameras and computers
have allowed the development of methods for
estimating GFR and ERPF without collecting
blood or urine samples. Commonly, calculations are made by using counts acquired from
the syringe containing the radiopharmaceutical
before injection and subsequent counts over the
kidneys after injection. Commercially available
software for camera-based clearances simplifies
corrections for patient and acquisition variables
and provides reasonably accurate computer-derived clearance values. Although camera-based clearances are not as accurate as are
those based on plasma samples, they are highly
reproducible and sufficiently reliable to be used
in clinical practice.

A renal functional measurement expressed
simply as *MAG3 clearance*, without a need
for corrections to estimate ERPF, is available using both single plasma sample-based
and camera-based techniques. MAG3 clearance may be used to follow the course of renal
disease and has proved useful in individual
laboratories in which its own range of normal
values can be determined. Both MAG3 clearance and GFR determination are as useful and
accurate measurements of renal function as is
creatinine clearance.

Anatomic (Cortical) Imaging

Renal cortical imaging is usually performed
for the evaluation of space-occupying lesions,
functioning pseudotumors such as cortical columns of Bertin (Fig. 9-5), or edema or scarring
associated with acute or chronic pyelonephritis, especially in children. These images of
the renal cortex are generally taken by using
^{99m}Tc-DMSA or glucoheptonate and by using
a pinhole or a high-resolution collimator, or
single-photon emission computed tomography
(SPECT).

CLINICAL APPLICATIONS
Diffuse Renal Disease

In the evaluation of diffuse renal diseases producing acute or chronic impairment of renal
function, such as acute pyelonephritis or chronic
glomerulonephritis, radionuclide techniques are
often sensitive but not disease-specific. Most
often, there is simply demonstration of unilaterally or bilaterally poor vascular perfusion and
poor radiopharmaceutical excretion (Fig. 9-6).
The renogram provides quantitative estimates
of the function of each kidney, information that
is not easily obtained by other methods. Generally, poor renal function results in flattening
of the renogram curve as concentration and
excretion of the radiopharmaceutical become
increasingly impaired.

In patients with *acute tubular necrosis* (ATN),
there may be normal or only modestly reduced
renal perfusion and preserved parenchymal
accumulation but bilaterally poor excretion of
^{99m}Tc-MAG3 (Fig. 9-7). This frequently presents as bilateral persistent nephrograms with
rising renogram curves. Reasonably good visualization of the kidneys indicates a favorable
prognostic outcome, whereas poor visualization
correlates with a prolonged or absent recovery.

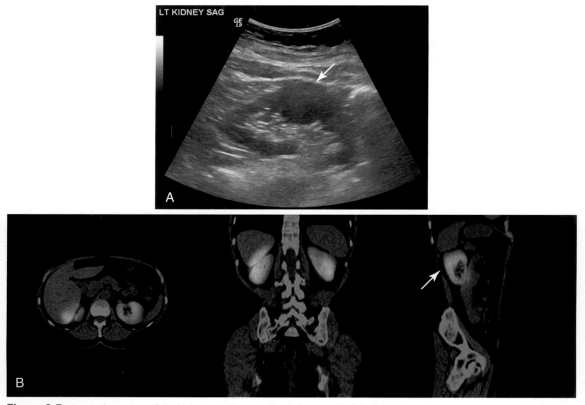

Figure 9-5. Cortical imaging of the kidneys. A, Longitudinal ultrasound of the left kidney shows an apparent midpole mass *(arrow).* **B,** SPECT/CT performed with 99mTc-DMSA shows that the area in question *(arrow)* has functional renal tissue and is a normal variant (column of Bertin). A renal cell cancer would not have demonstrated any activity. *CT,* Computed tomography; *DMSA,* dimercaptosuccinic acid; *SPECT,* single-photon emission computed tomography.

Vascular Abnormalities

Renal perfusion abnormalities may be encountered in patients evaluated for unexplained renal failure. Renal artery occlusion, avulsion or stenosis, venous thrombosis, and renal infarction can be demonstrated by nuclear techniques, but other radiographic studies remain the procedures of choice. The image presentations of these disorders and the detection rates are not significantly different from those demonstrated by conventional radiographic techniques.

In *acute renal vein thrombosis,* there is generally decreased or absent perfusion and delayed and diminished accumulation and excretion of 99mTc-MAG3 by an enlarged, engorged, edematous kidney.

Obstructive Uropathy

The diagnosis of urinary tract obstruction and assessment of its functional significance are common indications for radionuclide imaging in both adults and children. Obstruction may be suspected on the basis of clinical findings or as an incidental finding of a dilated renal collecting system on CT, ultrasound, or radionuclide renal imaging. Standard imaging techniques, such as ultrasonography, evaluate structure but do not depict urodynamics.

Routine Functional Imaging and Renography

With acute high-grade obstruction, routine radionuclide renal function imaging frequently discloses reduced renal perfusion. The renogram curve demonstrates a rising excretion slope determined by the severity of the hydronephrosis or the degree and duration (acute or chronic) of the underlying obstruction and by the amount of preserved renal function. To obtain an adequate image, there must be enough residual function to allow excretion of the radionuclide into the collecting system. The classic acute or subacute high-grade obstructive renogram is a steeply rising continuous arched curve with no definable excretion downsloping. In long-standing high-grade

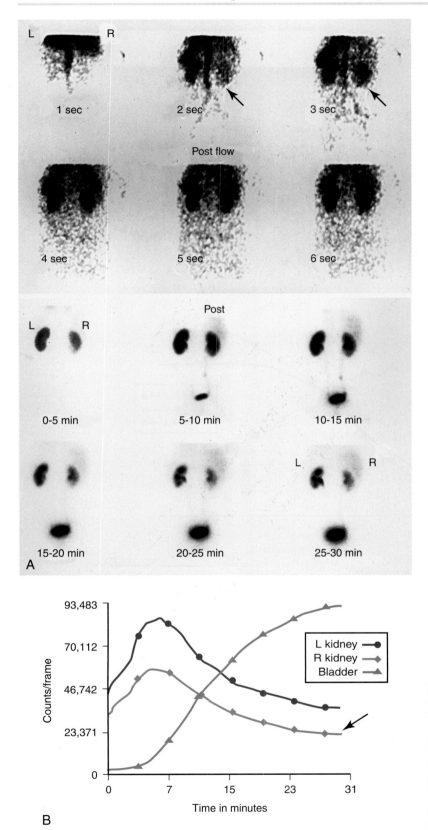

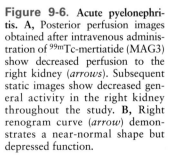

Figure 9-6. **Acute pyelonephritis.** **A,** Posterior perfusion images obtained after intravenous administration of ^{99m}Tc-mertiatide (MAG3) show decreased perfusion to the right kidney (*arrows*). Subsequent static images show decreased general activity in the right kidney throughout the study. **B,** Right renogram curve (*arrow*) demonstrates a near-normal shape but depressed function.

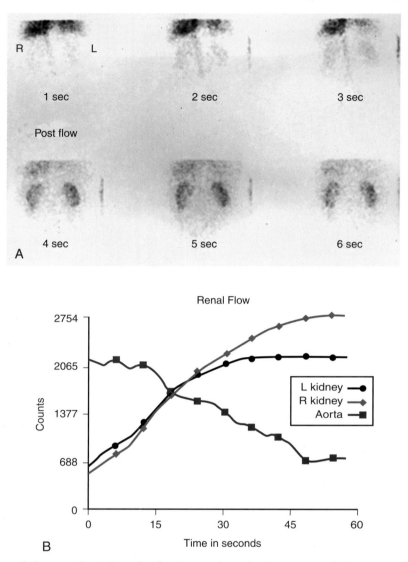

Figure 9-7. Acute tubular necrosis. A, Posterior flow images done after intravenous administration of ^{99m}Tc-mertiatide (MAG3) show symmetric and normal perfusion to both kidneys. **B,** Computer curves of blood flow during the first minute demonstrate a normal pattern, with aortic activity decreasing quickly after about 10 seconds and renal activity increasing rapidly up to about 30 seconds after injection, ultimately exceeding the peak aortic activity.

obstruction, no renal perfusion or function may be seen, and the renogram curve may be uniformly flattened.

Similar to anatomic imaging, however, routine renography may not differentiate obstructive collecting system dilatation from hydronephrosis of a nonobstructive nature, so that appropriate management can be instituted before significant renal damage occurs. In this setting, diuretic renography provides a noninvasive method to distinguish collecting system dilatation attributable to a true obstruction from that secondary to a patulous and atonic, but patent, collecting system.

Diuretic Renography

Diuretic renography has become an important diagnostic radionuclide test to distinguish between obstructive hydronephrosis and nonobstructive collecting system dilatation attributable to vesicoureteral reflux, urinary tract infection, congenital malformations, previous obstruction, or a noncompliant bladder. Generally, glomerular function declines earlier and more rapidly than does tubular function in response to ureteral obstruction. Thus radiopharmaceuticals excreted primarily by tubular secretion, such as ^{99m}Tc-MAG3, are the agents of choice for renography of patients

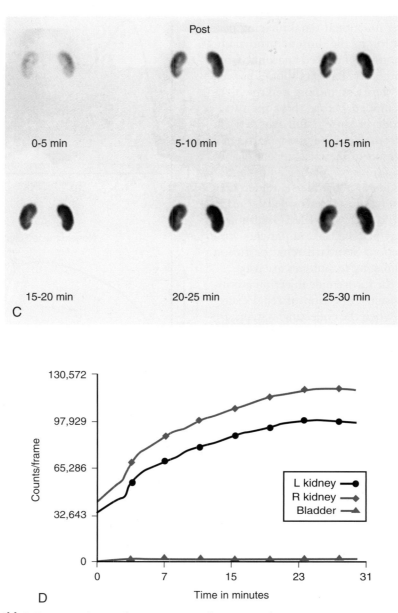

Figure 9-7. cont'd C, Renogram images demonstrate poor function on the 0- to 5-minute image and increasing parenchymal activity throughout the remainder of the study, with no obvious excretion. **D,** This is confirmed by the continuously rising renogram curves.

with suspected collecting system obstruction. However, ^{99m}Tc-DTPA may also be acceptable in more acute and less severe obstructions. Diuretic renography evaluates both renal function (obstructive nephropathy) and urodynamics (hydronephrosis) in a single test.

In patients with nonobstructive hydronephrosis and/or hydroureter attributable to vesicoureteral reflux, previous obstruction, or functional ureteropelvic disorders, the dilated intrarenal collecting system may fill but not reach pressures

sufficient to "open" the ureteropelvic junction to permit flow of urine under normal conditions of urine production. This may give the impression of a fixed anatomic abnormality rather than a functional abnormality. By increasing urine flow using a diuretic (such as furosemide), a functional obstruction may be overcome by increasing pressure in the renal pelvis and thus allowing urine to flow from the collecting system into the ureter to the bladder. A fixed, anatomic obstruction would not be expected to be overcome by the diuresis. Thus performing this maneuver during functional renal imaging permits documentation of the diuretic urodynamics and differentiation of a fixed anatomic from functional abnormality. Patients should be well hydrated before the examination, and the bladder should be emptied before the administration of furosemide because a full bladder can slow drainage from the upper part of the urinary tract and result in the false appearance of obstruction. In adults or infants who cannot empty their bladders, a bladder catheter may be used. The study is best performed by using 10 mCi (370 MBq) of ^{99m}Tc-MAG3, although ^{99m}Tc-DTPA may also be used in patients with good renal function. Standard renal perfusion and functional imaging techniques are used.

The timing of the furosemide injection is critical. Real-time visual inspection of renal excretion determines when the collecting systems are full. This usually occurs about 15 to 20 minutes after radiopharmaceutical injection but may occur later in hydronephrotic kidneys. Injection of the diuretic should be delayed until the dilated renal pelvis is full or the renogram curve is near its peak. At that time, an intravenous injection of furosemide, 40 mg for adults and 1 mg/kg to a maximum of 40 mg for children, should be administered. A larger dose, up to a maximum of 80 mg, may be required in patients with impaired renal function. Response to furosemide usually begins 2 to 5 minutes after injection; however, maximal diuresis is frequently not reached until 15 minutes after injection.

Renogram curves using regions of interest drawn over only the collecting systems or over the entire kidneys are obtained. Preference is generally given to collecting system regions of interest, which should also include the ureters if they appear to retain the radiopharmaceutical. Calculating the half-time excretion for diuretic renography is often performed either from the time of injection of the diuretic or at the beginning of the diuretic response. However, determination of the time of onset of the diuretic response can be subjective if the response is not discrete.

Interpretation of the data is generally performed by visual analysis of the renogram washout curve with assessment of the half-time excretion (Fig. 9-8). Dilated collecting systems secondary to either fixed or functional "obstruction" may produce continuously rising renogram curves before furosemide administration, with minimal

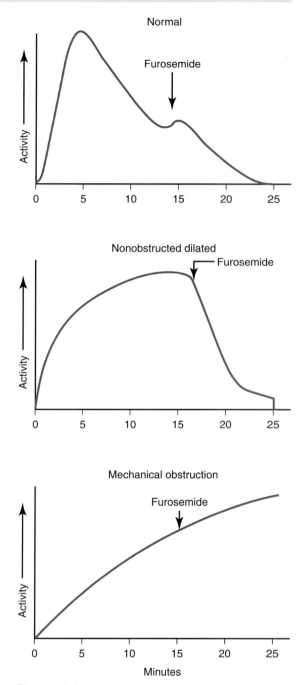

Figure 9-8. Characteristic time-activity curves in a diuretic renogram.

or no evidence of excretion downsloping. After furosemide administration, the curve is inspected for any change. In dilated, nonobstructed systems, furosemide causes increased urine flow through the collecting system, which washes out the initial increase in activity and causes a decline of the excretion slope in the computer-generated, time-activity curves (Fig. 9-9).

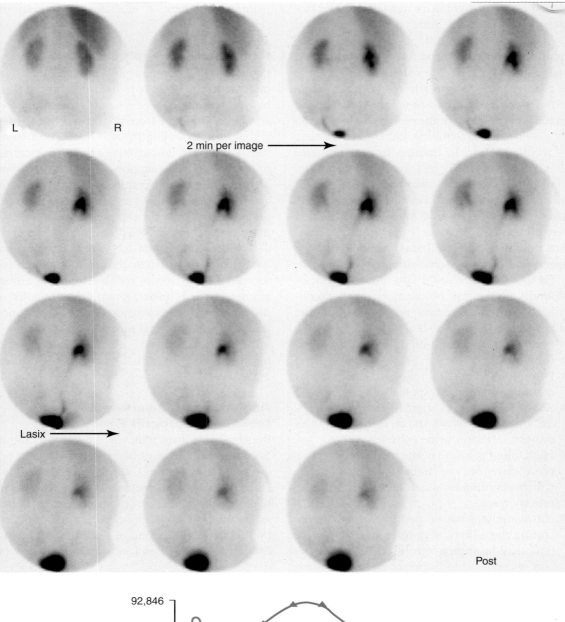

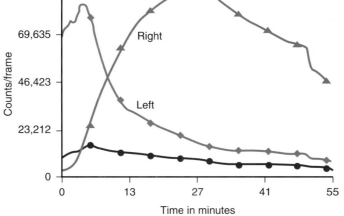

Figure 9-9. Nonobstructed patulous collecting system. A diuretic renogram *(top)* shows that activity in the collecting system of the right kidney decreases significantly after administration of furosemide (Lasix) at about 20 minutes.

In the case of significant mechanical obstruction, there is very little decrease in renal collecting system activity after furosemide administration, owing to the narrowed, fixed lumen of the ureter. The rising renogram curve is changed little or is unaffected (Fig. 9-10).

Assessment of the half-time excretion may aid in the interpretation of the renogram. In general, in a normally functioning kidney, a half-time of less than 10 to 15 minutes from the time of diuretic effect constitutes a normal response. Half-time values and renogram curves should always be considered in conjunction with the scintigraphic images and adequacy of existing renal function. Because a spectrum of renal function is encountered in clinical practice, a spectrum of diuretic responses is to be expected.

Factors that produce a false-positive impression of mechanical obstruction or that contribute to indeterminate results include the following:

■ Poor hydration, resulting in poor diuretic response
■ Poor underlying renal function, resulting in a diminished diuretic response
■ A noncompliant or rigid renal pelvis, producing increasing resistance to urine flow as diuresis increases urine volume
■ High filling pressure of the bladder as a result of a distended or noncompliant bladder, which may impair washout from the upper urinary tract
■ An overcompliant or patulous renal pelvis. During the diuretic response, increased urine flow may be sufficient to fill this large reservoir without being sufficient enough to wash out the tracer, producing a rising renogram curve.
■ A large hydronephrotic volume, especially in the presence of diminished function. With a larger volume in the system, a larger diuretic response is needed to clear that system of accumulated activity. This is the so-called *reservoir effect*.

Urinoma

Occasionally, activity on a renogram can be seen outside of the kidney or collecting system because of a urinoma (Fig. 9-11). Care should be taken to assess the images to see that the unusual collection of activity is increasing during the course of the examination because false positives can be the result of residual activity from prior nuclear medicine examinations (Fig. 9-12).

Pediatric Hydronephrosis

Perinatal ultrasonography has resulted in increased diagnosis of hydronephrosis and hydroureteronephrosis in newborns. Differentiation of obstructive from nonobstructive causes is therapeutically important. Obstruction commonly occurs in the regions of the ureteropelvic or ureterovesical junctions. Technetium-99m MAG3 diuresis renography appears to be reliable in the diagnosis of unilateral and bilateral ureteropelvic junction and ureterovesical junction obstruction (Fig. 9-13). In infants and children older than 1 month, glomerular filtration has usually matured to the level at which its measurement becomes reliable by using either glomerular or tubular agents. One difficulty is the diagnosis of coexisting ureteropelvic junction and ureterovesical junction obstructions—one or the other may be missed using this technique. See Appendix D for pediatric dosage guidelines.

Angiotensin-Converting Enzyme Inhibitor (Captopril) Renography

Renovascular hypertension constitutes about 1% to 4% of all cases of hypertension, but no discriminating findings allow its diagnosis on clinical grounds. In patients with renovascular hypertension, the most common cause of renal artery stenosis is atherosclerosis, predominant in the elderly; the second most common cause is fibromuscular dysplasia, occurring primarily in women younger than 35 years. When an angiotensin-converting enzyme (ACE) inhibitor is given to a patient with renal artery stenosis that has been compensated by the renal angiotensin mechanism, there is a decrease in GFR that is scintigraphically detectable. The test is highly specific for renal artery stenosis as a cause for the patient's hypertension, which may eliminate the need for diagnostic angiography.

Significant renal artery stenosis (60% to 75%) decreases *afferent* arteriolar blood pressure, which stimulates renin secretion by the juxtaglomerular apparatus. Renin elicits the production of angiotensin I, which is acted on by ACE to yield angiotensin II. Angiotensin II induces vasoconstriction of the *efferent* arterioles, which restores glomerular filtration pressure and rate. ACE inhibitors, such as oral

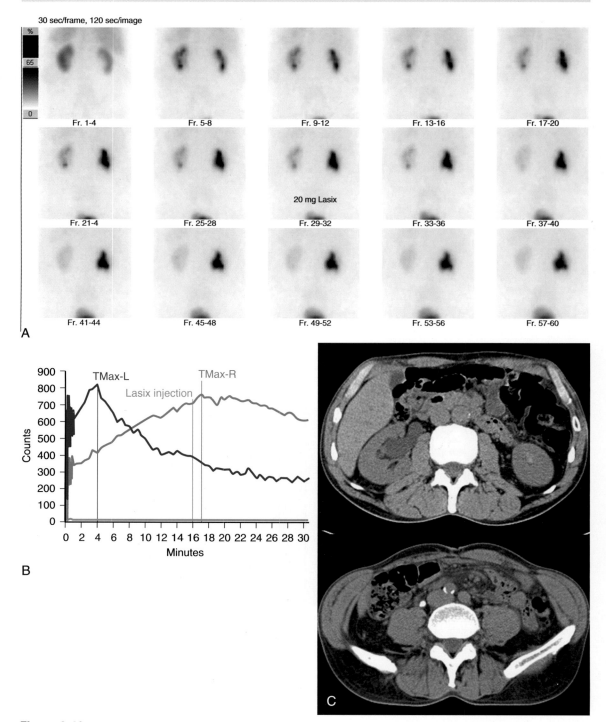

Figure 9-10. Abnormal diuretic renogram with obstruction. A, After intravenous administration of ^{99m}Tc-DTPA, the posterior 2-minute sequential images show a dilated collecting system of the right kidney. After administration of furosemide (middle of the second row of images), the activity in the collecting system on the left decreases normally; however, the activity in the right kidney decreases only slightly. **B,** Time-activity curves show the normal excretion on the left (*red curve*) and delayed excretion on the right (*green curve*). **C,** CT scan shows a dilated right renal pelvis and a mid-ureteral obstructing radiopaque stone. *TMax-L,* Time of maximum activity in left kidney; *TMax-R,* time of maximum activity in right kidney.

30 sec/frame, 120 sec/ image

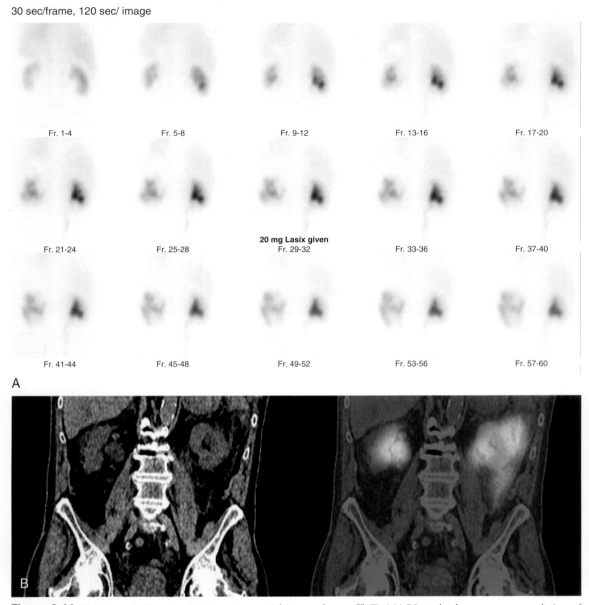

Figure 9-11. Urinoma. A, Posterior 2-minute sequential images from a ^{99m}Tc-MAG3 study show poor accumulation of activity in the collecting system of the left kidney. On later images, the outline of activity extends beyond the outline of the kidney seen on early images. **B,** SPECT/CT images show extension of activity lateral to the left kidney into the perirenal space and inferiorly.

captopril or enalapril and intravenous enala-prilat, prevent the production of angiotensin II, so that in patients with renal artery stenosis and compensated renal function, preglomerular filtration pressures are no longer maintained. This results in a significant sudden decrease in glomerular filtration. This induced decompensation can be documented by performing ^{99m}Tc-MAG3 or ^{99m}Tc-DTPA studies before and after the administration of captopril. Sensitivity and specificity may be higher with MAG3 than with DTPA, although excellent results

may be obtained with either radiopharmaceutical in most patients. A positive study indicates that a patient's hypertension is renin-dependent (renovascular hypertension), most commonly produced by renal artery stenosis, and that it is likely to be improved by renal revascularization.

ACE inhibition (ACEI) scintigraphy should not be used as a screening procedure for all patients with hypertension because it is not cost-effective and because screening a population with low prevalence for renal artery stenosis will lead to an unacceptably high false-positive

1 sec/frame

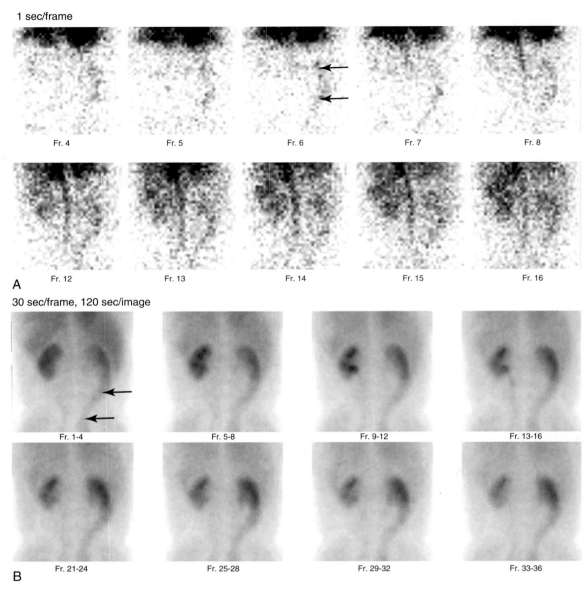

Figure 9-12. Retained activity from previous nuclear cardiac study. A, Posterior renal blood flow images from a ^{99m}-Tc-DTPA study show a vertical band of immediate activity in the right lateral abdomen. **B,** Two-minute delayed sequential images show this activity persists throughout the study (*arrows*). This might have been mistaken for a urinoma except that it was present on blood flow images before the kidneys were perfused. Investigation revealed that the patient had a ^{99m}Tc-sestamibi cardiac study 16 hours earlier, and this represents residual activity in the ascending colon.

rate and incite further unnecessary invasive testing. Patients should be selected carefully and limited to those with a moderate to high probability of renovascular hypertension. Selection criteria include the following:

■ Initial presentation of hypertension in patients older than 60 years or younger than 30 years
■ Severe or accelerated hypertension resistant to medication therapy
■ Hypertension previously well controlled but now difficult to manage medically

■ Hypertension in patients with other evidence of occlusive vascular disease
■ Unexplained renal dysfunction in patients with recent onset of hypertension
■ Unexplained hypertension in patients with abdominal or flank bruits

Patients taking ACE inhibitors therapeutically should have their medication halted for about 48 hours for captopril and for about 1 week for lisinopril or enalapril before the examination. The patient's ACEI medication may be maintained if it is deemed medically

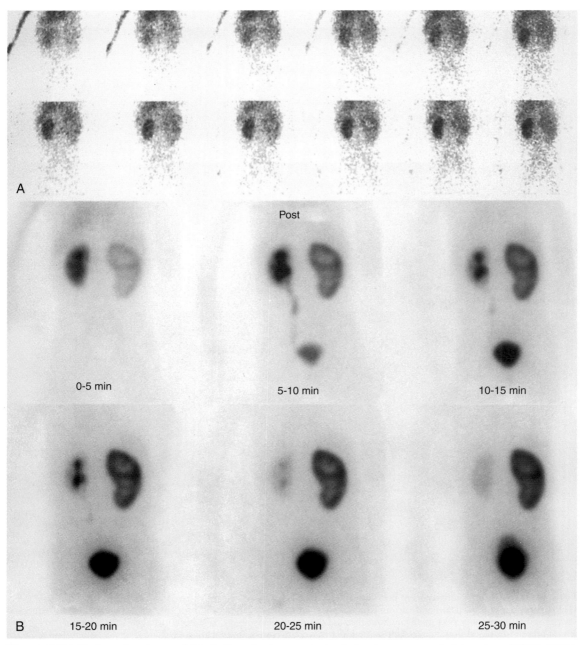

Figure 9-13. Hydronephrosis in a child. A, Posterior images obtained after intravenous administration of ⁹⁹ᵐTc-DTPA show decreased perfusion to an enlarged right kidney. **B,** Renogram shows a dilated collecting system of the right kidney.

necessary and inadvisable to halt administration for more than 24 hours. However,
the patient should refrain from taking ACEI
medication on the day of the study. Antihy-
pertensive drugs of non-ACE inhibitor classes
do not appear to affect the test results. The
patient should be fasting to allow for maximum absorption of oral captopril and should
be well hydrated.

Although ACEI scintigraphy protocols vary,
the basics of the examination are well defined
and include the following:

■ Twenty-five to 50 mg of oral captopril is
administered with sitting blood pressure
recordings at 15-minute intervals for 1 hour.
As an alternative, in patients with uncertain
gastrointestinal absorption of oral medication, intravenous enalaprilat (Vasotec),

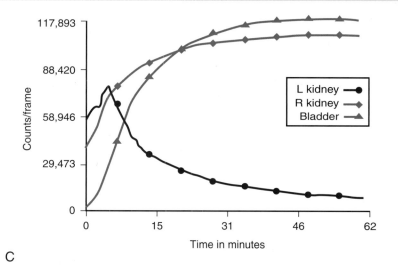

C

Figure 9-13. cont'd C, Computer-generated time-activity curves show that after administration of furosemide (at 15 minutes), there is no decrease in activity, indicating a high-grade obstruction on the right.

0.04 mg/kg up to a maximum of 2.5 mg, may be administered over 3 to 5 minutes.

■ One hour after captopril administration or 15 to 20 minutes after enalaprilat infusion, 10 mCi (370 MBq) of ^{99m}Tc-MAG3 (preferred in most patients, especially those with impaired renal function) or ^{99m}Tc-DTPA is administered intravenously, and routine renal scintigraphy with renography is performed. Some protocols use intravenous furosemide (40 to 60 mg) shortly after the administration of the radiopharmaceutical to clear the renal collecting systems of activity, which may interfere with the calculation of cortical indices. At the termination of imaging, a final blood pressure reading should be obtained before the patient leaves the imaging department.

In patients with unilateral renal artery stenosis and renal insufficiency, bilateral renal artery stenosis, or stenotic solitary or transplanted kidneys, captopril or enalaprilat should be used advisedly for diagnosis, especially if severe stenosis is known to be present. Under these circumstances, acute renal failure may be induced, which is generally self-limited, although persistent anuria may occasionally develop. Furthermore, in any patient undergoing captopril intervention studies, the possibility of severe hypotension induction exists. This complication usually responds to intravenous volume expanders (normal saline). Thus

it is prudent to maintain intravenous access throughout the study.

Two primary protocols may be used that comprise one- and two-stage examinations. Choice of the examination depends primarily on patient scheduling and department preferences. Because establishing a diagnosis of renal artery stenosis as a cause for hypertension depends on the induction or worsening of renal dysfunction after ACE inhibitor administration, a baseline study is extremely useful in assessing the effects of the medication on renal function.

The *single-day, two-stage protocol* consists of an initial baseline noncaptopril study, usually performed early in the day with a low radiopharmaceutical dose (1 to 2 mCi, 74 MBq of ^{99m}Tc-MAG3). This allows a repeat examination using captopril intervention several hours later, after clearance of the tracer from the kidneys and urinary tract. By administering 40 mg of furosemide during or after the first study to ensure good washout of residual activity, the waiting time between studies may be shortened further.

The *one-stage protocol* is generally performed on patients without evidence of preexisting renal dysfunction or failure. In this protocol, the captopril challenge study is performed first. If normal, a diagnosis of renovascular hypertension is unlikely (10% probability), and the baseline study is not needed.

The principal diagnostic criterion and the hallmark of renovascular hypertension is a postcaptopril renogram that becomes abnormal or more abnormal, usually unilaterally, than a baseline renogram in which an ACE inhibitor is not given. Using the glomerular agent ^{99m}Tc-DTPA, the principal finding is diminished uptake and excretion caused by a drop in glomerular filtration. There may also be prolonged parenchymal transit manifested by delay in time to peak activity of the renogram curve. If the fall in GFR is severe enough, there may be nonvisualization of a previously functioning kidney. Using the primarily tubular agent ^{99m}Tc-MAG3, reasonably adequate initial uptake and secretion are preserved. The reduced GFR, however, results in decreased urine production and flow and therefore in decreased washout of the secreted agent from the collecting tubules. This results in increased cortical retention, which is the principal finding (Fig. 9-14). This results in an abnormal renogram curve with an elevated cortical retention index (increased cortical activity at 20 minutes compared with the renogram peak). Occasionally, in very severe stenosis, early decreased uptake of ^{99m}Tc-MAG3 may also be identified.

A number of quantitative renogram parameters have been devised to assist in visual interpretation and to facilitate comparison of the baseline and the postcaptopril examinations. These criteria differ with respect to the radiopharmaceutical used. Several criteria frequently used to indicate an abnormality on ^{99m}Tc-MAG3 ACEI renography are as follows:

■ Percentage of renal uptake at 2 to 3 minutes by one kidney less than 40% of total uptake

■ Retained cortical activity at 20 minutes expressed as a fraction of peak activity differing from the contralateral kidney by more than 20%—or an increase from the baseline study of 0.15; normal is less than 0.3

■ Delay in the time to peak activity in the affected kidney of more than 2 minutes when compared with the baseline study or the unaffected kidney

These parameters have met with various levels of reported success and should be used only in conjunction with visual analysis of the renogram curves and review of the scintigraphic images.

In addition to unilateral renal artery stenosis, bilateral abnormalities produced or demonstrating worsening from baseline may be noted in bilateral renal artery stenosis, although detection becomes more difficult. Bilateral renal artery stenosis often behaves in an asymmetric fashion in response to ACEI renography and is therefore distinguishable from the usually symmetric appearance seen in patients with either essential hypertension or chronic parenchymal renal disease after captopril administration. Further, bilateral worsening of the renogram curves after ACEI administration may also be caused by hypotension induced during the study, dehydration, and bladder distention resulting in poor collecting system drainage. The diagnosis of renovascular hypertension resulting from segmental renal artery stenosis and after renal transplantation has been reported.

Both the sensitivity and specificity of ACEI renography surpass 90%. When strict attention is paid to patient preparation and examination protocol, false-positive studies are uncommon. As with most tests, however, its limitations should be recognized.

Scintigraphic abnormalities with captopril renography are best demonstrated in patients with renal artery stenoses of 60% to 90%. Abnormalities may not be demonstrated in stenoses of less than 60% because of the lack of significant renin-angiotensin compensation. Severe renal artery stenosis of greater than 90% may not be compensated sufficiently by the renin-angiotensin system at baseline to allow for a scintigraphically detectable change to occur after administration of ACE inhibitors. False-negative examinations may be caused by accommodation to the drug by patients receiving ACEI therapy, even with continued therapeutic response. This can be avoided by withholding captopril therapy for 2 to 4 days or the long-acting enalaprilat for 1 week before the study. In addition, using a patient's chronic medication regimen of ACE inhibitor to perform the ACEI renogram is not advisable.

The sensitivity and specificity of captopril renography may be diminished in patients with renal insufficiency, especially in those with small, poorly functioning kidneys. In patients with unilateral renal disease at baseline that does not demonstrate change after captopril administration, renal stenosis cannot be reliably differentiated from unilateral parenchymal disease. Also, asymmetric hydronephrosis or

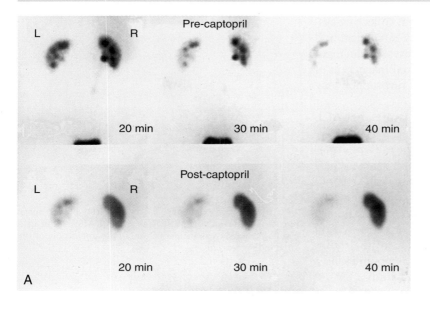

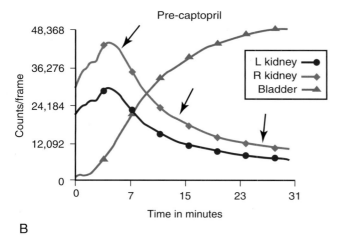

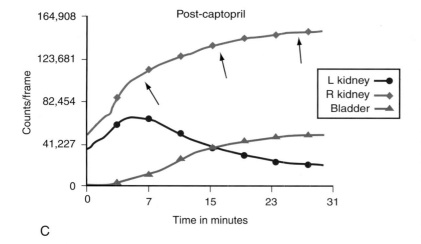

Figure 9-14. Right renal artery stenosis. A, Pre-captopril ^{99m}Tc-MAG3 renogram (*upper row*) shows slightly asymmetric activity. Post-captopril MAG3 renogram (*lower row*) shows markedly abnormal retention of activity in the right kidney as late as 40 minutes. **B,** Computer-generated curves before captopril administration show a normal right renogram curve (*arrows*). **C,** Curves after captopril administration (*arrows*) show markedly increasing activity owing to retention of ^{99m}Tc-MAG3 after administration of captopril.

poor drainage from an intrarenal collecting system may cause confusion between cortical and parenchymal retention of activity, producing a false-positive examination. Visual inspection of the images or administration of furosemide may prevent this problem.

A profound drop in blood pressure after ACE inhibitor administration may induce acute oliguria and cortical retention of the radiopharmaceutical not only in patients with renovascular hypertension, but also in patients with essential hypertension or even in normal control subjects, causing false-positive results. Poor hydration of patients may cause diminished urine formation and delayed transit and retention of the radiopharmaceutical in the renal cortex, mimicking a poststenotic kidney on the ACEI study.

Acute Pyelonephritis

The diagnosis of acute pyelonephritis in children based on clinical and laboratory observations is frequently difficult, even in the presence of fever, flank pain, or pyuria and a positive urine culture. CT and renal sonography have a low sensitivity and underestimate the degree of parenchymal involvement. Radionuclide renal cortical imaging is a highly sensitive technique for diagnosis of renal parenchymal infection and should be considered for the diagnosis of acute pyelonephritis in children. Normal cortical imaging effectively excludes a diagnosis of acute pyelonephritis. Imaging studies are usually not necessary for the diagnosis of acute pyelonephritis in adults.

Technetium-99m DMSA in a dose of 50 μCi (1.85 MBq)/kg is the radiopharmaceutical of choice, with a minimum administered dose of 500 μCi (18.4 MBq). Although ^{99m}Tc glucoheptonate (150 μCi [5.55 MBq]/kg) may be used, the lesser accumulation of activity in the bladder when using ^{99m}Tc-DMSA significantly reduces gonadal radiation dose and is therefore preferable in infants and young children. SPECT imaging may be used as needed.

In normal patients, cortical uptake of DMSA appears homogeneous throughout the kidneys on routine imaging, except for relative defects in the regions of the collecting systems. High-resolution magnified images, however, especially with the use of a pinhole collimator, may show heterogeneous uptake owing to prominent cortical columns and may provide better differentiation of the cortex from the medulla.

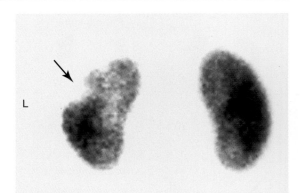

Figure 9-15. Pyelonephritis. The posterior planar image from a ^{99m}Tc-dimercaptosuccinic acid (DMSA) scan in a young child shows cortical defects in the upper pole of the left kidney (*arrow*).

Normal variants include smooth variations in cortical contour caused by fetal lobulation, which are distinguished from scars by preservation of cortical thickness.

In patients with acute pyelonephritis, there are three common patterns of presentation: (1) focal cortical defects (Fig. 9-15), (2) multifocal cortical defects, and (3) diffusely decreased activity.

In the acute phase, defects may be associated with edema presenting as a bulging renal contour. Because diminished activity of ^{99m}Tc-DMSA in areas of acute inflammation reflects early ischemia that precedes functional abnormalities, DMSA scans likely become positive before any significant tissue damage has occurred. These findings may resolve completely and return to normal within several months or may evolve into permanent damage with scar formation. If the disease progresses, scarring becomes prevalent, and the cortical defects become associated with contraction and volume loss. With significant infection or inflammation, edema can slow radionuclide uptake and excretion from the kidney(s). Occasionally, renal infections or inflammation can be visualized on ^{18}F-fluorodeoxyglucose (FDG) PET/CT scans (Fig. 9-16).

Renal Masses

Renal space-occupying lesions identified by sonography, CT, or magnetic resonance imaging (MRI) may occasionally warrant further evaluation with renal cortical imaging using ^{99m}Tc-DMSA or glucoheptonate to distinguish nonfunctioning from functioning renal tissue.

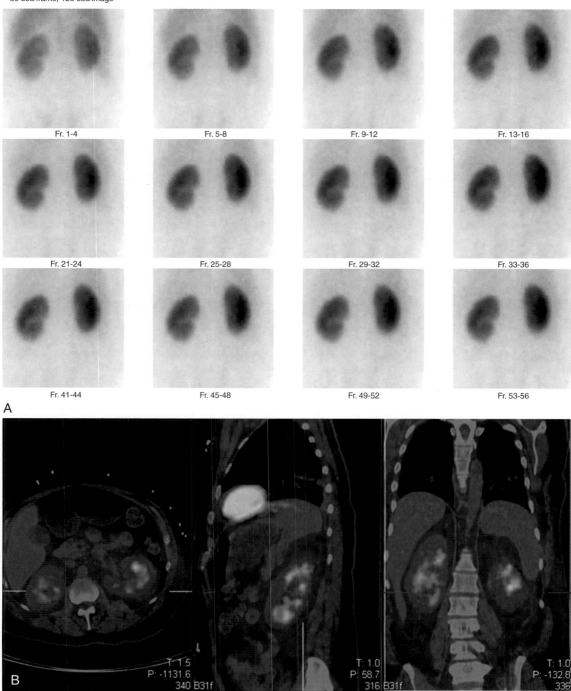

Figure 9-16. Interstitial nephritis. A, Sequential 2-minute images from a ⁹⁹ᵐTc-MAG3 scan in this oliguric renal failure patient show retention of activity in the kidneys. **B,** ¹⁸F-FDG PET/CT scan shows increased activity in the region of the papillae. *FDG,* Fluorodeoxyglucose.

Masses not representing renal parenchyma, such as neoplasms, abscess, cysts, hematoma, or infarcts, present as photopenic lesions in the renal parenchyma. Pseudotumors consisting of normally functioning renal tissue but simulating neoplasm may be caused by fetal lobulation, dromedary humps, and columns of Bertin, which are generally the most worrisome. These columns represent normal cortical tissue extending into the renal medulla between the renal pyramids and are frequently found at the junction of the upper and middle thirds of the kidney. Demonstration of functioning renal tissue in the region of the suspected mass confirms its benign nature.

Radionuclide Cystography

Radionuclide cystography is the technique of choice for the evaluation and follow-up of children with suspected vesicoureteral reflux. Radionuclide cystography is more sensitive than is iodinated contrast cystography, with reflux volumes as low as 1 mL being detected. There is also significantly less radiation exposure. For direct radionuclide cystography, 0.5 to 1 mCi (18.5 to 37 MBq) of ^{99m}Tc pertechnetate, ^{99m}Tc-DTPA, or ^{99m}Tc sulfur colloid is instilled through an indwelling bladder catheter, in a volume of normal saline sufficient to fill the bladder. A sample protocol and dosimetry are provided in Appendix E-1.

In normal patients, no radiopharmaceutical reflux from the bladder into the ureters or the kidneys is seen. When vesicoureteral reflux occurs, it may be identified during the bladder filling, voiding, or postvoid phases of the examination. For purposes of reporting, reflux is usually described as follows:

■ Minimal—confined to the ureter
■ Moderate—involving the pelvicalyceal system
■ Severe—reflux into the pelvicalyceal system accompanied by a dilated intrarenal collecting system or a dilated tortuous ureter

Minimal reflux is the most difficult to discern on images, and false-negative studies are not uncommonly those in which the reflux is confined to the distal ureter.

When required, residual urine volume in the bladder can be calculated by measuring the change in bladder count rate before and after voiding and comparing it to the voided urine volume. In addition, information concerning volume of reflux into the upper tracts also can be calculated by using regions of interest over the intrarenal collecting systems on computerized images.

Renal Transplant Evaluation

The transplantation of kidneys from living or cadaveric donors is a well-established organ transplantation procedure both surgically and medically. Transplants are placed in the anterior iliac fossa with vascular anastomosis to the hypogastric artery and the external iliac vein, and with ureteral anastomosis or implantation into the bladder. Ultrasound is usually the initial imaging procedure of choice. Radionuclide imaging using ^{99m}Tc-DTPA or ^{99m}Tc-MAG3 is a useful tool in evaluating the medical and surgical complications of renal transplantation. Imaging of renal transplants is performed with the patient supine. Anterior images are obtained over the iliac fossa containing the transplanted kidney. Baseline functional renal imaging and renography are generally performed shortly after surgery. Subsequent serial imaging may be obtained if abnormalities are noted on the baseline study to assess improving or deteriorating renal function or as medical or surgical complications are suspected.

In the normal transplant perfusion study, the radioactive bolus reaches the renal transplant at almost the exact time it is seen in the iliac vessels. As with a renogram of a native kidney, the maximal parenchymal phase is normally seen at 3 to 5 minutes, with bladder activity present at 4 to 8 minutes (Fig. 9-17). Immediately after transplantation and for up to 2 weeks, there may be fairly prominent visualization of the ureter, owing to edema at the ureterovesical anastomotic site.

Complications of renal transplantation are generally acute tubular necrosis (ATN), rejection, antirejection medication (cyclosporin) toxicity, and surgical mishaps.

ATN commonly occurs in cadaveric transplants and results from ischemia in the renal transplant after harvesting and before transplantation. The scintigraphic presentation of ATN consists of preserved or only mildly reduced perfusion but diminished renal function and progressive cortical retention of tubular agents, such as ^{99m}Tc-MAG3, with a consequent decrease in or absence of urine production (Fig. 9-18). ATN is generally observed during the first 3 to 4 days after surgery and usually resolves during the next several weeks.

Renal transplant rejection is primarily a small-vessel obliterative disease, with perfusion deteriorating faster and more severely than function in the early stages. The dynamic perfusion study often reveals poor perfusion, which usually worsens on serial examinations. The renogram is equally poor, demonstrating a diminished

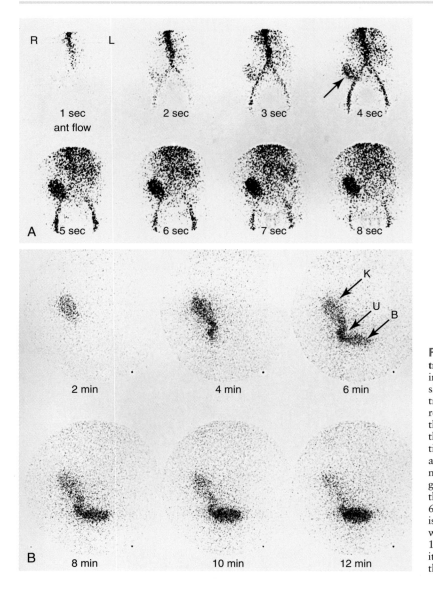

Figure 9-17. Normal renal transplant. A, Anterior perfusion images done with ^{99m}Tc-DTPA show prompt perfusion of the transplanted kidney in the right renal fossa (*arrow*). Note that in the early phases, the activity in the transplanted kidney is essentially equal to the intensity of activity in the iliac vessel directly next to the transplant. **B,** Renogram images show activity in the kidney (*K*) and ureter (*U*) by 6 minutes. Activity in the kidney is greatest at 4 minutes, and this washes out almost completely by 12 minutes, with most of the activity in the bladder (*B*) occurring at this time.

nephrogram phase and delayed appearance of bladder activity (Fig. 9-19), which may be largely due to the decreased perfusion and inability of the radionuclide to reach functional renal structures. Renal transplant rejection is usually classified according to its time of onset (hyperacute, acute, or chronic), with each form having a characteristic mechanism.

Hyperacute rejection occurs immediately (0 to 24 hours) after transplantation as a result of preformed antibodies in the recipient's blood. Hyperacute rejection produces rapid vascular thrombosis in the donor kidney, presenting as absent perfusion and severely reduced or absent function.

Acute rejection is a cell-mediated process characterized by lymphocytic infiltration. This generally occurs within the first 2 to 3 months after transplantation but may occur during the first several weeks. Acute rejection presents as decreased transplant perfusion with diminished radiopharmaceutical uptake and excretion. Acute rejection may also be imaged by using ^{99m}Tc sulfur colloid, which localizes in the rejecting transplant by trapping of the labeled colloid particles in fibrin thrombi. It appears to be less sensitive for detection of chronic rejection.

Chronic rejection is an antibody-mediated process that occurs 6 months to years after

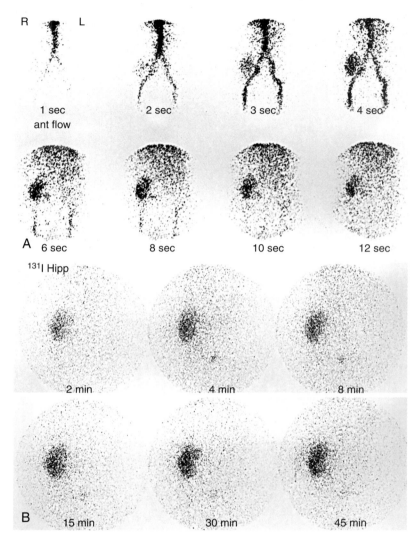

Figure 9-18. Acute tubular necrosis. **A,** Anterior perfusion images of the right iliac fossa transplant demonstrate normal perfusion. **B,** Renogram images done with iodine-131 Hippuran (a tubular agent similar to MAG3) show increasing parenchymal activity over 45 minutes, compatible with acute tubular necrosis.

transplantation. It is a slow process that produces a gradual obliteration of the renovascular bed with concomitant deterioration of renal transplant perfusion and function.

Cyclosporin nephrotoxicity (renal transplant toxicity from the antirejection drug cyclosporin) usually presents a scintigraphic appearance similar to that of ATN, with relatively good transplant perfusion and poor tubular function, which may result in progressive cortical retention of ^{99m}Tc-MAG3. Cyclosporin nephrotoxicity, however, characteristically occurs several weeks after transplantation when any ATN has resolved. The functional impairment associated with cyclosporin toxicity generally reverses after withdrawal of therapy.

Surgical complications include urine collections (urinomas), lymphoceles, hematomas,

ureteral obstruction, and vascular complications. Urinomas are caused by leakage from the ureteral anastomosis. This complication occurs shortly after surgery. If the leak of urine is significant, the excreted radiopharmaceutical may appear within the urine collection. If the leak is slow, the urinoma may present as a photopenic defect adjacent to the kidney or ureter. Photopenic defects in and around the renal transplant may also be a result of hematomas in the immediate postoperative period or lymphoceles, which commonly occur several months after transplantation.

Because a transplanted kidney has no venous collaterals, renal vein thrombosis produces deficient or absent perfusion and function in the transplanted allograft in a pattern identical to that seen with arterial obstruction. In the setting

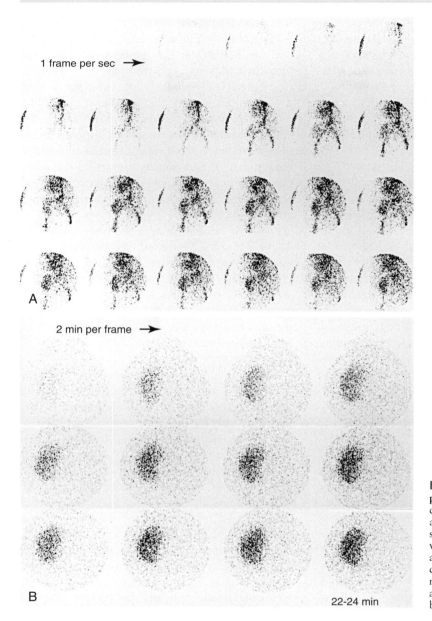

1 frame per sec →

2 min per frame →

A

B   22-24 min

Figure 9-19. Renal transplant rejection. **A,** ^{99m}Tc-diethylenetriamine pentaacetic acid (DTPA) flow study demonstrates poor flow to the transplant, which can be seen several seconds after the iliac vessels. **B,** Renogram demonstrates delayed parenchymal activity, with no evidence of activity in the collecting system or bladder.

of acute complete arterial or venous obstruction, the kidney presents as a photopenic reniform area outlined by background activity on radionuclide imaging. Postsurgical obstruction of the ureteral anastomosis may be diagnosed by radionuclide techniques in a similar fashion to native ureteral obstructions.

ADRENAL GLAND IMAGING
Adrenal lesions can present clinically with signs and symptoms of endocrine hyperfunction or as masses or adrenal enlargement on cross-sectional imaging. Incidental adrenal masses seen on CT or MRI are common. When clinically

warranted, nuclear medicine studies allow selection of patients for biopsy or surgical intervention. Although the sensitivity values of the studies are high, the specificity values depend strongly on the suspected pathology being evaluated.

Fluorodeoxyglucose (FDG) is only poorly accumulated in the normal adrenal glands raising the hope that PET/CT may be useful in assessing and characterizing adrenal masses in cancer patients as well as those "incidentalomas" encountered on CT scans done for other reasons. Up to 50% of adrenal masses in patients with a malignancy may be benign.

Adrenal uptake is usually taken to be positive if it is greater than or equal to that in the liver or has an SUV greater than 3.1. The accuracy of PET/CT to differentiate metastatic adrenal masses from benign lesions is about 90%, and false negatives can occur because of small lesions, hemorrhage, and necrosis. It is important to note that about 5% of adrenal adenomas are hypermetabolic.

Adrenal Medullary Imaging

Metaiodobenzylguanidine (MIBG) is a guanethidine analog similar to norepinephrine. It is taken up by chromaffin cells and is therefore useful for imaging normal and abnormal sympathetic adrenergic tissue, especially pheochromocytomas, whether located in the adrenal medulla or ectopically, and neuroblastomas. MIBG is localized in other neuroendocrine tumors to a lesser degree, including carcinoid, medullary thyroid carcinoma, and paraganglioma. In the settings of pheochromocytoma and neuroblastoma, the sensitivity and specificity of MIBG are high, approaching 90%.

The specific radiopharmaceutical used is radioiodinated MIBG labeled with 3 to 10 mCi (81 to 370 MBq) of iodine-123 (^{123}I). Iodinated MIBG is slowly metabolized; 75% to 90% is excreted by the kidneys as unaltered MIBG. Whole-body planar images or selected spot images of the regions of interest using a low-energy parallel-hole collimator are obtained serially over 24 to 72 hours, depending on the suspected pathology.

Radioiodinated MIBG appears normally in the salivary glands and liver, with faint activity apparent in the heart and thyroid gland. Because of renal excretion, there is renal and bladder activity. Nasal, neck muscle, diffuse lung activity, and bowel activity may be noted in some patients. The normal adrenal medulla is only occasionally visualized. It is seen best on delayed images in about 30% to 40% of patients, but the intensity is usually less than that of the adjacent liver and must be distinguished from the more intense abnormal accumulation seen in pheochromocytoma or neuroblastoma.

Clinical Applications

Pheochromocytoma. Imaging with whole-body ^{123}I-MIBG is the method of choice for pheochromocytomas. Scanning for pheochromocytomas is especially helpful in diseases with a high incidence of the neoplasm, including multiple endocrine neoplasms (MEN) types 2A and 2B, neurofibromatosis, von Hippel-Lindau disease, Carney triad, and familial pheochromocytoma. In addition to tumors of the adrenal medulla, ectopic pheochromocytomas are also imaged. The technique is sensitive in both adults and children.

Posterior adrenal images are obtained at 24, 48, or 72 hours, as needed. Whole-body planar imaging is useful if ectopic lesions are suspected. Pheochromocytomas imaged with radioiodinated MIBG present as focally increased activity whether the tumor is located in the adrenal medulla or ectopically (Fig. 9-20). Occasionally, some large tumors are not visualized because of extensive tumor necrosis.

Imipramine, insulin, reserpine, tricyclic antidepressants, and amphetamine-like drugs may inhibit localization of radioiodinated MIBG and thus interfere with tumor imaging. These should be withheld before imaging when practical.

Neuroblastoma. MIBG can be used to detect adrenal medullary neuroblastoma and its metastases in more than 90% of affected neonates and children. Whole-body imaging is performed 24 and 48 hours after administration. In normal subjects, the adrenal medulla may be seen on the more delayed images, and diffuse lung and gut activity can be prominent. Neuroblastomas and any metastases detected with MIBG present as foci of increased activity. Skeletal and marrow metastases are usually best seen on the 48-hour images. Aggressive chemotherapy may hinder the detection of some metastases.

Imaging of neuroblastomas and pheochromocytomas by using ^{111}In-pentetreotide (a radiolabeled somatostatin analog) and ^{18}F-FDG is further discussed in Chapters 10 and 11.

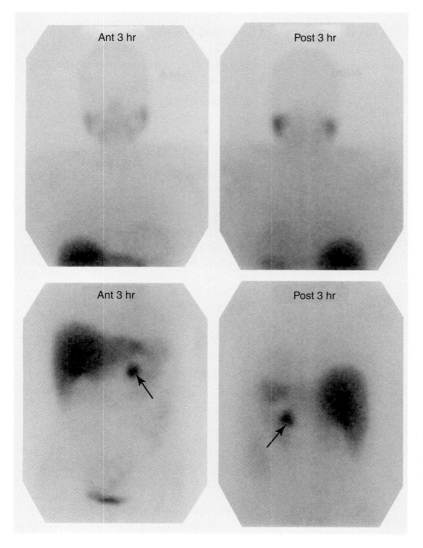

Figure 9-20. Pheochromocytoma. Anterior and posterior 3-hour images of the chest (*upper row*) and abdomen (*lower row*) done after administration of iodine-123 metaiodobenzylguanidine (MIBG) show a focus of abnormally increased activity (*arrow*) in the left adrenal gland.

PEARLS & PITFALLS

General

- The common indications for radionuclide scanning of native kidneys include allergy to iodinated contrast material, assessment of possible renal artery stenosis, and differentiation of obstruction from a flaccid collecting system. In children, cortical scanning agents are used for the evaluation of pyelonephritis.

- Technetium-99m DTPA reflects glomerular filtration (GFR). ^{99m}Tc-MAG3 is essentially a tubular agent and with a correction factor represents effective renal plasma flow (ERPF).

- Cortical binding agents bind to the proximal convoluted tubules. Technetium-99m-DMSA is a renal cortical binding agent (40% to 50%). Technetium-99m glucoheptonate is used to evaluate both renal cortical anatomy and the collecting system because it has both cortical binding (10% to 20%) and glomerular filtration.

- On blood flow images, normally perfused kidneys should have the same intensity of activity as is seen at the bifurcation of the aorta. Renal transplants should have the same intensity as the adjacent iliac artery.

PEARLS & PITFALLS—cont'd

- On serial 1- to 30-minute images of either normal native or transplanted kidneys, maximum parenchymal activity is seen at about 3 to 5 minutes, and bladder activity is seen by 4 to 8 minutes.

- On serial 1- to 30-minute images, the peak of renal activity represents the time when cortical uptake is equal to clearance. After the maximum renal activity peak, half of the renal activity should be cleared in about 8 to 12 minutes.

- On a postcaptopril renogram using Tc-99m-MAG3 as the imaging agent, the kidney that has delayed clearance with significant renal cortical retention should be the one with the renal artery stenosis. Bilateral delayed clearance can be caused by bilateral stenosis, obstruction, medical renal disease, dehydration, or hypotension.

- The usual dose of captopril (25-50 mg) only rarely produces systemic hypotension but, if this occurs, it requires prompt fluid administration to maintain intravascular pressure.

- Technetium-99m MAG3 or DTPA in a dilated intrarenal collecting system that does not clear by 20 to 30 minutes can be either a flaccid system or an obstruction. This can often be differentiated with a furosemide diuretic renogram. Rapid washout of activity after furosemide administration indicates a flaccid system as opposed to a fixed mechanical obstruction.

- In acute tubular necrosis (ATN), perfusion is usually normal with bilaterally increasing renal cortical activity and rising renogram curves when ^{99m}Tc-MAG3 is used.

- Always interpret the renogram curves in light of the scintigraphic imaging findings. When faced with abnormal time-activity curves, look at the images to see whether the problem is parenchymal or related to the collecting system.

Renal Transplant Imaging
- Common indications are to differentiate rejection from ATN. Occasionally, surgical complications may be suspected.

- ATN is usually seen within the first week after transplantation. It usually has preserved renal perfusion with progressive accumulation of tubular agents (^{99m}Tc-MAG3) in the renal parenchyma. It should improve with time.

- Occasionally, severe ATN can present with enough edema immediately after surgery to have reduced perfusion and therefore look similar to acute rejection.

- Cyclosporin toxicity can look like ATN but is usually not seen in the immediate postoperative period.

- Rejection usually has poor perfusion and poor tubular excretion.

- Look for photopenic defects around the transplant on the blood pool image that may be caused by urinomas, hematomas, and lymphoceles.

- There often is a low-grade ureterovesicular obstruction during the first few days after surgery as a result of edema at the anastomotic site.

Adrenal Imaging
- MIBG is a medullary adrenal imaging agent that effectively localizes in pheochromocytoma and neuroblastoma. It may also localize in carcinoid, medullary thyroid carcinoma, and paraganglioma.

SUGGESTED READINGS

Barron BJ, Kim EE, Lamki LM. Renal nuclear medicine. In: Sandler MP, Coleman RE, Patton JA, editors. Diagnostic Nuclear Medicine. 4th ed. New York: Lippincott Williams & Wilkins; 2003, p. 865-902.

Brown ED, Chen MYM, Wolfman NT, et al. Complications of renal transplantation: Evaluation with US and radionuclide imaging. RadioGraphics 2000;20:607-22.

Chong S, Lee KS, Kim HY, et al. Integrated PET-CT for the characterization of adrenal gland lesions in cancer patients: Diagnostic efficacy and interpretation pitfalls. RadioGraphics 2006;26:1811-26.

Dubovsky EV, Russel CD. Evaluation of renal and pancreatic transplants. In: Sandler MP, Coleman RE, Patton JA, editors. Diagnostic Nuclear Medicine. 4th ed. New York: Lippincott Williams & Wilkins; 2003, p. 1037-50.

Elaini AB, Shetty SK, Chapman VM, et al. Improved detection and characterization of adrenal disease with PET-CT. RadioGraphics 2007;27:755-67.

Fine EJ. Diuretic renography and angiotensin converting enzyme inhibitor renography. Radiol Clin North Am 2001;39:979-95.

Rossleigh MA. Renal cortical scintigraphy and diuresis renography in infants and children. J Nucl Med 2001;42:91-5.

Non-PET Neoplasm Imaging and Radioimmunotherapy

GALLIUM-67 IMAGING
  Clinical Applications
THALLIUM-201 CHLORIDE IMAGING
  Clinical Applications
TECHNETIUM-99M SESTAMIBI TUMOR
  IMAGING
NEUROPEPTIDE RECEPTOR IMAGING
  Somatostatin (Octreotide) Receptor Imaging
	ADRENAL TUMOR IMAGING
	LYMPHOSCINTIGRAPHY AND
	  INTRAOPERATIVE LOCALIZATION
	LABELED MONOCLONAL ANTIBODIES
	TREATMENT OF LYMPHOMA WITH
	  RADIOIMMUNOTHERAPY
	TREATMENT WITH INTRAVASCULAR
	  MICROSPHERES

In this chapter, tumor imaging using conventional gamma camera techniques is addressed. Thyroid cancer has been discussed in Chapter 4 and bone tumors and metastases in Chapter 8. Positron emission tomography (PET) imaging of neoplasms is discussed in Chapter 11. The affinity of various tumors for specific radiopharmaceuticals is shown in Box 10-1. The relative value of various imaging procedures for different tumors is shown in Chapter 11, Table 11-1. While some of these techniques have been largely supplanted by fluorine-18 fluorodeoxyglucose (^{18}F-FDG) PET/CT imaging, some are still useful in special settings. This is especially true of imaging with receptor-specific radiopharmaceuticals.

It has long been recognized that many routinely used radiopharmaceuticals may incidentally accumulate in neoplasms, but it was not until the introduction of gallium-67 (^{67}Ga) citrate as the first widely used tumor imaging agent that the noninvasive localization of primary and metastatic neoplasms using nuclear medicine techniques was realized. During the past decade, new biotechnologic advances have spurred the development of increasingly sensitive and specific tumor imaging agents for use in both single-photon and positron imaging.

Tumor-imaging radiopharmaceuticals may be divided into two broad groups: (1) those that have a nonspecific affinity for neoplastic tissue and may be used to image a range of tumors in various organs, including gallium-67 citrate (^{67}Ga), thallium-201 chloride (^{201}Tl), technetium-99m (^{99m}Tc) sestamibi, and fluorine-18 fluorodeoxyglucose (^{18}F-FDG); and (2) those designed to label specific tumor antigens, receptors, or metabolic processes, including monoclonal antibodies, peptides such as somatostatin (octreotide), and metaiodobenzylguanidine (MIBG). Both categories of radiopharmaceuticals are used in clinical nuclear medicine practice. Typical administered activities and radiation doses for tumor-seeking radiopharmaceuticals in current use are given as sample techniques in Appendix E-1.

GALLIUM-67 IMAGING

Gallium-67 citrate imaging was used for many years as a valuable diagnostic tool in the setting of neoplastic disease. Various aspects related to gallium have already been discussed in Chapter 1, and applications related to infection or inflammation are discussed in Chapter 12. With the development of newer, more tissue-specific radiopharmaceuticals and the widespread availability of computed tomography (CT), magnetic resonance imaging (MRI), and PET, most of the original applications of ^{67}Ga imaging are no longer routinely used.

The interpretation of ^{67}Ga images is complicated by marginal anatomic resolution and by interfering benign activity in the bowel, in postoperative sites of hematoma, infection, inflammation or wound healing, and in healing fractures. Thus careful attention to patient history and

Box 10-1 Radiopharmaceutical Affinity for Various Tumors

Gallium-67 Citrate
Hodgkin disease
Non-Hodgkin lymphoma (especially high-grade)
Hepatoma
Bronchogenic carcinoma
Melanoma
Seminoma
Rhabdomyosarcoma

Thallium-201 Chloride
Gliomas (high-grade)
Thyroid carcinoma
Benign tumors (usually fade over 2 hr)
Osteosarcoma
Lymphoma (especially low-grade)
Kaposi sarcoma (gallium-negative)

Technetium-99m Sestamibi
Cancer metastases
Breast cancer
Parathyroid adenoma
Gliomas
Lymphoma
Thyroid

Indium-111 Pentetreotide
APUD cell tumors
Pancreatic islet cell
Pituitary adenoma
Pheochromocytoma

Neuroblastoma
Paraganglioma
Carcinoid
Gastrinoma
VIPoma
Medullary carcinoma of thyroid
Small-cell lung cancer
Meningioma

Fluorine-18 Fluorodeoxyglucose
Most tumors (see Chapter 11)
Head and neck cancer
Esophageal cancer
Non–small-cell lung cancer
Melanoma
Lymphoma
Colorectal cancer
Breast cancer
Poorly differentiated neuroendocrine tumors

Iodine-123 or 131 Sodium Iodide
Thyroid cancer

Iodine-123 or 131 Metaiodobenzylguanidine
Pheochromocytoma
Neuroblastoma
Paraganglioma

Monoclonal Antibodies
Lymphoma

anatomic orientation and a thorough appreciation of the physiologic distribution of gallium and its excretion patterns are of utmost importance (Fig. 10-1). While renal activity is seen in the first 12 to 24 hours, 48 hours of the distribution of gallium activity is normally in osseous structures (bone and bone marrow), the nasopharynx, and variably in the lacrimal, salivary glands, and breasts (especially in lactating breasts). Activity in the salivary glands may be especially increased in patients who have undergone radiation or chemotherapy because of resultant sialadenitis.

Clinical Applications
Lymphoma
The malignant lymphomas constitute the neoplastic group in which gallium has been most extensively studied and was widely used before being largely replaced by ^{18}F-FDG PET imaging. The sensitivity of gallium in detecting lymphomatous disease depends greatly on the size,

location, and histology of the lesions. Lesions smaller than 1.0 cm are not often detected. Sites of involvement in the abdomen and pelvis may be difficult to identify because of interfering activity within the liver and colon and their often deep-seated location.

The sensitivity of ^{67}Ga imaging in untreated Hodgkin disease is more than 85% to 90%, with all histologic types showing some degree of gallium concentration (Fig. 10-2). The sensitivity of ^{67}Ga imaging in non-Hodgkin lymphoma (NHL) is less than that in Hodgkin disease and demonstrates variability related to histologic type. Gallium imaging is best reserved for higher-grade non-Hodgkin lymphomas because significantly lower detection rates are seen in low-grade lymphomas. Sensitivity ranges from about 90% in the histiocytic cell type to less than 60% with the lymphocytic well-differentiated type lymphoma. Success in imaging may be improved with high-dose single-photon emission computed tomography (SPECT) imaging. In addition to

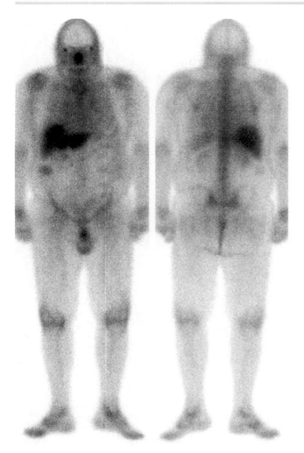

Figure 10-1. Normal gallium scan. Anterior (*left*) and posterior (*right*) images obtained at 48 hours. Some activity is seen in the lacrimal glands (upper outer aspect of the eyes), bone marrow, the nasopharynx, and the liver. In addition, there is some activity within the colon. This is normal physiologic excretion, which limits the usefulness of gallium in the abdomen.

soft-tissue disease, gallium scans can also identify osseous lymphoma. Thymic activity after chemotherapy or radiation can be confusing and can lead to a false-positive diagnosis of lymphoma recurrence (Fig. 10-3).

Hepatoma

In patients with a hepatic defect on a ^{99m}Tc colloid liver scan or a mass on CT that is suspected to be hepatoma, gallium uptake of greater intensity in the region of the abnormality than elsewhere in the liver is a strong indication of hepatoma (Fig. 10-4). When greatly diminished gallium uptake is identified in the suspect region, hepatoma is extremely unlikely. Gallium uptake in the anatomically abnormal region equal to that in the surrounding liver is equivocal and

may be found in regenerating nodules and hepatoma as well as in tumors of other causes, such as metastatic disease.

Other Neoplasms

Although the sensitivity of gallium imaging for bronchogenic carcinoma is about 90%, there is poor specificity because of the accumulation of gallium in a variety of non-neoplastic lesions, including infectious and inflammatory lesions and sarcoidosis. Therefore, gallium is not generally a useful tool in the differential diagnosis of pulmonary lesions. In general, melanoma, seminoma, and rhabdomyosarcoma are gallium-avid tumors, and gallium imaging displays excellent sensitivity for the detection of both primary and metastatic lesions within the limitations of the technique. Gallium studies exhibit low sensitivity for breast cancer, gastrointestinal tumors, and most genitourinary neoplasms and are of essentially no use in these settings. Gallium imaging is not recommended for the routine screening of patients with occult primary malignancies.

THALLIUM-201 CHLORIDE IMAGING

Thallium-201 chloride is a potassium analog that is avidly concentrated by some tumors. Long known for its use as a myocardial perfusion imaging agent, thallium has shown to be of value in the investigation of certain neoplastic diseases, including thyroid, lung, and breast cancer; glioblastomas; and bone and soft-tissue sarcomas. Compared with ^{67}Ga citrate, thallium generally shows less uptake in benign tumors, inflammatory processes, and remodeling bone. As with myocardial imaging, oncologic thallium imaging suffers the limitations of low administered activity, long half-life, and less than ideal, low-energy photon. After intravenous administration, ^{201}Tl localizes in the normal skeletal muscle, myocardium, liver, spleen, stomach, and colon, which may cause interference in the detection of certain lesions. Uptake is also seen in the choroid plexus, orbits, salivary glands, kidneys, and testes.

Tumor cell type, viability, and blood flow greatly influence the uptake of thallium in specific tumor masses. Thallium rapidly localizes in active, viable neoplasms, with peak uptake in tumors such as lymphoma and breast and lung carcinomas at about 10 to 20 minutes after

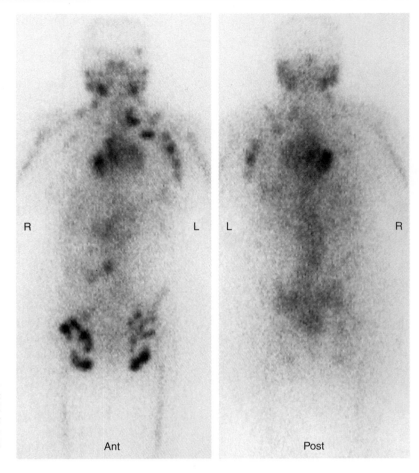

Figure 10-2. Lymphoma. Whole-body gallium scans performed at 48 hours demonstrate multiple foci of active disease in the neck, left axillary region, mediastinum central abdomen, and both inguinal areas.

injection. Imaging is usually performed 2 to 4 hours after administration to permit improved target-to-background ratios. Both 15- to 20-minute and 3-hour imaging may prove of value when the object is to distinguish benign from malignant masses. Early activity seen in benign lesions tends to decrease by 3 hours, whereas the activity in malignant lesions remains relatively constant. Lack of thallium uptake correlates with but is not diagnostic of a benign cause.

Clinical Applications
Brain Neoplasms
Thallium accumulates in malignant gliomas in proportion to the aggressiveness of the lesions. Low-grade lesions concentrate little or no thallium and may not be detected, whereas high-grade gliomas show markedly increased activity compared with normal brain tissue. Gliosis surrounding brain abscesses, however, may also demonstrate marked thallium accumulation, so that correlation with CT or MRI and clinical

findings is important in the differential diagnosis. Thallium imaging can be useful in distinguishing postradiation necrosis from recurrent tumor in patients with recurrence of symptoms and equivocal MRI findings. This topic is discussed more fully in Chapter 3.

Acquired Immunodeficiency Syndrome-Related Neoplasms
Kaposi sarcoma is thallium avid but does not take up gallium, whereas lymphoma concentrates both agents. Thus use of both agents may allow differentiation. Further, gallium uptake in a thoracic lesion without corresponding thallium uptake, or with mildly increased thallium uptake that fades on delayed images, suggests tuberculosis, *Mycobacterium avium-intracellulare,* or acute infection.

Other Adult Tumors
Although most lymphomas are thallium avid, the intensity of uptake is inversely proportional to the aggressiveness of the lesions. Low

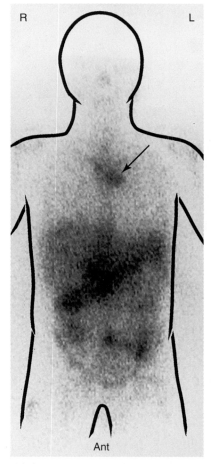

Figure 10-3. Reactive changes of the thymus. In this patient with known Hodgkin disease, a gallium scan was performed after radiation therapy of the thorax. A focus of activity is seen in the mediastinum slightly to the left of midline (*arrow*). This was not present on the gallium scan performed before radiation therapy. This benign reactive change can be seen in the thymus (and occasionally in the parotid glands) after radiation therapy or chemotherapy. It is important not to mistake this for recurrent disease.

metastatic or residual disease instead of radio-iodine. However, ^{18}F-FDG imaging is now the preferred method for imaging non-I-131-avid thyroid metastases. Thallium is also taken up by parathyroid adenomas, but ^{99m}Tc-sestamibi appears to be a better imaging agent and is more commonly used in this setting.

TECHNETIUM-99M SESTAMIBI TUMOR IMAGING

Although ^{99m}Tc-sestamibi concentrates in a number of tumors, including breast and thyroid cancers, it is primarily used to image parathyroid adenomas (discussed in Chapter 4). Although the exact mechanism of ^{99m}Tc-sestamibi uptake by tumor cells is uncertain, primary factors include its lipophilicity, which permits passive transport through tumor cell membranes, and its active uptake by mitochondria once intracellular. Cells with higher mitochondrial content show greater ^{99m}Tc-sestamibi concentration.

After intravenous injection, ^{99m}Tc-sestamibi distributes throughout the body in proportion to blood flow, localizing in the myocardium, thyroid, and salivary glands as well as in the spleen, kidneys, bladder, lungs, skeletal muscle, liver, gallbladder, and small and large intestines. Because sestamibi is used so frequently for cardiac imaging, incidental neoplasms can be apparent on the views of the chest and upper abdomen (Fig. 10-5).

Breast Cancer. Technetium-99m sestamibi concentrates in malignant breast tumors, with a mean contrast ratio approaching 6:1 when compared with normal breast tissue or surrounding fat. Dedicated high-resolution gamma cameras, some with dual heads, are used to image breast carcinomas. This has been termed breast-specific gamma imaging (BSGI) or molecular breast imaging. With this equipment, ^{99m}Tc-sestamibi has been reported to have a sensitivity and specificity of 80% to 90%. A negative scan in the presence of a palpable lesion is also significant, making breast cancer possible but unlikely. When used with judicious patient selection, this technique may be a valuable, non-invasive problem-solving adjunct to mammography and/or breast ultrasound. The addition of gamma imaging to mammography significantly increased the detection of node-negative breast cancer in dense breasts by 7.5 per 1000 women screened. In one study, the sensitivity of mammography alone was 27%, while the sensitivity

histologic grades tend to show marked thallium avidity, and higher-grade lesions display less or absent uptake. Thus this is the opposite of gallium avidity in tumors. Thallium may be useful in low-grade lymphomas, for which gallium imaging may demonstrate a somewhat lower sensitivity. Soft-tissue and skeletal sarcomas, including osteosarcoma, may concentrate thallium, and thallium imaging has been used to determine the success of preoperative chemotherapy and thus prognosis. Relapse rates are higher in patients exhibiting modest or no detectable change in thallium activity after treatment. Differentiated thyroid carcinoma is thallium avid and may be used in follow-up imaging for

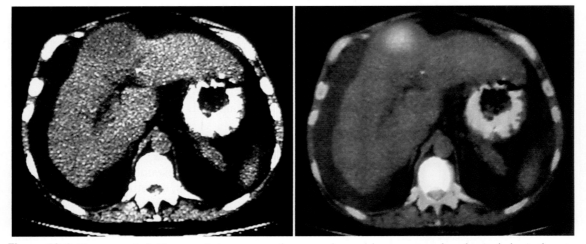

Figure 10-4. **Hepatoma.** *Left,* Narrow window computed tomography scan demonstrates a low-density bulge in the anterior aspect of this cirrhotic liver. *Right,* Gallium SPECT/CT fusion image shows increased gallium activity in this hepatoma.

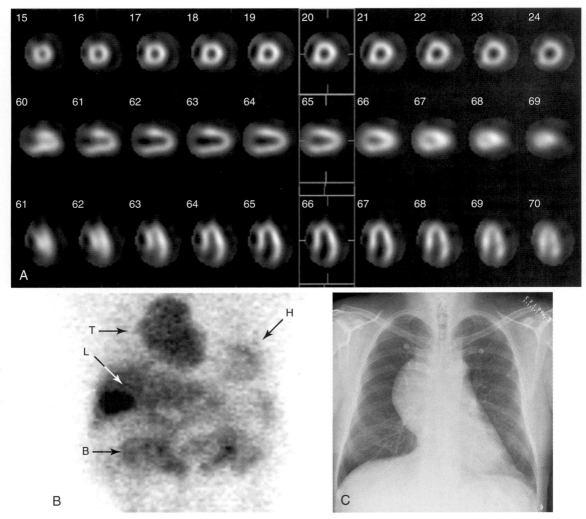

Figure 10-5. **Thymoma.** **A,** This patient had a ^{99m}Tc-sestamibi cardiac study that is normal. **B,** An astute technologist pointed out on the source image of the chest and abdomen that there was abnormal activity (*T*) in the chest and normal activity in the heart (*H*), liver (*L*), and bowel (*B*). **C,** Subsequent chest radiograph shows the large thymoma, which could have been easily overlooked if only the SPECT cardiac perfusion images had been reviewed.

of combined mammography and dedicated sestamibi imaging was 91% in at-risk women. Use of the technique as a screening procedure is not currently recommended.

Imaging of suspected breast cancer can be performed 10 to 20 minutes after the injection of 20 to 25 mCi (740 to 925 MBq) of ^{99m}Tc-sestamibi in an arm vein contralateral to the side of the suspected breast lesion. A foot injection is advised if both breasts are to be imaged. These original doses were based on standard gamma camera technology. Because of concerns regarding significant absorbed radiation dose to breast tissue with this technique, recent protocols have been developed using less than 10 mCi. This administered activity reduction has been made possible by the use of dual-headed dedicated cameras using pixilated detector digital technologies, such as position sensitive photomultiplier tunes (PSPMT) and cadmium zinc telluride (CZT) rather than single crystal sodium iodide analog detectors. Current high-resolution cameras which mimic conventional mammographic compression and place the breast in intimate contact with the detector, also offer improved sensitivity. Breast images are performed in standard mammographic projections, with special projections used as needed. Because there is little sestamibi washout from malignant lesions, imaging may be delayed, if needed, for up to 2 hours.

Technetium-99m sestamibi distributes homogeneously in the normal breast, regardless of the degree of breast density demonstrated on mammograms, and is usually of low intensity. A small number of patients exhibit diffusely increased activity in one or both breasts, which may be related to hormone levels at the time of imaging. This activity appears to be lowest at or about mid-cycle in premenopausal patients, especially those younger than 30 years. Although this is considered a benign finding, the increased background may obscure a lesion. A positive study presents as a discrete focus of increased activity in the breast or axilla that is greater than adjacent breast activity. The location of the abnormal focus should be carefully correlated with any palpatory and mammographic findings. Localization of nonpalpable foci for biopsy is now available using specialized localization systems.

While focally increased activity in the ipsilateral axilla in the presence of a primary lesion is strongly suggestive of axillary lymph node metastatic involvement, the sensitivity for axillary metastasis is variable and not sufficient to warrant use of the procedure for this purpose.

False-positive results may be related to benign fibroadenomas, fibrocystic change, or inflammation (including inflammatory fat necrosis) but have also been reported in benign conditions that confer a higher risk for developing carcinoma, including epithelial hyperplasia and complex sclerosing lesions. Imaging after recent needle or stereotactic biopsy may also be a cause of increased activity and thus a false-positive examination. False-negative results may occur with small (less than 1 cm), deep lesions or in tumors with less avidity for sestamibi.

NEUROPEPTIDE RECEPTOR IMAGING

Neuropeptides constitute a family of highly potent substances that consist of only a few amino acids. They are synthesized and released primarily by the brain (hence the name *neuropeptides*) and the gut and also by the endocrine system and lymphatic tissue. A number of neuropeptides and tissue receptors present as potential candidates for neuropeptide receptor imaging, including somatostatin, vasoactive intestinal peptide (VIP), α-melanocyte-stimulating hormone, and substance P receptors. Of these, radiolabeled somatostatin analogs have emerged as a prime example of the clinical utility of this approach.

Somatostatin (Octreotide) Receptor Imaging

Somatostatin is a naturally occurring neuropolypeptide that is synthesized and released by endocrine or nerve cells in various organs, especially the hypothalamus. It has a wide range of pharmacologic effects, including (as its name implies) the inhibition of secretion of growth hormone (somatotropin). Because a high density of somatostatin receptors is present in numerous neuroendocrine and some non-neuroendocrine tumors, radiolabeled somatostatin analogs can be used to image a variety of tumors, including primary and metastatic foci.

Neuroendocrine tumors are those derived from amine precursor uptake and decarboxylation (APUD) system cells, including carcinoid, pituitary adenomas, pancreatic islet cell neoplasms, medullary carcinoma of the thyroid, pheochromocytomas, neuroblastomas, paragangliomas, and small-cell lung cancers. Most of these are successfully imaged with radiolabeled somatostatin analogs with sensitivities approaching 80% to 100%. Exceptions are insulinomas (50% to 60% sensitivity) and medullary thyroid carcinoma (65% to 70% sensitivity). Some non-neuroendocrine tumors, including lymphomas, breast and lung carcinoma, gliomas (especially low-grade tumors), renal cell carcinoma and meningiomas, show variable and unpredictable uptake.

Because endogenous somatostatin has a biologic half-life of only a few minutes, radiolabeled analogs with greater in vivo stability have been developed. The eight-amino acid peptide iodine-123 (^{123}I) octreotide was the first to be used clinically. Subsequently, a cyclic structural modification of octreotide, ^{111}In-labeled pentetreotide (OctreoScan), was proven to have the additional advantages of greater stability and reduced hepatobiliary excretion (2%), with clearance primarily through renal elimination (90% at 24 hours). Less gastrointestinal activity allows for better visualization of abdominal tumor sites. However, considerable liver activity may obscure small hepatic metastases.

An intravenous imaging dose of 3.0 to 6.0 mCi (111 to 222 MBq) of ^{111}In-pentetreotide is used; the higher end of the dose range is preferred when SPECT is performed. Adverse effects from pentetreotide occur in less than 1% of patients. Imaging is performed at 4 and 24 hours, with 48-hour images acquired as needed to confirm a lesion suspected at 24 hours or when residual bowel or gallbladder activity is a problem. Planar images allow for survey of the whole body. SPECT/CT images are frequently helpful and may add to the sensitivity of the examination, especially in the upper abdomen, where interfering kidney, spleen, and often gallbladder activity may hamper imaging of the pancreas and duodenum. SPECT or SPECT/CT may also be useful in better evaluating suspect liver metastases. A detailed imaging protocol is presented in Appendix E-1.

Patient preparation is important for safe, effective imaging with ^{111}In-pentetreotide. Patients should be well hydrated to enhance renal clearance. A laxative should be used to decrease interfering bowel activity. In patients with diarrheal syndromes or insulinomas, laxatives should be prescribed only after consultation with the referring physician.

Because of its ability to inhibit the secretion of hormones, stable octreotide is helpful in controlling symptoms in patients with hypersecretion syndromes associated with metastatic carcinoid tumors, gastrinomas, insulinomas, glucagonomas, and vasoactive intestinal peptide-related tumors (VIPomas). Although somatostatin receptor-positive tumors may be visualized in patients receiving stable octreotide therapy, it is preferable to discontinue the drug temporarily for 24 to 48 hours before administration of ^{111}In-pentetreotide.

In a normal patient, ^{111}In-pentetreotide activity can be identified in the blood pool, normal thyroid gland, kidneys and bladder, liver, gallbladder, spleen, and, to a lesser degree, bowel on delayed images. The kidneys and spleen retain the most activity and therefore receive the highest absorbed doses. Because the radiopharmaceutical is in part retained by the renal parenchyma, the kidneys are seen even on delayed views (Fig. 10-6).

In abnormal images, primary neoplasms or metastases present as foci of increased activity. Because somatostatin receptors are expressed in some non-neoplastic, chronic inflammatory processes, such as granulomatous lesions (sarcoidosis, tuberculosis), Crohn disease, ulcerative colitis, and rheumatoid arthritis, these entities may serve as potential sources of false-positive results.

Indium-111 pentetreotide is primarily useful in evaluating neuroendocrine tumors, especially carcinoids (sensitivity, 85% to 95%) (Fig. 10-7) and gastrinomas (sensitivity 75% to 93%). A wider spectrum of tumors may be assessed with this radiopharmaceutical, however, including a number of nonendocrine solid tumors. Indium-111 pentetreotide is not useful in pancreatic carcinomas of exocrine origin because they do not express somatostatin receptors. The sensitivity of pentetreotide for imaging pheochromocytomas, neuroblastomas, and paragangliomas in extra-adrenal sites is over 85%.

Whole-body gamma camera imaging provides cost-effective screening of patients with suspected or known somatostatin receptor-containing tumors. The information obtained may disclose or confirm the presence of a lesion, detect metastases from a primary tumor, or characterize neuroendocrine conditions in

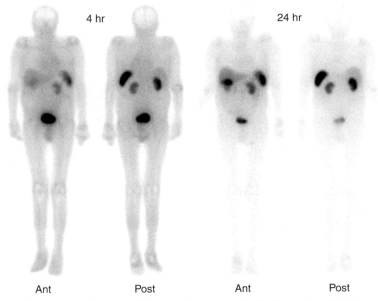

4 hr   24 hr

Ant   Post   Ant   Post

Figure 10-6. Normal ^{111}In-pentreotide (Octreotide) scan. Scans are typically done at 4 and 24 hours and are recognized by intense activity in the spleen, kidneys, and bladder.

which multicentric lesions may exist. In addition, because somatostatin receptor expression is seen more often in well-differentiated tumors, visualization may imply a more favorable prognosis. Patients with positive ^{111}In-pentetreotide images are also candidates for octreotide therapy because the documentation of somatostatin receptors provides a higher likelihood of controlling hormonal hypersecretion. Radionuclide therapy for octreotide-avid carcinoid tumors has been tried with various degrees of success using iodine-131 or yttrium-90 labeled octreotide.

ADRENAL TUMOR IMAGING

Iodine-123 or 131 MIBG imaging is useful and sensitive in the detection and evaluation of primary adrenal or extra-adrenal pheochromocytomas, neuroblastomas and their metastases, and of paragangliomas. Imaging adrenal neoplasms with radiolabeled MIBG is discussed in Chapter 9.

LYMPHOSCINTIGRAPHY AND INTRAOPERATIVE LOCALIZATION

Lymphoscintigraphy with ^{99m}Tc-sulfur colloid has been used to determine regional lymph node drainage pathways from malignant neoplasms, which may direct therapeutic management decisions, including radiation therapy fields and surgical approach. This technique has proved most useful in breast and skin malignancies, especially truncal and head and neck malignant melanomas.

The particles in standard colloid preparations are generally too large to be acceptable for most applications of lymphoscintigraphy. Thus the sulfur colloid is filtered to select a more appropriate particle size (less than 0.22 μm). The procedure involves several injections of small volumes (0.1 mL) of filtered ^{99m}Tc-sulfur colloid into the soft tissues at, or adjacent to, the tumor site. Generally, injection of the radiocolloid directly into the tumor is not advisable because this may significantly delay or even prevent migration into the lymphatic channels. For skin lesions such as melanoma, intradermal injections are used. For other tumors, subcutaneous or interstitial injections are performed. The detailed protocol is presented in Appendix E-1.

Once injected, the radiocolloid is removed from the area through lymphatic channels to reach regional lymph nodes, which receive lymphatic drainage from the primary lesion and thus have the potential of harboring metastases. Gamma camera imaging allows mapping of lymphatics and lymph nodes, especially sentinel nodes. The sentinel node is the first node to receive regional lymphatic flow from the tumor site and is a reliable biopsy indicator of the presence or absence of metastatic tumor in a lymph node group. If the sentinel node is free of tumor

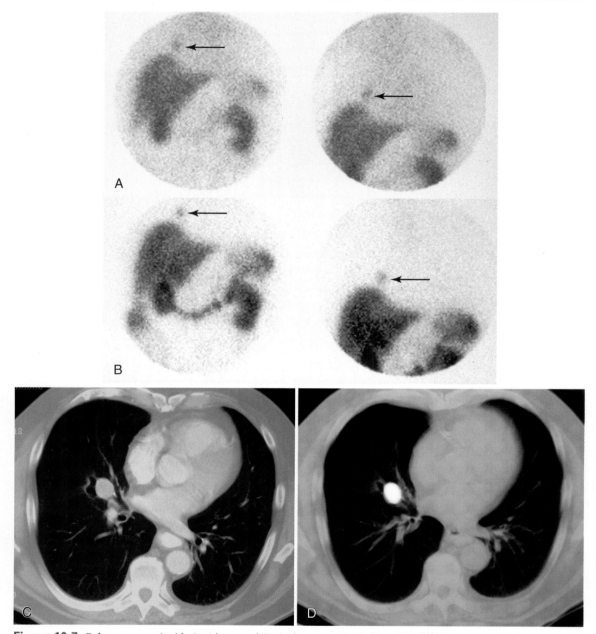

Figure 10-7. **Pulmonary carcinoid.** **A,** 4-hour and **B,** 24-hour anterior indium-111 (^{111}In) pentetreotide (somatostatin) images of the abdomen and chest show normal activity in the liver, kidneys, and bowel; however, an abnormal focus of activity is seen in the right lower chest (*arrow*). **C,** An abnormal enhancing lesion is seen on the CT scan. **D,** SPECT/CT fusion image clearly shows accumulation of ^{111}In pentetreotide by this carcinoid.

cells, the patient may be spared the morbidity and cost associated with elective dissection of the remaining lymph nodes in the chain.

Performing the procedure just before surgery also permits intraoperative identification of sentinel nodes for biopsy by using a hand-held gamma probe detector. Some authors have advocated the injection of radiocolloid in the operating room without the use of imaging. Use of a

gamma probe in the operating room can usually be performed 30 minutes to several hours after injection to help localize the sentinel node during surgery. The sentinel lymph node typically has 10 or more times the background count rate observed at a location remote from the injection site. Radiation doses to surgeons and pathologists from sentinel nodes are extremely low (well below the public dose

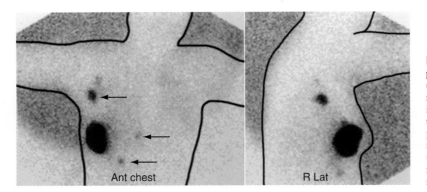

Figure 10-8. Lymphoscintigraphy. Anterior (*left*) and lateral (*right*) images after injection of radiocolloid around a cancer site in the right breast demonstrate that there are multiple routes of lymphatic drainage from this tumor, including into the right axilla (*upper arrow*), internal mammary node (*lower arrow*), and an inframammary node.

limit). Ninety percent of sentinel nodes have dose rates of less than 100 µSv (10 mrem)/hr at 3 cm.

A two-phase imaging technique is preferred that includes an early-phase series of static images or dynamic imaging to map visually the lymphatic channels followed by delayed static imaging to identify lymph node retention and to visualize sentinel nodes. The early or dynamic images permit a more exact identification of the first-draining node when more than one node is identified on the delayed images. The times of imaging are determined by the rate of migration of the radiocolloid from the site of injection.

In addition to normal pathways, abnormal patterns suggestive of tumor replacement of lymph nodes and lymphatic obstruction have been described. These include lack of migration of the radiocolloid through the lymphatic channels, decreased or absent nodal accumulation, and collateral channels. These findings may indicate the advisability of inclusion of the suspect nodes in radiation treatment fields and/or their surgical removal (Fig. 10-8).

When sentinel node biopsy is used for breast cancer staging, large studies have shown somewhat high false-negative rates (5% to 15% with less than 5% being desirable). The risk of missed disease after a negative sentinel node biopsy is 1% to 4% in patients with a T1 tumor and up to 15% in patients with a T3 tumor. These data point to the need for care in performing sentinel node mapping and some authors advocate dual mapping with separate injections of the radiotracer and isosulfan blue dye. Of interest is that patients with micrometastases or isolated tumor cell clusters in the sentinel node do not appear to have a worse disease-free survival than those patients with negative sentinel nodes.

In addition to oncologic settings, lymphoscintigraphy has been used in the diagnosis of the edematous extremity. Interdigital injection of the radiopharmaceutical in the involved extremity or a single injection on the dorsum of the hand or foot generally produces satisfactory visualization of the peripheral lymphatic channels and lymph nodes. Primary (congenital) lymphedema usually presents with only a few lymphatic channels, which are frequently unobstructed. Patients with secondary (obstructive) lymphedema may show evidence of obstructed lymphatics as evidenced by lack of migration of the radiocolloid from the injection site, diffuse dermal activity, or multiple tortuous collateral channels.

Recently, some centers have used needle introduction of a ceramic seed containing 0.1 to 0.3 mCi (3.7 to 11 MBq) of iodine-125 for intraoperative localization of nonpalpable breast lesions. The surgeon is guided to the lesion by using an intraoperative probe detector, similar to that used for sentinel lymph node detection with [99mTc]-filtered sulfur colloid lymphoscintigraphy. If this technique is used, the seed must be retrieved from the pathology specimen and returned to the supplier as radioactive waste.

LABELED MONOCLONAL ANTIBODIES

A number of monoclonal antibodies have been developed that target pancarcinoma antigens shared by various neoplastic lesions, such as carcinoembryonic antigen (CEA), or antigens specific to particular tumor types. These radiopharmaceuticals have met with mixed success in clinical application. The accuracy of the antibody depends in large part on the uniqueness of the antigen targeted and the specificity of the monoclonal antibody in recognizing the antigen. It is rare, however, to discover a monoclonal antibody that is specific to a particular normal or neoplastic tissue type. Cross-reaction with normal or other malignant tissues, with the resultant loss of specificity, is expected even under the best conditions.

The most recent generation of antineoplastic monoclonal antibodies includes indium-111 (^{111}In)- and ^{99m}Tc-labeled antibody fragments to particular tumor antigens. Imaging with these agents usually depends largely on delivering a sufficient number of labeled antibodies by the intravenous route to tumor sites to overcome background activity of various nontargeted normal tissue and organs (especially the liver, kidneys, and lungs), binding to antigens circulating in the plasma, and nonspecific leakage into the extravascular space.

Recent monoclonal imaging radiopharmaceuticals are largely focused on ovarian, prostate, and colon carcinomas. With progress in the development of monoclonal antibodies of higher specificity, an increasing number have achieved approval by the U.S. Food and Drug Administration (FDA). Unfortunately, even those with FDA approval are not widely used because of relatively low sensitivity and specificity in the range of only 50% to 70%. Perhaps the most widely used monoclonal radiopharmaceuticals used at this time are ibritumomab tiuxetan and tositumomab used for lymphoma therapy.

TREATMENT OF LYMPHOMA WITH RADIOIMMUNOTHERAPY

Treatment of lymphomas can be accomplished by labeling a monoclonal antibody against lymphoma antigens with radionuclides. The currently approved agents are ibritumomab tiuxetan (Zevalin) and tositumomab (Bexxar). Medications for the treatment of severe hypersensitivity reactions should be immediately available when using these drugs. Although general descriptions of the procedures are provided, FDA and manufacturers' information should be reviewed in detail before such therapeutic procedures are performed. Both treatments have a diagnostic step and a therapeutic step. In both steps, unlabeled or cold antibody is infused followed by the labeled antibody.

Yttrium-90 (^{90}Y)-labeled anti-CD20 murine (entirely mouse) monoclonal antibody (ibritumomab tiuxetan or Zevalin) has been developed for treatment of disseminated follicular

B-cell (NHL) refractory to stable rituximab therapy, and for treatment of patients with disseminated refractory or relapsed low-grade follicular or transformed B-cell NHL, including patients with rituximab refractory NHL. It is also now approved as a first-line therapy. The monoclonal antibody ibritumomab targets by specific binding of the IgG, kappa-monoclonal antibody to the C20+ antigen found on the surface of malignant as well as normal B lymphocytes. Radioisotopes (^{111}In for imaging or the pure beta emitter ^{90}Y for treatment) can be attached to ibritumomab by the chelating agent, tiuxetan. Yttrium-90 has a beta path length of 5 mm in soft tissue (about 100 to 200 cell diameters) and a physical half-life of 64 hours. The ^{111}In-labeled antibody is used for imaging the patient to determine that the biodistribution of the antibody is appropriate before administration of ^{90}Y-labeled therapeutic dose. The treatment has about a 75% overall response rate and works best in patients who have had fewer prior antineoplastic treatments. Plastic and acrylic materials are appropriate for shielding the syringe containing the beta-emitting ^{90}Y Zevalin, but lead shielding (appropriate for the ^{111}In Zevalin) should not generally be used because it will generate more penetrating bremsstrahlung radiation.

Yttrium-90 Zevalin therapy is appropriate for diffusely disseminated disease, and the procedure occurs over a period of about 1 week as follows. On day 1, the patient receives 650 mg of acetaminophen and 50 mg of diphenhydramine orally followed by unlabeled rituximab (Rituxan) intravenously (250 mg/m^2) at an initial test rate of 50 mg/hr followed in 4 hours by an imaging dose of 5.0 mCi (185 MBq) of ^{111}In-Zevalin injected intravenously over a period of 10 minutes. The purpose of the unlabeled rituximab is to saturate readily available C20 sites in the spleen and on normal circulating B cells. This improves the amount of ^{111}In-Zevalin available to image the tumor. The unlabeled rituximab should not be given as an intravenous bolus or push because deaths have been reported as a result of myocardial infarction, hypoxia, and acute respiratory distress syndrome.

Whole-body images of the ^{111}In-Zevalin are then obtained at 2 to 24 hours and again at 48 to 72 hours to assess biodistribution (Fig. 10-9). These are performed with a large-field-of-view gamma camera using the 172 and

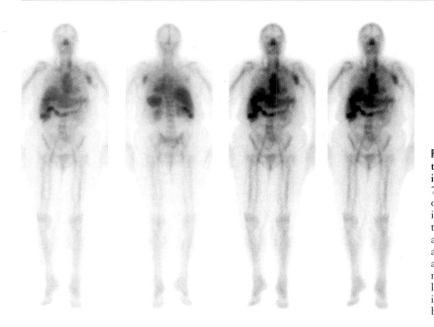

Figure 10-9. ¹¹¹In-ibritumomab tiuxetan (Zevalin) dosimetry images. Anterior and posterior 72-hour postinjection images are obtained to ascertain that there is normal biodistribution before therapy. In this case, expected activity is seen in the liver, bowel activity which changed with time, and tumor activity in the mediastinum and left axilla. Activity in the lungs or kidneys greater than that in the liver or fixed areas in the bowel would be abnormal.

247 keV photopeaks for ¹¹¹In with a 15% to 20% symmetric energy window. The expected biodistribution of Zevalin is easily detectable activity in the blood pool on the first day of imaging, decreasing on the second and third days; moderately high activity in the normal liver and spleen; and low or very low activity in normal kidneys, bladder, and bowel. Biodistribution is considered unacceptable if there is diffuse uptake of ¹¹¹In-Zevalin in the lungs that is more intense than the cardiac blood pool on the first day or more intense than the liver on the second- and third-day images, or activity in the kidneys that is more intense than the liver on the posterior view on the second and third days, or intense uptake throughout normal bowel comparable to the liver on the second- or third-day images. As expected, areas of tumor will also be visualized on these images.

If the biodistribution is acceptable, the ⁹⁰Y Zevalin therapeutic administration is performed on day 7, 8, or 9. On the day of treatment, an infusion of unlabeled rituximab is followed within 4 hours by 0.4 mCi (14.8 MBq)/kg of ⁹⁰Y Zevalin intravenously over a period of 10 minutes. The maximum administered activity is 32 mCi (1.18 GBq). Zevalin should not be administered to patients with a platelet count of less than 100,000/mm³. In patients with platelet counts between 100,000 and 149,000/mm³, the administered activity is reduced to 0.3 mCi (11.1 MBq)/kg. Response rates are about 75%,

but complete response is about 15% only. The most common adverse events are thrombocytopenia and neutropenia, which occur in about 90% of patients. There can be potentially fatal infusion reactions, and the treatment is contraindicated in patients with known type 1 hypersensitivity or anaphylactic reactions to murine proteins. Other infusion reactions include hypotension, angioedema, hypoxia, and bronchospasm.

The dose to caretakers and persons near a patient treated with Zevalin is less than 1 mrem (less than 10 μSv), and the patient can be released immediately after treatment without the need to measure dose rates or retained activity. Urinary excretion of Zevalin is about 7% during the first week. From the start of therapy and for a period of 1 week thereafter, it is recommended that a condom be used during intercourse and deep kissing should be avoided as should other transfers of bodily fluids. Patients are advised to wash their hands thoroughly after using the toilet. Despite the low radiation dose to others, patients are also advised to sleep apart for 4 to 7 days, drink plenty of liquids, wash laundry separately, avoid long trips with others, and limit time spent in public places.

Another anti-CD20 murine (entirely mouse) antibody radioimmunotherapeutic agent, tositumomab (Bexxar), labeled with iodine-131, has also proven useful in the treatment of patients with NHL, particularly those with chemotherapy-refractory disease. Like Zevalin, Bexxar has an initial dosimetric evaluation followed in 7 to 14 days by the therapeutic portion. Before receiving the antibody, the patient receives 650 mg of acetaminophen and 50 mg of diphenhydramine orally. In addition, the thyroid uptake of iodine-131 should be minimized by prior administration of potassium iodide (SSKI). For the dosimetric step, 450 mg of tositumomab in 50 mL of 0.9% sodium chloride is infused intravenously over 60 minutes. This is followed by 35 mg 5 mCi (185 MBq) of iodine 131 tositumomab in 30 mL of 0.9% sodium chloride over 20 minutes. Total body gamma camera counts and whole body images are obtained at 1 hour and before urination. Additional data are collected at 2 to 4 days and 6 to 7 days. Activity initially is seen in the blood pool and to a lesser extent in the liver and spleen. At later times, there is activity in the liver, spleen, thyroid, bladder, kidney, and tumor sites. Biodistribution is assessed. If abnormal, the therapy is not performed. Activity to be administered therapeutically is based upon total body residence time, body mass typically using supplied software and is calculated to give a whole body dose of 75 rads (0.75 Gy). I-131 tositumomab has demonstrated high response rates and long durations of response in patients with relapsed low-grade and transformed low-grade NHL. In clinical trials of Bexxar, the objective response rates ranged from 54% to 71% in pretreated patients. In newly diagnosed patients, the response rate has shown to be about 95%. Because this therapy is based upon the energetic gamma emitter iodine-131, regulations regarding release of patients are especially important.

TREATMENT OF HEPATOMA AND LIVER METASTASES WITH INTRAVASCULAR MICROSPHERES

Palliative treatment of nonresectable colorectal liver metastases and hepatoma with ^{90}Y-labeled glass or resin microspheres (TheraSphere and SIR-Spheres) has grown in use over the last several years. This technique offers more precise targeting of tumor volumes, decreased side effects and morbidity, and decreased radiation of normal tissues. The microspheres are 20 to 60 microns in diameter and are delivered via angiographic catheter into the hepatic artery.

The infusion is done very slowly to avoid reflux into the gastroduodenal artery. The majority of administered activity will localize in the capillary bed of the hypervascular tumor and to a lesser extent in normal parenchyma. The radiation dose is delivered locally because the penetration depth of the Y-90 beta particles is about 2.4 mm only. The lower size limit of the microspheres prevents the majority from passing through the tumor into the venous system, although some do pass through to the lung. The localized microspheres remain in the liver, do not degrade, and after placement are only retrievable by surgery. The product is usually delivered in 5-mL vials with an activity of about 81 mCi (3 GBq). The typical administered activity is about 40 to 70 mCi (1.5 to 2.5 GBq) and is calculated based on the desired absorbed radiation dose. However, the administered activity may be modified if there has been concomitant chemotherapy.

Initial patient assessment includes issues related to tumor resectability, extent of disease in the liver, extent of extrahepatic disease, hepatic vascular anatomy, arteriovenous shunting, liver and renal function, and the general constitutional status of the patient. Radiologic workup consists of a hepatic angiogram, combined angiogram CT scan, and embolization of the gastroduodenal artery or other vessel that might result in inadvertent delivery of microspheres. Before actual Y-90 microsphere delivery, an infusion is performed using ^{99m}Tc-macroaggregated albumin with imaging to assess any arteriovenous shunting through the tumor vascular bed and thus to the lungs or inadvertent delivery to other nontumor locations, as well to ensure proper positioning of the infusion catheter. If there is possible delivery of the microspheres through small arteries to the stomach, duodenum, or gallbladder, the procedure should be abandoned to avoid serious radiation damage to those organs. Treatment is questionable if there is a large amount of extrahepatic disease and the liver burden is not the life-threatening problem. If there is arteriovenous shunting of more than 10% to the lung, the dose must be reduced to prevent radiation pneumonitis, and shunting of greater than 20% is a contraindication to this form of therapy. Portal vein thrombosis is also a contraindication. After the microspheres are placed, it is possible to use SPECT imaging of

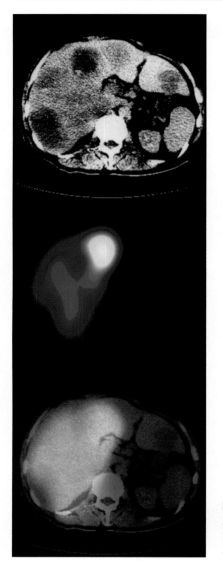

Figure 10-10. **Yttrium-90 (^{90}Y) microsphere therapy.** *Top,* CT scan in this patient with hepatoma shows multiple low density lesions. *Middle,* After hepatic artery injection of ^{90}Y microspheres, a SPECT image can be obtained by using the bremsstrahlung radiation. *Bottom,* SPECT/CT fusion image shows where the microspheres actually localized.

the bremsstrahlung radiation from the ^{90}Y to confirm localization (Fig. 10-10).

Environmental contamination with ^{90}Y microspheres should be taken seriously. The microspheres are very easily spread by foot traffic and hand contamination. Patients may travel home after the procedure, and at 5 hours after implantation, the dose rate at a distance of 0.5 m from a patient is about 1 mrem (10 μSv)/hr. No special precautions are required for linens and clothing, but there is a small amount of activity that may appear in the urine, and, as a result, for the first 24 hours, a toilet (not a urinal) should be used and flushed twice. Many jurisdictions have activity restrictions in the event of patient demise. Typical limits are set for autopsy (4 mCi [150 MBq]), cremation/burial (27 mCi [1 GBq]), and embalming (4 mCi [150 MBq]).

PEARLS & PITFALLS

- Gallium-67 scans are uncommonly performed. For inflammatory lesions, scans are performed 24 hours after injection and for tumors, at 48 to 72 hours.

- A gallium scan can most often be recognized by noting activity in the lacrimal glands, nasopharynx, liver, bowel, and skeleton. The images are usually count-poor (coarse).

- Lymphoma (especially Hodgkin and higher-grade lymphomas) and hepatoma are particularly gallium-avid tumors. Other tumors (such as lung cancer) also accumulate gallium. However, ^{18}F-FDG PET/CT scans are now generally preferred for staging and restaging lymphoma.

- Gallium-67 may localize in the parotid glands after radiotherapy or chemotherapy, and in the thymus after chemotherapy, especially in children and young adults. Reactive thymic changes should not be mistaken for recurrent mediastinal lymphoma.

- The commonly used cardiac perfusion agents thallium-201 and ^{99m}Tc-sestamibi accumulate nonspecifically in many tumors. Sestamibi accumulates avidly in cells with high mitochondria content.

- Many breast cancers, parathyroid adenomas, and metastatic thyroid cancers accumulate the cardiac agent ^{99m}Tc-sestamibi. Some benign breast conditions accumulate this agent.

- Indium-111 octreotide is avidly accumulated by tumors with somatostatin types 2 and 5 receptors, including pheochromocytoma, carcinoid, neuroblastoma, gastrinoma, islet cell tumors, pituitary adenomas, medullary thyroid cancer, and small-cell lung cancer. Most neuroendocrine tumors are well differentiated and slow growing and therefore have poor uptake on ^{18}F-FDG PET scans. Octreotide scans can be recognized by high activity in spleen and kidneys.

- ^{123}I-MIBG is accumulated by pheochromocytomas, paragangliomas, and neuroblastomas. MIBG scans can be recognized by activity in the liver, bowel, parotid glands, and sometimes the thyroid and heart.

- Kaposi sarcoma is thallium-avid but does not accumulate gallium. Lymphoma concentrates both agents.

- Lymphoscintigraphy is performed with intradermal or peritumoral injection of filtered ^{99m}Tc-sulfur colloid. The purpose is to identify the sentinel node, which is the lymph node most likely to be involved with metastatic tumor. Regardless of tumor quadrant location, the vast majority of sentinel nodes in breast cancer patients are located in the axilla.

SUGGESTED READINGS

Cole WC, Barrickman J, Bloodworth G. Essential role of nuclear medicine technology in tositumomab and 131-tositumomab therapeutic regimen for non-Hodgkin's lymphoma. J Nucl Med Technol 2006;34:67-73.

Intenzo CM, Jabbour S, Lin HC, et al. Scintigraphic imaging of body neuroendocrine tumors. RadioGraphics 2007; 27:1335-69.

Hindie E, Groheux D, Brenot-Rossi I, et al. The sentinel node procedure in breast cancer: Nuclear medicine as the starting point. J, Nucl. Med 2011;52:405-14.

Krynyckyi BR, Kim CK, Goyenechea MR, et al. Clinical breast lymphoscintigraphy: Optimal techniques for performing studies, image atlas, and analysis of images. RadioGraphics 2004;24:121-45.

Kwekkeboom DJ, Krenning EP. Somatostatin receptor imaging. Semin Nucl Med 2002;32:84-91.

Scarsbrook AF, Ganeshan A, Statham J, et al. Anatomic and functional imaging of metastatic carcinoid tumors. RadioGraphics 2007;27:455-76.

Schaffer NG, Ma J, Huang P, et al. Radioimmunotherapy in non-Hodgkin lymphoma: Opinions of U.S. medical oncologists and hematologists. J Nucl Med 2010;51:987-94.

Sharp SE, Shulkin BL, Gelfand MJ, et al. ^{123}I-MIBG scintigraphy and ^{18}F-FDG PET in neuroblastoma. J Nucl Med 2009;50:1237-43.

Society of Nuclear Medicine practice guideline for breast scintigraphy with breast specific gamma cameras. Version 1.0, approved 2010. http://www.snm.org. Accessed July 3, 2011.

Spies SM. Imaging and dosing in radioimmunotherapy with yttrium-90 ibritumomab tiuxetan (Zevalin). Semin Nucl Med 2004;34:10-3.

Wahl RL. Tositumomab and 131I therapy in non-Hodgkin's lymphoma. J Nucl Med 2005;46:S128-40.

Uren RF, Howman-Giles R, Thompson JF. Patterns of lymphatic drainage from the skin in patients with melanoma. J Nucl Med 2003;44:570-82.

Zhu X. Radiation safety considerations radioimmunotherapy with yttrium-90 ibritumomab tiuxetan (Zevalin). Semin Nucl Med 2004;34:20-3.

11

^{18}F-FDG PET/CT Neoplasm Imaging

INDICATIONS
PATIENT PREPARATION FOR ^{18}F-FDG IMAGING
NORMAL ^{18}F-FDG DISTRIBUTION
   AND VARIANTS

QUALITATIVE IMAGE INTERPRETATION
PET IMAGE QUANTITATION
WHOLE-BODY ^{18}F-FDG PET/CT NEOPLASM
   IMAGING

Positron emission tomography (PET) in clinical practice has been replaced by positron emission tomography/computed tomography (PET/CT). The most commonly used radiopharmaceutical is ^{18}F fluorodeoxyglucose (FDG). There are other PET agents for tumors, but they are not currently in mainstream clinical use. PET physics and basic properties of FDG have been discussed in Chapter 1, and PET/CT instrumentation and quality control (QC) have been presented in Chapter 2. Use of FDG for brain and thyroid neoplastic applications are also included in Chapters 3 and 4, respectively. FDG imaging in patients with infections and inflammatory conditions is covered in Chapter 12. PET/CT skeletal scintigraphy using ^{18}F sodium-fluoride is presented in Chapter 8.

This chapter is devoted to PET/CT imaging with ^{18}F-FDG and includes image interpretation and quantitation in the setting of neoplasm imaging. While FDG PET/CT is a powerful tool for neoplasm imaging, the sensitivity and specificity vary widely among tumor types. In addition, while many tumors are FDG-avid, in some cases, PET/CT may not be helpful in determining local staging, whereas, in other cases, PET/CT is helpful for staging but not for follow-up.

INDICATIONS

PET/CT in the setting of neoplasm is useful for a number of indications, especially when it replaces other conventional imaging procedures, guides, or obviates the need for invasive diagnostic or therapeutic procedures, or results in a change in patient management and/or treatment outcome.

Depending on the type of neoplasm, PET/CT may be used for diagnosis (such as with solitary pulmonary nodules and patients with metastases from unknown primary tumors), staging and restaging disease, monitoring therapeutic regimen, and in patient follow-up in a number of settings. Table 11-1 compares the relative values of common imaging procedures (including PET/CT) when diagnosing or assessing a neoplastic disease.

PATIENT PREPARATION FOR ^{18}F-FDG IMAGING

The biodistribution of ^{18}F-FDG is affected by blood glucose levels. Although there can be competitive displacement of the ^{18}F-FDG by high levels of blood glucose, the primary adverse effect of elevated serum glucose is the resultant elevation of insulin levels. Patients should fast for 4 to 6 hours before a scan (preferably overnight) so that basal insulin levels will allow for optimal images. Elevated insulin levels degrade scans by increasing muscle uptake of FDG. In general, serum glucose levels should be below 150 mg/dL, but glucose levels up to 200 mg/dL are usually acceptable for satisfactory image quality. Imaging diabetic patients can be especially challenging. In type 1 diabetes, insulin is not recommended, and imaging is usually performed in the morning after an overnight fast. In type 2 diabetes, short-acting insulin can be used, but this increases muscle uptake. If possible, regular insulin should not be used 2 to 4 hours before the examination. In fact, in general, the use of insulin is best avoided altogether.

Because there is significant excretion of ^{18}F-FDG via the kidneys (and ^{18}F-FDG is not reabsorbed as glucose is), good hydration is

TABLE 11-1 Relative Value* and Sensitivity of Various Imaging Procedures for Staging and Follow-Up of Various Tumors

TUMOR	18F-FDG PET/CT	99mTc-MDP or 18F-NaF	OTHER NM	RADIOGRAPHS	ULTRASOUND	CT OR MRI
Lymphoma	+++	Rare	Gallium +	Rare		+++
Prostate	Poor	+++		+	++	+
Melanoma	+++ For distant metastases; poor for local disease	+	Sentinel node ++	+		++ CT for small lung nodules
Lung (non-small cell)	+++	++		+		+++
Myeloma	++	+		++		+++ MRI
Ovary	++ 70%-90%				+++ Also for screening	+++ 95% MRI, 50%-90% CT
Uterus	++ 90%				+	+++ 90%
Cervix	++ 75%-90%					++
Colorectal	+++ Mostly for regional and distant metastases	Rare		Barium enema poor	Endoscopic +++	+++ MRI detects smaller hepatic metastases than PET/CT
Bladder	Poor	+				++
Kidney	+	+		++		+++
Thyroid	++	Rare	123I-NaI	++	++	+
Thyroid medullary cancer	+++ 96%		Octreotide 41%			++
Head and neck	+++	Rare		+		+++
Esophagus	++ Not for local spread; use for regional and distant disease				For T staging endoscopic +++	+++
Stomach	++ 50% Not for local spread; use for regional and distant disease	Rare		UGI poor	For T staging endoscopic +++	+++
Osteosarcoma	++	+++		++		+++
Breast	++ Not for primary or axillary disease; use for distant and chemotherapy response	+++	Sentinel node ++	+++ Mammography	+	+

Tumor					
Hepatoma	+ 30% have uptake at staging	Rare	Gallium +		+++
Pancreas	++	Rare		Endoscopic ++	+++
Carcinoid	Poor	90% for bone metastases	^{111}In-Octreotide 80%-95% / ^{123}I-MIBG 35%-85%		+
Gastrinoma			Octreotide 75%-93%		+
VIPoma	++		^{111}In-Octreotide 88%		+
Poorly differentiated neuroendocrine	++		No		
Benign pheochromocytoma	+ 60%		^{123}I-MIBG 85%-100% / ^{111}In-Octreotide 65%-75%		+++
Malignant pheochromocytoma	++ 75%-85%		^{123}I-MIBG 85%-100% / ^{111}In-Octreotide 87%		+++
Paraganglioma	++ 74%-88%		^{111}In-Octreotide 94% / ^{123}I-MIBG 57%-78%		95%-100% localized; 45% for metastases
Neuroblastoma	Stage 1 and 2 only	Stage 4	^{123}I-MIBG for bone and bone marrow disease		++

CT, computed tomography; ^{18}F-FDG, Fluorine-18 fluorodeoxyglucose; ^{18}F-NaF, fluorine-18 sodium fluoride; MRI, magnetic resonance imaging; NM, Nuclear medicine; PET, positron emission tomography; ^{99m}Tc-MDP, technetium-99m methylene diphosphonate.
*Value (+ [low] to +++ [high]) is the opinion of the authors, based upon clinical practice and the peer-reviewed literature.

recommended. Accumulation in the bladder has prompted some to recommend catheterization of patients with suspected pelvic pathology, but, in practice, this is usually unnecessary, especially if the patient has voided before beginning the scan and if interpretation includes using a three-dimensional rotating maximum intensity projection (MIP) display. Diuretics may be helpful in some patients when clearing activity from the kidneys and ureters is crucial.

The typical administered activity for ¹⁸F-FDG is in the range of 10 to 25 mCi (370-925 MBq) or about 0.14 mCi (5.5 MBq)/kg. Lower activities may be necessary on some older dedicated PET scanners (such as those using NaI detectors), which cannot process the higher count rates. The injection is intravenous, and the line should be flushed with 20 to 30 mL of saline. Portacaths or indwelling catheters should not be used unless absolutely necessary because retention in the reservoirs and catheter tips can cause errors in evaluation of the chest. If intravenous injection is not possible, ¹⁸F-FDG can be administered orally. If axillary or supraclavicular lymph node involvement is a consideration (e.g., breast cancer or upper-extremity melanomas), injection should be made in the upper extremity on the opposite side of the lesion. Imaging is typically performed 45 to 60 minutes after injection of ¹⁸F-FDG. However, a longer waiting period of up to 2 to 3 hours allows for better uptake in lesions, especially when imaging tumors are known to have a lower avidity for FDG, including treated lesions. The patient should not talk or chew gum for 30 minutes after injection of the ¹⁸F-FDG because this causes increased uptake in the muscles of the larynx and pharynx and the mastication musculature. For brain imaging, the patient should be injected in a dimly lit, quiet room to avoid excess brain stimulation, which will alter FDG distribution.

The patient should wear a gown and pajama pants, and all metallic objects should be removed. With dedicated PET scanners, the patient should normally be positioned supine with the arms down and knees at rest. The scan is obtained during shallow breathing. With PET/CT scanners, the patient is usually positioned with the arms up except when the suspected pathology is in the head or neck. In this case, the arms should be down. In some cases when pathology is suspected in both the neck and the chest, it may be necessary to perform scans with the arms in both positions to detect small lesions. In patients with neck muscle pain, muscle relaxants (e.g., Valium) may be useful to decrease interfering activity in neck musculature. While strenuous exercise just prior to ¹⁸F-FDG administration or during the uptake period may increase regional muscle activity, treadmill stress for myocardial perfusion scans performed approximately 4 hours before a PET/CT scan have shown no significant effect on the quality of the PET study.

NORMAL ¹⁸F-FDG DISTRIBUTION AND VARIANTS
General
The percentage of a ¹⁸F-FDG injected dose in major tissues is approximately as follows: urine (second hour) 20% to 40%, brain 7%, liver 4.5%, heart 3.3%, red marrow 1.7%, kidneys 1.3%, and lungs 0.9%. It is important to know the normal distribution and normal variants in ¹⁸F-FDG accumulation (Fig. 11-1) so as to not confuse them with actual pathology (Tables 11-2, 11-3, and 11-4).

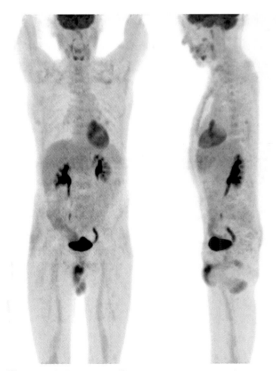

Figure 11-1. Normal ¹⁸F-FDG PET scan. On these anterior and right lateral MIP images, normal physiologic activity is seen in the brain, heart, urinary system, and, to a lesser extent, in other tissues. The high level of heart activity indicates the patient had not been fasting. *MIP,* Maximum intensity projection.

Brain

The gray matter of the brain (cortex, basal ganglia, and thalami) is always high in 18F-FDG uptake because the cells of gray matter have a high metabolic rate and use glucose as their primary substrate. When acquiring scans of the face and neck, it is important to exclude the brain from the acquisition to be able to see abnormalities that do not have as much activity as gray matter.

Vocal Cords

In the neck, activity near the vocal cords is seen if the patient was talking at the time of injection (Fig. 11-2). The activity can be minimized by having the patient remain silent during injection and during the early uptake of 18F-FDG. Speaking during the uptake period may also increase 18F-FDG

activity in the tongue. After lingual or laryngeal surgery, asymmetric activity can often be seen in the residual intact musculature and be difficult to differentiate from residual or recurrent tumor. An intense 18F-FDG focus in the lower neck just lateral to the midline may be caused by compensatory activation of an intact laryngeal muscle when the contralateral vocal cord is paralyzed because of any cause, but frequently by mediastinal tumor involvement of the recurrent laryngeal nerve.

Tonsils, Salivary Glands, and Thyroid

The tonsils (especially the palatine tonsils), lymphoid tissue at Waldeyer ring, and the parotid and submandibular glands can normally accumulate 18F-FDG. This activity usually decreases

TABLE 11-2 **18F-FDG Levels in Various Normal Tissues (SUV$_{mean}$ values where available)**

TISSUE LEVEL	COMMENT	TISSUE LEVEL	COMMENT
High Tissue Level		**Low Tissue Level**	
Brain (cerebellum) 8.2	High in gray matter, low in white matter	Thyroid 1.4	Can be high with Graves disease or thyroiditis
Tonsils 3.4-4.1		Stomach 1.6-2.3	Can be focally intense
Kidneys, ureters, bladder	Due to excretion	Pancreas 1.5	
Ascending colon (contents)	Usually tubular in distribution	Rectum and colon 1.0-1.6	Contents may be much higher
Myocardium 4.3	If fasting; if not fasting, SUV can exceed 20	Adrenal gland 1.4	
		Vertebrae 1.6	
Brown or USA fat	Frequently females and in cold environment	Red marrow 1.0	Can be high after stimulating agents
Uterus	During menses	Penis	
Moderate Tissue Level		Vagina	
Submandibular glands 2.2	Decreases with age	Ovaries	Depends on menstrual cycle; lowest after menstruation
Liver 2.1			
Blood 2.3		**No Activity Usually Seen**	
Testes 2.7		Skeletal muscle 0.9	Much higher if active or tense
Mild Tissue Level		Lung 0.4-0.7	
Aorta	Usually bandlike in thoracic aorta	Breast 0.6	More in young women and with lactation
Spleen 1.8		Lymph nodes	
Nasopharynx 1.7		Ovaries	Postmenopausal
Esophagus 1.9			

Adapted from Wang Y, Chiu E, Rosenberg J, et al: Standardized uptake value atlas: Characterization of physiological 18F-FDG uptake in normal tissues. Mol Imaging Biol 2007;9:83-90.
  USA, Uptake in the supraclavicular area.

TABLE 11–3 **Accumulation of ^{18}F-FDG in Abnormal Conditions**

TISSUE/ORGAN	ACTIVITY LEVEL	COMMENTS
Brain		
Ictal seizure focus	High	Very rarely done due to need to remain still and poor temporal resolution of PET
Interictal seizure focus	Low	Review temporal lobes
Radiation necrosis	Low	
Recurrent tumor	Variable	If increased activity suspect recurrence
Dementia—Alzheimer	Low posterior temporoparietal cortical activity	Often identical pattern to Parkinson dementia
Dementia—(FTLD-Pick)	Low frontal lobes	
Dementia—Multi-infarct	Scattered small areas of decreased activity	
Cerebellar diaschisis ("crossed")	Low area in one hemisphere	Low activity in cerebellum contralateral to supratentorial stroke, tumor, trauma, etc.
Huntington disease	Low activity in caudate nucleus and putamen	
Heart		
Infarct	Low	Minimal myocardial activity if patient has been fasting; very intense if meal with large amounts of glucose recently ingested
Hibernating	Normal or increased	
Stunned	Normal or increased	
Neoplasm		
Head and neck	Variable: with cell type	
Brain metastases	Low	Poor sensitivity against normal high activity of gray matter
Thyroid	Moderate	Especially helpful in poorly differentiated lesions with low or absent iodine-131 uptake
Lung	Moderate	Low in bronchoalveolar cell cancer, carcinoid, well-differentiated cancer, and mucinous metastases
Breast	Moderate	
Hepatoma	Variable: often low	
Esophagus	High	Usually focal, not linear or diffuse
Stomach	Variable	Interfering normal activity
Colorectal	High	Usually focal, not tubular
Melanoma	High	
Lymphoma	Variable	Higher in aggressive forms
Renal and bladder	Variable: often low	Interfering normal activity
Skeletal metastases	Variable	
Uterine	Variable	
Cervical	Variable	
Testicular	Variable	
Prostate	Low or absent	
Infection		
Pneumonia	Moderate to high	
Cellulitis	Moderate	
Osteomyelitis	High	
Granulomas		
Sarcoidosis	High	If active disease
Tuberculosis	High	If active disease
Trauma		
Recent surgery	Variable	
Fracture	Variable with age of onset	
Aortic graft	Moderate	
Radiation therapy	Moderate	May be increased for up to several months

FTLD, Frontotemporal lobe dementia.

TABLE 11–4 ^{18}F-FDG PET Imaging in Oncology

ANATOMIC REGION	NORMAL DISTRIBUTION	NORMAL VARIANTS	BENIGN LESIONS THAT MAY HAVE UPTAKE POTENTIAL FALSE (+)	LOW-UPTAKE LESIONS POTENTIAL FALSE (−)
Head/Neck	Brain: gray matter, cortex, basal ganglia Neck: soft palate, tongue, vocal cords, palatine tonsils, adenoids, parotids, salivary glands, thyroid Neck muscles: laryngeal, masticators, genioglossus	Head: extraocular muscles Neck: brown fat	Head: sinusitis Neck: thyroiditis, Graves disease, goiter, benign thyroid nodules, Warthin tumor, reactive lymph nodes	Brain metastases Low-grade gliomas
Chest	Mediastinum: heart muscle and atria, thymus in children and young adults, esophagus	Mediastinum: thymic rebound, base of ventricles, brown fat Axilla: lymph nodes (dose infiltration) Breast: premenopausal, hormone therapy	Aortic atherosclerosis Esophagitis, Barrett esophagus, after esophageal dilation procedure Hiatal hernia Empyema Pleurodesis Pneumonia Radiation pneumonitis Granulomatous diseases: tuberculosis, sarcoidosis, histoplasmosis, Aspergillosis, coccidioidomycosis, *Mycobacterium avium-intracellulare*, atypical mycobacteria Reactive lymph nodes Breast: inflammation, biopsy site, mastitis, fibroadenomas (low), gynecomastia	Lung: bronchioloalveolar cancer, carcinoid, solitary pulmonary nodule <1 cm Breast: lobular carcinoma, carcinoma in situ, tubular carcinoma
Abdomen	Kidneys Ureters Bladder Stomach Small bowel Colon Liver Spleen (low)	Brown fat: perinephric	Vascular bypass grafts Colonic Adenoma/polyps Adrenal hypertrophy Pancreatitis	MALT Liver: hepatocellular cancer (40%-50%), small lesions Kidney: renal cell cancer
Pelvis	Ureters Bladder Bowel Uterus (menses) Testes Penis (low)		Uterine fibroids Endometriosis Corpus luteum cysts Vascular bypass grafts	

Continued

TABLE 11-4	^{18}F-FDG PET Imaging in Oncology—cont'd			
ANATOMIC REGION	**NORMAL DISTRIBUTION**	**NORMAL VARIANTS**	**BENIGN LESIONS THAT MAY HAVE UPTAKE POTENTIAL FALSE (+)**	**LOW-UPTAKE LESIONS POTENTIAL FALSE (−)**
Skeleton/ Marrow	Skeletal muscle Brown fat: supraclavicular, paravertebral, intercostal	Marrow: G-CSF Tx (intense) Rad Tx (decreased)	Inflammation/infection Arthritis Phlebitis Spondylodiscitis Pigmented villonodular synovitis Benign bone lesions: fibrous dysplasia, Paget disease, nonossifying fibroma, giant-cell tumor, eosinophilic granuloma, aneurysmal bone cyst, enchondroma, osteomyelitis	Chondrosarcoma Plasmacytoma Low-grade sarcomas (osseous and soft tissue) Sclerotic metastases
Skin			Inflammation/infection Wound healing	
Any location		Percutaneous lines/tubes	Inflammation/infection Granulomatous diseases Postradiation change Wound healing Reactive lymph nodes Tense musculature Resolving hematoma Ostomies Vascular grafts Atheromatous disease Healing fractures Arthritis	Small lesions, nodal micrometastases Low-grade tumors, especially lymphomas (small lymphocytic cell) Metastases adjacent to fluorodeoxyglucose– avid primary cancer or high activity organs

with patient age and should be symmetric. Thyroid activity is normally not seen. However, mild diffuse activity can occasionally be seen in normal glands. Significantly increased activity can occur with thyroiditis or Graves disease (Fig. 11-3). An enlarged inhomogeneous gland should raise the possibility of a nodular goiter. An unexpected intense focal area raises the possibility of malignancy (20% to 30%), and further evaluation should be performed.

Thymus

Thymic activity can be seen normally in children but also occasionally in young adults up to the age of about 30 years. It is very uncommon in adults older than 30 years. Increased activity also can be seen as a result of thymic rebound after chemotherapy in children and young adults but also occasionally in older adults (Fig. 11-4).

Muscle and Brown Fat

In the resting skeletal muscle, ^{18}F-FDG uptake is usually low. Increased activity is often seen in the shoulder girdle (especially teres minor) and upper back if the patient was tense at the time of injection or within 30 minutes after injection. Muscle relaxants or antianxiety medications may be helpful in some patients, especially when imaging the neck, where the strap muscles often demonstrate increased activity. Heavy exercise within the 24 hours before the examination can increase muscle uptake as can elevated insulin levels (Fig. 11-5).

Activity can also be seen normally in the diaphragmatic crura, intercostal muscles, psoas muscles, thoracic paravertebral muscles, forearms, and muscles of mastication. In patients with severe dyspnea, there is often increased activity in intercostal muscles as a result of the increased work of breathing (see Fig. 11-2). At any location, symmetry and a diffuse or typical linear configuration are often helpful to distinguish normal muscle activity from pathology.

Activity in the supraclavicular region is typically a result of one of three causes: muscle activity, activity in lymph nodes resulting from pathology, or accumulation in fat. Muscle activity is seen in about 5% of patients and

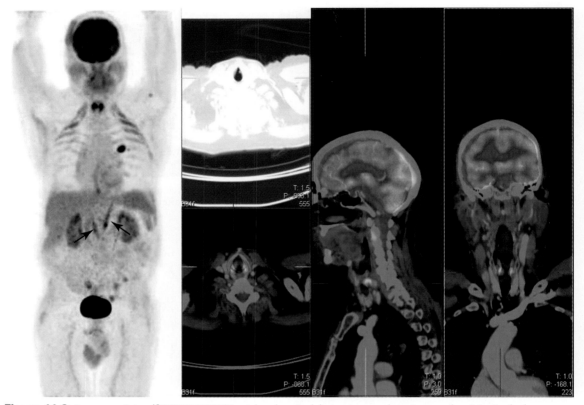

Figure 11-2. **Larynx activity.** ¹⁸F-FDG PET/CT axial and sagittal fusion images show increased activity in the larynx as a result of talking during or shortly after the injection. There is also activity from a left lung cancer and intercostal muscles as well as diaphragmatic crural activity (*arrows*) as a result of labored breathing caused by chronic obstructive pulmonary disease.

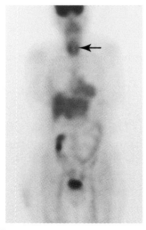

Figure 11-3. **Thyroid activity.** Coronal whole-body ¹⁸F-FDG PET image shows activity in the thyroid. This can occasionally be seen in normal glands, but significantly increased activity may occur in thyroiditis or Graves disease.

is usually linear and bilateral. Activity in fat occurs in about 2% to 5% of patients (mostly female) and in about 15% of children. The reason for uptake in fat in this location is unknown, but FDG is thought to accumulate in foci of brown fat (also called *USA-fat;* USA stands for *u*ptake in the *s*upraclavicular *a*rea). Uptake in this fat is typically symmetric, more often multifocal than linear, and located in low Hounsfield unit areas typical of fat on PET/CT images (Fig. 11-6). Standardized uptake values (SUVs) can range from 2 to 20, with the mean often about 7 or more (well above the threshold value worrisome for malignancy). Uptake appears to be related to adrenergic stimulation of muscles such as during periods of anxiety or shivering in response to ambient temperature and is seen more often with an acute lowering of temperature in the winter months or even in a cold, air-conditioned room. In patients with activity in neck fat, about one third will also show focal activity in perinephric fat, in mediastinal fat, and in paravertebral and posterior intercostal patterns (Fig. 11-7). Several interventions have been suggested to prevent uptake of FDG in brown fat, although with coregistered images of PET/CT, this is not necessary.

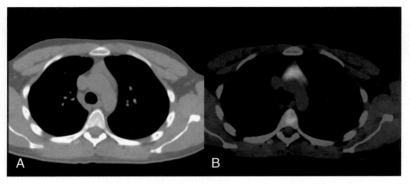

Figure 11-4. **Thymus activity. A,** The thymus is clearly seen anterior to the aortic arch on the CT scan. **B,** Increased FDG activity is evident on the PET/CT scan. In this case, it was a result of thymic rebound after chemotherapy.

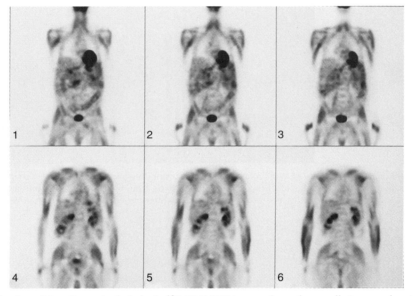

Figure 11-5. **Muscle activity.** Coronal whole-body ^{18}F-FDG PET images show abnormally increased activity in muscles of the arms and thighs as a result of increased insulin levels. This also can occur as a result of heavy exercise within 24 hours before the examination.

Heart

Left ventricular ^{18}F-FDG activity can be intense or faint. Although the myocardium uses fatty acids as its primary substrate, it will switch to glucose if high levels are available or if the patient has been exercising. A large amount of cardiac activity often means that the patient did not fast in preparation for the examination, and the heart is actively using glucose (see Fig. 11-1). Intense cardiac activity is usually not a problem but can interfere with a diagnosis of pathology located adjacent to the heart.

After 12 hours of fasting, the heart switches from glucose to fatty acid metabolism, and the activity becomes the same as the background blood pool. The switch from intense activity to faint activity is often not uniform, and the base of the heart tends to be the last section to convert from glucose metabolism. It is important not to interpret lack of activity near the left ventricular apex as an infarct without additional information. It is also important not to mistake isolated activity at the base of the heart for pathology such as abnormal mediastinal lymph nodes. The right ventricle usually has faint activity when compared with that of the left ventricle, unless there is right ventricular hypertrophy. Atrial activity is not infrequently noted, especially in the right atrium. This can be spotty and, again, should not be mistaken for abnormal lymph nodes.

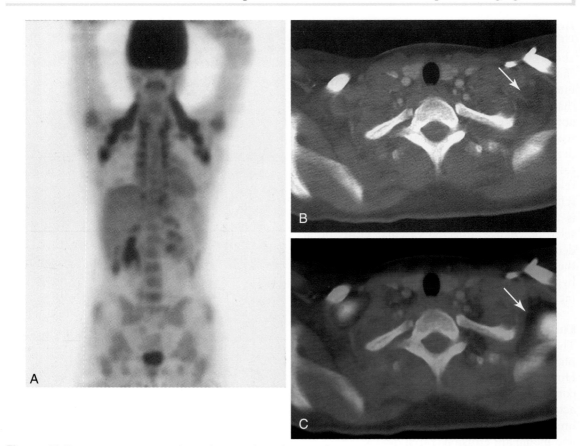

Figure 11-6. **Brown or USA (uptake in the supraclavicular area) fat. A,** Coronal whole-body ¹⁸F-FDG PET image in a young female shows intense (but normal) symmetric activity in the neck and axilla. This can be mistakenly diagnosed as lymphoma. **B,** Transaxial CT and **C,** ¹⁸F-FDG PET/CT fusion images show that the increased metabolic activity is in an area that is clearly fat density (*arrows*).

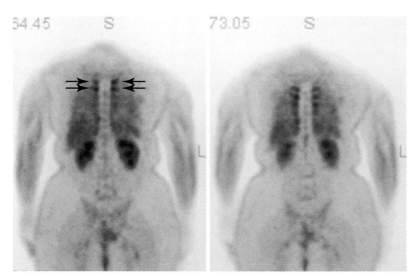

Figure 11-7. **Paraspinous fat.** Coronal whole-body ¹⁸F-FDG PET images show intense (but normal) activity in paraspinous fat (*arrows*).

Aorta

¹⁸F-FDG activity is seen in the aortic wall of about 60% to 70% of older adults. The uptake can be focal or bandlike and is usually more intense in the lower descending thoracic aorta than in the ascending portion or arch. Thoracic aortic uptake appears to be more common in women and patients with hyperlipidemia. The degree of activity appears to be unrelated to calcium deposition but has been shown to correlate with macrophage content in the atherosclerotic plaques. It is possible that the uptake is depicting the metabolic activity of atherosclerotic change. Infected vascular grafts often demonstrate increased activity, conforming to the shape of the grafts. However, aortofemoral bypass grafts routinely have some mild diffuse increased activity for years even if not infected.

Lungs

The lungs have relatively low uptake, appearing photopenic on attenuation-corrected images. However, on images that are not attenuation corrected, they will appear to have increased activity. Pleural effusions from congestive failure will not accumulate activity, but empyemas and malignant effusions often do.

Breast

Breast activity slightly above that in the blood pool is normal and is more common in young women and in postmenopausal women on hormone replacement therapy. It will be greater in lactating females (Fig. 11-8), but the activity is in the breast tissue and not in the milk. It is not necessary to discontinue breastfeeding in these patients. However, there may be significant dose concerns to the baby from direct gamma emission from the mother, and, as a result, some authors recommend that breastfeeding be suspended for 8 hours after the injection. The ¹⁸F-FDG activity in the breast is related to the glandular volume and density. As expected, fatty breasts have less activity than do dense breasts. However, even in dense breasts the SUV is almost always less than 1.5 (much below the 2.5 value that may suggest malignant tissue).

Gastrointestinal Tract

Activity in the bowel is exceedingly variable in terms of both intensity and location. The ¹⁸F-FDG activity in the bowel is located in the mucosa

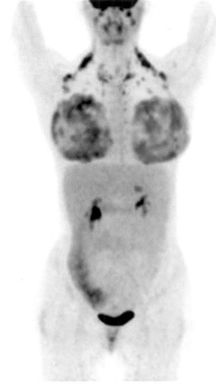

Figure 11-8. **Breast activity.** An anterior whole-body ¹⁸F-FDG PET image shows intense activity in both breasts in this lactating female. The activity is in the breast tissue and is not secreted in the breast milk. There is also incidental activity in "brown fat" in the supraclavicular and lower cervical region.

and not in the luminal contents. The FDG is not excreted by the liver and biliary system into the bowel. Low-level activity is sometimes seen in the normal esophagus and should be uniform throughout its length. Fusiform or focal esophageal activity should raise the possibility of pathology, including neoplasm, although esophagitis can produce a similar appearance.

Activity in the stomach is often greater than that in the liver, and a contracted normal stomach or hiatal hernia can appear very intense, causing difficulties in evaluation of esophagogastric junction and gastric neoplasms. Focal activity in the stomach should prompt a search for a gastric mass on the CT. Small-bowel activity is usually less than that seen in the colon and is commonly located in the lower abdomen or pelvis. Activity in the small bowel tends to be faint, but activity in the colon can normally be quite intense. It is often essential to view the rotating

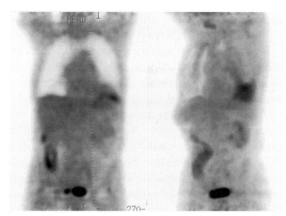

Figure 11-9. **Normal bowel activity.** *Left,* On an anterior whole-body image, the focus of ¹⁸F-FDG activity in the right lower quadrant (ascending colon) may be mistaken for pathology. *Right,* Oblique view taken from the rotating whole-body image shows the area of activity to be tubular in shape.

three-dimensional display (MIP image) to be able to distinguish normal colonic activity from pathology. The pattern of uptake in the colon may be diffuse, segmental, or nodular. It is usually highest in the cecum and ascending colon (Fig. 11-9) presumably because of the higher concentration of lymphocytes in this region. Diffuse activity is most often non-pathologic, whereas segmental uptake may imply inflammation. Nodular focal intense uptake is seen in about 1% of patients having studies for non-gastrointestinal reasons. This has a positive predictive value of 70% to 85% because of lesions such as polyps, villous adenomas, and carcinoma. Approximately 30% of such findings will prove to be malignant, and the majority of the remainder will be premalignant.

The liver typically has more activity than the background blood pool. Focal nodular hyperplasia can concentrate FDG. The gallbladder is not usually seen, and, if there is activity in this area, it should not be assumed to be normal or a normal variant. The pancreas is not normally seen.

Genitourinary Tract

Activity is almost always seen in the urinary tract because about 40% of the administered activity is excreted via the kidneys in the first 2 hours. The upper pole calyces, renal pelvis, and ureters are easily visualized on ¹⁸F-FDG PET scans (Fig. 11-10). Ureteral activity can be discontinuous because of peristalsis and can mimic pathologic foci. Bladder activity is

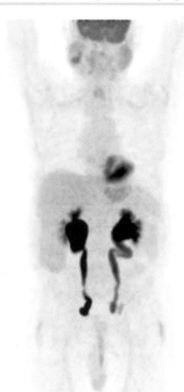

Figure 11-10. **Hydronephrosis.** Anterior whole-body ¹⁸F-FDG image shows marked activity in the renal collecting systems and ureters as a result of obstruction from a bladder cancer. Normal FDG excretion via the kidneys can severely limit FDG use for local evaluation of genitourinary malignancies.

usually intense. On a contrasted PET/CT scan, the heavier iodine contrast is usually dependent with the FDG layered anteriorly. In patients with suspected pelvic pathology, catheterization may be warranted to minimize or eliminate interfering bladder activity, but, in practice, this is usually not necessary. Activity can be present in the normal uterus (especially early in menstruation). Activity is also usually seen in the testes and, to a lesser extent, in the penis.

Bone Marrow, Lymph Nodes, and Spleen

Bone marrow activity is usually seen at levels that are slightly higher than the blood pool and about the same as the liver. Bone marrow activity can be increased in anemic patients or those who have had stimulatory therapy (e.g., granulocyte colony stimulation factor [G-CSF]) (Fig. 11-11). Increased marrow activity is highest at the end of chemotherapy and rapidly declines over 2 to 4 weeks. This may obscure marrow

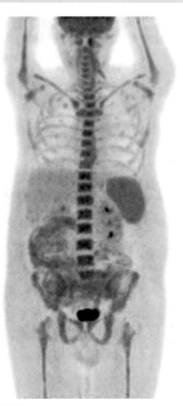

Figure 11-11. Bone marrow activity. Anterior whole-body ¹⁸F-FDG image in this severely anemic patient shows increased activity in the bone marrow. Similar activity can be seen after chemotherapy. This should not be interpreted as diffuse marrow metastases.

metastases, in some cases. Marrow activity will be decreased regionally in the treated area after radiation therapy.

Normal lymph nodes have very little activity. However, if an injection of the radiopharmaceutical into an arm vein was infiltrated, there may be activity in the axillary or supraclavicular nodes on the side of injection. Splenic activity is usually low but can be increased in anemic patients or those treated with G-CSF.

QUALITATIVE IMAGE INTERPRETATION

Commonly, the attenuation-corrected PET images are displayed simultaneously in three orthogonal planes: axial, coronal, and sagittal with the CT and as fused images. A three-dimensional (MIP) rotating display is also provided. Visual interpretation entails a review of these images to locate areas of suspected pathology. The MIP images can be especially helpful for an overview of radiopharmaceutical

distribution and for differentiating pathologic from physiologic foci.

Semiquantitative methods can also be used to aid interpretation. Suspicious or equivocal areas showing low or moderate activity can be further evaluated as needed using standardized uptake values (SUVs). A value above 2.5 should raise the possibility of malignancy. One should remember that if a lesion is small, the average measured SUV may be falsely low because of partial volume averaging. In this instance, the use of maximum pixel value may often be more reliable and reproducible. SUVs of obviously intense lesions may also be documented for future comparison with post-treatment follow-up scans.

Finally, a comparison of PET/CT images with other recent anatomic imaging (such as magnetic resonance imaging [MRI]), should be performed. Although most lesions will be seen on the attenuation-corrected images, if a lesion is known to be present or suspected on a CT scan and is not seen on the attenuation-corrected images, review of the non–attenuation-corrected images may be helpful. This is especially true if there are artifacts as a result of patient motion between the time of the transmission scan and the PET scan. However, it should be noted that lesions deep within the body are often less conspicuous on uncorrected images.

A thorough knowledge of physiologic distribution, normal variants, common causes of benign radiopharmaceutical uptake, and technical artifacts is essential for an accurate visual interpretation. The broad categories of benign conditions or lesions that can be associated with ¹⁸F-FDG accumulation include hyperplasia, ischemia, benign tumors, and any inflammation or infection producing focal infiltration of metabolically active host cells, including granulomatous diseases and fungal infections. In addition, a tailored, but rigorous clinical history is needed, including suspected or known lesion sites, tumor histology, type and timing of any treatment, as well as potentially interfering medications.

PET IMAGE QUANTITATION

In addition to obtaining cross sectional images, it is often helpful to quantify how much radioactivity is in a voxel or volume within the patient. When a PET camera is appropriately calibrated, it is able to assess the mCi/mL of tissue. Although there are a number of methods for quantifying uptake, the most common is the SUV, a semiquantitative index, defined by the following equation:

$$SUV = \frac{Mean\ ROI\ activity\ (mCi/mL)}{Activity\ administered\ (mCi)\ /body\ weight(grams)}$$
$$= grams/mL$$

where ROI is a user-specified region of interest. A conversion factor of 1.0 gram per milliliter is often used (assuming patients are essentially water), and this makes the SUV a simple number without units. Calculations can be done for the highest pixel in the object of interest (SUV_{max}) or an average value in the ROI (SUV_{mean}). Calculation of *SUV* does not require blood sampling. The imaging should take place at the same time point, if results are to be compared.

When ^{18}F-FDG is used, SUV measurements may be used to characterize a lesion with respect to its glucose metabolism. SUVs must be obtained using the attenuation-corrected (data) images. The SUV is determined by using special software by placing a region of interest (ROI) over the portion of the lesion with the greatest ^{18}F-FDG uptake and thus containing the maximum value pixel. SUVs based on maximal pixel values are commonly used rather than an average pixel value, although the latter has better reproducibility. An SUV would be 1.0 if the radionuclide was uniformly distributed throughout the body. The approximate normal SUVs for normal tissues are shown in Table 11-2. SUV measurements are typically obtained at 1 hour after injection even though activity in some lesions, such as neoplasms, may be slightly higher at 2 hours.

There are a number of factors that affect SUV measurements. Technical factors causing errors in SUV have been discussed at the end of Chapter 2. Body weight and composition are obvious factors, with obese patients having higher SUVs than do thin patients for both normal and malignant tissue. Typically SUVs are based on body weight. SUVs based on estimated lean body mass or body surface area are sometimes calculated. It should be noted that when performing serial scans on oncology patients, significant weight loss between studies may well affect SUVs, and increasing severity of illness may cause significant variation in serum glucose levels from earlier studies, even in diabetic individuals.

Because high serum glucose levels reduce tumor FDG uptake and thus SUVs, correction for glucose levels is helpful, especially when SUVs from serial studies are to be compared. The size of the ROI over an FDG-avid lesion will affect the average SUV, with smaller regions of interest resulting in higher average SUVs. However, as long as the ROI contains the maximum activity pixel, then the size of the ROI is irrelevant for determining that maximum value. Recent physical activity can elevate SUV in muscle, and inflammation in any tissue usually elevates the SUV. Because of partial volume effects, SUVs of lesions that are smaller than is the spatial resolution of the scanner will be underestimated. In addition, minor changes in scan technique can result in a change of 25% to 30% in measured SUV. When doing serial SUV measurements, it is important to standardize the time after injection because FDG accumulation in tumors, and therefore SUVs, continues to increase with time (up to at least 2 hours). SUV also depends on knowing exactly how much activity was injected and how much may have remained in the syringe. Any extravasation during injection will also affect calculated lesion SUV values. As a result of these many variables, many institutions do not actually calculate SUVs in every day practice but rather visually characterize lesions as having no visible activity or mild, moderate, or intense uptake.

It should be noted that, in practice, visual interpretation of the PET images often suffices, and obtaining SUVs is not necessary in every patient. When they are obtained to evaluate a lesion, caution is advised because benign lesions may be very FDG-avid, rendering high SUVs, whereas some malignant lesions may demonstrate little or no FDG activity, producing low uptake values. When monitoring tumor therapy, SUVs may be requested by treating physicians as a semi-objective index to aid in the assessment of therapeutic effects. In some institutions, a decline in SUV (max) after chemotherapy of more than 25% represents a favorable but partial metabolic response. A complete response is indicated by a decline in SUV to background.

WHOLE-BODY ^{18}F-FDG PET/CT NEOPLASM IMAGING

Cancer cells exhibit a number of aberrant characteristics compared with those of normal cells, which can potentially be used to image tumors.

Typically, there is increased glucose metabolism, increased DNA synthesis, increased amino acid transport, and overexpression of receptors and antigens. PET imaging with ^{18}F-FDG capitalizes on increased glucose metabolism in a wide variety of neoplasms to detect both primary lesions and their metastases.

Today, ^{18}F-FDG PET/CT scanning has become an integral tool in management of many tumor types. It is used for diagnosis, staging, restaging, and the evaluation of response to therapy. Use of PET/CT imaging in tumor staging results in a change of therapy in as many as 25% to 50% of patients. In about 10% to 15% of patients, unsuspected distant metastases will be found. In certain settings, PET can offer some insight into tumor biology, including tumor grade and prognosis.

Typically, the threshold for lesion detection is approximately 6 mm. Lesions greater than 1 cm are routinely detected, depending on the tumor histology. In general, ^{18}F-FDG PET is more sensitive for less well-differentiated cell types. Thus high uptake in a tumor is frequently, but not always, associated with a poorer prognosis. Conversely, well-differentiated lesions may occasionally be a source of false-negative scans because of diminished ^{18}F-FDG uptake. Although the degree of initial uptake in some neoplasms and/or their metastases may correlate inversely with response to therapy, this is not always the case.

Because of the complementary information of metabolic activity and anatomy supplied by PET and CT, respectively, together they offer unique advantages in the diagnosis, staging, and monitoring of malignancy. PET may often demonstrate that lymph nodes meeting normal CT criteria (less than 1 cm, short-axis) do indeed harbor metastases or, conversely, that enlarged lymph nodes, residual masses, postsurgical scarring, or anatomic distortion are not metabolically active and thus not likely malignant.

Uptake of ^{18}F-FDG after treatment may provide some information about tumor response. To monitor therapy response, a pretreatment scan is required as well as serial scans during therapy. It is important to standardize the protocol (fasting time, glucose level, hydration, etc.) to ensure that the scans will be comparable because evaluation involves both visual and quantitative assessments. The simplest quantitative method is the ratio of tumor to normal tissues or background, such as mediastinal blood pool, but a better method is determination of the SUV. The SUV reflects the glycolytic activity of the tumor and thus is an indirect marker of tumor growth rate. Thus any post-treatment alteration in the SUV may provide early evidence of tumor response as well as offer prognostic information regarding the success or failure of a particular treatment, allowing a change in therapeutic approach when appropriate.

Reduction or resolution of ^{18}F-FDG uptake is an early indicator of a favorable response. Although a response to therapy using CT or MRI is based upon changes in tumor volume, residual masses may persist even after the tumor cells have been excised or eradicated. Although a decrease in activity in lesions after treatment is a good indication of a favorable response, the resolution or absence of ^{18}F-FDG activity in a lesion after therapy should not be interpreted as eradication because PET cannot reliably detect residual microscopic disease. It is possible that some tumors are stunned by the initiation of chemotherapy so that FDG metabolism is reduced or absent for several weeks but then returns as the tumor cells recover. This may explain the reported inaccuracy of PET in the evaluation of neoadjuvant chemotherapy in some neoplasms. Thus patients should continue to receive the full course of therapy. A lack of response to treatment as measured by no significant change or a measurable increase in ^{18}F-FDG uptake may indicate that alternative therapies should be tried.

Interpretation of post-therapy scans can be challenging. Chemotherapy and radiation treatments can cause increased ^{18}F-FDG in both normal and neoplastic tissues. Post-treatment scans can be complicated by the presence of such inflammation, surgical site changes and wound healing, thymic rebound, or areas of infection occurring as a result of immune depression after chemotherapy. Thus a thorough knowledge of the patient's treatment history is mandatory.

PET imaging can be of considerable value in planning radiation therapy, especially when tumor anatomy and metabolism are mapped by using PET/CT. This more precise localization of disease extent, in turn, permits more accurate determination of planned treatment volumes. Irradiated neoplasms may initially show an increase in FDG uptake as well as increased uptake in the adjacent normal tissues because of inflammatory and granulation responses. In general, increased ¹⁸F-FDG uptake in post-irradiation regions resolves sufficiently in 2 to 3 months to permit reevaluation by PET/CT imaging, although significant uptake may persist for 6 months or more. Generally, a significant focus of FDG uptake more than 6 months after radiation treatment is indicative of tumor recurrence. Knowledge of the timing after therapy, the configuration of the radiation port, and comparison with a baseline scan all greatly assist in accurately interpreting scans in this setting. Postirradiation inflammation can sometimes be identified by its sharp demarcation, corresponding to the edges of the radiation port margins.

After chemotherapy, marrow rebound with or without G-CSF therapy, can produce intensely increased activity diffusely in the marrow. This activity generally returns to baseline levels in 2 to 4 weeks after therapy, so that a waiting period of 2 to 4 weeks before ¹⁸F-FDG PET imaging is usually sufficient to avoid interfering activity. In a few patients, marrow activity remains intense for months. Flare phenomena causing increased ¹⁸F-FDG activity in breast cancers shortly after hormonal therapy and some brain cancers shortly after chemotherapy have been reported and should not be mistaken for exacerbation of disease.

Head and Neck Cancers

Head and neck neoplasms constitute a heterogeneous variety of lesions. Some of the more common tumors, such as squamous cell carcinomas of the skin, nasopharynx, oral cavity, and larynx avidly accumulate ¹⁸F-FDG (Fig. 11-12). About half of basal cell carcinomas (mostly the nodular subtype) have identifiable FDG uptake. Assessment of the primary lesion with PET/CT is usually unwarranted. However, occasionally, an occult lesion presents as a metastasis to cervical lymph nodes, and PET imaging can be used as an adjunct to localizing a clinically unapparent primary tumor. However, such imaging can be challenging because of salivary gland excretion of FDG, asymmetric muscle activity, brown fat, pharyngeal muscle uptake, inflammation at biopsy sites and complex anatomy. ¹⁸F-FDG PET/CT has proven to be the imaging technique of choice for head and neck cancers.

A primary use of imaging is for staging head and neck cancers by identifying cervical and other regional lymph node metastases as well as distant disease, especially skeletal, hepatic, pulmonary, and distant nodal metastases. Early-stage tumors are treated and often cured by surgery or radiation therapy. Limited nodal

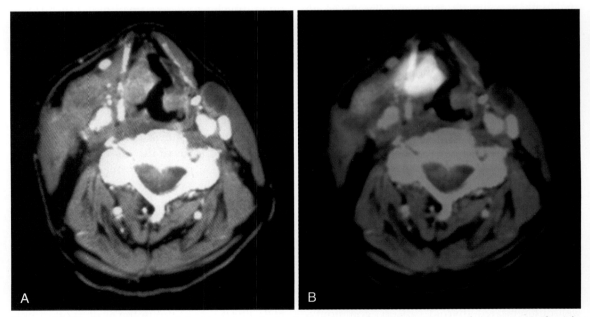

Figure 11-12. Laryngeal cancer. A, In this patient who has had a left neck dissection, a CT scan shows a mass in the right side of the larynx and adjacent adenopathy. The patient also had tiny pulmonary metastases detected on the CT scan only. **B,** Axial PET/CT ¹⁸F-FDG image shows marked activity in the tumor, but also activity laterally in a lymph node.

metastases are often amenable to surgical resection, whereas more extensive regional disease usually requires radiation therapy in addition to surgery. Scanning with ^{18}F-FDG/CT is more accurate (≈90%) for staging than is either CT or MRI. For restaging after treatment, detection of local residual or recurrent tumor is rendered challenging for all imaging modalities because of post-therapeutic change associated with altered anatomy and inflammation. PET has been shown to be sensitive (80% to 100%) for local recurrence, but its specificity is reduced by post-radiation inflammation. Radiation produces the most prominent changes in the epithelial surfaces of the oral mucosa, soft palate, paranasal sinuses, and palatine tonsils. To increase specificity, a minimum waiting period of 4 months after radiation has been recommended. At that time, there is both high sensitivity and specificity for the detection of recurrent primary tumor or for the development of nodal metastases.

Chemotherapy is a common first-stage treatment in advanced head and neck cancers. Scans with ^{18}F-FDG PET/CT are useful to evaluate response during therapy. In the neoadjuvant (induction) chemotherapy setting, ^{18}F-FDG PET can identify nonresponders, and additional surgical intervention or radiation therapy can be avoided in those patients who are unlikely to benefit. A decrease in ^{18}F-FDG activity (SUV) of about 80% to 90% is often associated with a complete remission. However, if the decrease is less than 40%, there is likely to be recurrent disease. The picture is somewhat complicated because, in some patients, the therapeutic response varies among different metastatic lymph node sites.

In patients with unilateral laryngeal nerve paralysis, asymmetric laryngeal muscle (posterior arytenoid muscle) activity on the functional unparalyzed side may mimic a metastatic lymph node. False-negative studies can result in patients with tumor deposits less than 6 mm. Small lung metastases are best identified by CT.

Thyroid Cancer

Thyroid cancer has been extensively discussed in Chapter 4. Radioiodines (iodine-131 [^{131}I] and iodine-123 [^{123}I]) are the most widely used radiopharmaceuticals used to evaluate and stage well-differentiated thyroid cancers, commonly papillary/follicular cell types. However, there are a number of thyroid cancers that do not accumulate radioiodine to a significant degree. These include poorly differentiated and medullary cancers. In addition, some thyroid cancers that are originally well-differentiated may recur as poorly differentiated cell types that do not readily accumulate radioiodines.

Patients with differentiated thyroid cancers are usually treated with a thyroidectomy and ^{131}I ablation of thyroid bed remnants and regional nodal disease. Follow-up uses serum thyroglobulin levels and whole-body radioiodine imaging if thyroglobulin levels are elevated. If radioiodine-avid lesions are identified by radioiodine whole-body imaging, then repeat ^{131}I therapy can be used. However, in some patients with elevated serum thyroglobulin levels, whole-body radioiodine scans are negative, suggesting less well-differentiated, more aggressive metastases. In this setting, ^{18}F-FDG PET imaging has significant value because it frequently demonstrates the recurrent lesions with an accuracy of about 90% (See Fig. 4-14). PET imaging is similarly useful in patients with medullary carcinoma of the thyroid treated with a thyroidectomy and who subsequently experience elevated serum calcitonin levels. Hürthle cell cancer, which is much more aggressive and more often metastatic than other thyroid cancers, usually has an intense ^{18}F-FDG uptake, and this may be the best imaging method for evaluating this cell type.

As with cancers of the head and neck, it is often difficult to detect small nodal metastases in the neck if the patient is scanned with the arms raised; it is often necessary to scan the patient with the arms up and then again with the arms down.

Many nonmalignant thyroid nodules accumulate ^{18}F-FDG. However, if there is a very intense focus of activity in the nodule, the probability of a malignant lesion is increased. An incidentally detected focus of increased FDG uptake in the thyroid on scans performed for unrelated reasons should be further evaluated to exclude carcinoma. Diffusely increased uptake commonly occurs in patients with thyroiditis and Graves disease.

Solitary Pulmonary Nodules and Lung Cancer

Solitary Pulmonary Nodule. Imaging with FDG PET/CT is useful in the evaluation of pulmonary nodules and masses (Fig. 11-13). The sensitivity and specificity of ^{18}F-FDG PET for

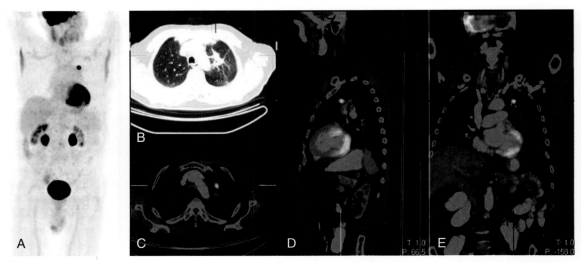

Figure 11-13. Non–small cell lung cancer. A, Anterior ¹⁸F-FDG image shows activity in the left upper lobe. **B,** CT scan demonstrates a left upper lobe spiculated mass. The patient did not want a needle biopsy. **C-E,** ¹⁸F-FDG PET/CT fusion images show markedly increased activity in the lesion (SUV of 10.3), indicating a high probability that this represents a malignancy. There is no evidence of regional or distant disease.

differentiating benign from malignant causes for solitary pulmonary parenchymal nodules that are greater than 1 cm is about 95% and 80%, respectively. Although CT has comparable sensitivity, its specificity is considerably lower, in the range of 40%. SUV reported for pulmonary nodules is typically an SUV_{max}. An SUV of 2.5 or greater usually indicates malignancy (positive predictive value [PPV] about 80%), and an SUV above 4.0 has a PPV of about 90%. Lesions with no uptake have a very low likelihood of being malignant (negative predictive value [NPV] of more than 95%). However, SUVs are not a binary distinguisher. For nodules with SUV greater than 0.6 to 0.8 and less than 1.5 to 2.0, the NPV is about 85% to 90%, and, for an SUV of 1.5 to 2.0, the NPV is about 80%.

False-positive studies may occur in inflammatory lesions and granulomatous diseases such a sarcoidosis, tuberculosis, and fungal infections (see Chapter 12). Such hypermetabolic lesions must be considered malignant until proved benign. Although non–FDG-avid lesions are highly unlikely to be malignant, false-negative studies may be seen in neoplasms with low metabolic activity such as a carcinoid tumor, a bronchioalveolar cancer, or a well-differentiated adenocarcinoma. Metastasis with low cellular density, such as mucinous lesions, may also show low ¹⁸F-FDG uptake. Primary lung cancers with low FDG levels usually represent stage 1 lesions with an excellent prognosis after resection.

It should be emphasized that lung nodules with suspicious CT characteristics and negative ¹⁸F-FDG PET scans should be monitored with serial CT scans or biopsied (see Table 11-5). Similarly, ¹⁸F-FDG negative small lung nodules less than 1 cm, especially in high-risk patients, warrant a CT follow-up because an average SUV of less than 2.5 may reflect a partial volume effect rather than the true metabolic activity of the nodule. It is important to note that with CT/PET fusion images, there may be a misregistration if the scans were not both done with shallow breathing. As expected, most benign pulmonary lesions such as hamartomas, adenomas, and inflammatory nodules are not FDG-avid as measured by the SUV.

Primary Lung Cancer. The most common primary lung cancers are ¹⁸F-FDG-avid, including both small-cell and non–small-cell types. However, because small-cell carcinoma is considered to be metastatic at the time of its diagnosis and because the initial treatment is systemic chemotherapy, primary staging with PET/CT imaging may not be warranted. Thus PET/CT imaging has largely been directed toward the evaluation of non–small-cell lung cancer.

After a diagnosis of non–small-cell carcinoma of the lung has been made, PET imaging can play an important role in staging, treatment planning, and restaging of the disease. Although CT is the preferred method of assessing primary tumor size and invasion, ¹⁸F-FDG

TABLE 11-5	Fleischner Society Recommendations for Newly Detected Incidental Pulmonary Nodule Follow-Up	
NODULE SIZE (MM)	**LOW-RISK PATIENT***	**HIGH-RISK PATIENT†**
<4	No follow-up needed	CT at 12 mo; if unchanged, no further follow-up‡
>4-6	CT at 12 mo; if unchanged, no further follow-up‡	CT at 6-12 mo; then at 18-24 mo if no change
>6-8	CT at 6-12 mo; then at 18-24 mo if no change	CT at 3-6 mo; then at 9-12 and 24 mo if no change
>8	CT at 3, 9, 24 mo, dynamic contrast-enhanced CT, PET/CT, and/or biopsy	Same as for low-risk patient

Adapted from Radiology 2005;237(2):395-400.
*Minimal or absent history of smoking and of other risk factors.
†History of smoking or other risk factors.
‡Nonsolid (ground-glass) or partly solid nodules may require longer follow-up.

PET can be helpful in evaluating patients presenting with pleural effusions by distinguishing malignant from benign effusions with an accuracy of 90%. PET may also aid initial CT assessment by distinguishing metabolically active primary tumor from adjacent atelectasis or postobstructive pneumonitis. Such differentiation can greatly aid in radiation treatment planning, allowing more precise determination of treatment volumes.

Scanning with ¹⁸F-FDG PET/CT has been shown to be superior to other forms of imaging for initial staging of non–small-cell lung cancer, particularly with regard to spread to regional lymph nodes, which is an important determinant of treatment options. Surgical resection of a primary lesion is often possible with ipsilateral, hilar, and mediastinal, as well as subcarinal lymph node involvement. But disease in the contralateral, hilar, and mediastinal nodes usually dictates nonsurgical treatment (Fig. 11-14). The CT criteria of size (greater than 1 cm) for abnormal lymph nodes are relatively insensitive (45% sensitivity, 85% specificity) for detecting metastatic disease to hilar and mediastinal lymph nodes. By using metabolic criteria, PET has a sensitivity and specificity of 80% to 90%. However, because the positive predictive value for mediastinal disease of an abnormal PET scan is only 65%, owing to false-positive studies caused by inflammatory lymph nodes, confirmation of metastatic disease should be sought before surgical treatment is denied. Importantly, the negative predictive value of an ¹⁸F-FDG PET scan for mediastinal metastases is about 95%.

Thus surgical treatment can proceed, based on a negative PET scan.

PET is an excellent technique for detecting distant metastases. About 10% of patients who have no evidence of metastatic disease on CT are subsequently shown to have metastases on ¹⁸F-FDG scans. PET can reliably differentiate benign from malignant causes of abnormal body CT findings and can help distinguish benign adrenal masses from metastases. Because of the high degree of FDG uptake in normal brain tissue, PET is less sensitive for detecting small cerebral metastases and is significantly less sensitive than is MRI.

The use of PET/CT scans to predict response to adjuvant therapies for non–small-cell lung cancer has not been extensively studied. However, an incomplete response of decreased ¹⁸F-FDG uptake after radiation or chemotherapy therapy appears to have almost the same poor prognosis as those who show no decrease in ¹⁸F-FDG uptake after treatment. The median survival of those patients with positive ¹⁸F-FDG scans at the completion of therapy is about 1 to 2 years, whereas those with negative results have about an 80% 3-year survival. Even in aggressively treated patients, the recurrence rate of intrathoracic and distant disease is high. Because of its high sensitivity and specificity, PET can be very useful in evaluating patients for suspected recurrence. In non–small-cell lung cancer, SUV has been shown to be an independent predictor of survival. Patients whose tumors exhibit high SUVs (more than 10 to 20) have significantly lower survival rates.

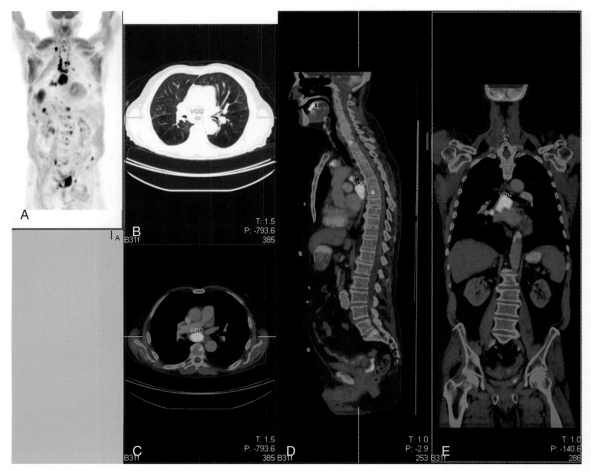

Figure 11-14. **Recurrent metastatic lung cancer.** **A,** Anterior whole-body ^{18}F-FDG PET image shows multiple foci of increased activity in the mediastinum, liver, and bones. **B,** On the axial CT image, the mediastinal nodes are difficult to appreciate. **C-E,** Axial, sagittal, and coronal PET/CT images provide much better spatial localization of the mediastinal and vertebral body metastases.

In the postsurgical patient, PET can reliably differentiate postsurgical scarring from metabolically active recurrent tumor. In patients undergoing radiation therapy, resultant radiation pneumonitis is often metabolically active, likely related to cellular inflammatory and macrophage reaction. This activity may obscure underlying persistent or recurrent viable tumor. Knowledge of the time of treatment and the position of the radiation field is essential to accurate interpretation. Generally, waiting at least 3 months after radiation therapy is completed before performing follow-up FDG PET/CT imaging is recommended. Radiation pneumonitis may remain metabolically active on PET scans for 6 months after treatment and, occasionally, up to a year or more.

Bronchioalveolar carcinoma, carcinoid lesions less than 1 cm in diameter, and, occasionally,

well-differentiated adenocarcinomas can have little ^{18}F-FDG uptake, resulting in false-negative scans. False-positive scans can occur as a result of benign processes with high metabolic rates, including granulomas, sarcoidosis, tuberculosis, histoplasmosis, coccidiomycosis, *Mycobacterium avium intracellulare,* and simple pneumonias. Increased ^{18}F-FDG uptake occurs in mesotheliomas. PET scanning has been reported to be superior to CT for staging this tumor, particularly in documenting the extent of pleural disease and detecting small involved mediastinal lymph nodes.

Lymphomas

Both Hodgkin and non-Hodgkin lymphomas of all types accumulate ^{18}F-FDG, although low-grade lymphomas do not accumulate activity as well as intermediate or high-grade lymphomas. Low-grade lymphomas, especially mucosa-associated

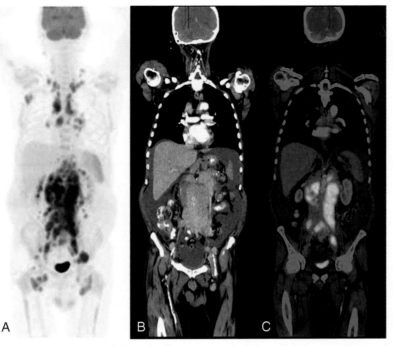

Figure 11-15. **Lymphoma.** **A,** Anterior whole-body ¹⁸F-FDG image performed for staging shows abnormal activity in para-aortic nodes and inguinal areas and mediastinum. **B** and **C,** Coronal images from the PET/CT clearly show the massive para-aortic adenopathy as well as mediastinal involvement.

lymphoid tissue (MALT), may produce false-negative results and may involve lymph nodes less than 1 cm in diameter, although these constitute about 25% of positive sites on a PET scan. False-positive studies may be caused by inflammation and infections involving lymph nodes, especially granulomatous infections.

Because the anatomic distribution of active disease is a major determinant of the mode of therapy used, PET/CT and other imaging modalities play an important role in the staging and restaging of lymphoma (Fig. 11-15). In general, ¹⁸F-FDG PET is more sensitive (85% to 95%) and specific (95%) than is CT for detecting nodal disease, as well as splenic and hepatic involvement. Existing information also indicates that PET is superior to gallium-67 (67Ga) single-photon emission computed tomography (SPECT) scanning for imaging lymphoma. Although marrow disease is accurately detected by using ¹⁸F-FDG PET, caution should be exercised when interpreting scans of patients who have received colony stimulating factors or who may be experiencing a post-chemotherapy marrow rebound.

Using PET to monitor therapy response requires a baseline ¹⁸F-FDG scan before treatment to compare with intra- or post-treatment images. In some settings, post-treatment scans are appropriate after one or two cycles of chemotherapy are completed. It is prudent to wait 1 to 2 weeks after therapy to avoid transient fluctuations in tumor metabolism. Scans done as early as 1 week after initiation of chemotherapy can show significant reduction in activity assessed both visually and using SUVs. The amount of reduction correlates with the ultimate outcome. About 80% to 90% of patients with residual activity after one cycle of chemotherapy will relapse, whereas about 80% to 90% of those with no activity at the same time will have much longer disease-free periods. In the treatment setting, false-positive scans can result from thymic rebound, reactive bone marrow, and inflammatory or infectious processes. Marrow activity is highest at the cessation of chemotherapy, declines quickly in 2 to 4 weeks but sometimes is not normal for many months. Thymic activity (See Fig. 11-4) is quite different with the lowest thymic uptake found at the end of chemotherapy and then increasing and reaching a peak at about 10 months post-therapy. Afterward, it slowly decreases over the next 12 to 24 months.

After therapy is completed, ¹⁸F-FDG/CT scanning can determine the overall response and can

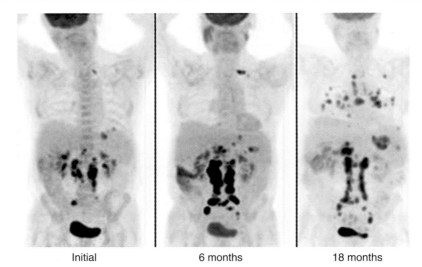

| Initial | 6 months | 18 months |

Figure 11-16. Progressive lymphoma. Multiple ¹⁸F-FDG whole-body images before therapy and 6 and 18 months post-chemotherapy show progressive disease extending above the diaphragm in spite of the treatment.

be very helpful in determining the significance of residual masses (Fig. 11-16). Relapse occurs in almost all patients who have a positive PET scan after the completion of therapy, whereas relapse occurs in about 25% of patients with residual masses on CT. The absence of disease on a post-treatment PET scan correlates with a low relapse rate. However, because a negative PET scan cannot exclude minimal residual disease, about 20% will suffer a relapse. Subsequent follow-up ¹⁸F-FDG scans have a sensitivity and specificity of about 80% to 90% for the detection of recurrent lymphoma. Although a low-grade lymphoma initially has a low SUV, an increase in the SUV on a follow-up scan suggests the possibility of transformation to a higher-grade tumor.

Even though the gray matter of the brain has high ¹⁸F-FDG activity, central nervous system involvement by lymphoma in patients with human immunodeficiency virus (HIV) disease is more avid. PET has been used in this setting to distinguish central nervous system lymphoma from infections, such as toxoplasmosis. Lymphomatous involvement of bone can be best imaged with either FDG PET or MRI. FDG allows a better assessment of current tumor activity (Fig. 11-17).

Breast Cancer

In the setting of breast cancer, whole body ¹⁸F-FDG PET/CT is used principally in the evaluation of locoregional recurrence, restaging, and response to therapy. There is currently no proven clinical role for FDG in screening for primary breast cancer or the evaluation of axillary lymph nodes. It should not be used as a replacement for either bone scintigraphy or diagnostic CT.

The sensitivity and specificity of whole body ¹⁸F-FDG PET for detection for primary breast cancer are both about 70% to 90%; however, these rates are markedly affected by tumor size. For lesions below 10 mm, the sensitivity is about 25%. False-negative studies may be caused by in situ, tubular and lobular carcinomas, as well as by ductal carcinomas in situ and small lesions. For lesions less than 2 cm in diameter, ¹⁸F-FDG scanning has a negative predictive value of only 50%, and, therefore it cannot reliably be used to defer or delay biopsy of a mammographically suspicious lesion. Advances in dedicated high-spatial resolution PET breast scanners (so-called positron emission mammography or PEM) have shown sensitivity rates for known breast cancers equivalent to MRI (about 90%). PEM has been shown to have a high PPV of 0.88. It can depict breast cancers not detected mammographically. In selected patients unable to undergo an MRI, PEM may provide an acceptable alternative.

Benign breast tumors usually have very low ¹⁸F-FDG uptake and are usually not a source of false-positive studies, although approximately 10% of fibroadenomas may show uptake of FDG. However, benign inflammatory processes may demonstrate significant FDG uptake.

Because ¹⁸F-FDG scanning cannot reliably detect small nodal metastases, it does not

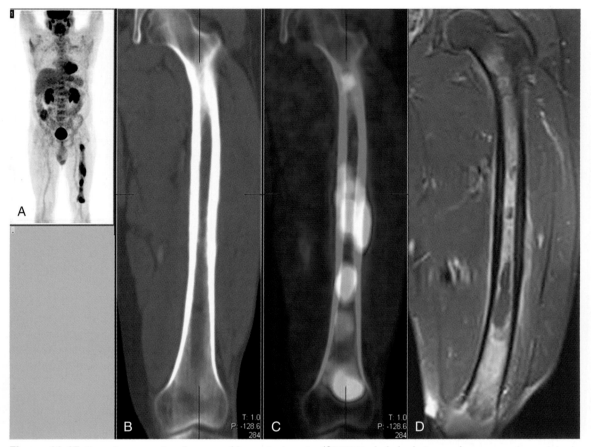

Figure 11-17. Lymphomatous involvement of bone. A, Anterior ¹⁸F-FDG whole-body image shows extensive activity in the left femur. **B,** CT scan is essentially normal. **C** and **D,** Both the PET/CT and MRI easily show the extent of disease as well as extension into soft tissue at the mid portion of the femur.

replace sentinel node biopsy or axillary node dissection for initial staging of breast cancer. PET/CT is useful as an adjunct to initial staging of large or locally advanced breast cancers to find distant disease. False-positive results can occur because of inflammatory changes shortly after biopsy or surgery.

PET/CT can be used to monitor response to therapy. Shortly after initiation of therapy with tamoxifen in patients with ER-positive breast cancers, there can be a "flare" phenomenon, during which uptake of ¹⁸F-FDG actually increases even though the tumor is responding favorably to therapy. When PET imaging is used to monitor early response of breast cancer to cytotoxic chemotherapy, favorable results can often be identified as early as a week or so after commencing treatment. As with other tumors, persistence of ¹⁸F-FDG activity after therapy carries a poor prognosis. A negative scan at the end of therapy is still associated with about a 25% recurrence

rate. This may be a result of nonvisualization of lesions less than 0.6 to 1.0 cm in size or when the lesion is well differentiated. For restaging, ¹⁸F-FDG PET has a relatively high sensitivity (90%) and specificity (80%) for the detection of recurrent disease, both locoregionally and at distant sites. It is especially useful to distinguish mature postsurgical scarring and fibrosis seen on CT from locally recurrent cancer.

Esophageal Cancer

Normal ¹⁸F-FDG uptake in the esophagus should be uniform. Because ¹⁸F-FDG will accumulate in both esophageal adenocarcinoma and squamous cell cancers, focally increased activity should raise the suspicion of malignancy (Fig. 11-18). However, focal activity can also be a result of benign processes such as esophagitis, hiatal hernia, Barrett esophagus, postprocedural changes from balloon dilatation procedures, and inflammatory changes from

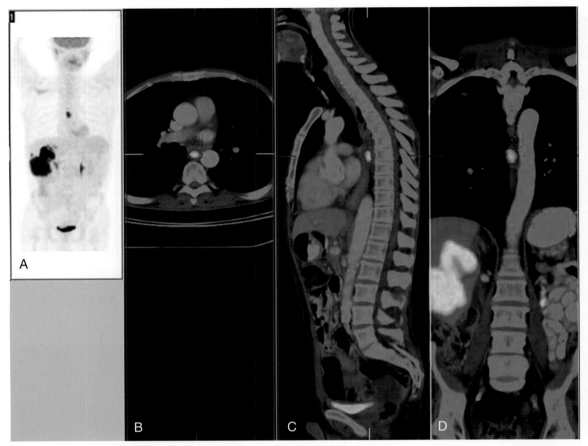

Figure 11-18. Esophageal cancer. A, ¹⁸F-FDG anterior whole-body image shows an intense focus of activity in the mid-esophagus. **B-D,** PET/CT scans show the esophageal lesion, but, more importantly, the distant hepatic metastases. There is normal physiologic activity in the renal collecting system and bladder.

radiation therapy, which reduces the specificity of such esophageal activity.

The limited resolution of PET scans compromises the evaluation of local invasion or regional lymph node metastases, and, therefore it is not appropriate for detecting and staging primary tumors. Primary tumor (T) staging of these tumors is done with endoscopic ultrasound. The insensitivity of FDG PET for detecting regional nodal disease is likely related to the proximity of involved nodes to the primary lesion, which makes differentiation difficult, and to the often microscopic nature of the nodal disease. However, when present, the finding of a discrete positive periesophageal or regional focus on PET imaging is highly predictive of metastatic nodal disease, with a specificity of about 90%. FDG PET/CT imaging of early stage (Tis or T1) disease is not recommended because of the low yield of positive results.

For PET/CT evaluation of tumors in the lower thoracic esophagus, it is important to differentiate between enlarged or FDG-avid nodes in the gastrohepatic ligament (resectable) and celiac nodes (unresectable). This can be difficult; however, gastrohepatic ligament nodes are slightly more cephalad and anterior to the origin of the celiac artery rather than adjacent to the celiac artery itself.

PET/CT scanning is primarily used to evaluate the possibility of stage 4 disease (distant metastases) and to identify those patients who are not candidates for surgical resection. PET is more accurate (80% to 90%) than is CT for the evaluation of cervical and upper abdominal nodal disease and spread to liver, lung, or bone. In patients treated by resection of the primary lesion, PET is very sensitive but not specific for recurrence at the anastomotic site. However, for the detection of distant recurrence outside of the surgical field, PET is both sensitive (95%) and specific (80%).

Reviews of the use of FDG PET for assessment of esophageal cancer response are mixed, and some authors feel that it is not sufficiently reliable to use in determining individual therapeutic response. Follow-up scans should not be performed less than 4 to 6 weeks after surgery and less than 8 to 12 weeks after completion of radiation therapy. Activity in the primary lesion may increase during the early course of radiation treatments, but responding lesions will ultimately show a decrease in FDG uptake later in the course. Further, esophagitis related to recent radiation therapy may cause interfering activity, which usually resolves after 4 to 6 weeks. False-positive results can occur also as a result of significant uptake in gastric mucosa near the esophagogastric junction or from reflux esophagitis. False-negative studies occur when the lesion is small or located in close proximity to other structures that avidly accumulate ^{18}F-FDG, such as the heart.

Gastric Cancer

In contrast to ^{18}F-FDG–avid esophageal carcinomas, the detection rate of ^{18}F-FDG for gastric cancer depends on the cell type (Fig. 11-19). Mucinous tumors, signet cell, poorly differentiated adenocarcinomas, diffuse tumors, and intestinal type tumors typically have low ^{18}F-FDG uptake. Interpretation is complicated by normal physiologic activity and unrelated inflammatory conditions. Endoscopic ultrasound is the most reliable method of preoperative determination of T stage. In addition, CT is more sensitive than PET in the detection of lymph node metastases in the perigastric region and along the gastric, common hepatic and splenic arteries because of better spatial resolution. FDG-PET can show metastases in more distant locations. Detection of primary gastric lymphoma varies by cell type, with uptake in more than 90% of

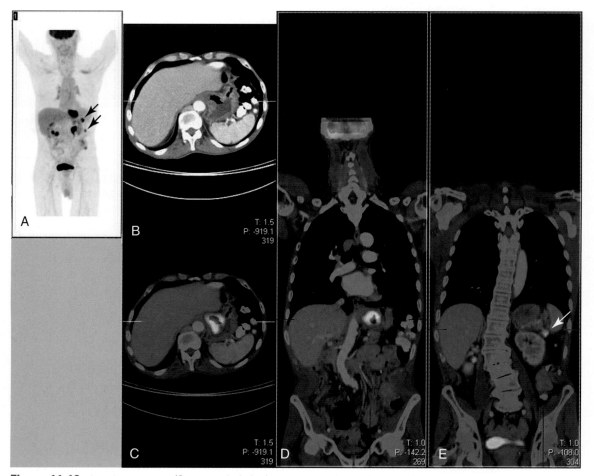

Figure 11-19. Gastric cancer. A, ^{18}F-FDG whole-body image scan shows abnormal focal activity near the gastric fundus but also two nearby FDG-avid lymph nodes (*arrows*). **B-D,** Axial CT and axial and coronal PET/CT images show the activity in the thickened gastric wall. **E,** Additional coronal PET/CT image shows the lymph node metastasis between the spleen and left kidney.

cases of aggressive non-Hodgkin lymphoma but much less uptake and intensity in cases of mucosa-associated lymphoid tissue (MALT).

Gastrointestinal Stromal Tumors

This uncommon tumor represents about 5% of all sarcomas. It most frequently occurs in the stomach, less often in the small intestine, and rarely in the colon. The sensitivity and positive predictive values are very high (85% to 100%) for both CT and ^{18}F-FDG PET. These tumors typically have high peripheral activity with central cold areas. Compared with CT, ^{18}F-FDG PET is better at predicting response after imatinib (tyrosine kinase inhibitor [Gleevec, Novartis]) therapy.

Colorectal Cancer

Although ^{18}F-FDG PET is very sensitive in the identification of primary colorectal adenocarcinomas (90% to 100%), the specificity (40% to 60%) is limited by the presence of physiologic bowel activity as well as activity accumulation in inflammatory lesions and benign colonic polyps. As was noted with stomach cancers,

mucinous cell type lesions and their metastases tend to have relatively low ^{18}F-FDG uptake.

The initial staging of colon cancer is predicated on endoscopic ultrasound, surgical, and pathologic findings. PET has a minor role in initial local and regional staging as sensitivity ($\approx$30%) is reduced in the presence of small quantities of malignant cells in pericolic lymph nodes and by the close proximity of the nodes to the primary tumor. However, when nodes are detected as FDG-positive, the specificity of the study is high (95%).

In detecting distant metastases, both nodal (internal iliac and retroperitoneal) and extranodal, PET is superior to CT in both sensitivity and specificity, at 95% and 75%, respectively (Fig. 11-20). In the liver, both modalities are limited and inferior to MRI in detecting lesions less than 1 cm in size. However, PET can play an important role in the selection of patients for curative resection or ablation of isolated hepatic metastases by determining the presence or absence of coexisting extrahepatic metastases. In this respect, PET offers significant incremental value to CT imaging, by identifying 10% to 20%

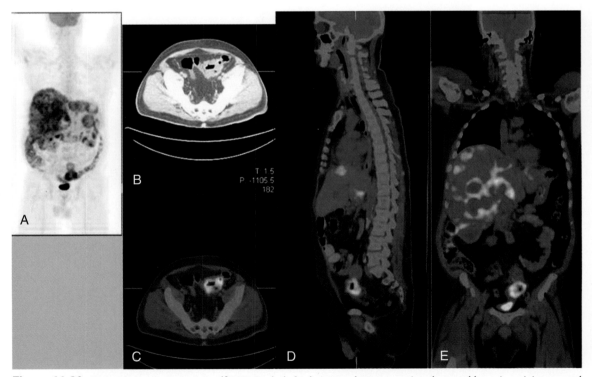

Figure 11-20. Sigmoid cancer. A, Anterior ^{18}F-FDG whole-body image shows extensive abnormal hepatic activity, normal physiologic colon activity, and a focal area of increased colon activity just above and to the left of the bladder, which could easily be mistaken for normal colonic activity. **B,** Axial CT and **C,** PET/CT images clearly show this activity to be in a focally thickened wall of the sigmoid. **D** and **E,** Sagittal and coronal PET/CT images also show the extensive and necrotic hepatic metastases.

additional extrahepatic sites of involvement than with CT alone. With respect to evaluation of treatment success after local ablative therapy of liver metastases from colorectal carcinoma, including cryotherapy, hepatic artery chemotherapy, and radiofrequency ablation, metabolic imaging with PET has been shown to be more accurate than is CT in differentiating post-therapy change from residual or recurrent tumor.

After initial treatment of colorectal carcinoma, PET offers significant information for restaging the disease: ^{18}F-FDG PET has been shown to be more sensitive than is CT or carcinoembryonic antigen (CEA) levels, and equally as specific as CEA levels for detecting recurrence. In this setting, PET is particularly useful for differentiating postsurgical and radiation change from recurrent disease, especially in the pelvis and presacral space. The ^{18}F-FDG scans are also valuable in cases in which there is a rising CEA titer and no obvious abnormality on CT. Positive ^{18}F-FDG follow-up scans should be correlated with CT findings to avoid false-positive etiologies such as sigmoid diverticulitis or even bladder diverticula. Both during and after radiotherapy and chemotherapy, tumor uptake of ^{18}F-FDG may increase even though the lesion is responding. This is somewhat similar to the flare phenomenon described for breast cancer. Follow-up scans are not usually performed during therapy, and post-therapy scans are usually delayed for about 2 months after the completion of therapy.

Hepatocellular Carcinoma (Hepatoma)

Although frequently hypermetabolic, hepatocellular carcinomas may contain high levels of phosphatases (as do normal hepatocytes), which can dephosphorylate FDG, permitting it to diffuse out of the tumor cells. Thus ^{18}F-FDG activity in hepatomas is variable, and only about 50% of hepatocellular carcinomas can be imaged with ^{18}F-FDG (Fig. 11-21).

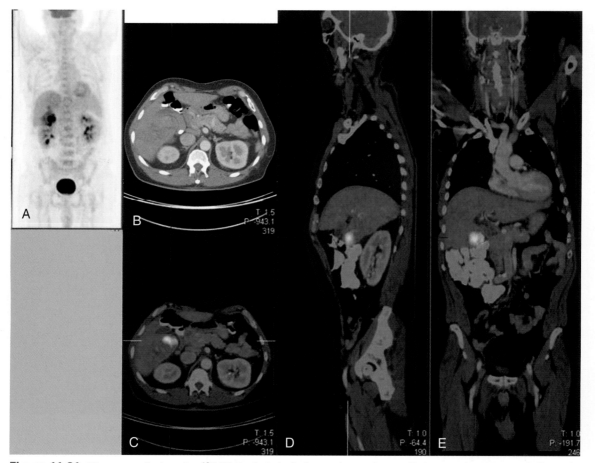

Figure 11-21. Hepatoma. A, Anterior ^{18}F-FDG whole-body image shows abnormally increased activity medially in the right lobe of the liver. **B,** Axial CT scan image shows a low attenuation lesion in this region. **C-E,** PET/CT axial, sagittal, and coronal images show activity in part of this hepatoma. Many hepatomas, however, do not show this level of uptake.

Therefore ¹⁸F-FDG PET is not useful as ultrasound or three-phase CT as a screening tool to detect small hepatocellular carcinomas or as CT for the detection of distant disease. Some authors have examined the potential utility of ¹¹C-acetate for the evaluation of hepatomas. Although the sensitivity is not as high as for ¹⁸F-FDG, ¹¹C-acetate may accumulate in those well-differentiated tumors that ¹⁸F-FDG does not. In general, for a hepatic lesion, if it accumulates both ¹⁸F-FDG and ¹¹C-acetate, a diagnosis of hepatoma should be favored. However, if the lesion accumulates only FDG and not acetate, a lesion other than hepatoma is likely.

Pancreatic Cancer

FDG PET/CT is sensitive and specific for the detection of primary pancreatic carcinoma. Thus it may be a useful adjunct to previous equivocal CT or endoscopic retrograde cholangiopancreatography (ERCP) examinations to establish the presence of a significant lesion (Fig. 11-22). However, because of the advanced stage and aggressive nature of this cancer, the role for PET/CT in staging and restaging pancreatic carcinoma or in directing management of patients awaits further definition.

Bone Tumors

Scanning with ¹⁸F-FDG PET is useful in evaluating the metabolic rate of osteosarcomas, their response to adjuvant and aggressive chemotherapy, and location of residual viable tumor. Because osteosarcomas are often heterogeneous (Fig. 8-46), the maximum SUV is a better indicator of the true malignant potential than is the average tumor SUV. In general, a higher maximum SUV correlates with a poorer prognosis. PET has been used to monitor response to therapy in both osteosarcoma and Ewing tumor. Decline in ¹⁸F-FDG uptake after therapy has been associated with an improved prognosis.

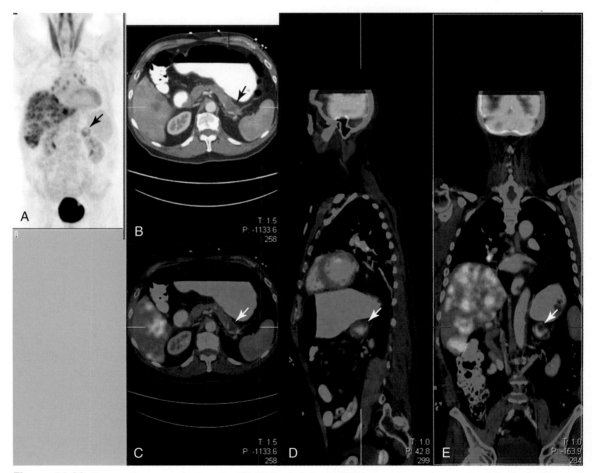

Figure 11-22. Pancreatic cancer. A, Anterior ¹⁸F-FDG whole-body PET image shows abnormal activity in the liver and mediastinum as a result of metastatic disease. **B,** Axial CT scan shows enlargement of the tail of the pancreas. **C-E,** Axial, sagittal, and coronal PET/CT images show that the pancreatic cancer itself (*arrows*) has mildly increased activity.

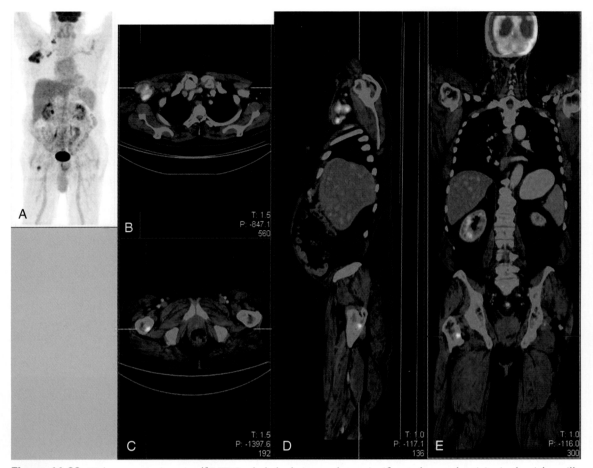

Figure 11-23. Melanoma. A, Anterior ¹⁸F-FDG whole-body image shows significant abnormal activity in the right axilla where a melanoma had been previously excised. There is also abnormal activity in the right lower cervical region and proximal right femur. **B,** Axial PET/CT images show clumped abnormal right axillary lymph nodes and **C,** a solitary skeletal metastasis in the right proximal femur. **D** and **E,** Sagittal and coronal PET/CT images confirm these findings.

For differentiation of residual masses after therapy, ¹⁸F-FDG PET is more reliable than either CT or MRI, and it is sensitive for the detection and evaluation of pulmonary metastases. A variety of benign and malignant bone neoplasms will accumulate FDG, and it should be noted that aggressive benign bone tumors (e.g., fibrous dysplasia and giant cell tumors) can have SUVs as high as or higher than those of osteosarcomas.

Malignant Melanoma

Scanning with ¹⁸F-FDG PET/CT is of limited use in initial staging of patients for spread to regional lymph nodes or in patients with primary lesions less than 1 mm in thickness and no evidence of metastases. Although melanoma typically exhibits marked FDG avidity, minimal nodal metastases may simply be too small to be detected. The sensitivity for detecting melanoma lesions greater than 1 cm is about

95%; for lesions 6 to 10 mm, about 80%; and for lesions less than 5 mm, less than 20% (Figs. 11-23 and 11-24). The replacement of PET with PET/CT does not appear to have affected overall node or metastasis staging with the exception of the detection of tiny pulmonary nodules on CT. ¹⁸F-FDG PET/CT scanning cannot replace lymphoscintigraphy to identify sentinel nodes for staging biopsy of regional lymph nodes.

However, PET/CT has proved to be useful in detecting distant metastases. Because of the wide variety of sites to which melanoma can metastasize, PET/CT is an efficient examination to detect such spread throughout the body. In addition, the detection of unsuspected distant metastases at initial staging or restaging has been shown to alter patient management in a significant percentage of patients, particularly those who are at a high risk for distant disease based on the extent of locoregional disease or

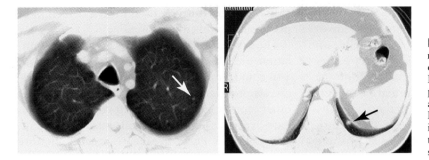

Figure 11-24. **Melanoma lung metastases.** Two axial CT images of the chest from the case shown in Figure 11-23 show multiple small pulmonary metastatic nodules that are below the resolution of the PET scan. This demonstrates the importance of carefully reviewing the lung CT portion of PET/CT scans.

those who have distant disease and are considering aggressive therapy. Because of the normally high uptake of ¹⁸F-FDG in the brain, an evaluation of central nervous system metastases is best done with MRI.

Gynecologic Cancers

Any ¹⁸F-FDG activity in the ovary of a postmenopausal woman should be considered suspicious for malignancy. For ovarian cancer located inside the pelvis, adding ¹⁸F-FDG PET scan to a CT scan does not improve accuracy of diagnosis even though the PET sensitivity and positive predictive values are about 70% to 90%. However, ¹⁸F-FDG PET does add marginally to the accuracy for lesions outside of the pelvis (such as the diaphragm, liver surface, omentum, and lymph nodes). For peritoneal carcinomatosis, sensitivity with ¹⁸F-FDG is only about 60%, but it is still higher than that with CT (≈45%). If either a nodular or diffuse pattern is seen in the peritoneum, the positive predictive value with PET is about 90%. ¹⁸F-FDG PET/CT can detect ovarian cancer recurrence in symptomatic patients with normal CA-125 levels; however, contrast-enhanced CT and PET/CT have similar accuracy in detecting recurrent ovarian cancer.

The value of PET/CT scanning in cervical cancer or endometrial cancers is yet to be fully defined. Cervical cancer can accumulate ¹⁸F-FDG with a sensitivity of about 70% to 90% and specificity of about 90%. Unfortunately, there is significant difficulty in differentiating tumor and nodal metastases from ¹⁸F-FDG activity in nearby bowel, bladder, and ureters. In these cases, the CT portion of the examination can be helpful.

Benign uterine tumors (including leiomyoma) usually have mild uptake of FDG. Leiomyosarcomas of the uterus usually have moderate to intense ¹⁸F-FDG uptake. Malignant uterine tumors usually have intense uptake, although small malignant tumors may have low uptake.

The sensitivity and specificity of ¹⁸F-FDG PET/CT for uterine cancer is about 90% to 95%. As with most other tumors, the sensitivity for gynecologic malignancy lesions less than 1 cm is reduced to about 30% to 50%, and for lesions less than 5 mm reported sensitivities are 0% to 20%. Sensitivity of FDG PET/CT for detecting pelvic and para-aortic lymph node metastases from endometrial cancer is about 50%. Compared to MRI, PET/CT is of limited usefulness for staging, although it can be helpful in detecting distant metastases.

Renal and Bladder Cancers

Renal and bladder cancers are both difficult to evaluate with ¹⁸F-FDG PET/CT. There is great variability of FDG uptake by renal cell cancers. Only 50% to 70% have sufficient ¹⁸F-FDG uptake to be imaged successfully. Oncocytomas have been reported to be FDG-avid. Interpretation can also be complicated by an occasional normal variant increase of ¹⁸F-FDG in the perirenal fat and in benign renal lesions, such as angiomyolipomas. However, the most significant issue is the large amount of urinary excretion of ¹⁸F-FDG, which can easily mask a tumor in the kidney or bladder. Further, activity in ureters segmented by peristalsis can mimic pathologic retroperitoneal nodes. FDG alone is not a useful tracer for the detection of primary bladder cancer, although the CT portion of a PET/CT can sometimes detect extravesicular extension. Sensitivity of FDG for nodal metastatic disease is about 75% and declines to 50% after chemotherapy.

Prostate and Testicular Cancers

The role of FDG PET/CT scanning in prostate cancer patients is extremely limited. MRI is the most sensitive and accurate (about 90% for both) imaging test. The sensitivity of ¹⁸F-FDG for the detection of prostate cancer is poor (≈50% to 65%). Even aggressive prostate cancers can be ^{18}F-FDG-negative. This may be a result of the low glucose metabolism of well-differentiated or slowly growing cells. An additional problem is the marked urinary excretion and accumulation in the bladder of the ^{18}F-FDG, obscuring nearby minimal or moderate uptake. A major problem is that ^{18}F-FDG uptake is not specific and cannot distinguish between benign prostatic hyperplasia, prostate cancer, and postoperative scarring.

Other tracers have recently been proposed, including ^{11}C-choline or ^{11}C-acetate. In early studies, ^{11}C-acetate appears to be significantly more sensitive than is ^{18}F-FDG but less specific because acetate accumulates substantially in hyperplastic tissue. Carbon-11 choline is known to be more sensitive than is FDG-PET for imaging prostate carcinoma but is limited by the inability to localize microscopic foci. As mentioned in Chapter 8, ^{18}F-NaF PET/CT bone

scans can be effectively used for the detection of prostatic osseous metastases.

The normal testes can show variable accumulation of FDG with SUVs ranging from about 1 to 6 and a mean of about 2.7. In testicular cancer, seminomas avidly accumulate FDG, whereas other nonseminomatous germ-cell tumors can have variable uptake. Teratomas may demonstrate low FDG uptake, especially mature teratomas, and PET using FDG cannot reliably differentiate post-treatment scar tissue from residual disease in mature lesions.

Miscellaneous Tumors

Multiple Myeloma. Disease status in myeloma is often difficult to assess. Imaging of multiple myeloma is most commonly done with skeletal survey and MRI (for marrow involvement). Radionuclide bone scans are frequently insensitive to focal lesions. FDG PET/CT is

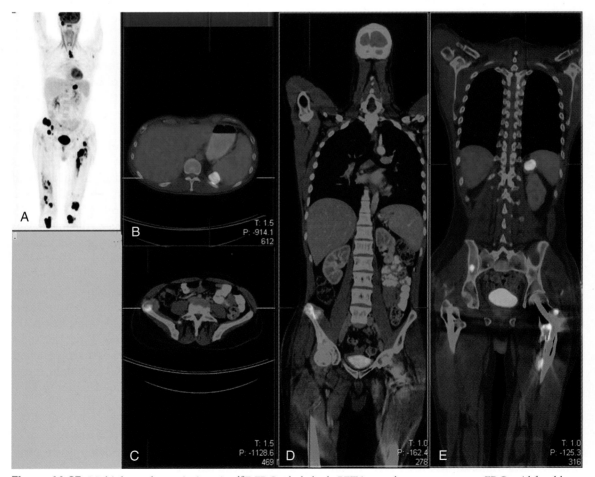

Figure 11-25. Multiple myeloma. A, Anterior ^{18}F-FDG whole-body PET image demonstrates many FDG-avid focal bone lesions. These were not visible on a radionuclide bone scan, but lytic lesions were seen on plain radiographs and CT. **B-E,** PET/CT images demonstrate the bone lesions but also clearly show focal increased activity medial to the spleen as a result of myeloma in the soft tissues.

more sensitive than skeletal radiograph and is as sensitive as MRI in detecting diffuse disease in the spine and pelvis. Although CT and MRI can identify lesions, they cannot differentiate active disease from inactive disease, posttreatment scarring, fractures, or benign lesions. Scans with ^{18}F-FDG can impact patient management by detecting sites of radiographically occult disease, recognizing disease progression, identifying extramedullary disease that worsens the patient's prognosis, and assessing the success of localized skeletal radiation therapy (Fig. 11-25). PET has shown to be useful in evaluating early-stage plasma cell dyscrasias (monoclonal gammopathy of undetermined significance), which may progress to multiple myeloma, to exclude the presence of more extensive disease.

Histiocytosis. FDG PET/CT scanning has been reported to be superior to CT, MRI, radionuclide bone scans, or plain films in the detection and response to therapy of Langerhans cell histiocytosis in the bones and soft tissues. A few reports also indicate that the lesions in Erdheim-Chester disease are often FDG-avid.

Neuroblastoma. Neuroblastomas and their metastases often accumulate ^{18}F-FDG. However, radioiodine-labeled metaiodobenzylguanidine (MIBG) is still felt to be superior, particularly for the detection of residual disease. Bone marrow involvement with neuroblastoma is often difficult to detect because of mild uptake and the presence of normal marrow activity.

Pheochromocytoma and Paraganglioma. PET agents, such as ^{18}F-fluorodopamine, ^{18}F-dihydroxyphenylalanine, and ^{11}C-hydroxyephedrine, have been shown to localize in pheochromocytomas. The detection rate with ^{18}F-FDG is about 70% (Fig. 11-26) and may be useful in patients

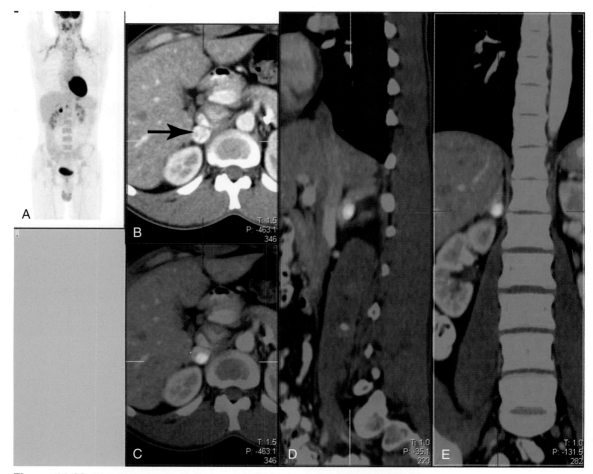

Figure 11-26. Pheochromocytoma. A, Anterior ^{18}F-FDG whole-body PET image shows increased activity in the right adrenal gland in this patient with anxiety, sweating, tremors, and heart palpitations. **B,** Axial contrasted CT scan shows the lesion to be very vascular (*arrow*). **C-E,** PET/CT images provide excellent spatial localization of the FDG within the right adrenal gland.

with MIBG-negative pheochromocytoma. Paragangliomas can be imaged with ¹⁸F-fluorodopamine (FDA), ¹⁸F-3,4-dihydroxyphenylalanine (DOPA), ¹²³I-MIBG, or ¹⁸F-FDG. Sensitivity rates for these agents are about 75% to 85%, although CT and MRI are better for non-metastatic disease.

Sarcomas and Soft Tissue Tumors. Soft-tissue sarcomas and rhabdomyosarcomas show variable degrees of ¹⁸F-FDG uptake, and sensitivity generally ranges from 80% to 90%. Ewing sarcomas are generally FDG-avid (90% sensitivity), and FDG scans can show metastases in lymph nodes and osseous metastases better than bone scintigraphy. FDG uptake does not appear to be reliable in determining Ewing responders from nonresponders to neoadjuvant treatment. Malignant fibrous histiocytomas typically show avid FDG uptake (Fig. 11-27). It should be noted that FDG uptake cannot be used to distinguish benign from malignant bone lesions. Benign lesions such as osteomyelitis and fibrous dysplasia can have intense uptake.

Bone Metastases

Excellent quality skeletal PET/CT images can be obtained using sodium ¹⁸F-fluoride (not ¹⁸F-FDG). These scans have a very high sensitivity for detecting skeletal metastases (see Chapter 8) and have at least as good, if not better, sensitivity for the detection of bone metastases as do technetium-99m (⁹⁹ᵐTc) diphosphonate scans.

Use of FDG scans for bone metastases can be somewhat difficult to interpret because of variation in normal marrow activity and diffusely enhanced marrow activity after the administration of granulocyte-stimulating factors. False-positive studies can be caused by focal benign processes such as vertebral compression fractures or sacral insufficiency injuries. If the SUV is above 2.0 in a skeletal lesion, malignancy should be included in the differential diagnosis.

Screening for Occult Tumors or Unknown Primary Tumors

The incidence of unknown primary tumors in oncologic patients is 0.5% to 7% at the time of initial diagnosis. In these cases, the primary

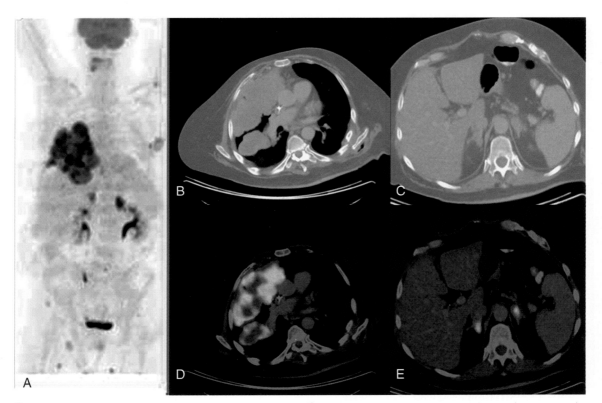

Figure 11-27. Malignant fibrous histiocytoma. A, Anterior ¹⁸F-FDG whole-body image shows abnormal activity in the right chest and adrenal glands. **B** and **C,** Axial CT and **D** and **E,** axial PET/CT images show the large multilobular lung lesion as well as the bilateral adrenal metastases.

tumor is detected in less than 40% of patients by using conventional diagnostic procedures. Scanning with ^{18}F-FDG PET has been used to evaluate the origin of these neoplasms and can detect the primary tumor in about 40% of cases. Overall, ^{18}F-FDG PET has an intermediate specificity and high sensitivity in this setting. This is expected because, although the procedure can easily identify many tumor types, there are a few common lesions (such as prostate cancer) that are not readily detected.

PEARLS & PITFALLS

- Abnormal ^{18}F-FDG activity may represent malignancy but is not pathognomonic and may represent inflammation, infection, or granulomatous disease.

- PET scans should not be read alone. The standard of care is PET/CT.

- The value of FDG PET/CT scans in staging most neoplasms is not in the evaluation of local disease but rather regional and distant disease.

- Diffuse FDG activity may be seen in the thyroid, but focal activity should raise the suspicion of thyroid cancer.

- Colonic activity is normal and usually is tubular and most intense in the cecum and ascending colon. Incidental focal colonic activity is seen in about 1% of patients has a positive predictive value of over 80% for a pathologically identifiable lesion and representing malignancy in about a third of those cases.

- An SUV above 2.5 is suggestive of malignancy but is not specific and should be used with caution. Cancers with a high SUV are generally more aggressive and have a poorer prognosis.

- Primary cancers that very avidly accumulate FDG are larynx, esophagus, non–small-cell lung, colorectal cancer, melanoma, and lymphoma.

- Malignancies that do not accumulate ^{18}F-FDG well are prostate, renal cell carcinoma, carcinoid, bladder, and mucinous cancers.

- Sometimes metastatic lesions are more FDG-avid than the primary tumor.

- Well-differentiated or mucinous tumors, carcinoid, and bronchoalveolar cell lung tumors may not be FDG-avid or may have SUVs well below 2.5.

- Focal, often symmetric ^{18}F-FDG activity in the neck, supraclavicular, and axillary regions should raise the suspicion of brown fat, particularly in females and during cold weather. It may also be present in the paraspinal and intercostal areas, usually symmetrically. Linear areas in the neck, shoulders, thighs, and arms may be from tense muscles.

- The limit of spatial resolution for PET scans is about 5 to 8 mm. Thus primary or metastatic FDG-avid lesions smaller than this may be present but not visualized. Specific care is needed to evaluate the CT portion of PET/CT scans for small metastatic lesions.

- To determine response, post-chemotherapy follow-up scans are often performed 3 weeks after the chemotherapy cycle.

- G-CSF therapy often causes diffusely increased bone marrow activity, which commonly persists for 2 to 4 weeks after cessation of chemotherapy. Increased thymic activity may occur weeks to months after chemotherapy. Increased activity is also seen for 2 to 3 months in body areas that received radiation therapy.

SUGGESTED READINGS

Bar-Shalom R, Yefremov N, Haim N, et al. Camera-based FDG PET and ^{67}Ga SPECT in evaluation of lymphoma: comparative study. Radiology 2003;227:353-60.

Basu S. PET and PET/CT in gastrointestinal stromal tumors: the unanswered questions and the potential newer applications. Eur J Nucl Med Mol Imaging 2010;37:1255-8.

Ben-Haim S, Ell P. ^{18}F-FDG PET and PET/CT in the evaluation of cancer treatment response. J Nucl Med 2009;50:88-99.

Buck A, Herrmann K, Stargardt T, et al. Economic evaluation of PET and PET/CT in oncology: evidence and methodologic approaches. J Nucl Med 2010;51:401-12.

Fletcher JW, Kymes SM, Gould M, et al. A comparison of the diagnostic accuracy of ^{18}F-FDG PET and CT in the characterization of solitary pulmonary nodules. J Nucl Med 2008;49:179-85.

Goethals I, Hoste P, DeVreiendt C, et al. Time-dependent changes in ^{18}F-FDG activity in the thymus and bone marrow following combination chemotherapy in paediatric patients with lymphoma. Eur J Nucl Med Mol Imaging 2010;37:462-7.

Grgic A, Yuksel Y, Groschel A, et al. Risk stratification of solitary pulmonary nodules by means of PET using ^{18}F-FDG and SUV quantitation. Eur J Nucl Med Mol Imaging 2010;37:1087-94.

Hustinx R, Lucignani G. PET/CT in head and neck cancer: an update. Eur J Nucl Med Mol Imaging 2010;37:645-51.

Jimez-Requena F, Delgado-Bolton RC, Fernandez-Perez C, et al. Meta-analysis of the performance of ^{18}F-FDG PET in cutaneous melanoma. Eur J Nucl Med Mol Imaging 2010;37:284-300.

Kazama T, Faria SF, Varavithya V, et al. FDG PET in the evaluation of treatment for lymphoma: clinical usefulness and pitfalls. RadioGraphics 2005;25:91-207.

Kim TJ, Kim HY, Lee KW, et al. Multimodality assessment of esophageal cancer: preoperative staging and monitoring of response to therapy. RadioGraphics 2009;29:403-21.

Kong G, Jackson C, Koh DM, et al. The use of ^{18}F-FDG PET/CT in colorectal liver metastases: comparison with CT and liver MRI. Eur J Nucl Med Mol Imaging 2008;35:1323-9.

Lim HS, Yoon W, Chung TW, et al. FDG PET/CT for the detection and evaluation of breast diseases: usefulness and limitations. RadioGraphics 2007;27:S197-213.

Lim SL, Yun MJ, Kim MJ, et al. CT and PET in stomach cancer: preoperative staging and monitoring of response to therapy. RadioGraphics 2006;26:143-56.

Lucignani G. FDG-PET in gynecological cancers: recent observations. Eur J Nucl Med Mol Imaging 2008;35:2133-9.

Prakash P, Cronin C, Blake M. Role of PET/CT in ovarian cancer: Review. Am J Roentgenol 2010;194(6):W464-70.

Rosen EL, Eubank WB, Mankoff D, et al. FDG PET, PET/CT, and breast cancer imaging. RadioGraphics 2007;27:S215-99.

Veit-Haibach P, Vogt FM, Jablonka R, et al. Diagnostic accuracy of contrast enhanced FDG-PET/CT in primary staging of cutaneous malignant melanoma. Eur J Nucl Med Mol Imaging 2009;36:910-8.

Zaheer A, Cho S, Pomper M. New agents and techniques for imaging prostate cancer. J Nucl Med 2009;50:1387-90.

12 Inflammation and Infection Imaging

RADIOLABELED LEUKOCYTES
   Mechanism of Localization
   Indium-111 Oxine Leukocytes
   Technetium-99m HMPAO Leukocytes
GALLIUM IMAGING
   Mechanisms of Localization in Inflammation/
     Infection
   Technique
   Clinical Applications

18F-FDG PET/CT IMAGING
FUTURE INFLAMMATION AGENTS

A variety of nuclear medicine imaging techniques provides effective methods for the detection and assessment of both clinically apparent and occult infectious and inflammatory conditions. Rather than representing organ-specific techniques, these procedures use radiopharmaceuticals that localize preferentially in inflamed or infected tissue in any location in the body. The available radiopharmaceuticals exhibit varying degrees of non-specificity and are best used with meticulous clinical correlation. The particular role of each of the readily available radiopharmaceuticals for infection imaging often depends on the clinical setting and the specific part of the body under scrutiny. Selection of the proper imaging agent is critical to the success of the procedure (Table 12-1). These agents include the following:

- Radiolabeled white blood cells
  - Indium-111 (^{111}In) leukocytes
  - Technetium-99m (^{99m}Tc) leukocytes
- Gallium-67 (^{67}Ga) citrate
- Fluorine-18 fluorodeoxyglucose (^{18}F-FDG)
- Radiolabeled monoclonal antibodies and antibody fragments
- Radiolabeled peptides

RADIOLABELED LEUKOCYTES

Leukocyte imaging using in-vitro labeling with ^{111}In-oxine or ^{99m}Tc-exametazime is currently the gold standard for diagnosing most infections in patients who are not immunocompromised.

Because leukocytes can be separated and labeled without significant loss of function, they can be used to image inflammatory processes. Both ^{111}In-oxine leukocytes and ^{99m}Tc-hexamethylpropyleneamine oxime (HMPAO) leukocytes have been shown to retain their innate function and have demonstrated relatively high sensitivity and specificity for acute infections. However, sensitivity may be somewhat lower for chronic infections. The procedure involves removing some of the patient's own leukocytes, labeling them, and reinjecting them before scanning. As with any autologous labeled biologic agent, extreme care must be taken to maintain the integrity of the blood sample and to ensure that reinjection of the labeled leukocytes is performed only in the patient from whom the cells were taken. Clinical studies comparing ^{99m}Tc and ^{111}In-leukocytes have not shown any intrinsic differences in sensitivity for infection when standard 24-hour imaging is performed. However, some notable differences between the two radiopharmaceuticals make one or the other preferable in certain clinical situations.

Mechanism of Localization

Radiolabeled leukocytes are attracted to sites of inflammation, where they are activated by local chemotactic factors and pass from the blood stream through the vascular endothelium into the soft tissues. The leukocytes then move toward the site of inflammation in a directed migration called *chemotaxis*. If the inflammation has an infectious

TABLE 12-1 Infection Imaging Radiopharmaceuticals

RADIOPHARMACEUTICAL AND ADMINISTERED ACTIVITY	TIME OF IMAGING	ADVANTAGES	DISADVANTAGES	COMMON USES
111In white blood cells 300-500 μCi (10-18.5 MBq)	12-24 hr	No interfering bowel/renal activity Delayed imaging possible Simultaneous 99mTc-sulfur colloid or 99mTc-diphosphonate bone imaging possible	Less sensitivity for nonbacterial and nonpyogenic infections 111In label not ideal for imaging Complex preparation	Bacterial infections Indolent inflammatory conditions: e.g., prosthetic joint infections Abdominal infections Prosthetic vascular graft infections Brain abscess Complicated osteomyelitis Extremity infections: e.g., diabetic foot Renal infections FUO: acute phase
99mTc-white blood cells 5-10 mCi (185-370 MBq)	0.5-4.0 hr	Early imaging Excellent early sensitivity 99mTc label ideal for imaging	Less sensitivity for nonbacterial and nonpyogenic infections Delayed imaging not ideal Early renal activity Bowel activity after 1-2 hr Complex preparation	Bacterial infections Acute inflammatory conditions: e.g., inflammatory bowel disease Complicated osteomyelitis Extremity infections: diabetic foot Osteomyelitis Prosthetic vascular graft infections
67Ga-citrate 5-10 mCi (185-370 MBq)	24-48 hr	A variety of infections detected, including opportunistic	Interfering bowel and renal activity Delayed imaging necessary 67Ga not ideal for imaging	Immunocompromised patients Uncomplicated osteomyelitis Chronic infections Diskitis/spinal osteomyelitis FUO: chronic phase
18F-FDG PET/CT 10 mCi (370 MBq)	1-2 hr	Excellent spatial localization Very sensitive	Not currently FDA approved for infections Non specific; also localizes in tumors	

FDA, Food and Drug Administration; *FUO,* fever of unknown origin

cause, the labeled neutrophils phagocytize and destroy any offending bacteria. Gamma camera imaging localizes these accumulations of radio-labeled leukocytes and thus reveals the site of inflammation or infection. Like gallium uptake, radiolabeled leukocyte uptake is not specific for infection and may occur in any inflammatory process that incites a leukocyte response. Occasional uptake in neoplasms may be noted.

Indium-111 Oxine Leukocytes

Compared with ^{67}Ga-citrate imaging, ^{111}In oxine–labeled leukocytes offer the following *advantages*:

- Less variable normal physiologic distribution from patient to patient
- Essentially no accumulation in the gastrointestinal tract, kidneys, or bladder, with less soft-tissue activity
- Less activity in noninfectious inflammation and tumors
- Greater concentration in abscessed tissues
- Earlier results, generally within 24 hours
  There are some *disadvantages*, however:
- Tedious, expensive labeling procedure that requires precautions associated with handling blood products
- Possibility that severely leukopenic patients may not permit labeling of an adequate number of leukocytes for successful imaging
- Less success in imaging some chronic infections
- Relatively high radiation dose

Labeling Principle

Imaging leukocyte distribution in the body became possible after the development of successful methods for labeling leukocytes with ^{111}In-oxine. Indium-111 oxine labels all cell types indiscriminately, including platelets and red blood cells. Thus the leukocytes are isolated from about 50 mL of anticoagulated blood before labeling, commonly through a process called *gravity sedimentation*, which simply consists of allowing the blood to sit for the time necessary for the red blood cells to settle to the bottom. Any red blood cells remaining in the supernatant may be either lysed by using hypotonic saline or ammonium chloride or removed by centrifugation.

Oxine forms a lipid-soluble complex with ^{111}In, which passively diffuses through the leukocyte cell membrane. Once this complex becomes intracellular, the ^{111}In separates from the oxine and binds to cytoplasmic components. The oxine then leaves the cell and is removed by washing the cells. A mixed population of leukocytes is usually labeled, although neutrophils constitute the majority. Labeling efficiencies are on the order of 95%. The patient's circulating granulocyte count should be at least 2000 cells/mL to have enough cells to label.

Minimal manipulation of the leukocytes is essential to the actual tagging procedure to avoid damage to the cells, which could diminish their viability and thus limit their effectiveness as an imaging agent. Failure to preserve normal physiologic leukocyte function may result in false-negative imaging study results.

Technique

About 0.5 to 1.0 mCi (18.5 to 37 MBq) of ^{111}In-oxine–labeled autologous leukocytes is administered intravenously. Care should be taken to avoid excessive agitation of the leukocytes because this may cause clumping, resulting in focal lung accumulation. Although some abscesses can be detected in the first few hours after the administration of labeled leukocytes, most imaging is performed 18 to 24 hours after administration. If the urgency of the clinical setting dictates, 4- to 6-hour images may be useful. A whole-body survey can be performed by using a medium-energy collimator, with gamma camera images obtained of specific areas of interest. Generally, both the 173- and 247-keV gamma emissions of ^{111}In are used. A sample imaging protocol and radiation dosimetry are presented in Appendix E-1.

Normal Scan

In the first few hours after administration of ^{111}In-leukocytes, activity is noted in the lungs (likely as a result of leukocyte activation), liver, spleen, and blood pool. The lung and blood pool activity decreases during the first few hours as spleen and liver activity increases. By 18 hours, no lung or blood pool activity is detected, but bone marrow activity is noted (Fig. 12-1).

Twenty-four hours after administration, the ^{111}In-leukocyte preparation may be found in the liver, spleen, and bone marrow, with the spleen providing the most prominent accumulation, significantly more than that in the liver. No renal or bowel activity is normally present. Damaged leukocytes that remain labeled may

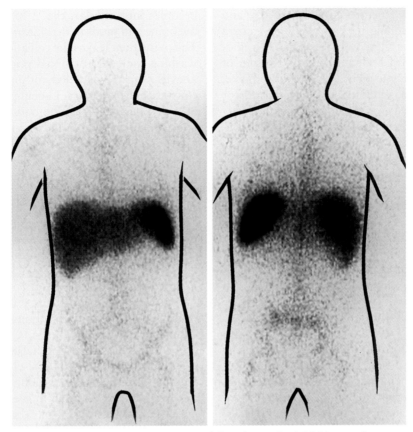

Figure 12-1. **Normal indium-111 leukocyte scan.** Anterior (*left*) and posterior (*right*) images demonstrate liver and splenic activity. The splenic activity normally is greater. A small amount of bone marrow activity is also identified.

provide increased activity in the liver, if slightly damaged, and increased lung activity if severely damaged.

Clinical Applications

General Considerations. Indium-111 leukocytes are taken up nonspecifically in sites of inflammation, inciting a leukocytic response, regardless of the presence or absence of infection (Box 12-1). The sensitivity (90%) and specificity (90%) are greatest for acute pyogenic infections of less than 2 to 3 weeks' duration. Their effectiveness for detecting more chronic infections is somewhat controversial, although sensitivity with mixed cell populations, which include lymphocytes and chronic inflammatory cells as well as neutrophils, generally appears high (80% to 85%). This may also be because some common bacterial infections may demonstrate significant levels of neutrophil infiltration for months. Labeled leukocytes are of no use in the detection of viral and parasitic infections. Factors that can theoretically reduce leukocyte

function, including antibiotics, steroids, chemotherapeutic agents, hemodialysis, hyperalimentation, and hyperglycemia, do not appear to diminish labeled leukocyte sensitivity for detecting infection.

Indium-labeled leukocytes are the preferred radiopharmaceutical for imaging abdominal infection, although in practice, a computed tomography (CT) scan is usually the initial imaging study ordered for abdominal pain or suspected infection. Because of the lack of normal bowel activity, ^{111}In-labeled leukocytes have a significant advantage over [67]Ga- and ^{99m}Tc-labeled leukocytes in diagnosing abdominal abscesses with high sensitivity (85% to 95%). As with gallium, however, the presence of considerable hepatic and especially splenic activity may hamper the detection of infection in the upper abdomen. Splenic bed abscesses with intense activity may even be confused with a normal spleen (Fig. 12-2). In this setting, ^{99m}Tc-colloid liver and spleen scans may be subtracted from the labeled leukocyte images to unmask

Box 12-1 Causes of Increased Activity on Labeled Leukocyte Images

Chest
Common Causes
Adult respiratory distress syndrome
Emphysema
Pleural tubes
Noninfected intravenous lines
Pneumonia

Uncommon Causes
Aspiration
Atelectasis
Cystic fibrosis
Graft infection
Herpes esophagitis

Abdomen
Common Causes
Enteric tubes
Ostomies
Phlegmon
Swallowed leukocytes
Wound infection

Uncommon Causes
Acute enteritis
Bowel infarction
Colitis

Crohn disease
Decubitus ulcer
Gastrointestinal bleeding
Graft infection
Pancreatitis
Transplant (with or without rejection)
Diverticulitis
Acute cholecystitis

Musculoskeletal And Skin Uptake
Common Causes
Intravenous site
Osteomyelitis
Sinusitis

Uncommon Causes
Lumbar puncture site
Rheumatoid arthritis
Septic arthritis

Any Body Part
Abscess
Cellulitis
Wound infection
Hematoma
Infected tumor

---

any adjacent abnormal activity. Uncomplicated pancreatitis is usually negative, but septic complications are usually imaged successfully.

Labeled leukocyte activity in the gastrointestinal tract is nonspecific and may indicate a number of pathologies, including Crohn disease, ulcerative colitis (Fig. 12-3), pseudomembranous colitis, diverticulitis, various gastrointestinal infections, fistulas, ischemic or infarcted bowel, and even vigorous enemazation before imaging. Increased activity in the bowel, especially the colon, may also be problematic in that activity may be found in the absence of true gastrointestinal disease. False-positive results are generally caused by swallowing of leukocytes in patients with endotracheal or nasoesophageal tubes, respiratory tract infections, sinusitis, or pharyngitis or in patients with gastrointestinal bleeding of any cause. In general, the more intense the bowel activity compared with liver activity, the more likely it is to indicate a true positive study.

Normal transient physiologic lung activity on early images (1 to 4 hours) severely limits usefulness of ^{111}In-leukocytes in evaluating pulmonary abnormalities. Increased lung activity is of low specificity at 24 hours as well because it may occur in numerous infectious and noninfectious processes, including atelectasis, congestive heart failure, pulmonary emboli, aspiration, pneumonia, and adult respiratory distress syndrome. Only one third of patients showing focal or diffuse uptake in the lungs have infectious causes, although focal uptake demonstrates a slightly better correlation with infection.

Fever of Unknown Origin (Occult Fever). In a genuine fever of unknown origin (FUO), the spectrum of possible pathology is extensive. The three major categories that account for most FUO are infections, malignancies, and noninfectious inflammatory disease. There is evidence which indicates that PET/CT with ^{18}F-FDG, while not specific for infection, may be the most efficient method for evaluation of FUO. The value of either ^{18}F-FDG or ^{67}Ga scanning in FUO is the ability to detect these pathologies rather than just infection. In occult fevers with a strong suggestion of a pyogenic cause, however, leukocyte scans may be the study of choice when CT or other anatomic imaging procedures cannot localize the disease.

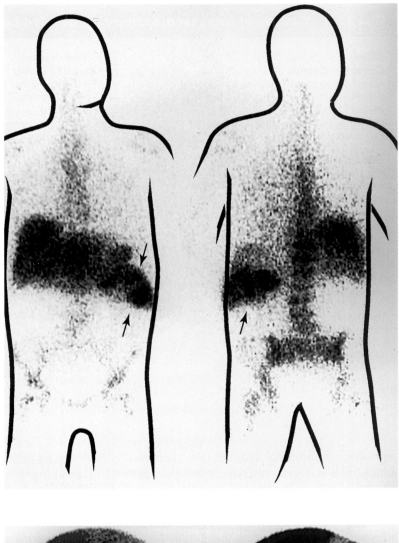

Figure 12-2. **Postsplenectomy abscess.** Anterior (*left*) and posterior (*right*) indium-111 leukocyte images demonstrate a focus of activity in the left upper quadrant (*arrows*) that might be mistaken for a slightly inferiorly displaced spleen, except that the spleen has been removed.

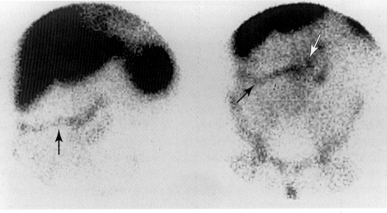

Figure 12-3. **Colitis.** Anterior views of the upper and lower abdomen demonstrate activity (*arrows*) in the ascending and transverse colon that is abnormal on indium-111 leukocyte scans. (Remember that there is normal physiologic colonic excretion with gallium scans.)

Immunocompromised Patients. Labeled leukocytes have significant limitations for imaging suspected infections in immunocompromised patients. They are not useful in the detection of viral or parasitic infections, demonstrate low specificity in the lungs, and are insensitive for determining active lymph node diseases such as lymphoma in these patients. False-negative examinations have been reported in tuberculous and fungal infections. In addition, the study may be technically difficult in severely leukopenic patients. However, ^{111}In-labeled leukocytes are often useful to evaluate suspected acute pyogenic infections, including sinusitis, bowel infections, and bacterial pneumonias in this setting.

Musculoskeletal Infections. Because labeled leukocytes are taken up by the bone marrow, normal, post-traumatic, or postsurgical variations in marrow distribution may produce confusing foci of increased activity owing to regionally increased marrow uptake. Such false-positive results in the marrow-bearing skeleton can be avoided by performing simultaneous marrow imaging with ^{99m}Tc-sulfur colloid (obtained on a separate photopeak) for comparison with labeled leukocyte distribution. Technetium-99m colloid activity 1 hour after injection is compared with ^{111}In leukocyte activity at 24 hours in the area of interest. Criteria for a positive study are (1) spatial incongruence (i.e., leukocyte activity in the absence of sulfur colloid activity) and (2) incongruence of intensity of activity (i.e., leukocyte activity considerably greater than corresponding colloid activity) (Fig. 12-4). Throughout the skeleton, false-positive results may also be produced by nonspecific uptake in recent fractures, heterotopic bone formation, recent radiation therapy, some neoplasms, and noninfectious inflammation, including that caused by gout and rheumatoid arthritis. Simultaneous bone scans may be of value in leukocyte imaging of the hands and feet to provide anatomic detail needed to separate soft tissue from bony activity.

Osteomyelitis. In uncomplicated acute osteomyelitis, especially with normal radiographs, a positive three-phase bone scan is definitive in most settings and obviates the need for further imaging with labeled leukocytes or magnetic resonance imaging (MRI). Use of planar technetium-99m-methylene diphosphonate (^{99m}Tc-MDP) for osteomyelitis has a sensitivity of greater than 80% and a limited specificity of about 50%. The specificity increases to more than 80% with use of single-photon emission computed tomography (SPECT)/CT. White blood cell (WBC) scanning has sensitivity and specificity above 90% and ^{18}F-FDG is reported to have a sensitivity of about 95% and a specificity of about 85%. Chronicity of infection does not appear to have a significant effect on sensitivity of

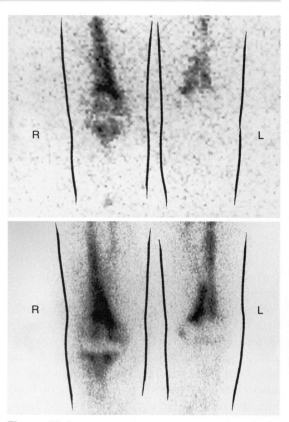

Figure 12-4. Expanded marrow. In this patient who has had a right knee joint replacement, there is a possibility of infection or loosening of the prosthesis. *Top,* Anterior views of an indium-111 leukocyte scan over both knees show asymmetric activity extending distal to the right knee joint. *Bottom,* Technetium-99m colloid scan over both knees demonstrates marrow activity, indicating, in this case, asymmetrically expanded marrow. The pattern of indium-111 leukocyte uptake is thus concordant with the marrow distribution and does not indicate infection.

leukocyte imaging, although false-negative results have occurred. Indium-111 leukocytes, however, have low sensitivity for spine infections, including osteomyelitis and diskitis. For uncertain reasons, more than half of spine infections appear as photopenic (cold) defects in the areas of involvement rather than as hot spots (Fig. 12-5). This focal photopenia, although suspicious for infection, is nonspecific and may be seen in numerous other entities, including tumor, compression fracture, avascular necrosis, radiation therapy, Paget disease, fibrous dysplasia, and myelofibrosis. In the setting of spinal infections, ^{67}Ga may be preferred. In the clinical circumstance of suspected osseous infection complicating disturbed or diseased bone in which radiographs and ^{99m}Tc-diphosphonate bone imaging are

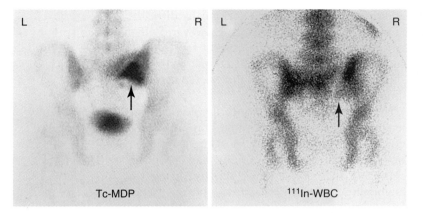

Figure 12-5. Osteomyelitis of the right sacroiliac joint. *Left,* Posterior view of the pelvis obtained on a bone scan demonstrates markedly increased activity (*arrow*) in the mid-portion of the right sacroiliac joint. *Right,* An indium-111 leukocyte scan in the same patient shows that the same area is relatively decreased in activity (*arrow*). This may be seen with ^{111}In leukocyte scans when the osteomyelitis is in the central portion of the skeleton, especially the spine. *MDP,* Methylene diphosphonate.

likely to be abnormal and nonspecific, ^{111}In-leukocytes provide an accurate tool to unmask or rule out osteomyelitis.

Post-Traumatic Infections. Indium leukocyte scans may be positive for several weeks in recent fractures in the absence of superimposed infection, although the uptake is usually faint. Intense focal uptake at a site of suspected osteomyelitis is indicative of bony infection. In this setting, sensitivity and specificity rates exceed 90%, which are significantly better than the rates for gallium imaging (50% to 60%).

Prosthetic Joint Infections. Combined leukocyte/marrow imaging is the radionuclide imaging procedure of choice for diagnosing prosthetic joint infection. Painful prosthetic joints may be attributable to loosening or infection. Bone scans may be falsely positive during the first year after surgery, owing to healing and bony remodeling, especially in the hip or knee. Although ^{111}In-leukocytes are very sensitive for periprosthetic infections, because labeled leukocytes may accumulate in the normal bone marrow adjacent to a prosthesis, including marrow in heterotopic bone formation, false-positive results may occur. To increase accuracy, the procedure of choice in this setting is a ^{111}In-leukocyte scan accompanied by ^{99m}Tc-sulfur colloid marrow imaging. The sulfur colloid study provides a map of postsurgical marrow distribution, whereas the leukocytes map both the distribution of marrow and any accompanying infection. Thus congruent images indicate that leukocyte uptake is likely related to normal marrow activity, whereas areas that concentrate leukocytes but not sulfur colloid indicate areas of infection. This combined study has a

sensitivity and accuracy in excess of 90%. In the hip, labeled leukocyte activity over the head of the prosthesis is strongly suggestive of infection, whereas activity in the region of the shank is less so because of a plug of marrow that may be pushed to the tip of the prosthesis when inserted.

Diabetic Foot Infections. Labeled leukocyte activity in normal bone marrow does not usually cause a problem in interpretation of images in the peripheral skeleton. Uptake of labeled leukocytes in adjacent ulcers or cellulitis, however, along with decreased resolution of anatomic detail using the ^{111}In label, may confound separation of soft tissue from bony uptake, especially in the hands and feet. In this setting, comparison of a simultaneous bone scan (obtained on a separate photopeak) with the ^{111}In leukocyte distribution may provide the anatomic information needed to distinguish between bone and soft-tissue activity. Leukocyte scans in this setting have an overall accuracy of about 80%.

Neuropathic Joint Infections. Infections may commonly complicate neuropathic joints. However, in early, rapidly progressing sterile neuropathia, both bone scans and ^{111}In-leukocyte scans are frequently positive because of associated inflammatory and destructive bony changes. Thus the findings on leukocyte and bone imaging may be indistinguishable from osteomyelitis. Faint, diffuse leukocyte activity that fades between the 4- and 24-hour images is suggestive of sterile disease, whereas more intense focal activity that is distinctly different in distribution from the bone scan activity and that increases over time suggests superimposed infection. In chronic forms of neuropathic osteoarthropathy, interpretation of the leukocyte and bone scans is simplified by the less avid inflammatory response and decreased soft-tissue background activity.

Active Arthritis. Arthritides, even those normally of a chronic nature, can have tremendous leukocyte responses. Thus leukocyte scans have been applied to diagnosing and monitoring the activity of rheumatoid arthritis. In this setting, 99mTc-labeled leukocytes show early positivity, improved image quality, and decreased radiation exposure compared with that of 111In-labeled leukocytes.

Vascular Graft Infection. Perigraft gas on a CT scan is diagnostic of infection; however, this is seen in only 50% of cases. In the setting of a negative or equivocal CT scan, 111In-leukocytes are useful in detecting vascular graft infections, including infections of dialysis access grafts. More than 90% of patients with positive scans have subsequently documented culture evidence of infection (Fig. 12-6). Causes of false-positive results are perigraft hematomas, graft thrombosis, and graft epithelialization, which occurs in the first several weeks after surgery.

Technetium-99m HMPAO Leukocytes

The role of 99mTc-HMPAO leukocytes in inflammation imaging can be better appreciated by a comparison with 111In leukocytes. Although they are similar in many respects, there are a few important differences:

■ The technetium label permits higher administered activity, which improves visualization of small-part anatomy, such as the hands and feet.
■ The shorter, 6-hour half-life of 99mTc limits delayed imaging, which can be important for optimal accumulation of labeled leukocytes in some processes.
■ Technetium-99m HMPAO leukocyte preparations display normal gastrointestinal tract, urinary tract, and gallbladder activity.
■ There is faster uptake of 99mTc-HMPAO leukocytes in sites of infection, permitting earlier imaging.
■ Low absorbed doses enhance suitability for imaging infants and children.

Otherwise, 99mTc-HMPAO leukocytes share most of the other advantages and disadvantages of 111In leukocytes.

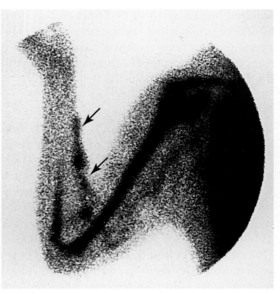

Figure 12-6. Graft infection. In this patient who was on renal dialysis, an infection of the dialysis graft was suspected. Technetium-99m leukocyte scan demonstrates normally expected activity in the bone marrow of the humerus and proximal forearm, but there is also markedly increased activity extending throughout and proximal to the graft site (*arrows*).

Labeling

The labeling process is similar in principle to that used in the 111In oxine procedure. A 99mTc-HMPAO lipophilic complex enters the separated leukocytes and is converted to a hydrophilic form, which is trapped inside the cells. The efficiency of this technetium label is less than that of indium. Unlike 111In oxine, which labels a mixed population of cells, HMPAO preferentially labels neutrophils.

Technique

Between 5 and 10 mCi (185 to 370 MBq) of 99mTc-HMPAO leukocytes are intravenously injected in adult patients. Technetium-99m leukocytes localize in sites of infection more rapidly than do 111In oxine leukocytes, with a maximal sensitivity at 30 minutes. The imaging sequence depends on the clinical setting. Early images are usually acquired at 0.5 to 4 hours by using a low-energy, high-resolution collimator or a low-energy, all-purpose collimator. The abdomen and pelvis are imaged first, before interfering normal bowel activity can accumulate. For whole-body imaging, views are obtained for 300,000 to 500,000 counts of the head, chest, abdomen, and pelvis, with extremity images obtained as clinically indicated.

Delayed images at 18 to 24 hours are obtained as needed, using a low-energy, all-purpose collimator if count rates are lower than expected. A sample imaging protocol is presented in Appendix E-1.

Normal Distribution

Indium-111 and ^{99m}Tc-leukocytes display identical biokinetics in the liver, spleen, and lung. Unlike ^{111}In-leukocytes, however, which show increasing bone marrow activity over 24 hours with constant activity thereafter, ^{99m}Tc leukocyte activity in bone marrow increases over the first 3 hours after injection but decreases over the next 24 hours. In addition, unbound ^{99m}Tc-HMPAO complexes from the leukocyte preparation are seen in the gastrointestinal tract, kidneys, and bladder and occasionally in the gallbladder. Bowel activity is likely related to biliary excretion. Renal activity is primarily attributable to urinary excretion, with a variable amount of parenchymal binding.

Clinical Applications

Thorax. Similar to their ^{111}In-labeled counterparts, ^{99m}Tc-leukocytes localize nonspecifically in lung inflammation or infection and play a limited role in chest disease. Uptake may be seen in pneumonias, systemic vasculitis, adult respiratory distress syndrome, *Pneumocystis carinii* pneumonia (PCP), or drug-induced pneumonitis. In bronchiectasis, preoperative ^{99m}Tc-leukocyte imaging may be used to determine which lesions noted on CT are active.

Abdomen/Pelvis. Early images for localization of abdominopelvic abscesses are sensitive because of the rapid accumulation of ^{99m}Tc-leukocytes in pyogenic foci. Sequential imaging at 1 and 4 hours is needed to differentiate abnormal leukocyte accumulations from nonspecific bowel activity and to avoid false-positive results caused by imaging at 4 hours only. For inflammatory bowel disease, 1-hour information with ^{99m}Tc is comparable to that seen on 3-hour ^{111}In images, with ^{99m}Tc providing better visualization in the small bowel. Bowel segments showing increased activity at 1 hour that increase in activity at 4 hours provide a higher specificity of diagnosis than does activity appearing for the first time at 4 hours or remaining at the same intensity. Technetium-99m leukocytes can be used to establish a diagnosis, identify diseased segments, confirm

relapse, identify complications of Crohn disease such as mural abscess, and quantify disease. The distribution of activity in the colon allows a distinction between Crohn disease and ulcerative colitis with a high degree of certainty. Rectal sparing, small-bowel involvement, and "skip" areas suggest Crohn disease, whereas continuous involvement from the rectum without small-bowel involvement suggests ulcerative colitis. A false-positive appearance on early images may be caused by oozing from recent anastomoses or active gastrointestinal bleeding. With ^{99m}Tc leukocytes, renal infections and hepatobiliary sepsis may be difficult to distinguish from physiologic activity, and ^{111}In-labeled leukocytes may be preferable in these settings.

GALLIUM IMAGING

Gallium-67 imaging accumulates nonspecifically in inflammatory and infectious diseases, as well as neoplastic diseases. The nonspecificity of gallium has caused it to be supplanted for the imaging of many infectious processes by more specific imaging agents such as radiolabeled leukocytes. However, gallium has been used for over 3 decades as an infection imaging agent and continues to be a limited use radiopharmaceutical for the detection and localization of certain inflammatory lesions.

Mechanisms of Localization in Inflammation/Infection

The mechanisms of gallium citrate localization in inflammatory tissues are likely different in some respects from the mechanisms associated with localization in neoplasms. The process is complex, but a few basic principles are known to be associated with such concentration: (1) gallium forms complexes with plasma transferrin that act as carriers for ^{67}Ga to sites of inflammation; (2) gallium is also incorporated into leukocytes, bound by intracellular lactoferrin, which then migrate to inflamed areas; and (3) gallium may be taken up by pathogenic microorganisms themselves by binding to siderophores produced by the bacteria.

Technique

The technique used for gallium imaging in the setting of inflammation and infection is in many ways similar to that used when imaging neoplasms. The major difference is the temporal sequence for obtaining images. Initial images are obtained earlier in cases of suspected inflammatory disease, usually 18 to 24 hours after injection. Images are subsequently obtained at 24-hour intervals as needed to allow for improved target-to-nontarget ratios and for the possible differentiation of normal bowel activity from accumulations in pathologic entities. Suggested imaging protocol and dosimetry are presented in Appendix E-1.

Clinical Applications

The significance of an abnormal accumulation of gallium increases with the intensity of the focus as seen on appropriate images. In general, however, any abnormal gallium activity equal to or greater than that seen in the liver may be considered significant.

Abdominal and Retroperitoneal Inflammation and Infection

In general, the proper interpretation of gallium images in the abdomen hinges on the differentiation of physiologic activity from abnormal accumulations of the radiopharmaceutical. A common problem in image interpretation in the abdomen is the presence of gallium in the bowel, which may mimic lesions or mask disease. Bowel activity is particularly prominent in the colon and may be diffuse or focal. Frequently, activity is seen in the regions of the cecum, hepatic and splenic flexures, and rectosigmoid. These accumulations may appear as early as a few hours after injection. The progress of excreted gallium through the colon over time may provide the best evidence of physiologic activity, whereas persistence of gallium in a given area of the abdomen should be viewed as abnormal.

Abscesses in the retroperitoneum are frequently related to associated renal infection. Persistence of more than faint renal activity after 24 hours, progressively increasing activity, and unilateral discrepancy in gallium activity in the kidneys should be considered abnormal. However, abnormally increased activity in one or both kidneys can occur in nonspecific pathologic and physiologic states and may therefore present a difficult problem of differential diagnosis. The differential includes urinary obstruction, nephritis, acute tubular necrosis, diffuse infiltrative neoplasm, vasculitis, parenteral iron injections, blood transfusions, and perirenal inflammatory disease.

Thoracic Inflammation and Infection

Gallium accumulates nonspecifically in tumors and in a variety of inflammatory abnormalities, including pyogenic and viral pneumonias, PCP, early radiation pneumonitis, acute respiratory distress syndrome, granulomatous and fungal diseases, vasculitis, idiopathic pulmonary fibrosis, pneumoconioses, lymphangitis metastases, connective tissue diseases, and drug reactions (amiodarone, busulfan, cyclophosphamide methotrexate, procarbazine, vincristine). The degree of gallium activity has been used to determine whether a pulmonary process is in an active or a quiescent stage. In general, increasing degrees of gallium activity correlate with increasing activity of disease. Acute inflammatory diseases of the heart and pericardium may also produce positive gallium images. In both the chest and abdomen, hematomas and healing wounds, both sterile and infected, may demonstrate gallium uptake.

Fever of Unknown Origin

Initial imaging for an FUO should begin with labeled leukocytes or CT scan and followed with an ^{18}F-FDG or gallium study, if necessary. Although gallium is reasonably sensitive for localized pyogenic disease (80% to 90%), it is less sensitive than are radiolabeled leukocytes, especially in the abdomen, where about one third of infections responsible for FUO are found. In addition, a gallium study should be used with caution in patients who have been treated with systemic antibiotics because false-negative results may occur under these circumstances.

Immunocompromised Patients

Because its sensitivity for detection of infection does not depend on acute pyogenic response, gallium imaging can sometimes be a useful radionuclide procedure for detecting and evaluating the varied opportunistic pulmonary infections and adenopathies common in patients with compromised immune systems resulting from acquired immunodeficiency syndrome (AIDS), antineoplastic chemotherapy, or immunosuppression after organ transplantation.

In immunocompromised patients, gallium scans of the thorax should always be interpreted in comparison with recent chest radiographs, which add specificity to the examination. A normal gallium scan with a normal chest radiograph essentially excludes an infectious process. A normal gallium scan in the presence of a focal mass or infiltrate on the chest radiograph, however, suggests the diagnosis of Kaposi sarcoma, which does not accumulate gallium.

Bilateral intense diffuse homogeneous pulmonary uptake of gallium is the classic appearance of PCP and occurs in 60% to 70% of cases. The gallium scan is frequently positive before chest radiographs become abnormal. Gallium imaging is 90% sensitive for the disease, and, although not specific, diffuse pulmonary activity in this population should prompt investigation or treatment of the offending organism. The specificity of a diffusely positive scan is greater when the chest radiograph is negative and the pulmonary activity is intense (equal to or greater than liver activity) (Fig. 12-7).

Treatment of PCP or prophylaxis with aerosolized pentamidine may alter the classic appearance of diffuse uptake in active or recurrent infections. Because aerosol deposition is less efficient in the upper lobes, the resultant relative undertreatment may restrict recurrent disease to the upper lung zones. In addition, with early aggressive therapy, patients can survive long enough to develop chronic airway and parenchymal changes, which may further alter the distribution of successful treatment and thus the

distribution of recurrent disease. Under these circumstances, positive gallium scans may appear as nonhomogeneous or even focal areas of increased activity. Successful treatment of PCP is generally reflected by decreasing intensity of gallium uptake or a return to a normal appearance.

In patients with AIDS, lymph node involvement by a variety of diseases is common. Gallium uptake in the generalized lymphadenopathy associated with AIDS and AIDS-related complex is variable in occurrence and degree of activity, which may be minimal. Increased gallium uptake equal to or greater than liver activity in hilar, mediastinal, periaortic, or supraclavicular nodes suggests the diagnoses of malignant lymphoma, *Mycobacterium tuberculosis*, or *M. avium-intracellulare*. However, this nodal activity is nonspecific, and other less common infectious processes cannot be excluded.

In the abdomen, abnormal gallium accumulation may be seen in bacterial abscess and gastrointestinal infections, as well as in regional lymph nodes affected by *M. avium-intracellulare* or lymphoma. The usefulness of gallium for the detection and evaluation of AIDS-related diseases of the gastrointestinal tract is limited by interfering physiologic bowel activity and the lack of correlation of abnormal uptake with specific

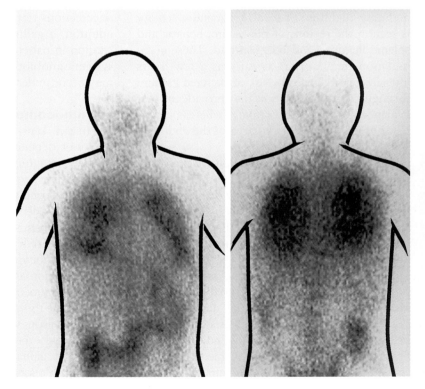

Figure 12-7. Pneumocystis pneumonia. Anterior (*left*) and posterior (*right*) 24-hour gallium images demonstrate normal physiologic excretion in the colon; however, there is markedly abnormal increased activity in both lungs. Note the negative cardiac defect produced by the intense lung activity.

pathogens, as is seen in thoracic disease. Intense colonic activity (greater than liver activity) that persists unchanged over 72 hours of imaging is suspicious, but not diagnostic, of infectious colitis and should be interpreted with caution.

Combined imaging with thallium-201 (^{201}Tl) and ^{67}Ga may add to the diagnostic specificity of gallium imaging in the setting of immunocompromised patients. With some exceptions, this type of combined imaging has yielded the following results: Kaposi sarcoma is gallium-negative but thallium-positive. Lymphoma is both gallium- and thallium-positive. Acute infections, tuberculosis, and M. *avium-intracellulare* are usually gallium-positive and thallium-negative but may show faint thallium uptake.

Osteomyelitis

The initial imaging test of choice for osteomyelitis is a routine radiograph. If this is negative, triple-phase bone imaging with ^{99m}Tc-diphosphonates combined with leukocyte imaging is the radionuclide procedure of choice for the diagnosis of uncomplicated osteomyelitis, with a sensitivity of greater than 90%. But this test is nonspecific. In some circumstances, gallium imaging may increase the specificity of a positive bone scan and suggest the presence of osteomyelitis, especially in situations such as vertebral osteomyelitis and osteomyelitis superimposed on underlying bone disease. In these settings, the following apply:

- Osteomyelitis is likely if gallium activity exceeds bone scan activity in the same location (spatially congruent images) or when the spatial distribution of gallium exceeds that of the bone scan (spatially incongruent images).
- Osteomyelitis is unlikely if gallium images are normal, regardless of bone scan findings or when gallium distribution is less than bone scan activity on spatially incongruent images.
- Because gallium is a weak bone agent in addition to being an inflammatory marker, a gallium scan may be considered nondiagnostic for osteomyelitis when the distribution and activity of the gallium and bone scan activity are the same.

Triple-phase bone scans are often difficult to obtain in the spine because of overlying vascular and blood pool structures, and routine bone scans are nonspecific for infection. In addition, radiolabeled leukocyte studies have a high false-negative rate for infection in the spine. Gallium

imaging in conjunction with a bone scan provides improved sensitivity for the diagnosis of both tuberculous and nontuberculous vertebral osteomyelitis, with an accuracy of more than 85% when both studies are positive.

Sarcoidosis

The lesions of active sarcoidosis are quite gallium avid, especially in the chest. Both nodal and parenchymal lung involvement can be detected. In the early stages, gallium images are frequently positive before any radiographic abnormalities are noted. The finding of increased gallium activity in intrathoracic lymph nodes (right paratracheal and hilar) in a pattern resembling the Greek letter lambda (λ) is suggestive of sarcoidosis. However, a *lambda sign* in combination with a so-called *panda sign*, produced by symmetric increase in activity in the lacrimal, parotid, and salivary glands, represents a highly specific pattern for sarcoidosis (Fig. 12-8). Similarly, the panda sign by itself is not specific and may be seen in a significant percentage of patients with radiation sialoadenitis, primary Sjögren syndrome, and in patients with AIDS.

In the presence of gallium-avid adenopathy in the mediastinal and hilar regions, the diagnosis of lymphoma or infectious disease, especially in human immunodeficiency virus (HIV)-positive patients, must also be considered. In malignant lymphomas, however, the adenopathy is frequently asymmetric.

In the later stages of sarcoid lung disease, a diffuse increase in lung activity with or without gallium-avid adenopathy is common. In this setting, gallium can be used to distinguish active parenchymal disease from inactive sarcoidosis or chronic fibrosis. Diffuse increased activity (equal or greater than liver activity) correlates with active disease, whereas normal lung activity (equal to soft-tissue background activity) is compatible with remission. In extensive sarcoidosis, periaortic, retroperitoneal, and pelvic nodal activity may be seen, but this is more commonly found in patients with lymphoma.

^{18}F-FDG PET/CT IMAGING

The uses of ^{18}F-FDG positron emission tomography (PET)/CT scanning for neoplasms have been discussed in Chapter 11. It was pointed out that increased FDG activity while sensitive for many diseases is nonspecific. Active inflammation

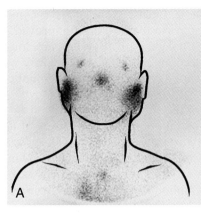

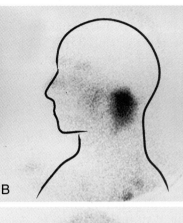

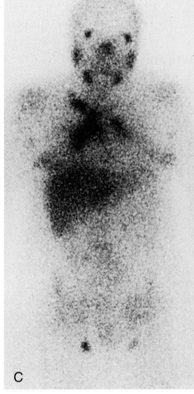

Figure 12-8. Sarcoidosis. **A** and **B**, 48-hour anterior and lateral images of the head and neck from a gallium-67 (^{67}Ga) scan in this 25-year-old woman show symmetrically increased activity in the parotid glands, salivary glands, and lacrimal glands (*panda sign*). **C**, ^{67}Ga scan in a different patient also shows the lambda sign of lymph nodes in the mediastinum as well as a panda sign. Either sign alone is suggestive of sarcoidosis, but together they offer high specificity for the diagnosis. Note also the active inguinal nodes.

or infection in almost any tissue will result in increased ^{18}F-FDG accumulation as a result of overexpression of glucose transporter isotypes and overproduction of glycolytic enzymes. Such uptake can cause problems in distinguishing a lung abscess or pneumonia (Fig. 12-9) from a lung cancer or in distinguishing reactive from metastatic disease in hilar or mediastinal lymph nodes in patients with chronic inflammatory lung disease and lung cancer. FDG is not currently approved by the U.S. Food and Drug Administration (FDA) for use in infection imaging, but it is used for this purpose in a number of institutions.

Increased activity is also present in active granulomatous infections (tuberculosis and sarcoidosis) (Figs. 12-10 and 12-11). With regard to the evaluation of sarcoidosis, ^{18}F-FDG PET/CT scanning is more sensitive than ^{67}Ga-citrate and provides better quality images. ^{18}F-FDG scanning can be helpful in distinguishing a noncalcified inactive granuloma (Fig. 12-12) from an active granuloma or lung cancer. Increased activity after radiation therapy can be problematic, especially when following response to therapy. Most uptake related to radiation therapy is slightly greater than blood pool, although

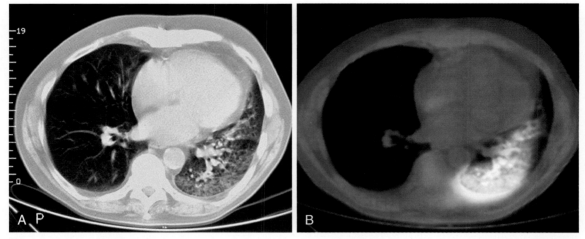

Figure 12-9. Pneumonia. A, CT scan of the chest demonstrates an alveolar infiltrate in the left lower lobe. **B,** ¹⁸F-FDG PET/CT scan shows increased metabolic activity in the pneumonia. *FDG,* fluorodeoxyglucose.

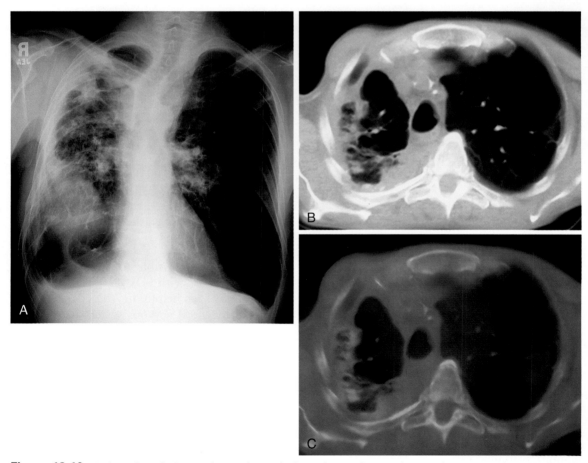

Figure 12-10. Active tuberculosis. A, Chest radiograph shows hyperinflation (chronic obstructive pulmonary disease) but also a right upper lobe cavitary infiltrate with hilar and mediastinal retraction. **B,** Chest CT confirms the findings but is unable to assess activity. **C,** ¹⁸F-FDG PET/CT fusion image shows increased metabolic activity.

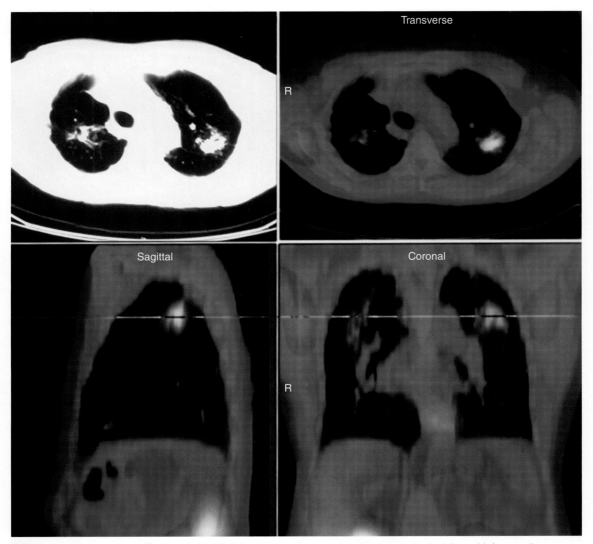

Figure 12-11. Sarcoidosis. ^{18}F-FDG PET/CT fusion images show increased activity in both right and left upper lung zones.

radiation pneumonitis can be very intense. Increased uptake has also been reported in the lymph nodes, lung, and pleura-related inflammation in patients with occupational lung disease.

Virtually any active infection of inflammatory change in the abdomen can demonstrate increased uptake, including hepatic abscesses (Fig. 12-13), inflammatory bowel disease (Fig. 12-14), renal abscess, pancreatitis, or pyelonephritis (Fig. 12-15). Increased ^{18}F-FDG accumulation also may be secondary to recent wounds, ostomies, infected indwelling catheters (Fig. 12-16), hematomas, thrombus, mycotic aneurysm (Fig. 12-17) healing fractures, osteomyelitis, gastritis, thyroiditis, colitis, rheumatoid arthritis, radiation therapy (up to 2 years), and HIV-associated adenopathy (Fig. 12-18).

It is not always possible to distinguish infection from tumor with FDG PET/CT. One area where it has been helpful in AIDS patients is to distinguish central nervous system (CNS) lymphoma (metabolically active) from CNS toxoplasmosis (not metabolically active). Studies with FDG have shown that in HIV-1 patients, the infection first involves the upper torso and later the lower torso and that the degree of uptake relates to the viral load. Vascular grafts also have been associated with increased ^{18}F-FDG uptake, but this does not necessarily indicate infection.

Osteomyelitis. With acute simple fractures, ^{18}F-FDG accumulation can be initially high, but, after about 8 weeks, it should resolve considerably. In chronic benign vertebral fractures, the standardized uptake value (SUV) is usually

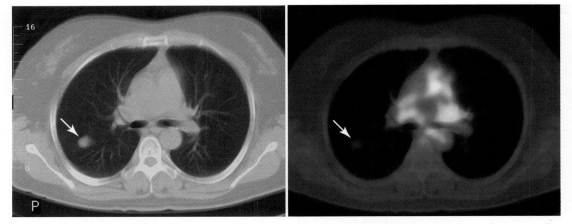

Figure 12-12. Inactive granuloma. *Left,* A solitary pulmonary nodule was identified on chest radiograph. CT scan shows the nodule to be noncalcified. *Right,* ¹⁸F-FDG PET/CT image does not show any metabolic activity. An active granuloma can have uptake and would not be possible to differentiate from a malignancy.

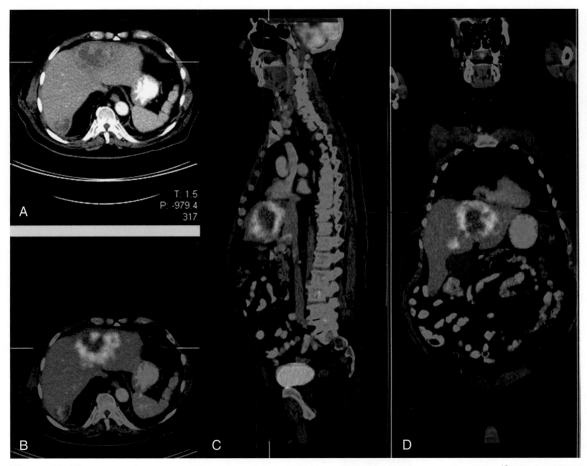

Figure 12-13. Hepatic abscess. A, CT scan shows two areas of irregularly decreased attenuation. **B-D,** ¹⁸F-FDG PET/CT fusion images show increased metabolic activity in the same regions.

less than 2, whereas pathologic fractures caused by neoplasm often have SUVs greater than 2, usually about 4. Degenerative joint disease can also result in increased ¹⁸F-FDG uptake, and there can be occasional nonspecific focal

uptake in anterior rib ends. Increased activity is seen in osteomyelitis, and ¹⁸F-FDG scanning has been reported to be more accurate than either three-phase ⁹⁹ᵐTc-methylene diphosphonate or gallium-67 (⁶⁷Ga)-citrate imaging

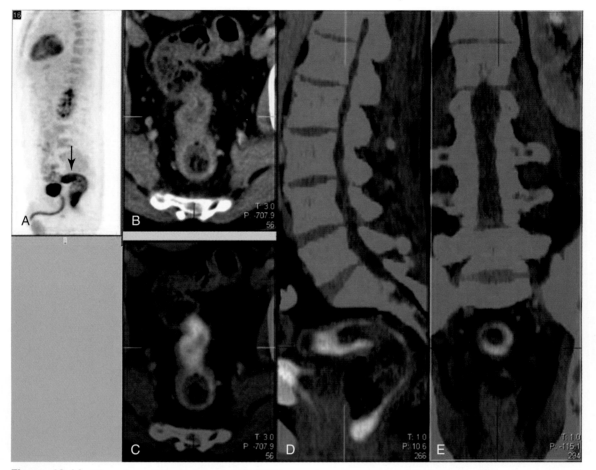

Figure 12-14. **Ulcerative colitis. A,** Lateral MIP PET image shows increased activity in the rectum and rectosigmoid (*arrow*). **B,** CT scan shows bowel wall thickening, and **C-E,** 18F-FDG PET/CT images show increased activity. *MIP,* Maximum intensity projection.

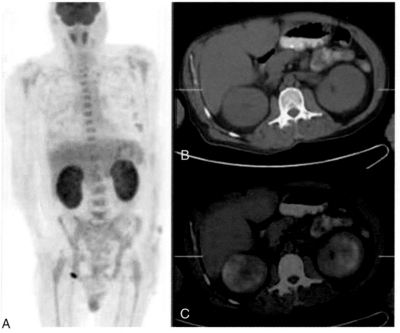

Figure 12-15. **Pyelonephritis. A,** Anterior MIP PET image shows diffuse activity in both kidneys much greater than would be normally expected. **B,** CT scan shows bilaterally enlarged kidneys. **C,** 18F-FDG PET/CT image shows that the activity is diffuse throughout both kidneys.

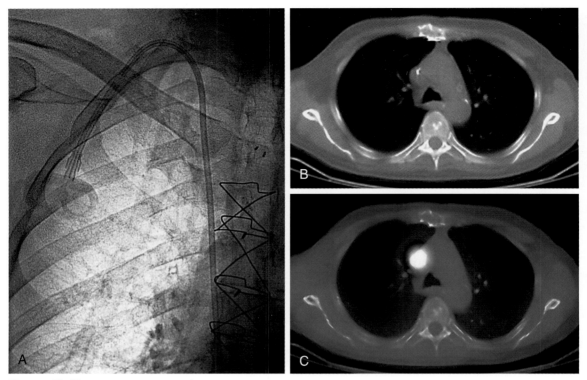

Figure 12-16. Infected central catheter. A, Radiograph shows a chemotherapy catheter suspected of being infected. **B,** Chest CT shows the catheter tip in the superior vena cava. **C,** ^{18}F-FDG PET/CT image shows markedly increased activity.

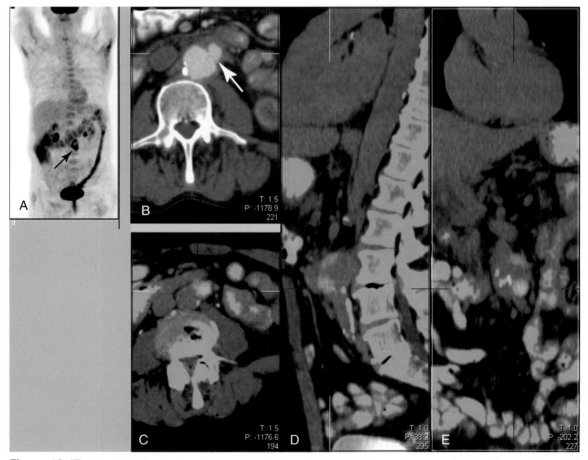

Figure 12-17. Mycotic abdominal aortic aneurysm. A, Anterior MIP PET image shows an abnormal focus of increased activity in the central abdomen (*arrow*). **B,** Contrasted CT scan shows contrast filling a focal abdominal aortic aneurysm (*arrow*). **C-E,** ^{18}F-FDG PET/CT images show increased metabolic activity in the mycotic aneurysm.

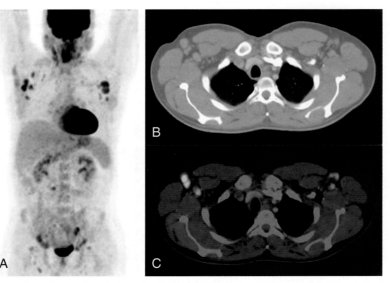

Figure 12-18. HIV-reactive adenopathy. **A,** Anterior MIP PET image shows increased activity in both axilla and pelvis. **B,** CT scan of the axilla shows enlarged lymph nodes. **C,** 18F-FDG PET/CT image shows the increased metabolic activity to be within the nodes. The differential diagnosis, in this case, would include lymphoma.

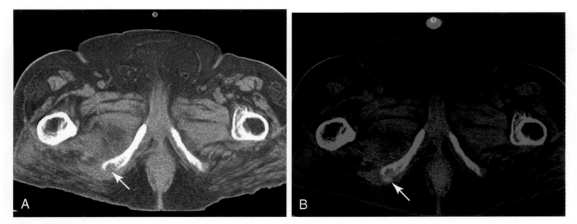

Figure 12-19. Osteomyelitis of the ischium. **A,** CT scan of the lower pelvis shows bone erosion of the ischium (*arrow*) and surrounding stranding edema. **B,** 18F-FDG PET/CT image shows increased metabolic activity within the bone.

for chronic osteomyelitis (Fig. 12-19). Unfortunately, if there is a question of cellulitis versus chronic osteomyelitis, differentiation can be difficult because of the hypermetabolism associated with either entity and lack of accurate spatial localization to bone. The situation is improved with use of PET/CT. Associated bone erosion on the CT portion of the PET/CT scan is very helpful to confirm the diagnosis. A negative 18F-FDG scan can be very helpful in excluding chronic osteomyelitis. Septic or active inflammatory arthritis is also associated with increased uptake (Fig. 12-20). Use of 18F-FDG for evaluation of painful prostheses

shows somewhat promising results, but currently combined leukocyte-marrow scanning remains the procedure of choice.

Fever of Unknown Origin. Limited prospective data indicate that 18F-FDG PET imaging may play a role as an adjunctive study in the evaluation of patients with FUO because it detects a wider spectrum of diseases than labeled white blood cells and appears to be more sensitive than gallium-67 imaging. In these studies, the PET scan contributed to the final diagnosis in 25% to 70% of the patients. In infectious causes of FUO, thoracoabdominal and soft tissue infection, as well as chronic

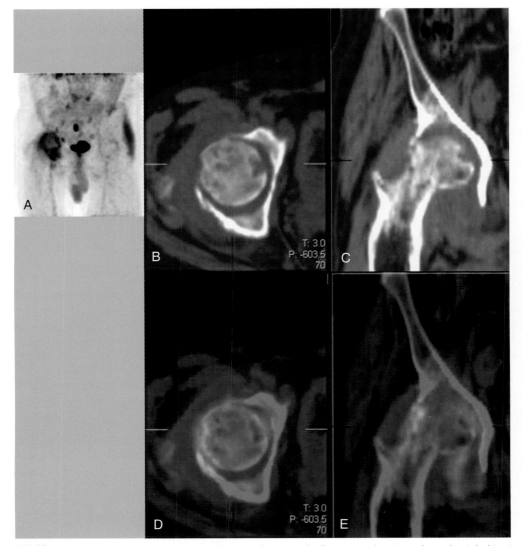

Figure 12-20. Septic arthritis. A, Anterior MIP PET image shows markedly increased activity about the right hip. **B** and **C,** CT scan shows mottled destruction of the right femoral head. **D** and **E,** Corresponding ^{18}F-FDG PET/CT images show the increased metabolic activity to be centered in the joint space.

osteomyelitis, can be diagnosed with a high degree of certainty. A negative ^{18}F-FDG PET scan essentially excludes orthopedic prosthetic infections. In patients with noninfectious inflammatory diseases, ^{18}F-FDG PET seems to be of value in detecting other diseases, such as inflammatory bowel disease, large vessel vasculitis, and sarcoidosis. With respect to neoplastic causes, Hodgkin disease, aggressive non-Hodgkin lymphoma, colorectal cancer, and sarcomas are usually readily detected. It is likely that when hybrid PET/CT is used, enhancement of the specificity of the examination will further advance the diagnostic impact of ^{18}F-FDG PET in the diagnosis of FUO.

FUTURE INFLAMMATION AGENTS

Potential new inflammation imaging agents include peptides, liposomes, and nanocolloids. A number of radiolabeled chemotactic and antimicrobial peptides with a high affinity for inflammatory cells that bind in vivo to both circulating granulocytes and those already present at the site of inflammation have been identified as potential imaging agents. A number of these are bacterial products that initiate leukocyte chemotaxis by binding to high-affinity receptors on the surfaces of inflammatory cells. Other interesting approaches involve the use of ^{99m}Tc multilamellar liposomes, which are phagocytized by leukocytes at sites of inflammation, and the use of ^{99m}Tc-labeled nanometer-sized human serum albumin colloids (nanocolloids), which leave the circulation and enter the extravascular spaces because of discontinuity of the vascular endothelium at sites of inflammation.

PEARLS & PITFALLS

- Leukocyte imaging with ^{111}In-oxine or ^{99m}Tc-exametazime (HMPAO) is the gold standard for diagnosing most infections in the immunocompetent patients. Combined leukocyte/marrow imaging is the radionuclide imaging procedure of choice for diagnosing prosthetic joint infection.

- Gallium-67 citrate and ^{111}In leukocyte scans are usually photon poor, and the images are coarse or grainy.

- Technetium-99m HMPAO leukocyte scans have more counts, and the images appear less grainy and smoother.

- Gallium-67 photon energies are essentially 90, 190, 290, and 390 keV.

- Gallium-67 activity is normally seen in the skeleton, lacrimal glands, nasopharynx, and liver. Liver activity is usually greater than that in the spleen. Colon activity is normal on delayed images.

- Labeled leukocyte activity is normally seen in the bone marrow, liver, and spleen, with the spleen having more intense activity than the liver. Patchy lung activity may be the result of leukocytes damaged during labeling.

- Colonic activity is normal on ^{67}Ga citrate and ^{99m}Tc-leukocyte scans but not on ^{111}In-leukocyte scans.

- Renal activity may be seen normally on ^{67}Ga images during the first 24 hours and on ^{99m}Tc-HMPAO leukocyte images, but not on ^{111}In-oxine leukocyte scans.

- ^{111}In-oxine labels neutrophils, lymphocytes, monocytes, and, to some extent, erythrocytes and platelets. ^{99m}Tc-HMPAO binds to neutrophils.

- ^{99m}Tc-leukocytes are usually imaged at 1 to 4 hours and ^{111}In-leukocytes at 24 hours.

- ^{18}F-FDG localizes in sites of infection, aseptic inflammation, autoimmune diseases, fractures, as well as many tumors. It is very sensitive although nonspecific. The mechanism of localization is increased expression of glucose transporters in activated inflammatory cells by cytokines and growth factors.

- Focal areas of uptake on ^{67}Ga scan are nonspecific and can represent either tumor or inflammation. Indium-111-leukocytes have been reported to localize in some neoplasms, although this is an uncommon occurrence.

- On ^{67}Ga imaging, sarcoidosis and lymphoma may have a similar appearance. Both may show mediastinal and lymph node involvement. Sarcoidosis is suggested by the presence of the lambda sign (increased activity in the right paratracheal and bilateral hilar regions) and the panda sign (symmetrically increased activity in the lacrimal, parotid, and salivary glands). Abdominal involvement is more common in lymphoma.

- Diffuse lung activity on ^{67}Ga scan is often caused by PCP in patients with AIDS.

- Acute fractures and hematomas can show mildly increased activity on leukocyte and FDG scans.

- Focal activity in the abdomen on a leukocyte scan may be a result of an abscess or inflammatory bowel disease (such as Crohn disease). Activity in the colon can be seen in ulcerative colitis or cytomegalovirus.

- Osteomyelitis in the axial skeleton (especially the spine) produces cold defects in up to half of the cases using labeled leukocytes. The scan may also have a normal appearance. Gallium is preferred to labeled leukocytes in the setting of suspected spinal osteomyelitis or diskitis.

SUGGESTED READINGS

Braun J, Kessler R, Constantinesco A, et al. ^{18}F-FDG PET/CT in sarcoidosis management: review and report of 20 cases. Eur J Nucl Med Molec Imaging 2008;35:1537-43.

Gotthardt M, Bleeker-Rovers C, Boerman O, et al. Imaging of inflammation by PET, conventional scintigraphy, and other imaging techniques. J Nucl Med 2010;51:1937-49.

Kwee T, Kwee R, Alavi A. FDG-PET for diagnosing prosthetic joint infection: systematic review and metaanalysis. Eur J Nucl Med Molec Imaging 2008;35:2122-32.

Love C, Marwin SE, Palestro CJ. Nuclear medicine and the infected joint replacement. Semin Nucl Med 2009; 39(1):66-78.

Love C, Palestro CJ. Radionuclide imaging of infection: continuing education. J Nucl Med Tech 2004;32:47-57.

Love C, Tomas MB, Tronco GG, et al. FDG PET of infection and inflammation. RadioGraphics 2005;25:1357-68.

Meller J, Sahlmann CO, Scheel AK. ^{18}F-FDG PET and PET/CT in fever of unknown origin. J Nucl Med 2007; 48(1):35-45.

Palestro CJ. Radionuclide imaging of infection: in search of the grail. J Nucl Med 2009;50(5):671-3.

Rini J, Bhargava K, Tronco G, et al. PET with FDG labeled leukocytes versus scintigraphy with ^{111}In-oxine labeled leukocytes for detection of infection. Radiology 2006;238:978-87.

Sathekge M, Goethals I, Maes A, et al. Positron emission tomography in patients suffering from HIV-1 infection. Eur J Nucl Med Molec Imaging 2009;36:1176-84.

13 Authorized User and Radioisotope Safety Issues

OVERVIEW

Regulatory requirements and radiation safety issues are important in the daily operation of a nuclear medicine section or department. There are a number of specific designations in the U.S. Nuclear Regulatory Commission (NRC) regulations related to performance and qualifications for various aspects of nuclear medicine practice. The personnel recognized by the NRC as having particular responsibilities in nuclear medicine are required to complete and document regulation-specified training and experience in order to be deemed "authorized" on facility radioactive materials licenses. A nuclear medicine practitioner should be familiar with these personnel classifications.

Authorized User

Nuclear medicine activities in any department or outpatient imaging center take place under the supervision and authorization of an *authorized user*, also referred to as an *AU*. An AU is a physician (medical or osteopathic), dentist, or podiatrist who is licensed to practice and who meets specific requirements and is identified as an AU on the institution's license or permit. Other physicians and technologists may work with byproduct material under the supervision of an AU. All radiopharmaceuticals dispensed or administered must be pursuant to an order (e.g. prescription) of an AU. For most diagnostic radiopharmaceuticals this does not need to be done for each patient individually but can be accomplished with standing orders. For radiopharmaceuticals used for therapy, and in some other circumstances detailed later in this chapter, a *written directive*, which may only be issued by an AU, is required for each treatment.

Institutions with a broad scope license may have AUs designated by the Radiation Safety Committee, but they are not listed on the license. With a limited scope license, which constitutes the majority of licenses, the AU must be listed on the license. Training requirements for an AU vary, depending on the type of procedure. The training requirements are covered in several following sections. Some items with which an AU should be very familiar are shown in Box 13-1.

Radiation Safety Officer

A *radiation safety officer* (RSO) is typically a health physicist or medical physicist who must meet substantial additional training and experience requirements. Every radioactive materials license must list one (and only one) permanent RSO. An RSO is responsible for implementing the radiation safety program and ensures that activities are being performed in accordance with approved procedures and regulatory requirements. The RSO must meet the training requirements outlined in the Federal Regulations 10 CFR, Part 35.50.

Duties of the RSO include investigating overexposures, accidents, and other mishaps and collecting or establishing written policies and procedures relative to purchasing/ordering, receipt and opening, storage, inventory, use, and disposal of byproduct material. The RSO is also responsible for performing checks of survey instruments and other safety equipment, training of personnel, performing radiation surveys, retaining copies of reports and policies, briefing management once each year, and establishing investigational levels of personnel exposure, which when exceeded, initiates an investigation by the RSO and taking emergency action if control of radioactive material is lost. For up to 60 days each year, a licensee may permit one or more AUs or individuals qualified to be an RSO to function as an RSO.

Other Authorized Personnel

An *authorized medical physicist* is an individual who is predominantly involved with high energy external beam radiotherapy, brachytherapy, and stereotactic radiosurgery and who has little

---

Box 13-1 Typical Items with Which an Authorized User Should Be Familiar

Duties and responsibilities of an authorized user
Public and occupational dose limits
Personal dosimeters (requirements, types, and use)
Signage and required posting of rooms and packages
Receipt, survey, and wipe testing of packages
Dose calibration before administration of radionuclides
Written directive (authority, requirements, and contents)
Administration of therapy with unsealed radionuclides
Release of patients after therapy with unsealed radionuclides
Survey and wipe tests of areas in the department
Radioactive spills, major and minor, definition and management
Waste disposal (methods and labeling)
Medical event, definition, and reporting requirements
Radiation protection measures (clothing, gloves, syringe shields, etc.)
Approximate doses to persons near patients
Record keeping and record retention
Pregnancy (patients and staff)
Breastfeeding restrictions
Where to get help and additional information

---

involvement with most diagnostic nuclear medicine operations. Specific training requirements can be found in 10 CFR, Part 35.51. An *authorized nuclear pharmacist* is identified as such on the facility license or permit and must meet requirements specified in 10 CFR, Part 35.55. These individuals are usually employed in commercial or large institutional radiopharmacies.

The remainder of the chapter is devoted to information with which the nuclear medicine physician and technologist should be familiar and which should be easily accessible. Patient dosimetry from specific procedures can be found in Appendix E. Issues related to pregnancy and breastfeeding are in Appendix G. Items related to release of radionuclide therapy patients are in Appendix H, and emergency procedures for radioactive spills can be found in Appendix I.

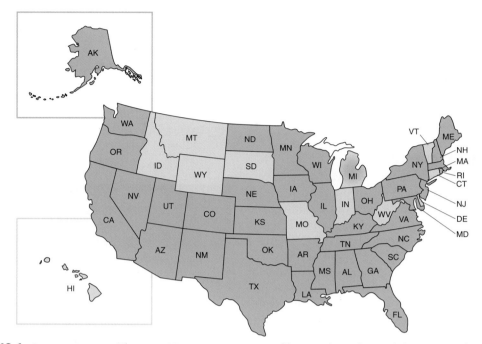

Figure 13-1. Agreement states. There are 37 agreement states (*in blue*). Michigan has withdrawn its application as of August 2011.

REGULATORY AGENCIES

Radioactive materials and radioactive exposures are regulated by the NRC, other federal agencies, and/or the states. The NRC regulates special nuclear material (enriched uranium and plutonium), source material (uranium and thorium), and byproduct material. Byproducts are materials made radioactive by exposure to radiation in a nuclear reactor or from the decay products of uranium and thorium. In 2005, the definition of byproduct material was expanded to include discrete sources of naturally occurring radionuclides (such as radium-226) and accelerator-produced radioactive material. The NRC or the individual states are now responsible for possession and use of these materials. The states are also responsible for radiation-producing instrumentation such as x-ray machines and particle accelerators. Byproduct material encompasses the radionuclides used in diagnostic radiopharmaceuticals, including positron emission tomography (PET), and therapeutic agents.

NRC regulations govern most nuclear medicine operations and may be found in the Code of Federal Regulations (10 CFR, Parts 20, 30, and 35). Part 20 is concerned with standards for protection against radiation, including permissible dose limits, levels, concentrations, precautionary procedures, waste disposal, posting in radiation areas, and reporting theft of radioactive materials. Part 35 is concerned with the medical use of byproduct material, including the *ALARA* (*as low as reasonably achievable*) program, licensing, required surveys, instrumentation, and training requirements. In addition to the ALARA policy, the NRC also has a safety culture policy which emphasizes "safety first" without being a regulation. This refers to an organization's collective commitment to emphasize safety as an overriding priority to guarantee protection of people and the environment. Specified training for AUs (including physicians practicing nuclear medicine) is also given in Part 35.

Many states have an agreement with the NRC to accept the responsibility for regulating byproduct, source, and special nuclear materials within their jurisdiction. These are known as *agreement states* (Fig. 13-1), and their regulations are at least as strict as those of the NRC. The agreement states regulate all sources of radiation in the state (with the exception of federally controlled sites, such as the Department of Veterans Affairs [VA] facilities and military bases).

The philosophy of a radiation protection program required by the NRC is that of ALARA. This is designed to keep radiation doses *as low as reasonably achievable*. To satisfy requirements of ALARA, administrative personnel, the RSO, and all AUs must participate in an ALARA program as requested by the facility's radiation safety committee (RSC) or RSO. The program must also include notice to the workers of the program's existence and the worker's responsibility to participate in this philosophy.

TYPES OF LICENSES

NRC regulations describe two types of specific licenses for the medical use of byproduct materials. There are specific licenses of broad-scope and specific licenses of limited scope. Broad-scope licenses are described in NRC regulations, Part 33 (10 CRF 33.11) and are usually reserved for large hospitals and academic institutions. There are type A, B, and C broad-scope licenses, depending on the amount of byproduct material in possession. Type A broad-scope licensees are typically the largest licensed programs. Broad-scope licensees have significant decision-making authority.

Part 35 specific licenses of limited scope are usually for small hospitals and office practices. Human research is usually conducted under a broad-scope license but is also possible with a limited scope license. Specific Part 35 licenses are related to the particular use or uses of byproduct materials, as addressed in the specific sections of the regulations, as follows:

■ CFR 35.100—the use of radiopharmaceuticals for uptake, dilution, and excretion studies
■ CFR 35.200—the use of radiopharmaceuticals, generators, and reagent kits for imaging and localization studies
■ CFR 35.300—the use of radiopharmaceuticals for unsealed radiopharmaceutical therapy
■ CFR 35.400—the use of radioisotope sealed sources in brachytherapy and for teletherapy
■ CFR 35.500—the use of radioisotope sealed sources for diagnosis

There is also an NRC "Master Materials" license. Formerly, the NRC issued individual licenses to the U.S. Veterans Affairs (VA) medical centers. Under the master materials license, the VA system is authorized to issue individual permits to each of its VA medical centers replacing the previous NRC licenses. The license requires use of NRC licensing and inspection criteria. Finally, there is a general in-vitro license for clinical or laboratory tests not involving administration of byproduct material to humans.

DOSE LIMITS

NRC dose limits are shown in Box 13-2. Radiation dose is expressed in several forms. Absorbed dose is energy deposited in tissue and is expressed in units of rads or Gray (Gy). Absorbed organ dose can be multiplied by a radiation weighting factor to account for the effectiveness of different types of radiation. The radiation weighting factor of photons and

---

Box 13-2 Nuclear Regulatory Commission Dose Limits (2004), Part 20

A. Occupational exposures (annual)
  1. Whichever is more limiting:
    a. Total effective dose equivalent, or 5 rem (50 mSv)
    b. Sum of deep dose equivalent and committed dose 50 rem (500 mSv) equivalent to any organ/tissue except lens of the eye (nonstochastic)
  2. Eye dose equivalent 15 rem (150 mSv)
  3. Shallow dose equivalent to skin/extremity 50 rem (500 mSv)
  4. Minors (occupational under the age of 18 years) 10% of the above
B. Public exposure
  1. Total effective dose equivalent (annual) 0.1 rem (1 mSv)
  2. Dose in unrestricted area (in any 1 hr) 2 mrem/hr (0.02 mSv/hr)
C. Embryo/fetus exposures
  1. Total dose equivalent (after pregnancy declared) 0.5 rem (5 mSv)
D. Planned special occupational exposure
  1. In any year as in A, above
  2. In individual's lifetime 5 × A, above
E. Required notification of NRC* from a single event dose exceeding the following:
  1. Immediate (telephone)
    a. Total effective dose equivalent 25 rem (0.25 Sv)
    b. Eye dose equivalent 75 rem (0.75 Sv)
    c. Shallow dose equivalent 250 rem (2.5 Sv)
  2. Within 24 hours (telephone)
    a. Total effective dose equivalent 5 rem (0.05 Sv)
    b. Eye dose equivalent 15 rem (0.15 Sv)
    c. Shallow dose equivalent 50 rem (0.5 Sv)
  3. 30 days any doses in excess of occupational, public, or embryo/fetus limits

*If in a Nuclear Regulatory Commission state. If in an agreement state, reporting to the state may vary but is usually very similar.

x-rays is 1.0. This yields an equivalent dose, which is expressed in units of rem or Sievert (Sv). The equivalent dose can be multiplied by a defined tissue weighting factor, which accounts for different potential detriment from the exposure of various tissues. This quantity is called *effective dose*. Effective dose is also expressed in units of rem and Sv. Dose limits for organs are equivalent dose, and dose limits for the whole body are effective dose.

Occupational

Occupational dose is that received in the course of employment in which the individual's assigned duties involve exposure to radiation or radioactive material from licensed and unlicensed sources of radiation whether in the possession of the licensee or other person. Occupational dose does *not* include doses from (1) natural background radiation, (2) medical exposures of the individual, (3) exposure to persons who have been administered radioactive material and released, (4) voluntary participation in medical research, or (5) as a member of the public.

A licensee must demonstrate that unmonitored individuals are not likely to receive in 1 year a radiation dose in excess of 10% of the allowable occupational limits or they must monitor external and/or internal occupational radiation exposure to such individuals. Practically speaking, this 10% rule governs who should wear a film badge (or other monitoring device) in a nuclear medicine facility.

Public

Public dose is that received by a member of the public from exposure to radiation or to radioactive material released by a licensee. Public dose does *not* include (1) occupational exposure, (2) medical exposures the individual has received, (3) exposure to natural background radiation, (4) any medical exposure from another person who has received radioactive material and been released, or (5) voluntary participation in biomedical research.

Embyo/Fetus

An embryo/fetus is subject to a dose equivalent limit of less than 0.5 rem (5 mSv) during the entire pregnancy from occupational exposure of a woman who has declared her pregnancy. This is true even though the mother may be subject to higher occupational exposure limits in her employment. If the dose equivalent to the fetus is found to have exceeded 0.5 rem (5 mSv) or is within 0.05 rem (0.5 mSv) of exceeding this dose by the time the woman declares the pregnancy to the licensee, the licensee is in compliance as long as the additional dose equivalent to the embryo/fetus does not exceed 0.05 rem (0.5 mSv) during the remainder of the pregnancy. It should be noted that there is no fetal dose limit if the pregnancy is not declared to the employer.

Breastfeeding

Breastfeeding cessation is not regulated, but there are NRC guidelines. Cessation is not needed for ^{18}F-FDG, and cessation times for technetium radiopharmaceuticals range from 0 to 24 hours. Breastfeeding is usually discontinued for a week or more for thallium-201, gallium-67, and indium-111 pharmaceuticals. Breastfeeding is contraindicated for several months after radioiodine therapy (see Appendix G).

Family and Caregivers

In 1997, the NRC amended its regulations for the release of patients receiving treatment with radioactive materials from an activity-based limit to a dose-based limit. The regulation was based on the maximally exposed individual (including family or caregivers) not being likely to exceed an effective dose equivalent of 0.5 rem (5 mSv) from this single radioisotope treatment (see Appendix H). Compliance with the dose limit is demonstrated by (1) using a default table for activity or dose rate or (2) performing a patient-specific dose calculation. If the total effective dose equivalent to any other individual is likely to exceed 1 mSv (0.1 rem), written radiation safety guidance (instructions) to reduce this dose through ALARA practices is required to be given to the patient. There is no specific guidance with regard to radiation exposure of pregnant women through contact with the treated patient, but it does indicate that written instructions must be provided if a nursing child of the patient is likely to exceed an effective dose of 100 mrem (1 mSv). These instructions must include (1) guidance on interruption or discontinuation of breastfeeding and (2) the potential consequences of not following this guidance.

RADIATION SAFETY COMMITTEE

This requirement varies in accordance with the type of license granted to a facility. Under NRC regulations, each medical institution with a type A broad-scope license is required to have an

RSC. The committee membership must include an AU of each type of use permitted by the licensee—the RSO, a representative of the nursing service, and a representative of management who is not an AU or an RSO. Other members may be included as appropriate. Institutions with type B or C broad-scope licenses or those with program-specific licenses are not required to have an RSC.

The committee must meet at intervals not to exceed 6 months, and, at a minimum, at least half of the members (including the RSO and management representative) must be present. Minutes must include the date of the meeting; a listing of those present and absent; a summary of deliberations, discussions, and recommended actions; and an ALARA program review. The committee is required to maintain a copy of the minutes for the duration of the license.

The committee also reviews for approval or disapproval those who wish to become AUs, the RSO, and /or other staff members requiring approval. They also review audits, reviews, and inspections; evaluate the results; and specify necessary corrective actions. The committee must review every 6 months the summary of occupational radiation dose records and any health and safety issues or possible radiation safety program deviations from regulatory compliance or required practices. There must be an annual review of the radiation safety program. Other duties include review and approval of changes to training, equipment, physical plant or the facilities, radiation safety procedures, or practices. The RSC also has duties relative to research involving licensed byproduct material. They must evaluate human subject research and coordinate with the institutional review board to ensure that for research requiring ionizing radiation, the informed consent process has been followed.

NRC TECHNICAL REQUIREMENTS
Dose Calibrators and Survey Instruments
If radiopharmaceuticals and patient dosages are prepared on-site, the licensee must possess and use instrumentation to measure the activity of unsealed byproduct material before it is administered to each patient. The instrument (dose calibrator) must also be calibrated according to nationally recognized standards or the manufacturer's recommendations. Survey instruments must also be calibrated before first

use, annually, and after repair. All scales with readings up to 1000 mrem (10 mSv) must be checked for accuracy by obtaining two separate readings on each scale, and the indicated exposure must be within 20% of the calculated exposure. Dates of calibration must be indicated on the instrument. Records of the information, including serial number of instruments, names of those performing the calibration, and dates must be kept for 3 years.

Determination and Records of Dosages
The licensee needs to determine and record the activity of each dosage before medical use. For patient unit doses supplied by a commercial radiopharmacy, there must be direct measurement or a decay correction based on the activity determined by the licensed preparer. For other than unit doses (usually multidose vials), determination of activity for each individual patient dosage must be made by direct measurement (dose calibrator), a combination of measurement and mathematical calculations, or combinations of volumetric measurements and mathematical calculations. Unless specified by the AU, a licensee may not use any dosage if it falls outside of the prescribed dosage range or differs from the prescribed dosage by more than 20%. Records of dosage determination must be retained for a period of 3 years and must contain the name of the radiopharmaceutical, patient's or subject's name or identification number, the prescribed dosage or a notation that the total activity is less than 30 µCi (1.1 MBq), date and time of administration of the dosage, and the name of the individual who determined the dosage.

Calibration, Transmission, and Reference Sources
In addition to patient imaging and treatment, radioisotope sources are used for instrument calibration and quality control purposes as well as for transmission images. Any person authorized for medical uses of byproduct material may receive, possess, and use byproduct material for check, calibration, transmission, and reference use. This includes sealed sources not exceeding 30 mCi (1.11 GBq) provided or redistributed in original packing by a licensed manufacturer. Possession also includes byproduct material with a half-life of not longer than 120 days in

individual amounts not to exceed 15 mCi (0.56 GBq) or byproduct material with a half-life of longer than 120 days not to exceed the smaller of 200 µCi (7.4 MBq) or 1000 times the quantity in Appendix B of Part 30 of 10 CFR. One can also possess technetium 99m (^{99m}Tc) for these purposes in amounts as needed.

Labeling of Vials and Syringes

Each vial or syringe that contains unsealed byproduct material must be labeled to identify the radiopharmaceutical. Each syringe shield and vial shield must also be labeled unless the label on the syringe or vial is visible when shielded.

Survey of Ambient Exposure Rate

The licensee is required to perform surveys in the nuclear medicine facility with a radiation detection survey instrument at various intervals, but at least once a month. Surveys must be done weekly in areas of radionuclide use or storage and waste storage. A daily survey is required to be done of all areas where byproduct material requiring a written directive (treatment dosages) was prepared or administered. A daily survey is not required of a hospital room if the patient is confined to the room. Records must include the instrument used, the name of the individual making the survey, and the date; these records must be retained for 3 years.

TRAINING REQUIRED FOR USE OF UNSEALED BYPRODUCT MATERIAL

Uptake, Dilution, and Excretion Studies (Written Directive Not Required)

Except for quantities that require a written directive, a licensee may use any unsealed byproduct material for uptake, dilution, or excretion studies if it is obtained from a licensed manufacturer, prepared by an authorized nuclear pharmacist, is used by a physician who is an AU, or used in accordance with a radioactive drug research committee or investigational new drug protocol accepted by the U.S. Food and Drug Administration (FDA).

An AU for these purposes is a physician who meets the following specific requirements of 10 CFR, Part 35.190:

A. Is certified by a medical specialty board whose certification process has been recognized by the NRC or an agreement state and who meets the requirements listed in the following item C

B. Be an AU for imaging or therapeutic studies before October 24, 2005, or

C. Has completed 60 hours of training and experience, including a minimum of 8 hours of classroom and laboratory training in radionuclide handling techniques applicable to the use

Imaging and Localization Studies (Written Directive Not Required)

This category of byproduct use encompasses the major components of diagnostic nuclear medicine practice. Training for this category requires that the AU be a physician who meets one or more of the following criteria (10 CFR, Part 35.290):

A. Is certified by a medical specialty board whose certification process has been recognized by the NRC or an agreement state and who meets the requirements listed in item C of the following (This includes American Board of Radiology (ABR) certificates in Diagnostic Radiology from June 2006 forward with the words "AU eligible" appearing above the ABR seal.)

B. Was an AU of procedures requiring a written directive before October 24, 2005, and has experience with radiopharmaceutical preparation or

C. Has completed 700 hours of training and experience, including a *minimum* of 80 hours of classroom and laboratory training in basic radionuclide handling techniques applicable to use of unsealed byproduct material for medical use not requiring a written directive (The training must include, at a minimum: (a) classroom and laboratory training in radiation physics, instrumentation, radiation protection, mathematics pertaining to the measurement of radioactivity, chemistry of byproduct material for medical use, radiation biology; and (b) supervised work experience under an AU of at least this level, in ordering, receiving, and unpacking radioactive materials and making necessary surveys, calibrating instruments to determine activity of dosages and operation of survey meters, calculating, measuring and safely administering doses, prevention of medical events and cleanup of spills, elution of generator systems, testing the eluate for radionuclidic purity, preparing reagent kits with the eluate, administering radioactive materials to patients or research subjects *and* written attestation from a preceptor AU regarding fulfillment of requirements and the individual's ability to function independently for these uses.)

Unsealed Byproduct Material (Written Directive Required)

A written directive is a written order by an AU for the administration of byproduct material or radiation from byproduct material to a specific patient or human research subject. A written directive is required before the administration of ^{131}I sodium iodide greater than 30 μCi (1.11 MBq), any therapeutic dosage of unsealed byproduct material, or any therapeutic dose of radiation from byproduct material. If the patient's life is in danger, the written directive can be delayed up to 48 hours. The written directive must include (a) the patient's or research subject's name, (b) the dosage, (c) the AU's signature, (d) date, and (e) the route of administration (except for radioiodine). Copies of written directives must be retained for 3 years.

These uses include the therapeutic administration of oral sodium iodine-131 for hyperthyroidism, thyroid ablation, and differentiated thyroid cancer metastases as well as the intravenous therapies with beta-emitting radionuclides such as the labeled monoclonal antibodies, including Bexxar, Zevalin, and others.

Required Training

Training for this category requires that the AU be a physician who meets one or more of the following criteria (10 CFR, Part 35.390):

A. Is certified by a medical specialty board whose certification process has been recognized by the NRC or an agreement state and who meets the requirements listed in the following item C (This includes certificates issued by the American Board of Nuclear Medicine with the words "United States" under the certification number, and the American Board of Radiology in Radiation Oncology with the words "AU eligible" appearing above the ABR seal, from June 2007 forward.)

B. Was an AU of procedures requiring a written directive before October 24, 2005, or

C. Has completed 700 hours of training and experience, including a *minimum* of 200 hours of classroom and laboratory training in basic radionuclide handling techniques applicable to use of unsealed byproduct material for medical use requiring a written directive (The training must include, at a minimum: (a) classroom and laboratory training in radiation physics, instrumentation, radiation protection, mathematics pertaining to the measurement of radioactivity, chemistry of byproduct material for medical use, radiation biology; and (b) supervised work experience under an AU of at least this level, in ordering, receiving and unpacking radioactive materials and making necessary surveys, calibrating instruments to determine activity of dosages and operation of survey meters, calculating, measuring, and safely administering doses, prevention of medical events and cleanup of spills, administering of radioactive drugs to patients or research subjects *and* written attestation from a preceptor AU regarding fulfillment of requirements and the individual's ability to function independently for these uses.)

The training (under the previous item C also requires training in administering doses to a minimum of three patients/subjects in each of the following categories for which the user is requesting user status: (a) oral administration of less than or equal to 33 mCi (1.22 GBq) of sodium iodide-131 for which a written directive is required, (b) administration of greater than 33 mCi (1.22 GBq) of sodium iodide-131, (c) parenteral administration of any beta emitter or photon emitting radionuclide with an energy of less than 150 keV, for which a written directive is required; and/or (d) parenteral administration of any other radionuclide for which a written directive is required. There also must be written attestation regarding competency from a preceptor AU who meets all of the training requirements or was an AU of this type before October 24, 2005.

Related Procedures

For those procedures requiring a written directive, the licensee must have procedures to assure with high confidence that the patient's or subject's identity is verified, that the administration is in accordance with the patient's treatment plan, and that manual and/or computer-generated dose calculations have been performed before dosage administration.

Safety instruction also must be provided initially and at least annually to personnel caring for patients or research subjects who cannot be released in the guidance contained in Appendix G. The training must include issues related to patient and visitor control, contamination and waste control, and notification of the RSO. Records of this training must be kept for 3 years. When patients cannot be released because of the amount of radioactivity or ambient dose rate, the patient must be in a private room with a private sanitary facility. Two such patients, however, may be in the same room. The door to the room must have a radioactive materials sign, and there must be an indication as to how long visitors may stay. The RSO must be notified if the patient has a medical emergency or dies.

Oral Therapeutic Administration of ^{131}I-sodium Iodide (Written Directive Required)

These sections of the NRC regulations addressing ^{131}I use refer to those users who wish to use only ^{131}I for therapeutic purposes rather than the full spectrum of beta-emitting radionuclides as described previously. A written directive is still required. The activity levels of ^{131}I used in treatment define two training and experience categories for AUs: (a) less than or equal to 33 mCi (1.22 GBq) for hyperthyroidism treatment and (b) greater than 33 mCi (1.22 GBq) for thyroid ablation and thyroid cancer metastases.

Less Than or Equal to 33 mCi (1.22 GBq) Iodine-131

The training requirements (10 CFR, Part 35.392) are similar to those described previously to be an AU for procedures requiring a written directive except that the required training is 80 hours only, and the training is specific to ^{131}I-sodium iodide. In addition, case experience with oral administration of less than or equal to 33 mCi (1.22 GBq) of ^{131}I to three patients or research subjects is required.

Greater Than 33 mCi (1.22 GBq) Iodine-131

Training requirements (10 CFR, Part 35.394) for users in this category are as specified in the preceding paragraph except that the case experience with oral administration of greater than 33 mCi (1.22 GBq) of ^{131}I to three patients or research subjects is required.

The board certification pathway for the use of ^{131}I in quantities less than or equal to 33 mCi (1.22 GBq) includes the American Board of Radiology certificate in Diagnostic Radiology with the words "AU eligible" appearing above the ABR seal from June 2006 forward. Uses of ^{131}I in quantities greater than 33 mCi (1.22 GBq) in addition to quantities less than or equal to 33 mCi are covered by American Board of Radiology certificates if issued from June 2011 forward.

TRAINING FOR SEALED SOURCES FOR DIAGNOSIS

An AU of sealed sources for diagnosis must be a physician, dentist, or podiatrist who (a) is certified by a specialty board that includes the following as part of the training or (b) has had 8 hours of classroom and laboratory training in handling techniques specific to the device to be used. Training must include radiation physics and instrumentation, radiation protection, mathematics pertaining to the use and measurement of radioactivity, radiation biology, and training in the use of the device for the uses requested.

MEDICAL EVENTS AND REQUIRED REPORTING

A *medical event* occurs when a patient intervention using byproduct material results in unintended radiation exposure. Formerly, the term *misadministration* was used, although it was defined somewhat differently. A medical event must be reported if it is

A.

1. A dose that differs from the prescribed dose or dose that would have resulted from the prescribed dose by more than 5 rem (0.05 Sv) effective dose equivalent, or 50 rem (0.5 Sv) to an organ, tissue, or shallow dose equivalent to the skin *AND*

   the total dose delivered differs from the prescribed dose by 20% or more, *OR*

   the total dosage delivered differs from the prescribed dosage by 20% or more or falls outside of the prescribed dose range,

OR

the fractionated dose delivered differs from the prescribed dose, for a single fraction by 50% or more.

2. A dose that exceeds 5 rem (0.05 Sv) effective dose equivalent,

OR

50 rem (0.5 Sv) to an organ, tissue, or shallow dose equivalent to the skin from any of the following:

- an administration of a wrong radioactive drug containing byproduct material
- an administration of a radioactive drug by the wrong route of administration
- an administration of a dose or dosage to the wrong individual or research subject
- an administration of a dose or dosage by the wrong mode of treatment
- a leaking sealed source

3. A dose to the skin or an organ or tissue other than the treatment site that exceeds by 50 rem (0.5 Sv) to an organ or tissue and 50% or more of the dose expected from the administration defined in the written directive

B. Any event resulting from an intervention in a patient or human research subject in which the administration of byproduct material or radiation from byproduct material results or will result in *unintended* permanent functional damage to an organ or a physiologic system, as determined by a physician.

For any of the previous items, the licensee in an NRC state must notify by telephone the NRC operations center no later than the next calendar day after the discovery of the medical event. If a licensee is in an agreement state, the report is made to appropriate regulatory agency in that state. In addition, a written report must be submitted to the NRC regional office within 15 days after the discovery of the medical event. The report must include the licensee's and prescribing physician's name; a description of the event; what effect occurred, if any; why the event occurred and subsequent actions taken; and certification that the individual or relative was notified and, if not, why not. The name or identifying information of the exposed individual is not to be included. The referring physician and the exposed individual also must be notified within 24 hours or as soon as possible, unless the referring physician indicates that he or she will inform the person or responsible relative or guardian unless the referring physician based on medical judgment feels that telling the individual would be harmful. A copy of the report to the NRC with the patients' names added must be provided to the referring physician no later than 15 days after discovery of the event. A record of the medical event is not required to be retained, although it is probably a good idea. In the VA, reports are made by the hospital to the central VA office under its Master Materials license.

Reports and notification must also be made in circumstances of an unintended dose to an embryo/fetus or a nursing child that is greater than 5 rem (0.05 Sv) dose equivalent, resulting from administration of a byproduct material to the mother or from external radiation from a byproduct material. Notification and reports are not required if the dose was specifically approved in advance by the AU.

MAINTENANCE OF RECORDS

Required records must be kept for various specified periods of time and are specified in 10 CFR Part 35, subpart K. They must be legible for the entire period, and there must be provisions to prevent loss or tampering. Records may be kept in electronic format. A copy of the authorities, duties, and responsibilities of the RSO (with signatures of the RSO and management), and records of procedures for administrations requiring a written directive must be kept for the duration of the license. Records of actions taken by management relative to the radiation protection program need to be kept for 5 years. Most other records need to be kept for 3 years.

TRANSPORTATION OF RADIOACTIVE MATERIALS

Interstate transportation of radioactive materials usually is controlled by regulations of the Department of Transportation (DOT). The NRC requires that DOT regulations be observed when radiopharmaceuticals are returned to a manufacturer or transported between offices, laboratories, or hospitals, with the exception of materials transported by a physician for medical practice.

Hazard levels: The DOT has assigned hazard levels to radionuclides based on their radioactive toxicity. Transport group I is reserved for

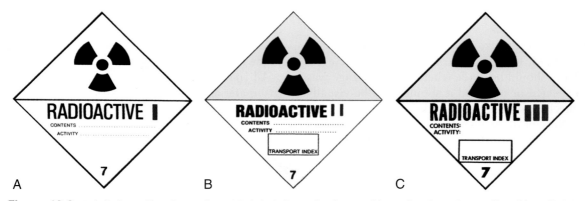

Figure 13-2. Labels for radioactive packages. Labels indicate the degree of hazard and maximum allowable radiation emitted from the package. **A,** Radioactive-white I label means that the maximum allowable surface dose rate is less than 0.5 mrem (5 μSv) per hour. **B,** Radioactive-yellow II label has a maximum surface dose rate of 50 mrem (0.5 mSv) per hour and a maximum dose rate at 1 meter of 1 mrem (10 μSv) per hour. **C,** Values for Radioactive-yellow III are 200 mrem (2 mSv) per hour and 10 mrem (0.1 mSv) per hour, respectively.

very hazardous radionuclides, such as plutonium-239 (^{239}Pu) and americium-241 (^{241}Am), whereas transport group VI includes radionuclides of very low hazard, such as uncompressed krypton-85 (^{85}Kr) gas. Radionuclides used in nuclear medicine are in transport groups III and IV.

Packaging: The type and amount of radionuclide determine the hazard level of the material and therefore the type of packaging required. Packaging of medical radionuclides is of two common forms: type A packaging is designed to prevent loss or disbursement of a limited amount of radioactive material under normal conditions during transport and during minor accidents. Type B packaging is for higher-activity radioactive material and is designed to survive severe accidents. Most radionuclides used in nuclear medicine come in Type A packaging.

Labeling: Packages of radioactive materials must be labeled according to one of the three following categories (Fig. 13-2):

- *Radioactive-white I:* No special handling is required. Surface dose rate must not exceed 0.5 mrem/hr (5 μSv/hr).
- *Radioactive-yellow II:* Special handling is required. Surface dose rate may not exceed 50 mrem/hr (0.5 mSv/hr), and dose rate may not exceed 1 mrem/hr (10 μSv/hr) at 1 meter from any external surface.
- *Radioactive-yellow III:* Surface dose rate exceeds 50 mrem/hr (0.5 mSv/hr) but is less than 200 mrem (2 mSv)/hr, and dose rate may not exceed 10 mrem/hr (0.1 mSv/hr) at 1 meter from any external surface.

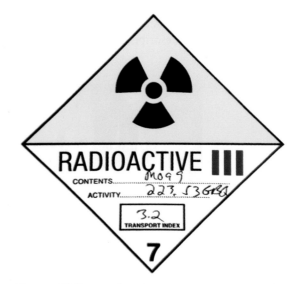

Figure 13-3. Specific information contained on radioactive package label. This is a label from a package containing a ^{99}Mo-^{99m}Tc generator. The contents specify the radionuclide as Molybdenum-99. The activity contained in the package is 223 GBq (6 curies). The transportation index is 3.2, indicating the measured dose rate at 1 meter from the intact package should be 3.2 mrem (32μSv)/hr.

- *Transportation index (TI):* The transportation index should be displayed on the label. The TI is the number of millirems per hour measured at 1 meter from the package (Fig. 13-3). The maximum TI for packages transported by common and contract carriers in open vehicles is 10. If the TI is above 10, the package must be in a closed exclusive use vehicle.

RECEIPT OF RADIOACTIVE SHIPMENTS

When any package of radioactive material is received, it should be placed in a secure area. Note should be made whether the package was expected or not, and it should then be visually checked for damage or leakage.

Receipt of the package must be registered in a log and then stored in an appropriate, shielded area. Although many materials being received at a nuclear medicine laboratory are not required to be monitored, it is certainly a good idea to do so.

Monitoring: All packages with radioactive labels must be monitored at their external surfaces unless the radioactivity is in the form of a gas or certain other forms as defined in the regulations, or unless activity levels are less than Type A quantities as defined in 10 CFR 71.4. (Note: Type A activity is different from Type A packaging described previously.) Most packages being received in nuclear medicine departments are not in excess of Type A activities. Type A packages typically contain activity in the range of curies (TBq).

All packages known to contain radioactive materials should be monitored if there has been degradation of package integrity, such as crushed, wet, or damaged packaging. In these cases, in addition to external dose rate motoring, removable contamination should be assessed using a wipe test. Packages requiring monitoring must be assessed within 3 hours of receipt or within 3 hours of the next business day.

External measurements should be made at 1 meter from the package with a survey meter (Fig. 13-4) and compared with the mrem/hr expected indicated by the TI on the package label. Some facilities then survey the package almost at surface contact. If measurements are excessive, an external wipe test should be performed to assess for contamination.

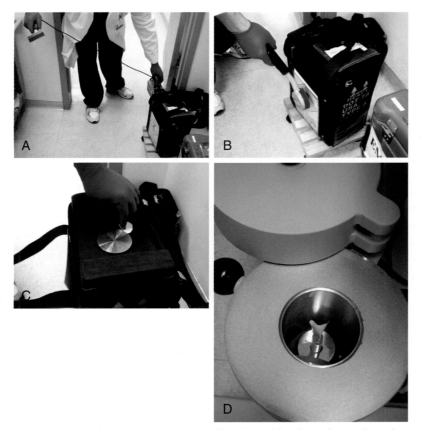

Figure 13-4. Survey upon receipt of a package containing radioactivity. After the package is brought to a secure area and logged in, the dose rate is measured at 1 meter and compared to the TI. **A,** Many survey meters have a cord between the probe and meter that is 1 meter long, allowing an easy measurement. In this case, the pancake detector probe has a red plastic cover. **B,** Next, a surface measurement is made. **C,** The wipe test is done and **D,** the wipe is placed in a well counter for measurement. All results are recorded in a log or computer. *TI,* Transportation index.

To perform a contamination test for removable activity from the surface of the package, an absorbent paper is usually wiped over an area of about 300 cm² and counted. Some laboratories wipe over about 100 cm² (about 4 × 4 inches) and then multiply that value by 3. The wiping paper is then placed in a well counter for analysis. If contamination of any package is suspected, such a test should be performed.

Notifications: The licensee must immediately notify the final delivery carrier and the NRC Operations Center by telephone (a) if removable contamination is in excess of 6600 disintegrations/minute over 300 cm² (about 7 × 7 inches) or otherwise specified in section 71.87 of the NRC regulations, or (b) if external radiations levels exceed certain limits.

Recordkeeping: A shipment of arriving radioactive material should be recorded in both a receiving report and the radionuclide logbook. The receiving report should indicate the shipment identification, including supplier's name, the radionuclide and lot number, as well as the package survey results, including the measured external radiation level and the results of any surface and internal package wipe tests for removable contamination. Also to be recorded are the amount and type of radionuclide as indicated by the manufacturer or supplier, as well as the nuclear medicine laboratory confirmation of this information.

SAFE HANDLING AND ADMINISTRATION OF RADIOPHARMACEUTICALS

Unshielded radioactive materials should never be picked up directly with the fingers because very high doses may result. Instead, these materials should be handled with clamps, forceps, or other holding devices. When time and distance are not adequate or practical for radiation protection, shielding must be used. It is important to remember that when dealing with beta radiation, a shield should be made of a low-atomic-number material. If a high-atomic-number material, such as lead, is used, the interaction between the beta particles and the lead may cause the emission of bremsstrahlung radiation, which is highly penetrating. Plastic shielding is usually sufficient for beta-emitting radionuclides.

When using ^{99m}Tc, lead shielding is sufficient. The half-value layer, which is the amount of lead required to reduce the radiation exposure by half, is 0.2 mm of lead for ^{99m}Tc. A thickness of 2.5 mm of lead attenuates radiation from ^{99m}Tc by a factor of about 1000. Radionuclides with more energetic gamma rays may require much more shielding. High-energy positron emitters are usually shielded with tungsten shielding.

Shielding is of two general types: (a) bench top shields and (b) syringe or vial shields. Bench top shields are frequently constructed of lead bricks and usually have a viewing portal of lead glass to shield the face and eyes. Direct handling of unshielded thin-walled plastic syringes containing short-lived radionuclides can cause skin exposure in the range of 500 to 1000 mrad/hour/mCi (0.14 to 0.27 mGy/hour/MBq). Although brief handling of unshielded radionuclides is usually well within permissible limits, syringe shields reduce exposure levels by a factor of at least 3.

Syringe shields should be used when preparing a radiopharmaceutical kit or performing a radiopharmaceutical injection unless the use of the shield is contraindicated for that patient (Fig. 13-5). It is not necessary to use a syringe shield for drawing up a dose. If vials are used,

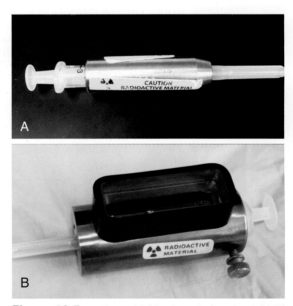

Figure 13-5. Syringe shields. A typical syringe shield (**A**) can be made from lead or tungsten. It may or may not have a lead glass window. **B,** Some shields may be made entirely from leaded glass. A syringe shield for positron emitters must be much thicker because of the higher energy of the photons. Such PET syringe shields can weigh up to 2.5 pounds. Plastic shields are appropriate for beta-emitters.

the vials must be kept in radiation shields, and the shield must be labeled with the radiopharmaceutical name.

Because the basis of imaging procedures is the detection of radiation emanating from the patient, the patient is by definition a source of exposure. Estimates of typical exposure to technologists from standard imaging procedures range from 0.4 to 3 mrem (4 to 30 µSv)/hr (Table 13-1). Between 50% and 90% of the dose that technologists receive usually come from being with the patient while the patient is imaged rather than from the radiopharmaceutical preparation, assay, or injection. Although radiation from the patient constitutes a measurable level, these levels are not high enough to be used as an excuse to keep the technologist and physician from providing the patient with the best medical care.

For diagnostic clinical procedures, it is not necessary to follow the package inserts in the use of a radiopharmaceutical. The only restriction is that the chemical form must not be changed. This allows the AU to administer an approved radiopharmaceutical to patients in a different physical state, such as gas instead of liquid; by a different route of administration; or in a different administered activity without filing a notice of claimed investigational exemption for a new drug.

PERMISSIBLE MOLYBDENUM CONCENTRATION

A licensee may not administer a radiopharmaceutical that contains more than 0.15 µCi (55 kBq) of molybdenum-99 (^{99}Mo) per mCi (MBq) of ^{99m}Tc. Persons using ^{99}Mo/^{99m}Tc generators are required by the NRC to measure the ^{99}Mo concentration in the first eluate after receiving the generator; however, SNM guidelines indicate this must be done for every elution. Records must include the ^{99}Mo/^{99m}Tc ratio, time and date of the measurement, and the name of the individual who made the measurement. The record must be retained for 3 years.

PET RADIATION SAFETY

With the higher energies associated with positron-emitting radionuclides, there have been concerns about the radiation safety aspects of positron emission tomography (PET) scanning. Significant sources of occupational exposure may be associated with handling radiopharmaceuticals before patient injection

TABLE 13-1	Approximate Radiation Dose Rates at 1 Meter from Nuclear Medicine Patients			
STUDY	**RADIOPHARMACEUTICAL**	**ADMINISTERED ACTIVITY, mCi (mBq)**	**TIME AFTER ADMINISTRATION (hr)**	**DOSE RATE, mrad/hr (µGy/hr)**
Bone	^{99m}Tc-MDP	20 (740)	0	0.9 (9)
		20 (740)	3	0.35 (3.5)
Blood pool	^{99m}Tc red blood cells	20 (740)	0	1.4 (14)
Heart	^{201}Tl-chloride	20 (740)	0	2 (20)
	^{99m}Tc-sestamibi	20 (740)	0	0.9 (9)
Liver	^{99m}Tc sulfur-colloid	4 (148)	0	0.2 (2)
Tumor/ infection	^{67}Ga citrate	3 (111)	0	0.35 (3.5)
Tumor	^{18}F-FDG	10 (370)	0	30 (300)
	^{18}F-FDG	10 (370)	0-1	10 (100)
	^{18}F-FDG	10 (370)	1	5 (50)
Thyroid cancer therapy	^{131}I-sodium-iodide	100 (3700)	0	22 (220)
	^{131}I-sodium-iodide	100 (3700)	12	12 (120)
	^{131}I-sodium-iodide	100 (3700)	24	11 (110)
	^{131}I-sodium-iodide	100 (3700)	72	1.8 (18)

Adapted from sources and magnitude of occupational and public exposures from nuclear medicine procedures: Report no. 124. Bethesda, Md.: National Council on Radiation Protection and Measurements; 1996.
DTPA, Diethylenetriamine pentaacetic acid; *^{18}F-FDG,* fluorine-18 fluorodeoxyglucose; *^{67}Ga,* gallium-67; *^{111}In,* indium-111; *MDP,* methylene diphosphonate; *^{99m}Tc,* technetium-99m; *^{201}Tl,* thallium-201.

and with repetitive close contact with patients shortly after injection. These exposures are potentially significantly higher than are those experienced with routine handling and administration of technetium-99m (^{99m}Tc) radiopharmaceuticals.

When compared with 10 mCi (370 MBq) of ^{99m}Tc, the same activity of ^{18}F will result in a dose rate about sixfold higher or 35 versus 199 mR/hour (0.31 versus 1.74 mSv/hour) at a distance of 20 cm (8 inches) from the source. This is the distance corresponding to handling a vial of radionuclide with tongs. Syringe shields used for ^{99m}Tc are usually about 0.32 cm (⅛ inch) of lead or equivalent, but this is inadequate for positron emitters. Because increasing the lead thickness by a factor of 16 (to achieve the same protection) is impractical, use of tungsten, which has a higher atomic number (Z) and electron density, is preferred. It provides about 1.4 times the shielding as an equivalent thickness of lead. Dose rates from patients recently injected with Fluorine-18-fluorodeoxyglucose (^{18}F-FDG) may also be a significant source of occupational exposure and exposure to other patients. Typically, shielded quiet rooms are provided for the patients to relax between their injection and scanning (Fig. 13-6). Immediate absorbed doses at 1 meter from patients injected for ^{18}F-FDG scans are about 30 mrem/hr (300 μSv/hr). By the time they leave the department, the dose rates are reduced to less than 2 mrem/hr (20 μSv/hr).

ALARA AND DOSES TO PATIENTS

Nuclear medicine accounts for a significant portion of the radiation dose received by the U.S. population. There has been extremely rapid growth in nuclear medicine procedures over the last decade, and, in 2007, there were just under 20 million nuclear medicine examinations, which accounted for about 5% of the number of all diagnostic medical radiation procedures but about 25% of the total dose. The annual per capita effective dose in the United States from nuclear medicine is approximately 0.8 mSv. The total annual per capita effective dose from all sources (including natural background) is 5.7 mSv. Table 13-2 provides the effective dose from common nuclear medicine procedures. The *effective dose* is a general measure of radiation detriment and can be

used to compare potential detriment from different procedures and practices. It should be noted that published values for effective doses from specific radiopharmaceuticals vary somewhat because of differences in initial assumptions, metabolic models, and tissue weighting factors.

The nuclear medicine physician has a duty to the patient to obtain diagnostic quality images while keeping the radiation dose to the patient (and resultant doses to technologists) as low as reasonably achievable (ALARA). While many nuclear medicine physicians have specified a given activity for a certain examination, it is sometimes necessary to adjust administered activities depending on the patient size and condition. Suggested administered activities for various procedures on pediatric patients are presented in Appendix D, and suggested adult doses are given in Appendix E.

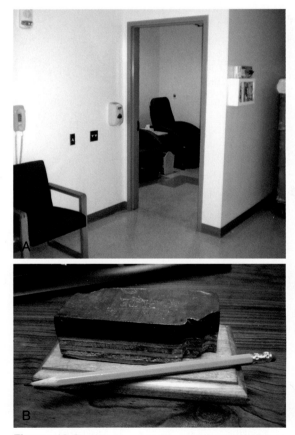

Figure 13-6. PET post injection patient waiting room. **A,** Because of the high energy and dose rate of PET radionuclides, patients are usually placed in a special, low-light quiet, waiting area while waiting for their PET/CT scan. **B,** Such areas often require substantial lead shielding in the walls.

TABLE 13-2	Representative Patient Effective Doses for Various Nuclear Medicine Examinations

EXAMINATION	ADMINISTERED ACTIVITY (MBq)*	mSv/MBq†	EFFECTIVE DOSE (mSv)
Brain (Tc-99m HMPAO/exametazime)	740	0.0093	6.9
Brain (Tc-99m ECD/Neurolite)	740	0.0077	5.7
Brain (F-18 FDG)	740	0.019	14.1
Thyroid scan (NaI-123)	25	0.075 (15% uptake)	1.9
Thyroid scan (Tc-99m pertechnetate)	370	0.013	4.8
Parathyroid scan (Tc-99m sestamibi)	740	0.009	6.7
Cardiac stress-rest (thallium)	185	0.22	40.7
Cardiac rest–stress (Tc-99m sestamibi 1 day protocol)	1100	0.0085 (0.0079 stress–0.0090 rest)	9.4
Cardiac rest–stress (Tc-99m sestamibi 2-day protocol)	1500	0.0085 (0.0079 stress–0.0090 rest)	12.8
Cardiac rest–stress (Tc-tetrofosmin)	1500	0.0076	11.4
Cardiac ventriculogram (Tc-99m RBCs)	1110	0.007	7.8
Cardiac (F-18 FDG)	370	0.019	7.0
Lung perfusion (Tc-99m MAA)	185	0.011	2.0
Lung ventilation (Xe-133)	740	0.00074	0.5
Lung ventilation (Tc-99m DTPA)	1300 (40 actually inhaled)	0.0049	0.2
Liver–spleen (Tc-99m sulfur colloid)	222	0.0094	2.1
Biliary (Tc-99m DISIDA)	185	0.017	3.1
GI bleeding (Tc-99m RBCs)	1110	0.007	7.8
GI emptying (Tc-99m, solids)	37	0.024	0.9
Renal (Tc-99m DTPA)	370	0.0049	1.8
Renal (Tc-99m MAG3)	370	0.007	2.6
Renal (Tc-99m DMSA)	370	0.0088	3.3
Renal (Tc-99m glucoheptonate)	370	0.0054	2.0
Bone (Tc-99m MDP)	1110	0.0057	6.3
Gallium-67 citrate	150	0.100	15
Pentetreotide (In-111)	222	0.054	12
White blood cells (Tc-99m)	740	0.011	8.1
White blood cells (In-111)	18.5	0.360	6.7
Tumor (F-18 FDG)	740	0.019	14.1

DISIDA, Diisopropyl iminodiacetic acid; *DMSA*, dimercaptosuccinic acid; *DTPA*, diethylenetriamine pentaacetic acid; *ECD*, ethyl cysteinate dimer; *F*, fluorine; *FDG*, fluorodeoxyglucose; *HMPAO*, hexamethylpropyleneamine oxime; *In*, indium; *MAA*, macroaggregated albumin; *MAG3*, mercaptoacetyltriglycine; *MDP*, methylene diphosphonate; *NaI*, sodium iodide; *RBCs*, red blood cells; *Tc*, technetium; *Xe*, xenon.
*Recommended ranges vary, although most laboratories tend to use the upper end of suggested ranges.
†ICRP Publication 80 Annals of the ICRP 28(3), 1998. Note: Published values for effective doses for a given radiopharmaceutical vary somewhat. Effective doses are primarily used to compare radiation and potential detriment from different examinations rather than to calculate individual risk.

RELEASE OF INDIVIDUALS AFTER ADMINISTRATION OF RADIONUCLIDES

A patient may be released if the total effective dose equivalent to any other individual (family or caregiver) is not likely to exceed 0.5 rem (5 mSv). If the total effective dose to any other individual is likely to exceed 0.1 rem (1 mSv), then the patient must be given instructions (including written) on actions to maintain doses to others following ALARA principles. See also Appendices G, H, and I for further information.

Patients receiving diagnostic nuclear medicine examinations do not emit enough radiation to have effective doses to other persons that approach 0.5 rem (5 mSv) and therefore the patients can be released without any calculations. For therapy patients, the situation can be substantially different. The NRC provides guidance on release of these patients based upon (1) a certain amount of administered activity (e.g., 33 mCi [1.2 GBq] or less of iodine-131), or (2) dose rate (7 mrem [70 μSv]/hr or less at 1 meter for iodine-131) (see Table H-1A). These values are based on very conservative assumptions. Patients also can be released with much higher activities based on patient-specific calculations and if the effective dose to a maximally exposed other person is not likely to exceed 0.5 rem (5 mSv). For a useful calculator, see http://www.doseinfo-radar.com/ExposureCalculator.html. In general, if another person will not exceed 25% of exposure time at 1 meter from the patient after release, then administered activities of over 50 mCi (1.85 GBq) to hyperthyroid patients and 200 mCi (7.4 GBq) to thyroid cancer patients may be administered with subsequent release of patients. These patients should be given instructions on maintaining distance from other persons, sleeping arrangements, minimizing time in public places, precautions to reduce the spread of radioactive contamination, and the length of time each of the precautions should be in effect. The exact instructions vary from institution to institution. A typical example is shown in Box 13-3. If using patient-specific calculations, the home environment to which the patient returns should be assessed, specifically with respect to the presence of infants and children (who are at most risk). Patients are also strongly discouraged (but not prohibited) from staying at hotels immediately after treatment.

Box 13-3 Typical Precautionary Release Instructions for Patients Treated with Iodine-131*

Avoid public transport, if possible, for the first day. If it must be used, try to limit time to less than several hours.

Strongly discourage patient from staying in a hotel immediately after treatment.

Try to stay about 1 meter away from others for 1 week.

If possible, stay home from work for several days. Depending on the nature of the job, this might range from 0-5 days.

Minimize contact with children for 2 weeks. If possible, have them stay elsewhere for 1 week.

Do not kiss children or infants for 2 weeks.

Minimize contact with pregnant women, and, in the first 24 hours, stay at least 1 meter away.

Promote frequent fluid intake to help excrete unbound radioiodine.

Sleep separately for 4-7 days, and for 24 days if partner is pregnant.

Limit sexual activity and kissing for several days.

Do not share a bathroom, if possible, for several days. Use separate towels.

Shower or bathe daily. Rinse sink or tub after use.

Avoid urine spill by urinating while sitting, and flush toilet 2-3 times.

Wash hands frequently.

Sharing food or eating utensils should be avoided. If preparing food for others, use gloves.

Clothing and linens should be laundered separately.

Carry your radioiodine treatment form for 3 months.

Breastfeeding must be discontinued for several months.

*Unless otherwise specified, these precautions should last for about 5-7 days. None of these is absolute.

Because of the threat of terrorism, radiation detectors have been installed in many airports, border crossings, public buildings, and even subways. These devices are very sensitive and can easily detect most nuclear medicine patients for several days (e.g., bone and thyroid scans), weeks (e.g., thallium-201 cardiac scans), or even several months (e.g., therapies containing iodine-131 [^{131}I]) after the procedures. As a result, the NRC has recommended that all nuclear medicine patients be advised that they

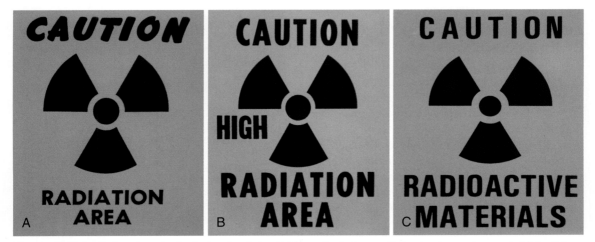

Figure 13-7. Radiation signs. A "Radiation Area" sign (**A**) is required where radiation levels are >5 mrem (>0.05 mSv) per hour at 30 cm from a source or from any surface through which radiation penetrates. A "High Radiation Area" sign (**B**) is required where radiation levels are >100 mrem (>1 mSv) per hour at 30 cm from a source or from any surface through which radiation penetrates. A "Caution Radioactive Materials" sign (**C**) is required at the entrance to a room when radioactive materials exceed 10 times the amounts listed in Appendix C of CFR, Part 20.

may activate radioisotope security alarms and that they receive written information documenting their treatment for potential law enforcement use. It should contain (1) patient identification, (2) nuclear medicine facility contacts, and (3) a statement that the radiation received by the patient is allowed by NRC medical use regulations and poses no danger to the public with specifics to include the name and date of the nuclear medicine procedure, the radionuclide, its half-life, and administered activity.

RESTRICTED AREAS, RADIATION AREAS, AND SIGNAGE POSTING

Nuclear medicine laboratories are generally divided into restricted and unrestricted areas. Examples of unrestricted areas are offices, file space, patient waiting areas, and nonradiation laboratory space. These areas must have dose rates of less than 2 mrem/hour (20 μSv/hour) and of less than 100 mrem (1 mSv) over total of 7 consecutive days. If these limits are exceeded, control of the area is required. A restricted area is one in which the occupational exposure of personnel is under the supervision of a person in charge of radiation protection. Access to the area is restricted, and working conditions within it are regulated. Restricted areas are not accessible to the general public. Examples of restricted areas are those dedicated to radiopharmaceutical preparation, dispensing, administration, and storage, as well as the imaging areas.

Signage is required for various areas (Fig. 13-7). A *radiation area* is one that has levels that could result in dose equivalent in excess of 0.005 rem or 5 mrem (0.05 mSv) in 1 hour at 30 cm from the radiation source. A *high radiation area* is one in which there are levels that could result in a dose equivalent of over 0.1 rem or 100 mrem (1 mSv) in 1 hour at 30 cm from the source. All radiation areas require posting with a conspicuous sign. Posting is also required for areas where there is likely to be airborne radioactivity. Areas where licensed radioactive material (exceeding 10 times the quantity specified in 10 CFR Appendix C to Part 20) is used or stored must have a *caution radioactive materials* sign. If a patient who has received radioactive material is in a hospital room and that patient could have been legally released (based on activity or dose rate levels), posting is not required.

FACILITY RADIATION SURVEY POLICIES

Surveys for contamination and ambient radiation exposure are covered in NRC guidelines, 10 CFR 20.1101, 20.1402, and 35.70. Policies regarding surveys of working areas vary among institutions (Fig. 13-8). It is important to follow whatever written procedures are in place in the facility. Model procedures for area surveys are provided by the NRC (Appendix R, NUREG 1556, Vol 9, Rev 2). Many institutions will perform daily radiation surveys of all areas of

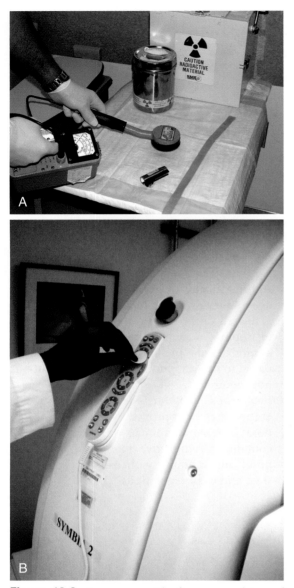

Figure 13-8. Area surveys. The frequency and type of periodic radiation and contaminations surveys vary among departments, but they should be specified in written policies. **A,** These often include surveys with an instrument as well as wipe tests (**B**) of specified equipment and areas. The one specific requirement is that daily surveys must be performed in all areas used for the preparation and administrations of radiopharmaceuticals for which a written directive is required.

elution, preparation, assay, and administration and weekly surveys in all areas of use (imaging areas), storage, and waste storage.

A licensee is required to survey all areas in which radiopharmaceuticals requiring a written directive are prepared and administered at the end of each day (except where patients are confined, such as hospital rooms, and cannot

be legally released). In addition, for procedures requiring a written directive, if the patient is kept in the hospital, items removed from a patient's room must be either monitored or treated as radioactive waste.

A licensee possessing sealed sources must leak test the source every 6 months. If more than 0.005 µCi (185 Bq) of removable activity is on a wipe sample, the source is said to be leaking. This procedure is not required if the materials (a) have less than a 30-day half-life, (b) are gases, or (c) consist of less than 100 µCi (3.7 MBq) of beta- or gamma-emitting radionuclide. It is also not required of alpha-emitting radionuclides of less than 10 µCi (0.37 MBq) or sources stored and not being used. Semiannual inventory of all sealed sources and survey of all stored materials in sealed sources are required.

Survey records must also contain the instrument used to make the survey and the initials of those persons performing such a survey. In addition, if a licensee uses radioactive gases, such as xenon-133, there is a requirement to check the operation of the traps or collecting systems each month and to measure ambient ventilation rates in areas of use every 6 months. For areas in which radioactive gas is used, the licensee must calculate and post the time needed after a spill of radioactive gas to reduce the concentration in the room to the occupational limit. A record of the calculations and assumptions must be retained as long as the area is used. Negative pressure in the rooms (compared with surrounding rooms) is no longer required but is recommended, if feasible.

WASTE DISPOSAL

The following methods are available for radioactive waste disposal:

Transfer to an authorized commercial facility for burial: Waste must be packaged and shipped according to appropriate regulations.

Burial: Burial in the soil may be approved by the NRC or an agreement state. This method is usually not available to nuclear medicine laboratories.

Return to supplier: Some nuclear medicine laboratories return residual spent dosages, contaminated syringes, and multidose vials to the supplying commercial radiopharmacy for disposal. In this case, the hospital should have a written agreement with the supplier that they will accept the responsibility of being the shipper for the return. If this is not done, the hospital will be held responsible for all DOT and NRC shipping requirements.

Release into sewer system: If the material is readily soluble or dispersible in water, it may be released in the following amounts:

Ten times the limit specified in Appendix C of 10 CFR 20, or the quantity of radioactive material that, when diluted by the average daily amount of liquid released by the hospital into the sewer system, results in an average concentration no greater than the amount specified in Appendix B, Table 3, column 2 of 10 CFR 20. The greater of these two values is permitted.

Monthly: The amount of radioactive material that when diluted by the average monthly total amount of liquid released into the sewer system results in an average concentration of no greater than the amount specified in Appendix B, Table 1, column 2 of 10 CFR 20.

Yearly: A total of no more than 1 Ci (37 GBq) of NRC-licensed or other accelerator-produced materials.

NOTE: Excreta from people who have received radioactive materials for medical diagnosis or therapy are not regulated by the NRC, and disposal in the sewer system in any amount is allowed.

Decay in storage: A licensee may hold byproduct material with a physical half-life of less than 120 days for decay in storage before disposal without regard to the amount of radioactivity if (a) monitoring at the surface cannot distinguish any difference from natural background, and (b) labels are removed or obliterated and a record of each disposal is maintained for 3 years.

Venting: Many nuclear medicine laboratories use xenon-133 (^{133}Xe) for pulmonary ventilation studies. Although direct venting into the atmosphere of certain amounts of this material is permissible (for limits, see CFR, Part 20.1101d) and gives the least dose to the technologists, it often requires physical plant remodeling for adequate air flow. Another means of disposing of ^{133}Xe is storage and decay using commercially available, activated charcoal traps. Negative pressure in rooms in which radioactive gases are administered (including xenon-133) compared to the surrounding rooms is useful but not required.

Other disposal methods: Methods such as incineration may be approved by the NRC for disposal of research animals or organic solvents containing radioactive materials. Such disposal must comply with existing applicable state and local regulations.

PEARLS & PITFALLS

- All packages with radioactive labels must be monitored for surface contamination upon receipt. If the package is damaged or contains very large activities (in excess of Type A DOT amounts), both contamination and dose rate monitoring are necessary.

- The amount of activity in a diagnostic unit dose from a radiopharmacy does not need to be measured and can be calculated from the labeled activity and decay time. If doses are prepared in-house or unit doses are modified or split, the activity must be measured in a dose calibrator.

- Typical dose rates to the hands from holding radiopharmaceutical syringes range from 0.5 to 1.0 rad/hr/mCi (0.14 to 0.27 mGy/hr/MBq). Syringe shields are recommended and usually reduce the dose by a factor of about 3. All vials, syringes, and syringe shields must be labeled with the radiopharmaceutical name unless the label can be seen through the shield.

- Typical doses from patients soon after injection of most diagnostic radiopharmaceuticals at 1 meter are about 1 mrem (10 μSv) per hour but for ^{18}F-FDG patients, the dose rate is

PEARLS & PITFALLS—cont'd

5 to 30 mrem (50 to 300 μSv) per hour. From iodine-131 therapy patients, the dose rates are about 5 and 30 mrem (50 and 300 μSv) per hour for hyperthyroidism and cancer, respectively.

- Annual occupational dose limits are 5 rem (50 mSv) effective dose, 50 rem (0.5 Sv) to any organ or tissue, and 15 rem (150 mSv) to the eye. Public dose limits are 0.1 rem (1 mSv) annually or 2 mrem (20 μSv) per hour. The fetal dose limit is 0.5 rem (5 mSv) after the pregnancy is declared.

- Personal dosimeters need to be used on individuals who are likely to receive in excess of 10% of the allowable occupational dose limits.

- A written directive is not required for most diagnostic procedures. A written directive is required for diagnostic procedures exceeding 30 μCi (1.1 MBq) of iodine-131 and all therapy procedures. Daily surveys are required in areas where written directive procedures are administered and performed.

- The permitted variation for an administered dose from the prescribed dose is ± 20%.

- A medical event refers to a patient intervention that results in unintended radiation exposure. For nuclear medicine, this generally means that there was an effective dose in excess by 5 rem (50 mSv) or an absorbed dose in excess by 50 rem (0.5 Sv) to a tissue or organ *and* (a) that differs from the prescribed dose by 20% or more *or* (b) that the excess dose was caused by administration of the wrong radiopharmaceutical, the wrong route of administration, or to the wrong patient. The NRC must be notified of a medical event and a written report filed. While deplorable, administration of a wrong radiopharmaceutical, or by the wrong route, or to the wrong patient is not a NRC reportable medical event if the doses previously listed are not exceeded.

- Medical events often occur because there are errors attributable to inattention in the administered quantities (mCi vs. μCi), lack of dose calibration, or patient identification.

- Release of nuclear medicine patients is allowed under NRC regulations based upon a certain amount of administered activity or dose rate (e.g., 33 mCi [1.2 GBq] or less of iodine-131 or 7 mrem [70 μSv] per hour or less at 1 meter for iodine-131). Patients also can be released with much higher activities based on patient-specific calculations and if the effective dose to a maximally exposed other person is not likely to exceed 0.5 rem (5 mSv). For a useful calculator, see http://www.doseinfo-radar.com/ExposureCalculator.html.

- Patients receiving radionuclide therapy, especially with iodine-131, should be advised that they may activate radioisotope security alarms, especially when traveling through airports or crossing international borders. Thus patients should receive written information documenting their treatment for law enforcement use.

- Breastfeeding cessation is not regulated but there are guidelines. Cessation is not needed for ^{18}F-FDG, and cessation times for technetium radiopharmaceuticals range from 0 to 24 ours. Breastfeeding is usually discontinued for a week or more for thallium-201, gallium-67, and indium-111 pharmaceuticals. Breastfeeding is contraindicated for several months after radioiodine therapy (see Appendix G).

- Major radiation spills are based on activity released (greater than 100 mCi [3.7 GBq] of ^{99m}Tc or ^{210}Tl, 10 mCi [370 MBq] of ^{67}Ga and ^{111}In, and 1 mCi [37 MBq] of ^{131}I). For minor spills, efforts should be directed at containment, decontamination, and notification of the RSO. All major spills require the presence of the RSO (see Appendix I).

- Radioactive materials can be stored and decayed. If the material no longer can be distinguished from background radiation, it may be disposed of as in-house waste. Any generators or other material being returned to the supplier must meet DOT packaging and labeling requirements.

- Excreta from people who have received radioactive materials for medical diagnosis or therapy are not regulated by the NRC, and disposal in the sewer system in any amount is allowed.

SUGGESTED READINGS

Ionizing radiation exposure of the population of the United States. Report 160. Bethesda, Md.: National Council on Radiation Protection and Measurements; 2009.

Radiation Dose Assessment Resource. RADAR Medical Procedure Radiation Dose Calculator and Consent Language Generator. http://www.doseinfo-radar.com/RADARDoseRiskCalc.html, February 22, 2011; Accessed February 22, 2011.

Radiation protection for medical and allied health personnel. Report no. 105. Bethesda, Md.: National Council on Radiation Protection and Measurements; 1989.

Society of Nuclear Medicine. Procedure guideline for the use of radiopharmaceuticals 4.0. http://www.snm.org/guidelines, July 4, 2011; Accessed on July 4, 2011.

Sources and magnitude of occupational and public exposures from nuclear medicine procedures. Report no. 124. Bethesda, Md.: National Council on Radiation Protection and Measurements; 1996.

United States Nuclear Regulatory Commission. Consolidated guidance about materials licenses. Program-Specific Guidance About Medical Use Licenses NUREG-1556, Vol 9, Rev 1, May 2005, Washington, DC. (This has model procedures and is available at http://www.nrc.gov.)

United States Nuclear Regulatory Commission. NRC Regulations, Title 10, Code of Federal Regulations. http://www.nrc.gov/reading-rm/doc-collections/cfr/; Accessed February 22, 2011.

Unknown Case Sets

The following case sets have been designed to assess your overall knowledge in nuclear imaging. Each set contains 11 cases, and almost all sets have an example of central nervous system, thyroid, cardiac, respiratory, gastrointestinal, musculoskeletal, tumor, or abscess and positron emission tomography (PET) cases. This is a common review format. In addition, there are several questions regarding each case. You should be able to recognize most of the examinations, know the radiopharmaceutical used, understand the technique, give a differential diagnosis of one to three entities, and in some cases, discuss management. Table 1 in this set may help you differentiate and recognize different types of whole-body scans. By challenging yourself on all of the case sets, you will have covered many of the most common entities in nuclear medicine. Answers to all of the cases and additional questions are given after Case Set 7. If you have trouble with a case, go back to the chapter and specific text on that topic and review it. Good luck.

TABLE 1 Normal Distribution of Activity on Various Types of Whole-Body Scans

RADIOPHAR-MACEUTICAL	LIVER	SPLEEN	GU	BOWEL	BONE MARROW	SALIVARY	THYROID	OTHER
^{18}F-FDG	+	+	+++	++ usually colon	+	+	+/−	Brain+++ Heart++/− Larynx+/− Muscle+/−
^{111}In-WBC	++	+++			+			
^{99m}Tc-WBC	++	+++	+	+	+			
^{67}Ga-citrate	++	+	+ 0-1 day	+++ usually colon	+	+		Lacrimal+/−
^{123,131}I sodium iodide	+		++	++ stomach, colon		+	If present or remnant	Nasal+
^{111}In-octreotide	++	+++	+++	+			+	
^{123,131}I-MIBG	+		++	+		+	+	Heart+ Nasal+ Lung+
^{99m}Tc-sulfur colloid	+++	++			+			
^{99m}Tc-sestamibi	+	+	+	++			+	Heart++ Gallbladder
^{201}Tl-chloride	++	++	+	++		+		Muscle++ Heart++ Testis++
^{131}I-NP-59	++			++				Gallbladder
^{111}In-Zevalin	++	++	+	+	+ 2-3 days			Blood pool 0-1 days

Adapted from table of Harry Agress Jr., MD.
+, ++, +++, Degree of uptake of the radiopharmaceutical in the tissue specified.

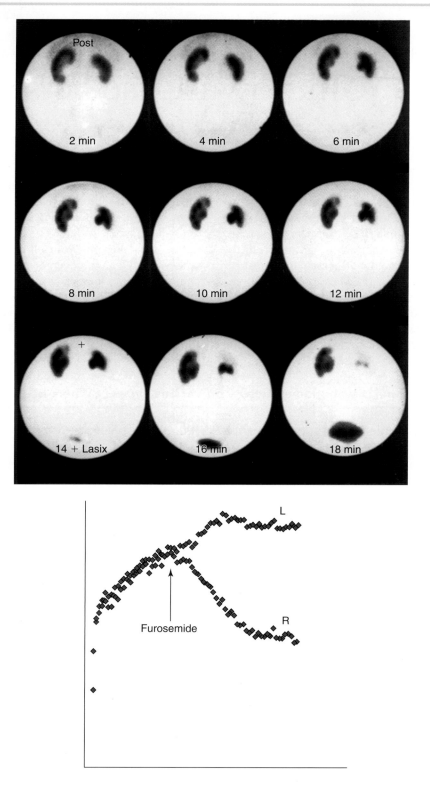

CASE 1-1

1-1a. What is the diagnosis?

1-1b. Could this study be done with ^{99m}Tc-DMSA?

1-1c. After Lasix, how fast should the DTPA or MAG3 activity in a normal kidney decrease?

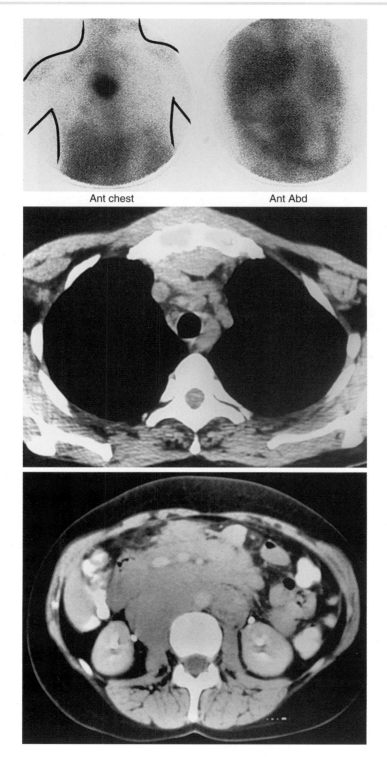

Ant chest   Ant Abd

CASE 1-2

1-2a. What is the diagnosis?

1-2b. What radiopharmaceutical was used?

1-2c. What is the approximate photon energy of this radiopharmaceutical's gamma emissions?

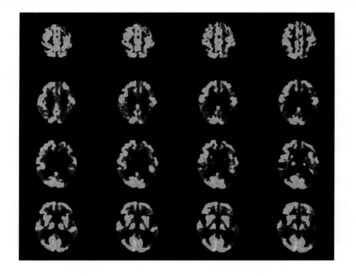

CASE 1-3

1-3a. What is the diagnosis?
1-3b. What would be the expected findings in Lewy body dementia?
1-3c. What is crossed cerebellar diaschisis, and is it present in this patient?

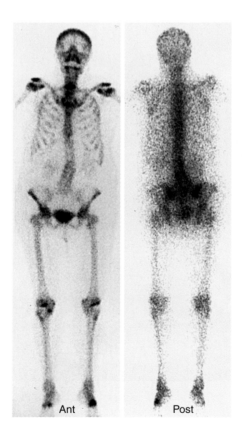

CASE 1-4

1-4a. What is wrong on this scan?
1-4b. What energy window should be used?
1-4c. How often should the energy resolution ("peaking") be checked?

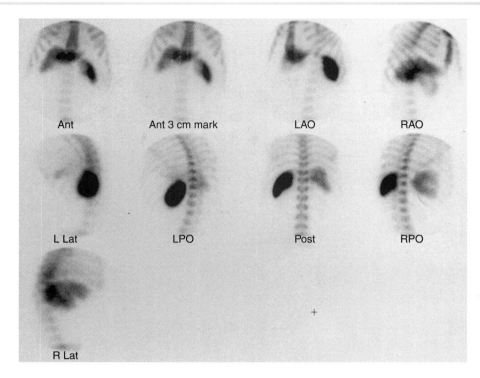

CASE 1-5

1-5a. What type of scan is this?

1-5b. What is the diagnosis?

1-5c. What are the pertinent findings?

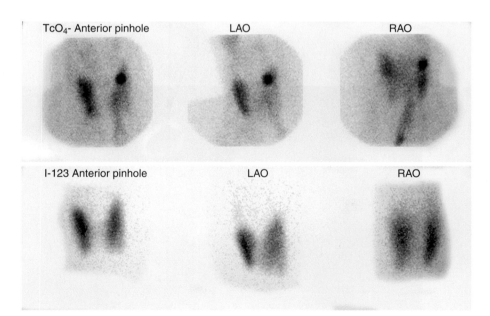

CASE 1-6

1-6a. What are the findings in this patient with a palpable left upper lobe thyroid nodule?

1-6b. Does this finding warrant further follow-up?

1-6c. On the ^{99m}Tc-pertechnetate RAO image, what is the activity below the thyroid gland?

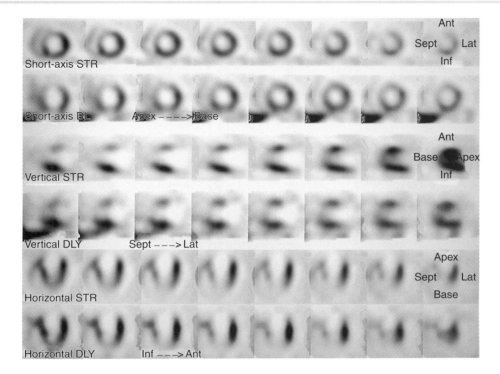

CASE 1-7

1-7a. What is the diagnosis?

1-7b. Are there important ancillary findings?

1-7c. What is the route of excretion of ^{99m}Tc-sestamibi?

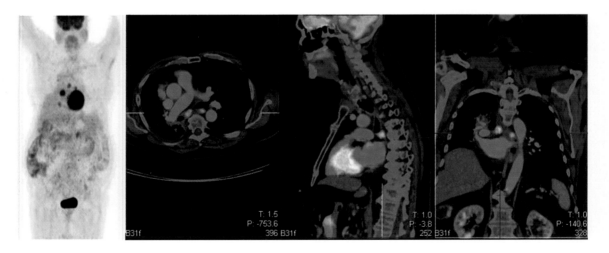

CASE 1-8

1-8a. What is the most likely primary pathology?

1-8b. Is this patient amenable to surgery?

1-8c. Is bronchoalveolar cancer typically FDG-avid?

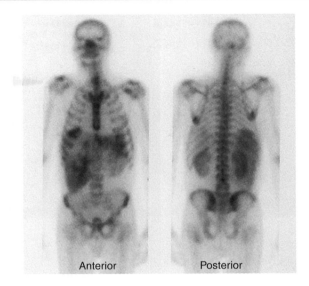

Anterior   Posterior

CASE 1-9

1-9a. What type of scan is this?

1-9b. What tumor types would be suspected?

1-9c. What are some other causes of soft tissue uptake on bone scans?

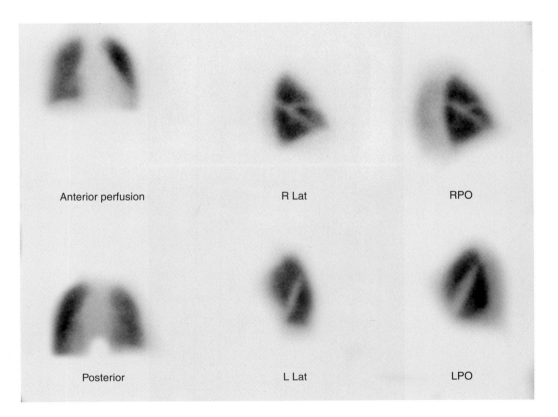

Anterior perfusion   R Lat   RPO

Posterior   L Lat   LPO

CASE 1-10

1-10a. Assuming that the ventilation scan is normal and the chest radiograph shows hyperinflation, what is the probability of pulmonary embolism?

1-10b. Does this appearance have a specific name?

1-10c. What is the "stripe" sign and what is its significance (if any)?

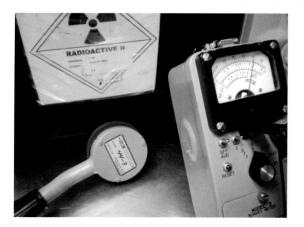

CASE 1-11

1-11a. What procedure is being performed?

1-11b. What is the exposure rate from the package?

1-11c. If the package is visibly damaged or leaking, what should you do?

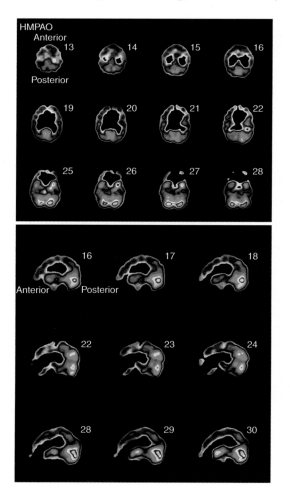

CASE 2-1

2-1a. What are the findings?

2-1b. What are the differential possibilities?

2-1c. Does the distribution of activity represent regional metabolism or regional blood flow?

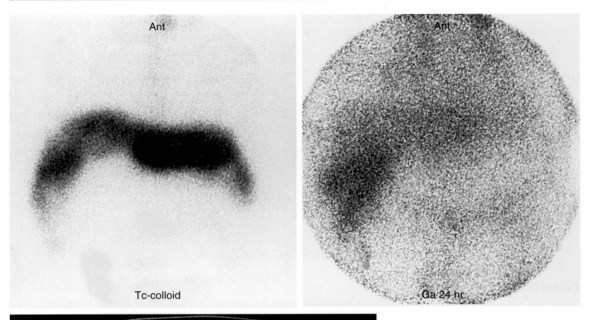

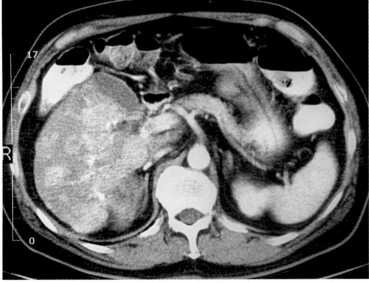

CASE 2-2

2-2a. What is the diagnosis?

2-2b. What other liver lesions may accumulate gallium?

2-2c. What are appearances of hepatic adenoma and focal nodular hyperplasia on a ^{99m}Tc-sulfur-colloid liver scan?

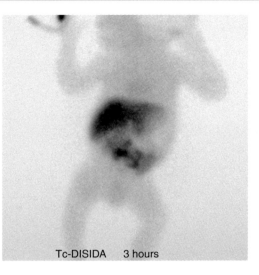

Tc-DISIDA   3 hours

CASE 2-3

2-3a. What type of scan is this?

2-3b. What is the diagnosis?

2-3c. In an effort to keep radiation doses low to children, what administered activity should be given to this 2-kg infant?

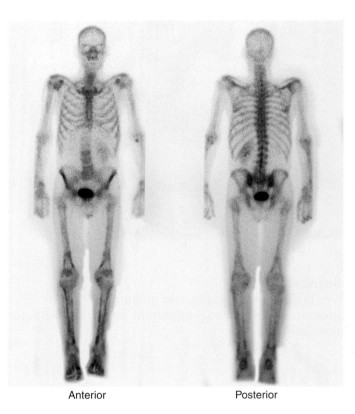

Anterior   Posterior

CASE 2-4

2-4a. What is the diagnosis?

2-4b. Is there an incidental finding?

2-4c. What is another radiopharmaceutical that can be used for bone scans besides ^{99m}Tc-MDP?

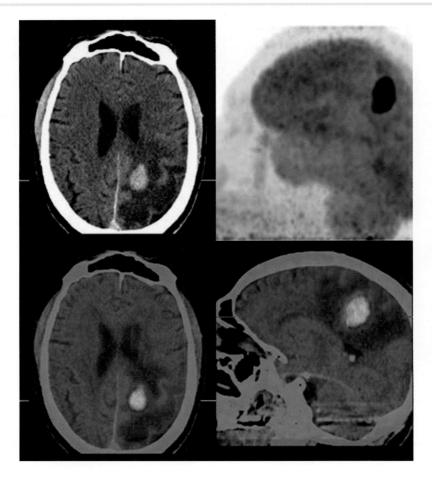

CASE 2-5

2-5a. What is the most likely diagnosis?

2-5b. How would an area of central necrosis have changed your diagnosis?

2-5c. How useful is this test in a patient with suspected CNS metastases from lung cancer?

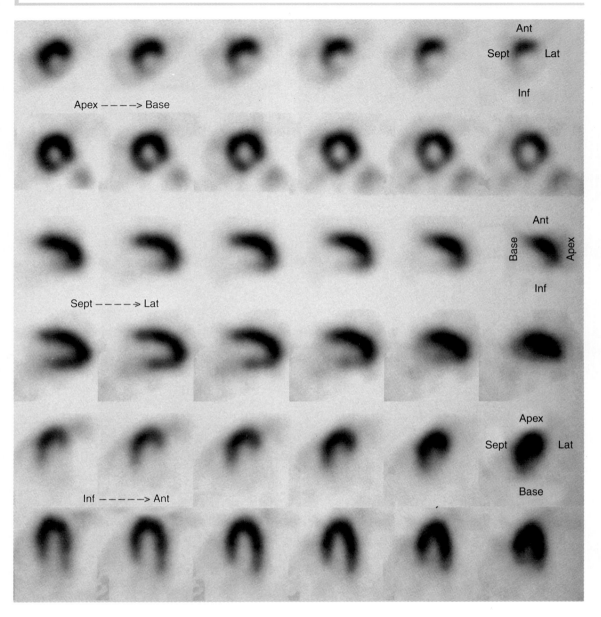

CASE 2-6

2-6a. What is the diagnosis?

2-6b. What vessels are involved?

2-6c. Where is the left ventricular apex on a bull's eye (polar map) image?

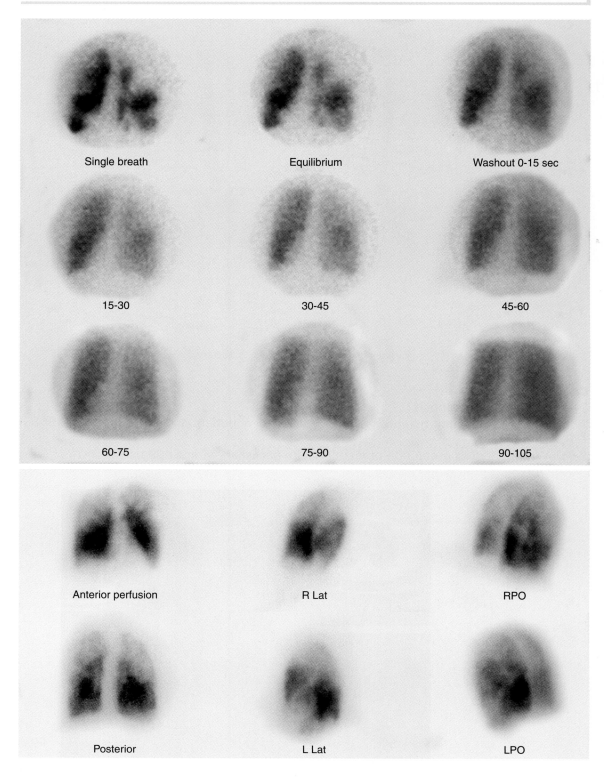

Single breath

Equilibrium

Washout 0-15 sec

15-30

30-45

45-60

60-75

75-90

90-105

Anterior perfusion

R Lat

RPO

Posterior

L Lat

LPO

CASE 2-7

2-7a. What is the diagnosis?

2-7b. What category is this, according to modified PIOPED II criteria?

2-7c. A lot of central deposition on a ^{99m}Tc-DTPA aerosol scan is an indication of what entity?

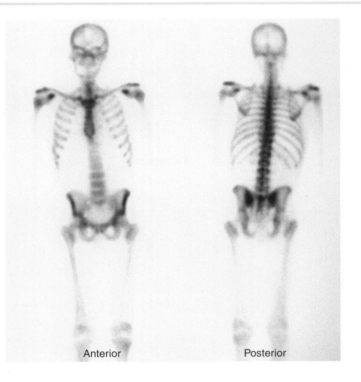

Anterior   Posterior

CASE 2-8

2-8a. What is the diagnosis?

2-8b. Under what circumstances would you treat a patient with strontium-89 (Sr-89) chloride?

2-8c. What radiation protection precautions are necessary after Sr-89 treatment?

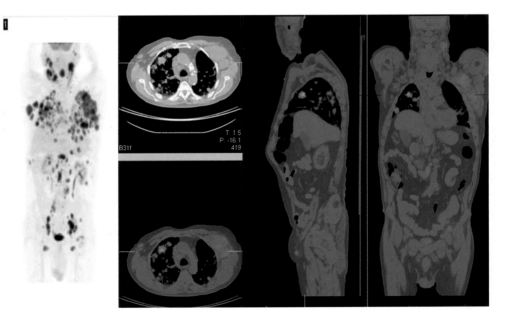

CASE 2-9

2-9a. What is the most likely diagnosis?

2-9b. What is/are the main use(s) for FDG PET/CT in lymphoma?

2-9c. Are MALT lymphomas typically FDG-avid?

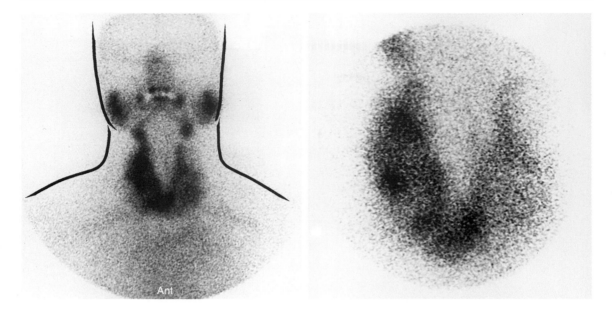

CASE 2-10
2-10a. What is the diagnosis?
2-10b. Is fine needle aspiration biopsy warranted?
2-10c. With what radiopharmaceutical was this scan performed?
2-10d. In treating toxic MNG with I-131, is the administered activity generally more or less than when treating Graves disease?

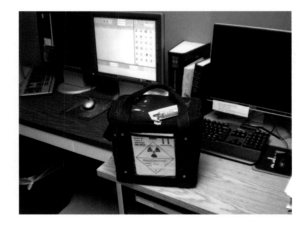

CASE 2-11
2-11a. Is there a problem with delivery of this package containing radioactive material?
2-11b. What are the requirements concerning transport of a radioactive package?
2-11c. What are the requirements concerning delivery?

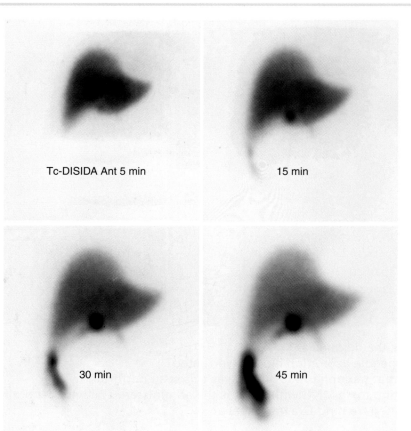

Tc-DISIDA Ant 5 min

15 min

30 min

45 min

CASE 3-1

3-1a. What is the diagnosis?

3-1b. Is the gallbladder present?

3-1c. What special views can be helpful?

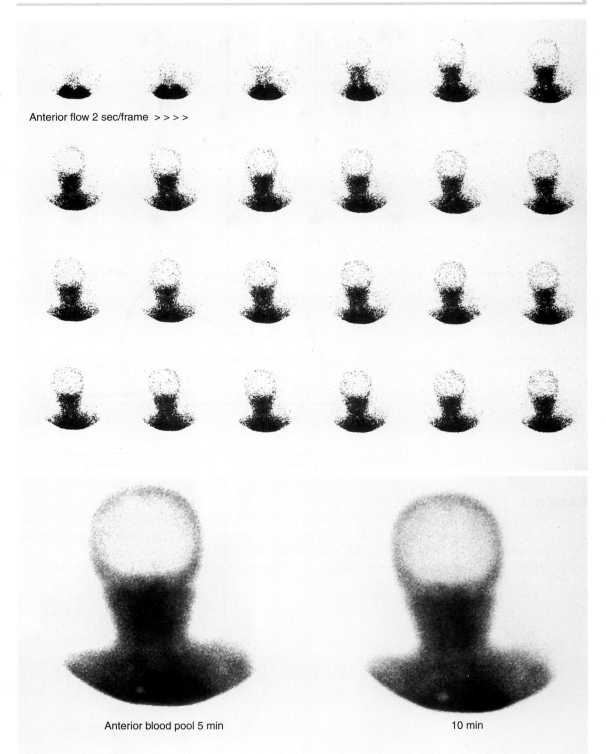

Anterior flow 2 sec/frame > > > >

Anterior blood pool 5 min   10 min

CASE 3-2

3-2a. What is the diagnosis?

3-2b. Can this study be done with ^{99m}Tc-hexamethylpropyleneamine oxime (HMPAO)?

3-2c. What would be the significance of activity in the sagittal sinus activity in a patient without obvious arterial phase activity?

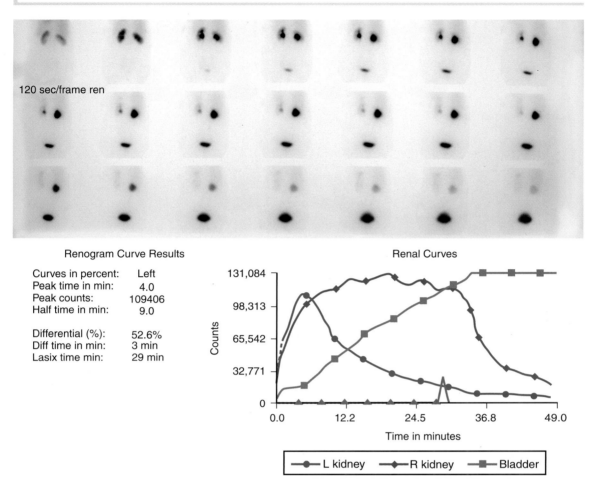

Renogram Curve Results

Curves in percent:	Left
Peak time in min:	4.0
Peak counts:	109406
Half time in min:	9.0
Differential (%):	52.6%
Diff time in min:	3 min
Lasix time min:	29 min

120 sec/frame ren

Renal Curves

— L kidney   — R kidney   — Bladder

CASE 3-3

3-3a. What is the diagnosis?

3-3b. If 370 MBq (10 mCi) of $^{99m}TcO_4^-$ had been administered to the patient inadvertently instead of ^{99m}Tc-MAG3, would it constitute a reportable "medical event"?

3-3c. What is the difference in mechanism of renal excretion between DTPA and MAG3?

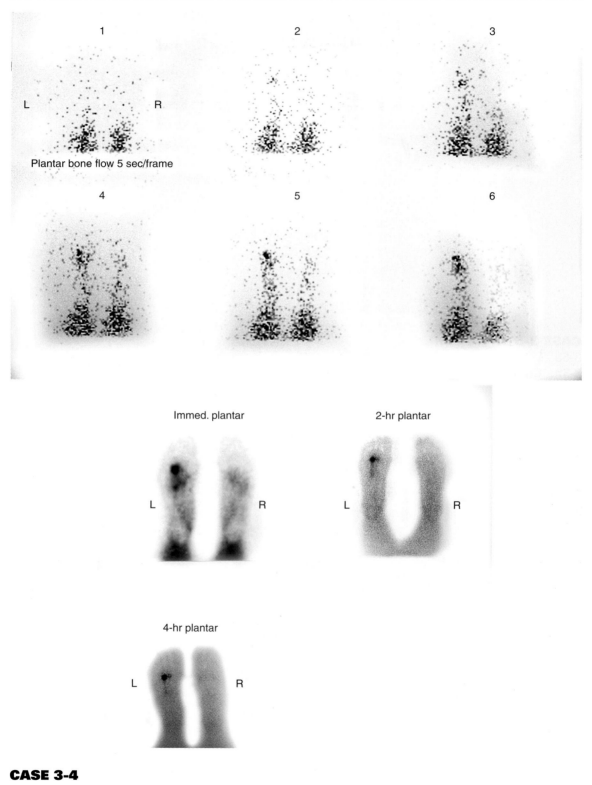

1 2 3

Plantar bone flow 5 sec/frame

4 5 6

Immed. plantar 2-hr plantar

L R L R

4-hr plantar

L R

CASE 3-4

3-4a. What is the diagnosis?

3-4b. Can osteomyelitis or an acute fracture have this appearance?

3-4c. If this were an acute fracture, how long would increased activity be expected?

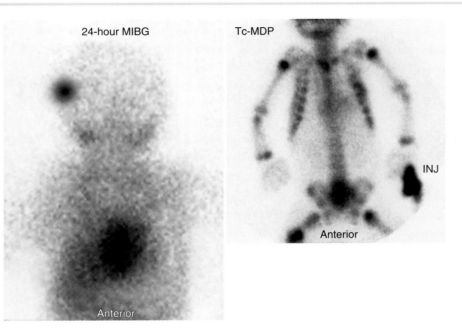

CASE 3-5
3-5a. What is the diagnosis?
3-5b. Could the tumor have been imaged with indium-111 pentetreotide?
3-5c. What other tumors could be imaged with indium-111 pentetreotide?

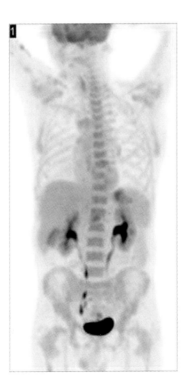

CASE 3-6
3-6a. What type of scan is this?
3-6b. What is the major finding?
3-6c. What are possible reasons for this finding?

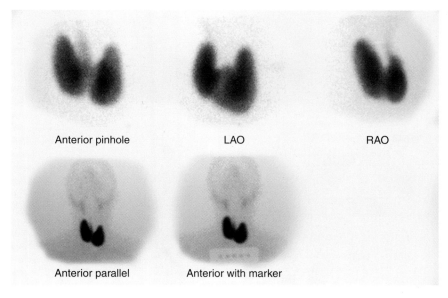

Anterior pinhole   LAO   RAO

Anterior parallel   Anterior with marker

CASE 3-7

3-7a. What is the diagnosis?

3-7b. Comparing technetium-pertechnetate with iodine-123 for scanning, how is the radiopharmaceutical administered and when should the patient be scanned?

3-7c. If the 24-hour iodine uptake were 65%, and the patient had a known cardiac disease, would you treat this patient, and if so, how?

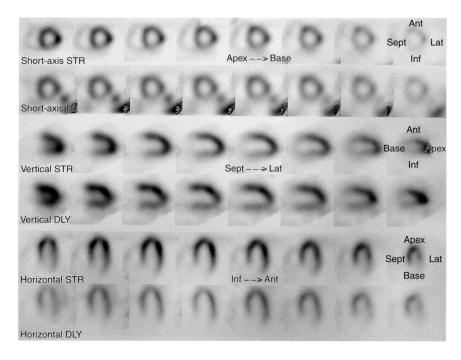

Short-axis STR   Apex – – > Base

Short-axis DLY

Vertical STR   Sept – – > Lat

Vertical DLY

Horizontal STR   Inf – – > Ant

Horizontal DLY

CASE 3-8

3-8a. What is the diagnosis?

3-8b. What type of artifact may be caused by left bundle branch block?

3-8c. What produces the areas of focally increased activity on the short-axis images at about the 2 o'clock and 7 o'clock positions?

Rotating display images

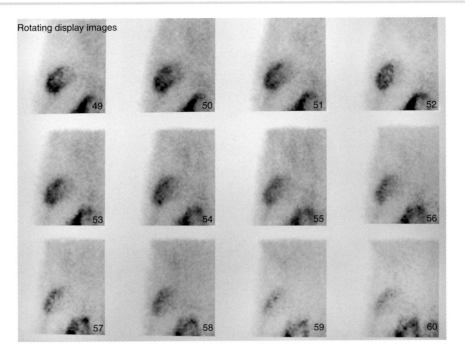

CASE 3-8, cont'd

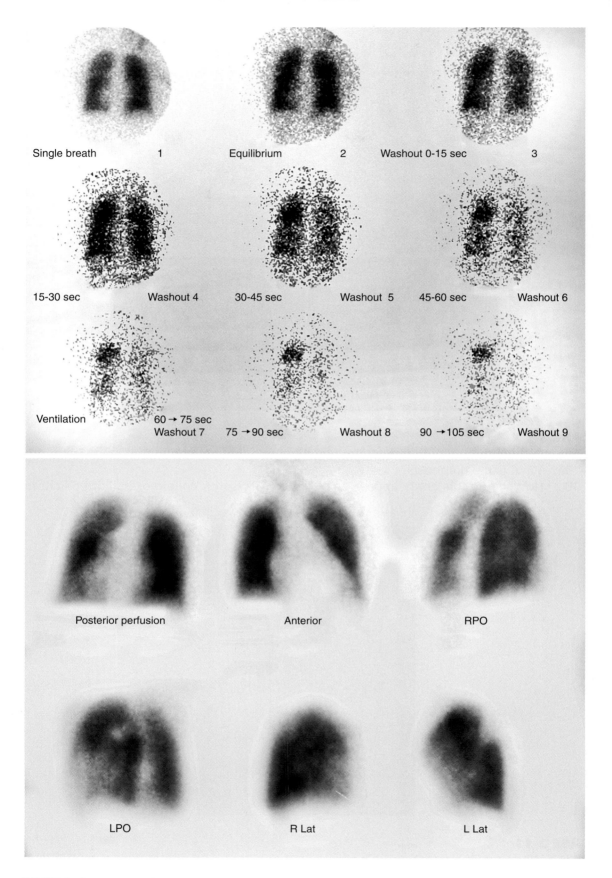

Single breath   1

Equilibrium   2

Washout 0-15 sec   3

15-30 sec   Washout 4

30-45 sec   Washout 5

45-60 sec   Washout 6

Ventilation   60 → 75 sec   Washout 7

75 → 90 sec   Washout 8

90 → 105 sec   Washout 9

Posterior perfusion

Anterior

RPO

LPO

R Lat

L Lat

CASE 3-9

3-9a. In what projection is a xenon-133 scan typically performed, and why?

3-9b. Where does the xenon go when the patient exhales?

3-9c. What is the diagnosis?

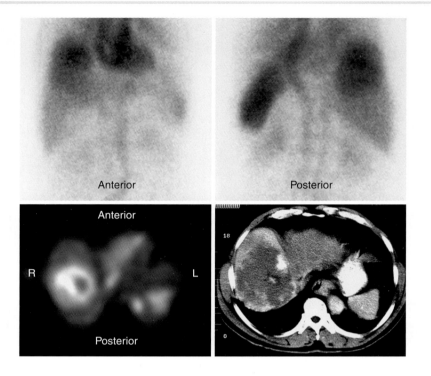

Anterior

Posterior

Anterior

R   L

Posterior

CASE 3-10

3-10a.   What is the radiopharmaceutical used in this examination?

3-10b.   What is the diagnosis?

3-10c.   How would this entity appear on either a ^{99m}Tc-sulfur colloid or gallium-67 citrate scan?

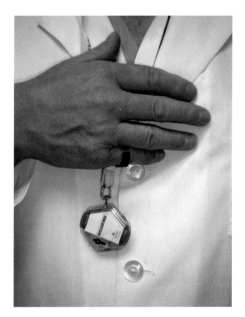

CASE 3-11

3-11a.   When are dosimeters required?

3-11b.   What are the annual dose limits for the whole body and hands?

3-11c.   Do occupational dose limits include either background or personal medical exposure received by a technologist?

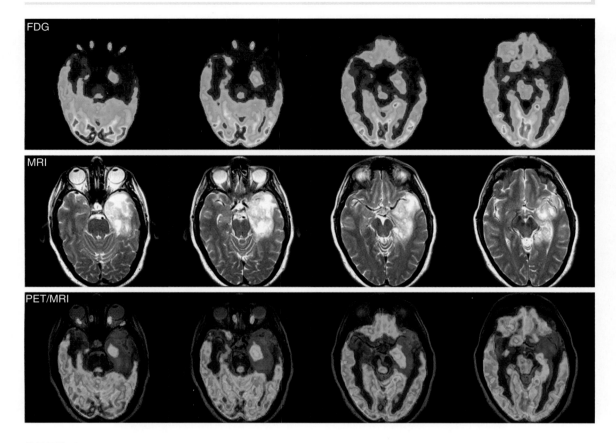

CASE 4-1

4-1a. What is the most likely diagnosis?

4-1b. What findings would be expected on thallium-201 and technetium-99m HMPAO brain scans done to distinguish recurrent tumor from radiation necrosis?

4-1c. What is the significance of increased ^{18}F-FDG activity in an area of a previously known low-grade glioma?

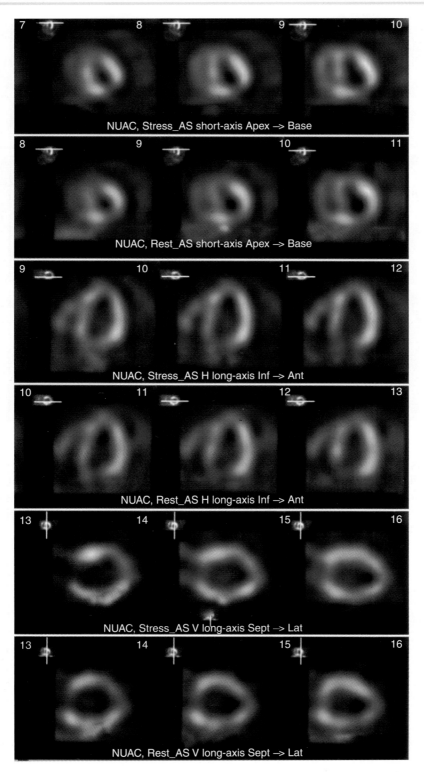

NUAC, Stress_AS short-axis Apex –> Base

NUAC, Rest_AS short-axis Apex –> Base

NUAC, Stress_AS H long-axis Inf –> Ant

NUAC, Rest_AS H long-axis Inf –> Ant

NUAC, Stress_AS V long-axis Sept –> Lat

NUAC, Rest_AS V long-axis Sept –> Lat

CASE 4-2

4-2a. What is the diagnosis?

4-2b. What is the top normal left ventricle (LV) end-diastolic volume?

4-2c. What does the myocardial uptake of the PET imaging agents ^{13}N-ammonia (^{13}NH$_3$) and rubidium-82 (^{82}Rb) indicate?

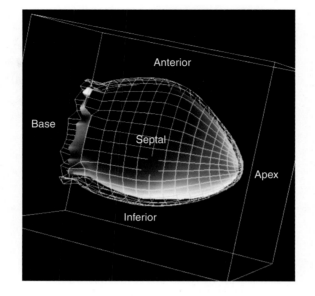

CASE 4-2, cont'd

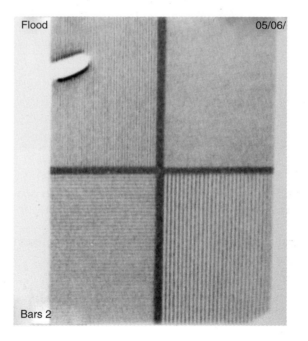

CASE 4-3

4-3a. What is the diagnosis?

4-3b. How was this image obtained?

4-3c. How often is this type of image obtained?

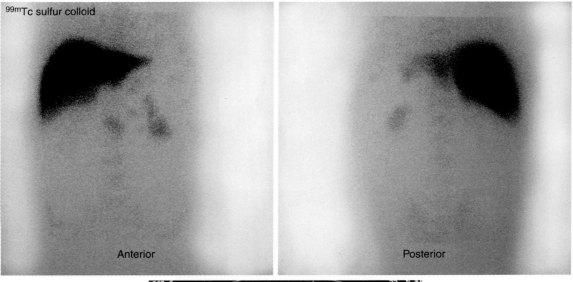

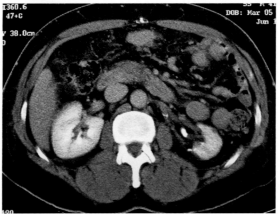

CASE 4-4

4-4a. What is the diagnosis in this patient who was in an auto accident 5 years earlier?

4-4b. What radiopharmaceutical besides technetium-99m sulfur colloid can be used to make this diagnosis?

4-4c. What other entities can cause nonvisualization of the spleen on a ^{99m}Tc-sulfur colloid scan?

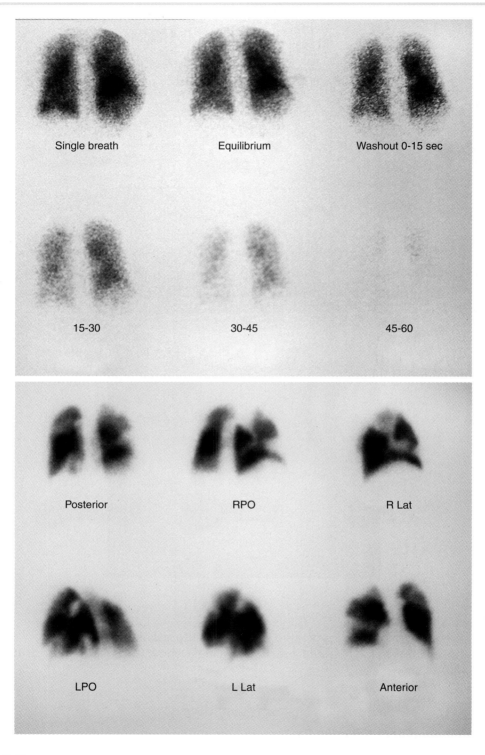

Single breath	Equilibrium	Washout 0-15 sec
15-30	30-45	45-60
Posterior	RPO	R Lat
LPO	L Lat	Anterior

CASE 4-5

4-5a. What is the diagnosis?

4-5b. What is the approximate number and size of ^{99m}Tc-MAA particles administered?

4-5c. If this patient has pulmonary hypertension, what is the likelihood that pulmonary emboli are the cause, and why is this information important?

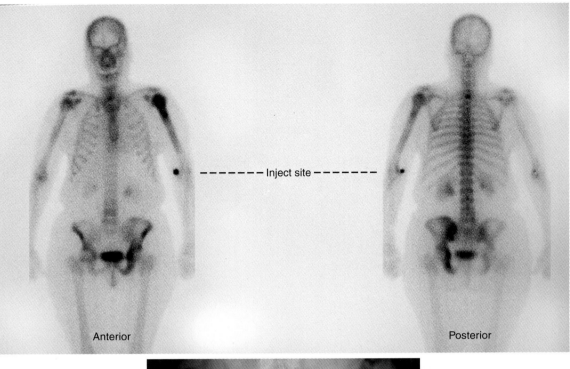

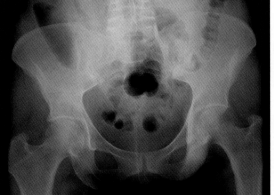

CASE 4-6

4-6a. What is the diagnosis?

4-6b. What are the pertinent associated findings on the pelvis radiograph?

4-6c. Do the lytic lesions associated with Paget disease show increased radionuclide uptake on a bone scan?

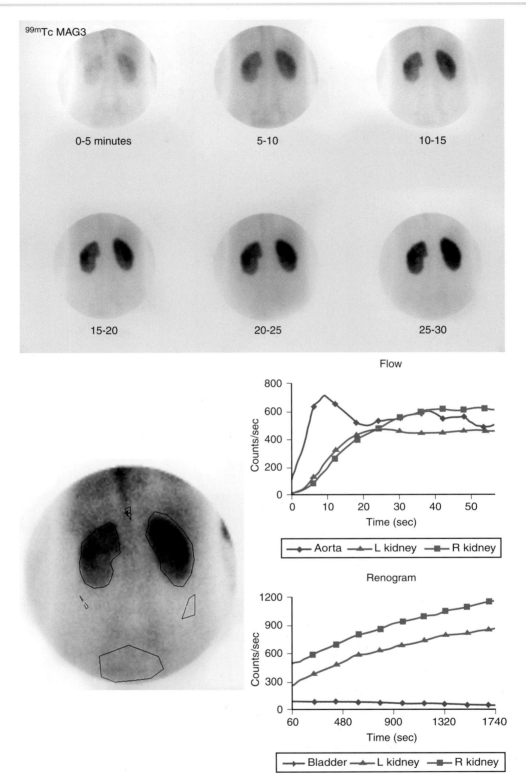

99mTc MAG3

0-5 minutes   5-10   10-15

15-20   20-25   25-30

Flow

Renogram

CASE 4-7

4-7a. What is the diagnosis?

4-7b. Could dehydration produce the same pattern?

4-7c. Would chronic renal disease produce the same pattern?

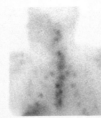
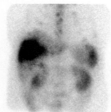
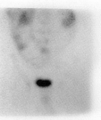

Ant chest 6 hr   Ant abd. 6 hr   Ant pelvis 6 hr

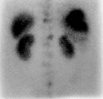
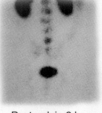

Post chest 6 hr   Post abd. 6 hr   Post pelvis 6 hr

CASE 4-8

4-8a. What type of scan is this?

4-8b. What is the diagnosis?

4-8c. What other pathologic entities show increased activity with this radiopharmaceutical?

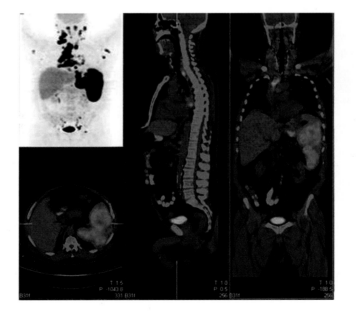

CASE 4-9

4-9a. What is the likely diagnosis?

4-9b. What is the significance of the splenic activity?

4-9c. What is the size threshold for the detection of a lesion on FDG PET?

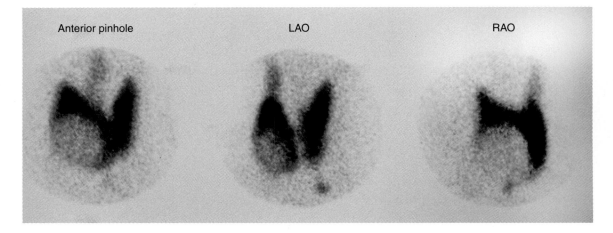

Anterior pinhole   LAO   RAO

CASE 4-10

4-10a. What is the most likely diagnosis?
4-10b. What is the differential diagnosis?
4-10c. What is the next step in management?

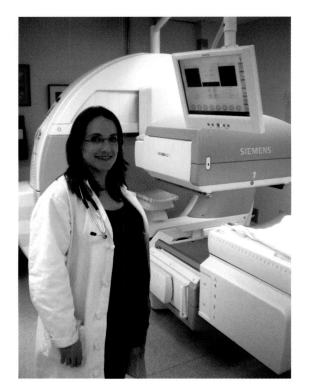

CASE 4-11

4-11a. Can a pregnant technologist or physician be actively involved with nuclear medicine patients?
4-11b. Under the ALARA principle, what procedures would you consider restricting the technologist from performing?
4-11c. What are the dose limits for the embryo/fetus?

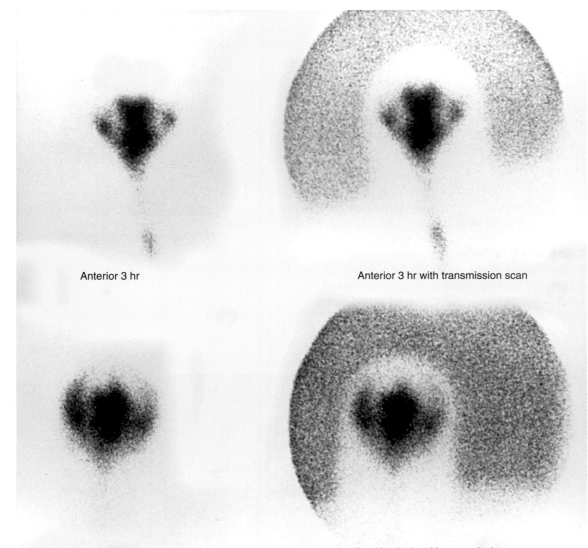

Anterior 3 hr

Anterior 3 hr with transmission scan

Anterior 24 hr

Anterior 24 hr with transmission scan

CASE 5-1

5-1a. What is the likely diagnosis?

5-1b. What characteristics differentiate this from a normal study?

5-1c. Identify the anatomy on these images.

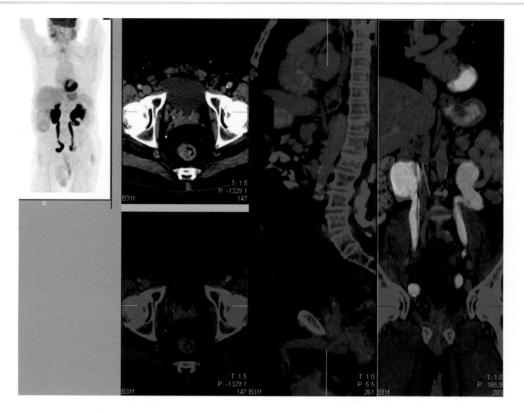

CASE 5-2

5-2a. What is the major finding?

5-2b. What is the likely cause?

5-2c. What is the value of ^{18}F-FDG PET in this entity?

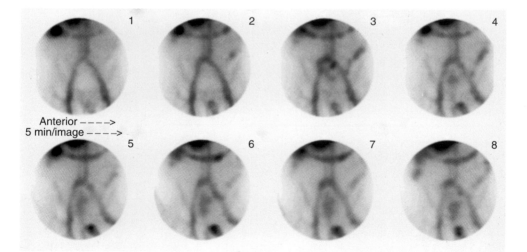

Anterior – – – –>
5 min/image – – – –>

CASE 5-3

5-3a. What is the finding?

5-3b. What bleeding rate is necessary to reliably detect the bleeding with angiography and scintigraphy?

5-3c. If the study had been negative, what would be the next step in management?

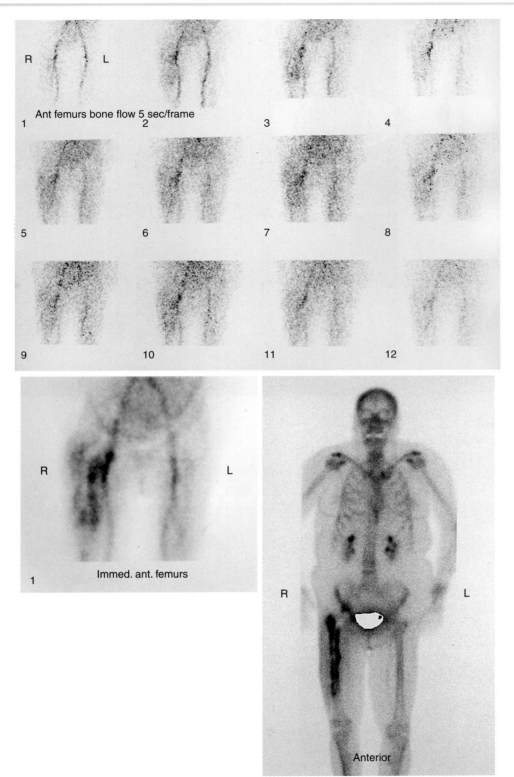

R   L

Ant femurs bone flow 5 sec/frame

1   2   3   4

5   6   7   8

9   10   11   12

R   L

Immed. ant. femurs

1

R   L

Anterior

CASE 5-4

5-4a. What is the diagnosis?

5-4b. What other nuclear medicine techniques are more appropriate in this setting?

5-4c. What is the pattern typically seen on MDP scans with hip prosthesis loosening?

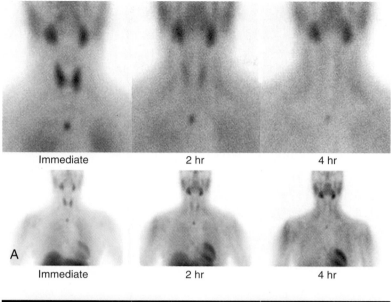

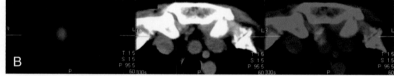

CASE 5-5

5-5a. What type of examination is this?

5-5b. What is the most likely diagnosis?

5-5c. What other entities might this represent?

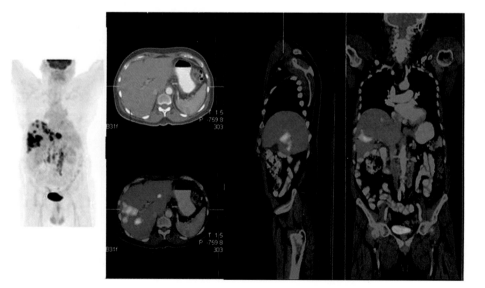

CASE 5-6

5-6a. What is the diagnosis in this patient with a rising CEA?

5-6b. What is the best test for suspected liver metastases from colon cancer?

5-6c. What is the role of FDG PET/CT in staging colorectal cancer?

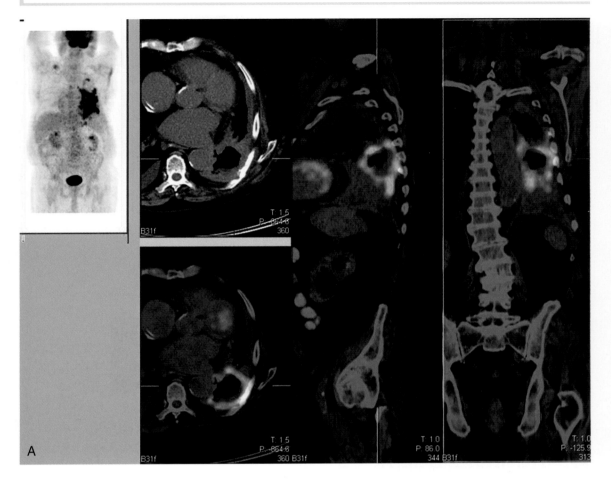

CASE 5-7

5-7a. What is the diagnosis?

5-7b. What is the hot spot in the right supraclavicular region?

5-7c. Which set of images is not attenuation-corrected?

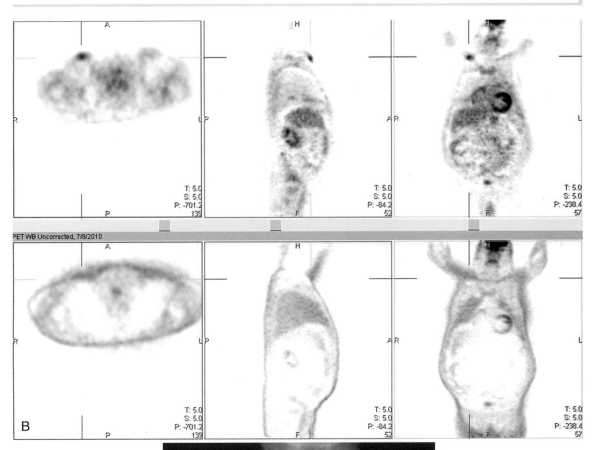

PET WB Uncorrected, 7/8/2010

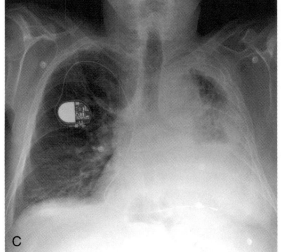

CASE 5-7, cont'd

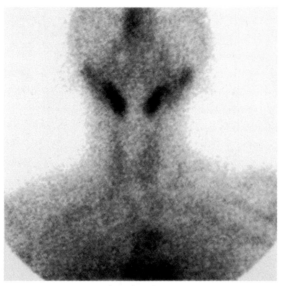

Anterior planar

CASE 5-8

5-8a. What is included in the differential diagnosis?

5-8b. Would this pattern likely be due to prior stable iodine ingestion?

5-8c. What scan patterns might be seen with chronic forms of thyroiditis?

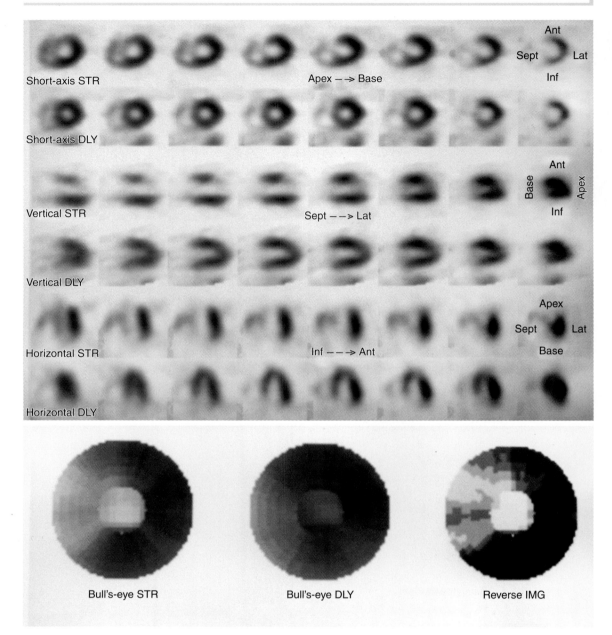

Short-axis STR

Apex — → Base

Ant
Sept — Lat
Inf

Short-axis DLY

Vertical STR

Sept – – → Lat

Ant
Base — Apex
Inf

Vertical DLY

Horizontal STR

Inf – – → Ant

Apex
Sept — Lat
Base

Horizontal DLY

Bull's-eye STR   Bull's-eye DLY   Reverse IMG

CASE 5-9

5-9a. What is the diagnosis?

5-9b. What would be the implications if the left ventricle dilated on the stress images?

5-9c. What is the mechanism of transient ischemic dilatation?

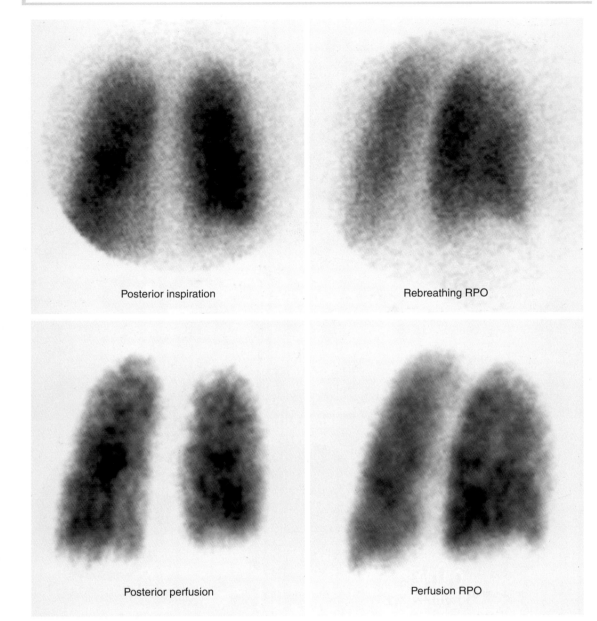

Posterior inspiration

Rebreathing RPO

Posterior perfusion

Perfusion RPO

CASE 5-10

5-10a. Assuming a normal chest radiograph, what is the diagnosis?

5-10b. What modified PIOPED II probability category would this represent?

5-10c. What is the differential diagnosis in this case?

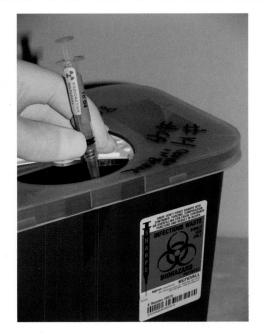

CASE 5-11

5-11a. What methods are used for the disposal of radioactive syringes?

5-11b. Is the method shown here appropriate?

5-11c. How long is storage required?

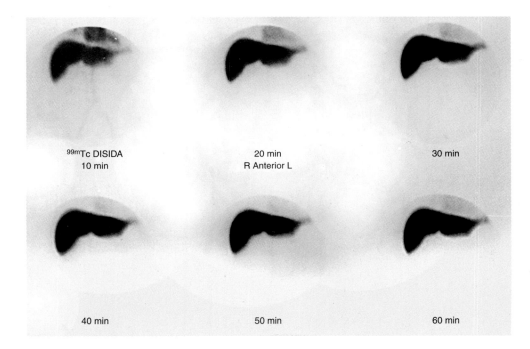

CASE 6-1

6-1a. What type of scan is this?

6-1b. What is the diagnosis?

6-1c. Is this radiopharmaceutical conjugated by the liver?

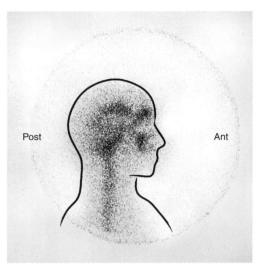

CASE 6-2

6-2a. What is the diagnosis in this post-traumatic patient?

6-2b. How is the patient prepared for this procedure?

6-2c. With normal images, can a "normal" diagnosis be made for this procedure?

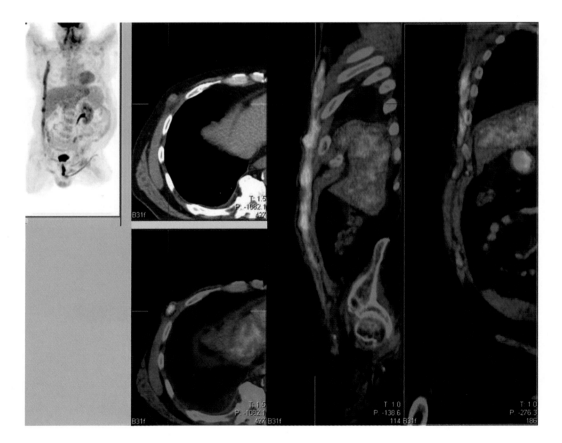

CASE 6-3

6-3a. What is the diagnosis?

6-3b. What criteria should be used in making the diagnosis?

6-3c. What is the value of ^{99m}Tc-WBC compared with FDG PET/CT in this setting?

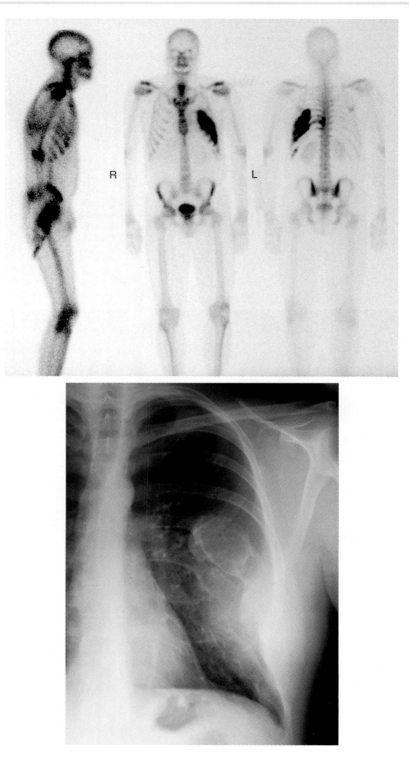

CASE 6-4

6-4a. What is the diagnosis?

6-4b. Are multiple enchondromas typically "hot" on a bone scan?

6-4c. What physiologic factors cause increased activity on bone scans?

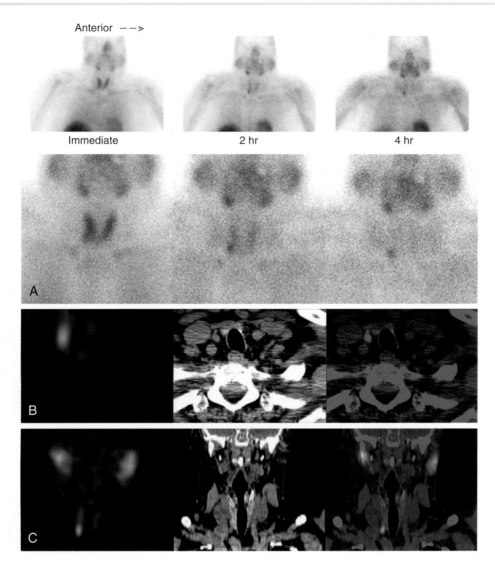

Anterior — —>

| Immediate | 2 hr | 4 hr |

CASE 6-5

6-5a. What is the most likely diagnosis?

6-5b. Could this lesion be a thyroid adenoma?

6-5c. What method could be used to help locate the lesion at surgery, and how would the patient be prepared?

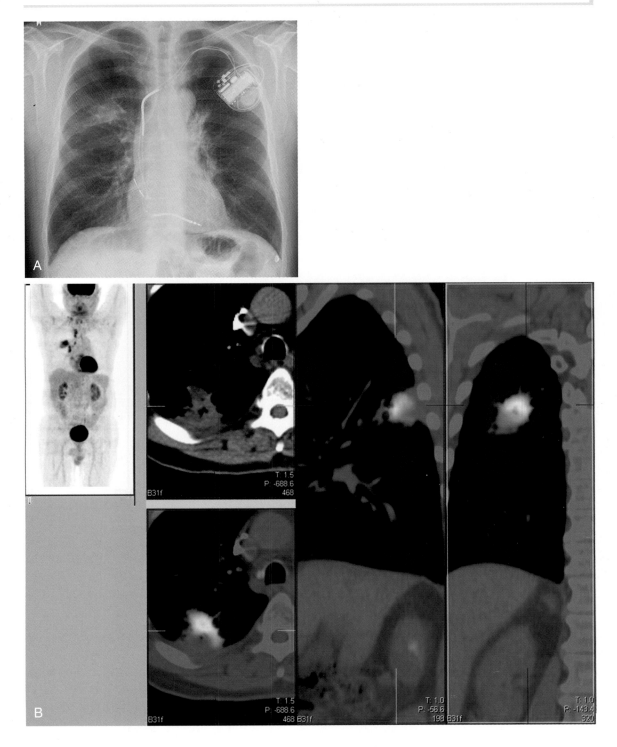

CASE 6-6

6-6a. What is the diagnosis?

6-6b. Is metastatic disease present?

6-6c. What is the role of ^{18}F-FDG PET/CT in infection?

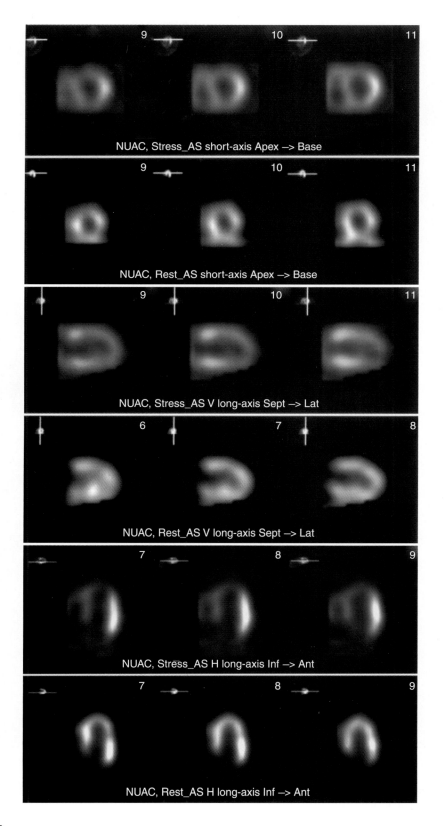

NUAC, Stress_AS short-axis Apex –> Base

NUAC, Rest_AS short-axis Apex –> Base

NUAC, Stress_AS V long-axis Sept –> Lat

NUAC, Rest_AS V long-axis Sept –> Lat

NUAC, Stress_AS H long-axis Inf –> Ant

NUAC, Rest_AS H long-axis Inf –> Ant

CASE 6-7

6-7a. What is the diagnosis?

6-7b. What parameters are used to determine whether physical exercise stress was adequate in this patient?

6-7c. What degree of coronary artery stenosis is important?

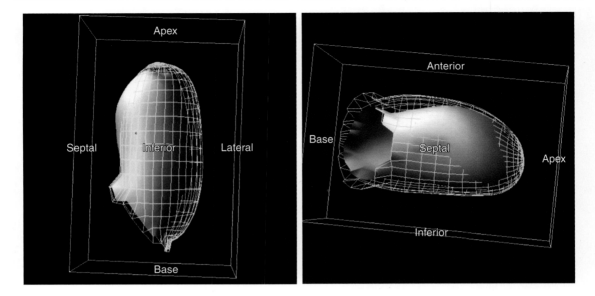

CASE 6-7, cont'd

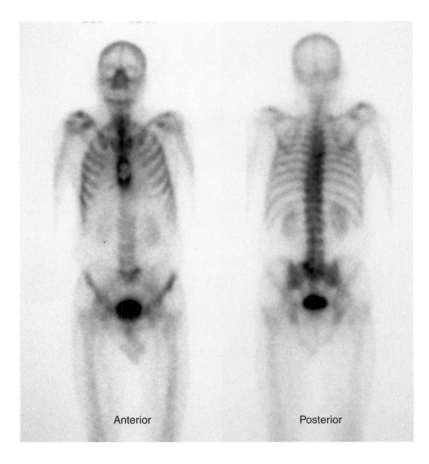

CASE 6-8

6-8a. What is the diagnosis?

6-8b. What cancer types often produce predominantly lytic bone metastases?

6-8c. What tumor type most often causes single sternal metastases?

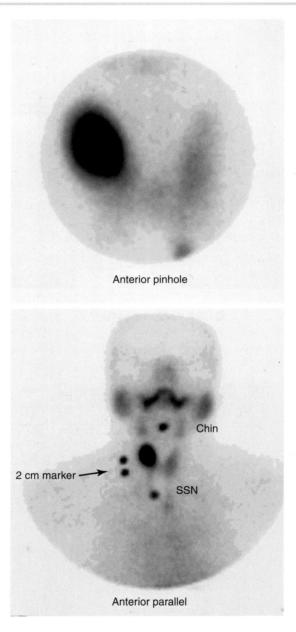

Anterior pinhole

2 cm marker →

Chin

SSN

Anterior parallel

CASE 6-9

6-9a. What is the most likely diagnosis?

6-9b. Could this lesion be malignant?

6-9c. Does the remainder of the gland appear normal?

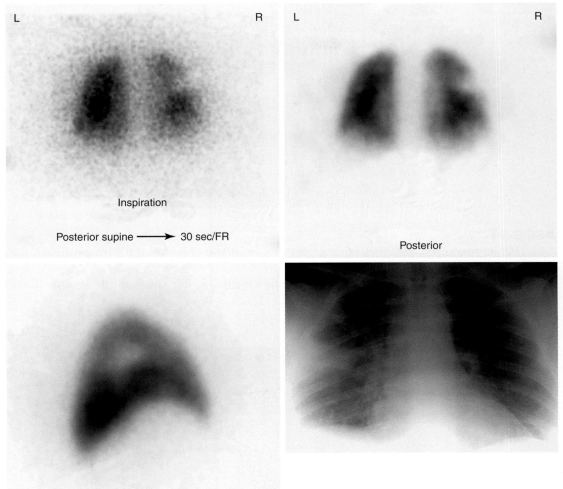

Inspiration

Posterior supine 30 sec/FR

Posterior

R Lat

CASE 6-10

6-10a. What is the diagnosis?

6-10b. What is meant by the term "triple match"?

6-10c. What probability of PE is associated with a triple match?

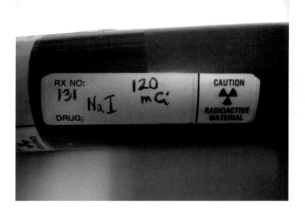

CASE 6-11

6-11a. What specific paperwork is required to administer this radiopharmaceutical?

6-11b. Who must supervise the administration?

6-11c. Under what conditions can a patient be released after therapeutic administration of I-131?

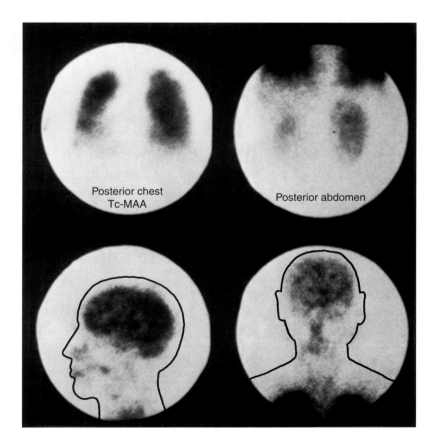

CASE 7-1

7-1a. What is the diagnosis?

7-1b. If you suspected such a shunt was present, should you have done this procedure at all or modified the procedure?

7-1c. What causes "hot spots" in the lung on a ^{99m}Tc-MAA perfusion scan, and are they clinically significant?

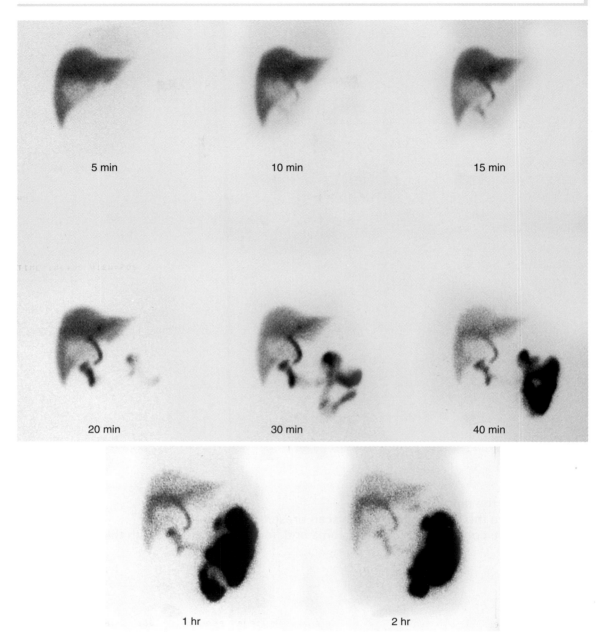

5 min   10 min   15 min

20 min   30 min   40 min

1 hr   2 hr

CASE 7-2

7-2a. Is this likely to represent chronic cholecystitis?

7-2b. Is there a need to alert the clinician, and if so, why?

7-2c. Is there an advantage to slow infusion of CCK over more than 10 minutes in performing a gallbladder ejection fraction study?

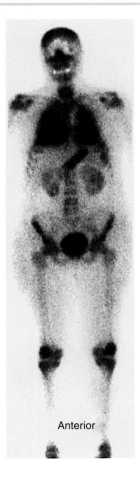

Anterior

CASE 7-3

7-3a. What is the diagnosis?

7-3b. What are the two common bone scan presentations of this entity?

7-3c. What are common clinical symptoms and findings associated with this entity?

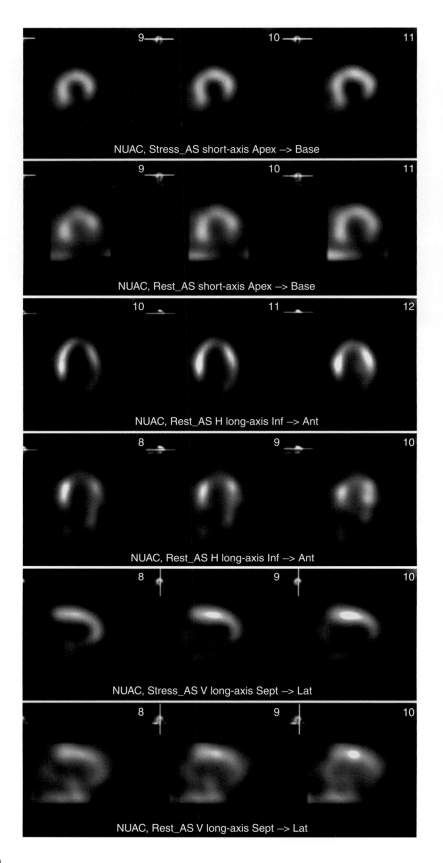

NUAC, Stress_AS short-axis Apex –> Base

NUAC, Rest_AS short-axis Apex –> Base

NUAC, Rest_AS H long-axis Inf –> Ant

NUAC, Rest_AS H long-axis Inf –> Ant

NUAC, Stress_AS V long-axis Sept –> Lat

NUAC, Rest_AS V long-axis Sept –> Lat

CASE 7-4

7-4a. What is the diagnosis?

7-4b. What is hibernating myocardium?

7-4c. What is stunned myocardium?

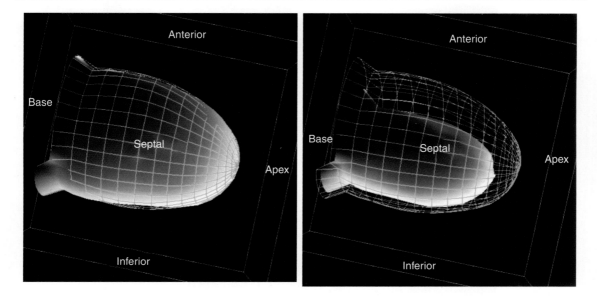

CASE 7-4, cont'd

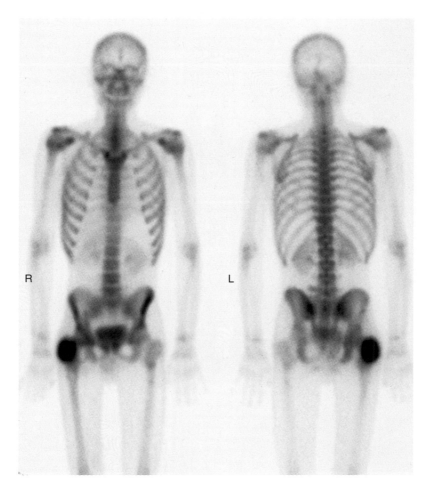

CASE 7-5

7-5a. What is the diagnosis?

7-5b. What would a septic hip look like on a bone scan?

7-5c. What are other diagnostic considerations?

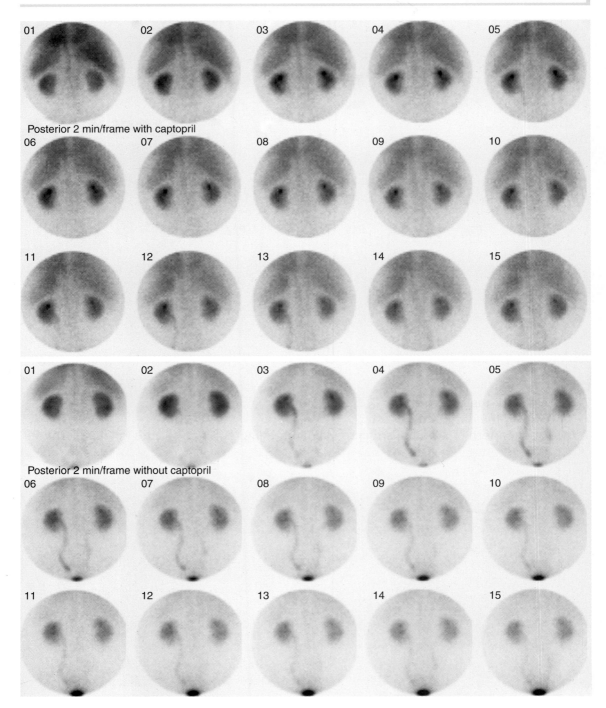

Posterior 2 min/frame with captopril

Posterior 2 min/frame without captopril

CASE 7-6

7-6a. What is the diagnosis?

7-6b. What is the mechanism by which captopril works?

7-6c. Is a known severe renal artery stenosis a relative contraindication to this procedure?

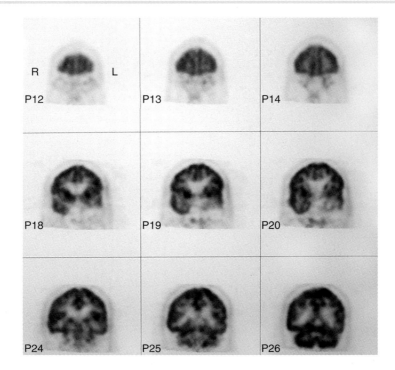

CASE 7-7

7-7a. What are the findings?

7-7b. What is the differential?

7-7c. What pattern of metabolism is seen with imaging during a seizure (ictal imaging)?

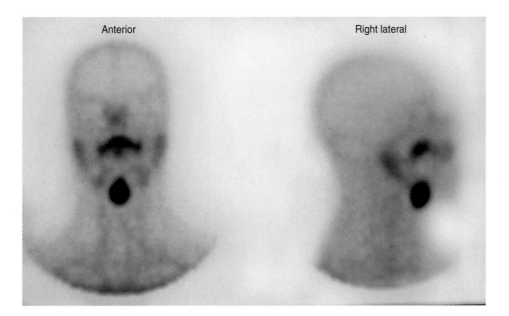

CASE 7-8

7-8a. What is the diagnosis?

7-8b. What is the usual thyroid function status in these patients?

7-8c. What is the pathogenesis of this entity?

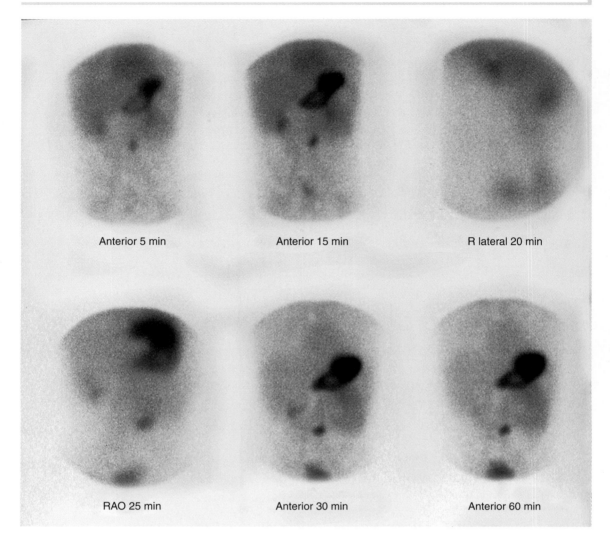

Anterior 5 min	Anterior 15 min	R lateral 20 min
RAO 25 min	Anterior 30 min	Anterior 60 min

CASE 7-9

7-9a. Is this a GI bleeding study?

7-9b. Does a negative result mean that there is no Meckel diverticulum present?

7-9c. What premedication(s) can increase the sensitivity of this procedure?

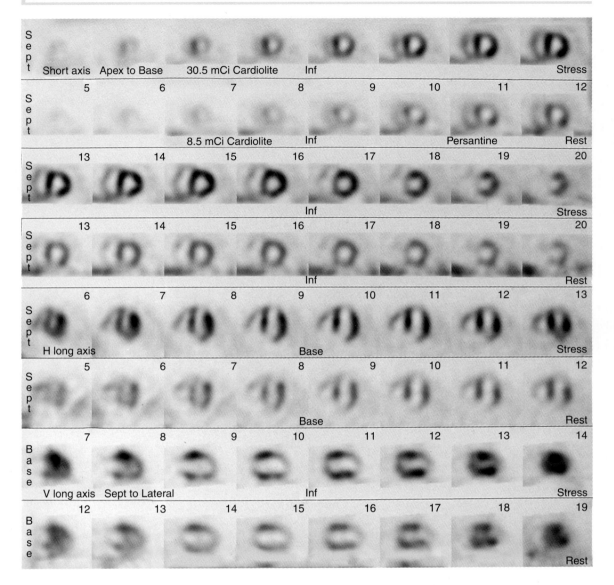

CASE 7-10

7-10a. What is the diagnosis?

7-10b. What are the adverse reactions associated with dipyridamole pharmacologic stress, and how are they treated?

7-10c. What are the side effects and method of treatment for adverse reactions to adenosine stress?

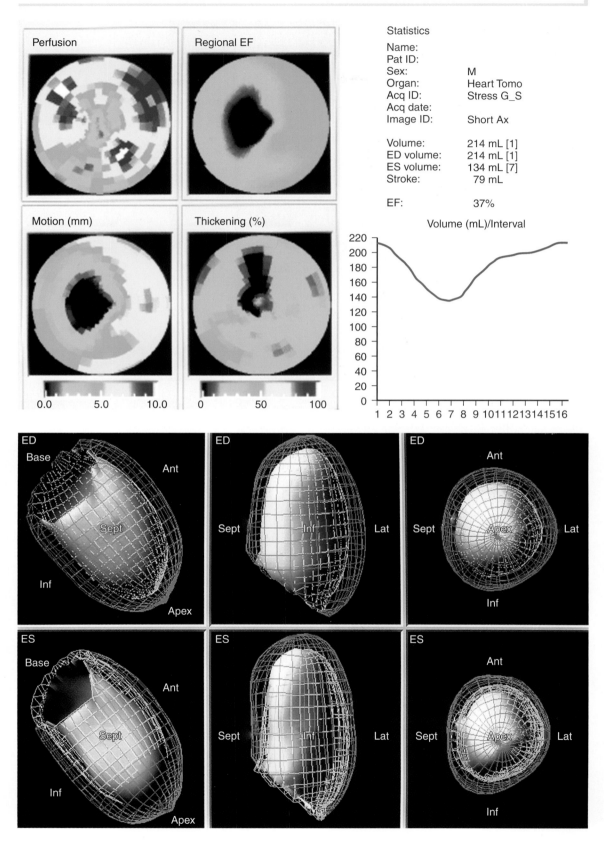

Perfusion

Regional EF

Motion (mm)

0.0   5.0   10.0

Thickening (%)

0   50   100

Statistics

Name:	
Pat ID:	
Sex:	M
Organ:	Heart Tomo
Acq ID:	Stress G_S
Acq date:	
Image ID:	Short Ax
Volume:	214 mL [1]
ED volume:	214 mL [1]
ES volume:	134 mL [7]
Stroke:	79 mL
EF:	37%

Volume (mL)/Interval

220 200 180 160 140 120 100 80 60 40 20 0

1 2 3 4 5 6 7 8 9 10 11 12 13 14 15 16

ED — Base — Ant — Sept — Inf — Apex

ED — Sept — Inf — Lat

ED — Ant — Sept — Apex — Lat — Inf

ES — Base — Ant — Sept — Inf — Apex

ES — Sept — Inf — Lat

ES — Ant — Sept — Apex — Lat — Inf

CASE 7-10, cont'd

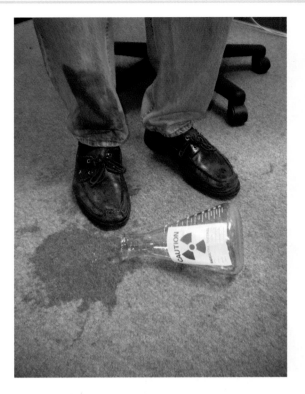

CASE 7-11

7-11a. The beaker contained 370 MBq (10 mCi) of iodine-131. What category spill is this?

7-11b. What are the actions that need to be taken?

7-11c. Are additional actions potentially needed because of the nature of this radiopharmaceutical?

Answers to Unknown Case Sets

CASE 1-1

1-1a. What is the diagnosis? Lasix renogram and time-activity curves demonstrating high-grade obstruction of the left kidney and a nonobstructed extrarenal pelvis on the right.

1-1b. Could this study be done with ^{99m}Tc-DMSA? No, DMSA is a cortical agent with essentially no urinary excretion.

1-1c. After Lasix, how fast should the DPTA or MAG3 activity in a normal kidney decrease? Half should be excreted in 7 to 10 minutes. For suspected high grade obstruction, MAG3 is preferred because of its tubular secretion component.

CASE 1-2

1-2a. What is the diagnosis? Lymphoma. Chest and abdominal scans showing accumulation of the radiopharmaceutical in both mediastinal and abdominal nodal masses.

1-2b. What radiopharmaceutical was used? Gallium-67-citrate, as evidenced by the relatively poor image quality, liver greater than spleen activity, as well as physiologic bowel activity. While gallium is sensitive for lymphoma assessment and follow-up, it has been replaced by PET/CT in many institutions.

1-2c. What is the approximate photon energy of this radiopharmaceutical's gamma emissions? 90, 190, 290, 390 keV. Two or more of these are generally used.

CASE 1-3

1-3a. What is the diagnosis? Alzheimer disease, as evidenced by symmetrically decreased metabolism in the parietotemporal regions bilaterally.

1-3b. What are the expected findings in Lewy body dementia? Changes similar to Alzheimer disease but with less occipital sparing.

1-3c. What is crossed cerebellar diaschisis and is it present in this patient? It is seen as hypometabolism in the cerebellar hemisphere contralateral to a supratentorial cerebral lesion such as tumor, stroke, or trauma. It is not present in this patient.

CASE 1-4

1-4a. What is wrong on this scan? There is degenerative disease but no evidence of metastatic disease on this ^{99m}Tc- methylene diphosphonate (MDP) bone scan with loss of resolution on posterior image. This was caused by the posterior camera head being off-peak (not set for the correct energy window for ^{99m}Tc). A camera head that is too far from the patient, poor radiopharmaceutical labeling, or camera electronic malfunctions may also produce this appearance.

1-4b. What energy window should be used? 140 keV. Often a 20% window (± 14 keV) is used.

1-4c. How often should the energy resolution ("peaking") be checked? At least daily. Many new cameras do this automatically for each examination.

CASE 1-5

1-5a. What type of scan is this? ^{99m}Tc-sulfur colloid liver-spleen scan.

1-5b. What is the diagnosis? Hepatic cirrhosis.

1-5c. What are the pertinent findings? Small liver displaced from the ribs as a result of a large amount of ascites, increased splenic activity relative to the liver on the posterior view, and markedly increased shift of colloid to the bone marrow.

CASE 1-6

1-6a. What are the findings in this patient with a palpable left upper lobe thyroid nodule? Discordant thyroid nodule, as evidenced by increased activity on the technetium scan but not on the radioiodine scan.

1-6b. Does this finding warrant further follow-up? Yes. A small number of these are thyroid carcinomas.

1-6c. On the ^{99m}Tc-pertechnetate RAO image, what is the activity below the thyroid gland? Swallowed saliva. How can you be sure? This can be checked by having the patient drink water and by reimaging.

CASE 1-7

1-7a. What is the diagnosis? Large anterior-apical infarct.

1-7b. Are there important ancillary findings? Yes. The diverging ventricular walls (the "trumpet sign") indicate an aneurysm is likely present.

1-7c. What is the route of excretion of ^{99m}Tc-sestamibi? Biliary to bowel. Nearby liver, biliary, and bowel activity must be taken into account in timing the images to minimize artifact. The organ receiving the largest absorbed dose is the gallbladder.

CASE 1-8

1-8a. What is the most likely primary pathology? Lung cancer.

1-8b. Is this patient amenable to surgery? No, because there are contralateral mediastinal metastases.

1-8c. Is bronchoalveolar cancer typically FDG-avid? No.

CASE 1-9

1-9a. What type of scan is this? A bone scan. What is the abnormality? Diffuse uptake in an enlarged liver consistent with hepatic metastases. Hepatic necrosis could also be considered but is much less common.

1-9b. What tumor types would be suspected? Mucinous tumors of the colon, ovary, and breast.

1-9c. What are some other causes of soft tissue uptake on bone scans? Infarcts, malignant ascites and malignant pleural effusions, lymphoma, lung cancer, meningioma, osteogenic sarcoma, dystrophic calcification, uterine fibroids, amyloidosis, dermatomyositis, calcific tendonitis, renal failure, hyperparathyroidism, mastitis, hematomas, soft-tissue inflammation, diffuse or focal.

CASE 1-10

1-10a. Assuming the ventilation scan is normal and the chest radiograph shows hyperinflation, what is the probability of pulmonary embolism? Low probability for pulmonary embolism.

1-10b. Does this appearance have a specific name? This is a "fissure sign" (right major and minor fissures) seen with pleural fluid or pleural thickening (often seen in patients with COPD).

1-10c. What is the "stripe" sign and what is its significance (if any)? The stripe sign is different from the fissure sign. The stripe sign refers to a stripe of activity between a perfusion defect and the lung periphery. It is characteristic of COPD and indicates a very low probability of pulmonary embolism.

CASE 1-11

1-11a. What procedure is being performed? Surveying package used for transport of radioactive materials.

1-11b. What is the exposure rate from the package? Cannot tell because the selector knob is on "battery check." The dial, however, indicates that the battery is good.

1-11c. If the package is visibly damaged or leaking, what should you do? Secure it and call the radiation safety officer (RSO).

CASE 2-1

2-1a. What are the findings? Decreased activity in the frontal and frontotemporal regions on a ^{99m}Tc-HMPAO SPECT brain scan.

2-1b. What are the differential possibilities? These findings are characteristic of Pick disease but can also be seen in schizophrenia, depression, and supranuclear palsy. Atypical or early Alzheimer disease may uncommonly present in this manner.

2-1c. Does the distribution of activity represent regional metabolism or regional blood flow? HMPAO is a marker of regional blood flow, not metabolism.

CASE 2-2

2-2a. What is the diagnosis? Hepatoma. Gallium-67 is very sensitive for the detection of hepatocellular carcinoma. However, the test of choice if a hepatoma is suspected is a three-phase CT scan.

2-2b. What other liver lesions may accumulate gallium? Abscess, lymphoma, and metastasis, with sensitivity varying with the primary tumor type.

2-2c. What are appearances of hepatic adenoma and focal nodular hyperplasia on a ^{99m}Tc-sulfur-colloid liver scan? The adenoma will typically appear cold, whereas FNH may appear the same activity as the liver or even increased.

CASE 2-3

2-3a. What type of scan is this? Hepatobiliary. Why is it typically performed in this patient age group? Hepatobiliary scan is done to differentiate biliary atresia from neonatal hepatitis.

2-3b. What is the diagnosis? Neonatal hepatitis, as evidenced by small bowel activity. Premedication for 5 to 7 days with oral phenobarbital (2.5 mg/kg bid) may be used to improve hepatic excretion and test accuracy.

2-3c. In an effort to keep radiation doses low to children, what administered activity should be given to this 2-kg infant? 1.0 mCi (37 MBq). Nobody expects you to remember this, but you should know where to look it up. See Appendix D.

CASE 2-4

2-4a. What is the diagnosis? Hypertrophic pulmonary osteoarthropathy.

2-4b. Is there an incidental finding? Yes, right nephrectomy.

2-4c. What is another radiopharmaceutical that can be used for bone scans besides ^{99m}Tc MDP? PET/CT bone scans can be done with ^{18}F-sodium fluoride. It is very sensitive but has about a seven-fold higher cost and a sevenfold higher radiation dose than does MDP.

CASE 2-5

2-5a. What is the most likely diagnosis? ^{18}F-FDG-avid brain lymphoma seen as a homogeneously enhancing hypermetabolic mass.

2-5b. How would an area of central necrosis have changed your diagnosis? An area of necrosis would be common in a high grade astrocytoma.

2-5c. How useful is this test in a patient with suspected CNS metastases from lung cancer? This would be a poor choice because most metastases are less metabolic than normal brain tissue and may not be apparent on FDG PET imaging. An enhanced MRI is the best test.

CASE 2-6

2-6a. What is the diagnosis? Small inferior and lateral left ventricular infarct with a large area of peri-infarct ischemia.

2-6b. What vessels are involved? Circumflex and right coronary.

2-6c. Where is the left ventricular apex on a bull's eye (polar map) image? In the center.

CASE 2-7

2-7a. What is the diagnosis? Chronic obstructive pulmonary disease (COPD). There are multiple matched ventilation/perfusion abnormalities bilaterally with delayed clearance of xenon-133 from the lungs.

2-7b. What category is this according to PIOPED II criteria? Very low.

2-7c. A lot of central deposition on a ^{99m}Tc-DTPA aerosol scan is an indication of what entity? COPD.

CASE 2-8

2-8a. What is the diagnosis? Superscan with diffuse skeletal metastases.

2-8b. Under what circumstances would you treat a patient with strontium-89 chloride? Blastic metastases should be present, and the WBC and platelet counts should be above 2400/µL and 60,000/ µL, respectively. Optimally, renal function should be normal or the administered dose should be reduced to accommodate a renal dysfunction, depending on its severity.

2-8c. What radiation protection precautions are necessary after Sr-89 treatment? Because of beta (and no gamma) emission, few restrictions are necessary. Excretion is urinary and, to a lesser extent, fecal, which requires some instructions regarding frequency of urination to reduce bladder dose, sitting to urinate, and flushing the toilet twice afterward. Life expectancy should be at least 3 months because many states have restrictions on cremation, etc.

CASE 2-9

2-9a. What is the most likely diagnosis? Lymphoma based upon extensive adenopathy and multiple lung lesions. Metastatic melanoma and diffuse infection in an immunocompromised patient also would be possibilities.

2-9b. What is/are the main use(s) for FDG PET/CT in lymphoma? It is useful for staging, determining response to therapy, and detection of recurrence.

2-9c. Are MALT lymphomas typically FDG-avid? No.

CASE 2-10

2-10a. What is the diagnosis? Multinodular goiter.

2-10b. Is fine needle aspiration biopsy warranted? In general, no, because the cold areas commonly are a result of nonfunctioning or poorly functioning adenomas and are much less likely to be cancer than is a solitary cold nodule. A dominant nodule or MNG in a child deserves further characterization.

2-10c. With what radiopharmaceutical was this scan performed? Significant activity in the salivary glands indicates that it was performed with technetium-99m pertechnetate.

2-10d. In treating toxic MNG with I-131, is the administered activity generally more or less than when treating Graves disease? More.

CASE 2-11

2-11a. Is there a problem with delivery of this package containing radioactive material? Yes, it is not in a secured location, and the office almost certainly has no sign indicating "radioactive materials."

2-11b. What are the requirements concerning transport of a radioactive package? Material must be in an approved, usually Type A, container with a label indicating the transport index (TI) as well as the radiopharmaceutical and contained activity.

2-11c. What are the requirements concerning delivery? Packages must be secured, examined, monitored, and logged in. Examination of the package should be performed within 3 hours of receipt if it is received during normal working hours.

CASE 3-1

3-1a. What is the diagnosis? Bile leak with activity in the porta hepatis and right paracolic gutter.

3-1b. Is the gallbladder present? No. In this case, the patient has had a cholecystectomy. Leaking bile commonly pools in the porta hepatis, gallbladder fossa, or around the liver (the "reappearing liver" sign). Obtaining a history of prior surgery is critical.

3-1c. What special views can be helpful? Right lateral decubitus views and pelvic views can often be useful.

CASE 3-2

3-2a. What is the diagnosis? Brain death, as evidenced by no intracranial perfusion on the technetium-99m (^{99m}Tc) pertechnetate study. The actual diagnosis of brain death should not be made by nuclear imaging tests alone but requires consideration of clinical parameters.

3-2b. Can this study be done with ^{99m}Tc-hexamethylpropyleneamine oxime (HMPAO)? Yes.

3-2c. What would be the significance of activity in the sagittal sinus activity in a patient without obvious arterial phase activity? The significance is somewhat controversial, but most of the patients have a grave prognosis, and slight activity does not contradict the diagnosis of brain death.

CASE 3-3

3-3a. What is the diagnosis? Unobstructed patulous collecting system of the right kidney with prompt washout of activity from the collecting system after Lasix.

3-3b. If 370 MBq (10 mCi) of ^{99m}TcO$_4^-$ had been administered to the patient inadvertently instead of ^{99m}Tc-MAG3, would this constitute a reportable "medical event"? No. An administration of a wrong radiopharmaceutical is reportable only if it causes an effective whole body dose exceeding 0.05 Sv (5 rem) or 0.5 Sv (50 rem) to any organ. This does not occur with most diagnostic doses.

3-3c. What is the difference in mechanism of renal excretion between DTPA and MAG3? DTPA is predominantly filtered whereas MAG3 is excreted by proximal tubules with minimal filtration.

CASE 3-4

3-4a. What is the diagnosis? Stress fracture of third metatarsal.

3-4b. Can osteomyelitis or an acute fracture have this appearance? Yes. Both can be "hot" on all three phases.

3-4c. If this were an acute fracture, how long would increased activity be expected? For at least a few months and often up to a year.

CASE 3-5

3-5a. What is the diagnosis? Neuroblastoma with activity in the lower chest on both iodine-131 metaiodobenzylguanidine (^{131}I-MIBG) and technetium-99m methylene diphosphonate (^{99m}Tc-MDP) scans. A skull metastasis is also present.

3-5b. Could the tumor have been imaged with indium-111 pentetreotide? Yes.

3-5c. What other tumors could be imaged with indium-111 pentetreotide? Other neuroendocrine APUD tumors, including carcinoid, medullary thyroid cancer, pituitary adenomas, pancreatic islet cell tumors, paragangliomas, and small-cell lung cancer. Some non-APUD tumors can have variable uptake, including lymphoma, breast cancer, low grade gliomas, and meningiomas.

CASE 3-6

3-6a. What type of scan is this? ^{18}F-FDG, as evidenced by the brain activity, renal excretion, and whole-body images with arms over the head.

3-6b. What is the major finding? Increased marrow activity.

3-6c. What are possible reasons for this finding? This occurs as a result of prior treatment with chemotherapy or G-CSF and typically decreases rapidly in 2 to 4 weeks, but, in some patients, increased activity can persist for 18 to 36 months. Increased marrow activity can also be seen in patients with anemia.

CASE 3-7

3-7a. What is the diagnosis? Graves disease.

3-7b. Comparing technetium-pertechnetate with iodine-123 for scanning, how is the radiopharmaceutical administered and when should the patient be scanned? Intravenous administration and imaging at 15 to 30 minutes for technetium pertechnetate and oral administration and 3 to 24 hours imaging for iodine-123.

3-7c. If the 24-hour iodine uptake were 65% and the patient had known cardiac disease, would you treat this patient, and if so, how? The patient's circulating thyroid hormone levels and TSH should be checked. The patient can be treated usually with about 10 to 20 mCi (370 to 740 MBq); however, with such a medical history, it may be advisable to pretreat the patient with antithyroid medications.

CASE 3-8

3-8a. What is the diagnosis? Fixed LV inferior wall defect. This is proved to be a diaphragmatic attenuation artifact, as evidenced by the moving extracardiac cold defect (projecting over the inferior ventricular wall on some views) on the rotating raw data images.

3-8b. What type of artifact may be caused by left bundle branch block? A reversible septal defect mimicking ischemia.

3-8c. What produces the areas of focally increased activity on the short-axis images at about the 2 o'clock and 7 o'clock positions? Insertions of the papillary muscles.

CASE 3-9

3-9a. In what projection is a xenon-133 scan typically performed, and why? In the posterior projection because the energy of xenon-133 is relatively low, and there is less attenuation of the photons by the heart and overlying soft tissue. Further, more pulmonary segments are assessed on the posterior image.

3-9b. Where does the xenon go when the patient exhales? It should go into a xenon "trap," which has a canister filled with activated charcoal. This needs to be replaced periodically.

3-9c. What is the diagnosis? Left upper lobe focal air trapping with a smaller perfusion abnormality. In this case,

it was due to a mucous plug. Other obstructing lesions such as lung cancer should also be considered.

CASE 3-10

3-10a. What is the radiopharmaceutical used in this examination? ^{99m}Tc-labeled red blood cells.

3-10b. What is the diagnosis? Hepatic cavernous hemangioma in the dome of the right lobe.

3-10c. How would this entity appear on either a ^{99m}Tc-sulfur colloid or gallium-67 citrate scan? Hemangiomas would be "cold" and have no activity on either scan.

CASE 3-11

3-11a. When are dosimeters required? When there is a likelihood that an employee would be exposed to more than 10% of the occupational dose limit, dosimetry is required.

3-11b. What are the annual dose limits for the whole body and hands? 5 rem (50 mSv) effective dose for the whole body and 50 rem (0.5 Sv) equivalent dose for the hands.

3-11c. Do occupational dose limits include either background or personal medical exposure received by a technologist? No.

CASE 4-1

4-1a. What is the most likely diagnosis? ^{18}F-FDG PET/MRI scan demonstrating findings consistent with a low-grade temporal glioma.

4-1b. What findings would be expected on thallium-201 and technetium-99m HMPAO brain scans done to distinguish recurrent tumor from radiation necrosis? Both entities would show decreased HMPAO activity but with recurrent tumor, thallium activity is increased.

4-1c. What is the significance of increased ^{18}F-FDG activity in an area of a previously known low-grade glioma? This would suggest anaplastic transformation. FDG activity in primary brain tumors is generally inversely correlated with survival.

CASE 4-2

4-2a. What is the diagnosis? Dilated cardio-myopathy with global hypokinesia.

4-2b. What is the top normal left ventricle (LV) end-diastolic volume? The value used is somewhat variable and dependent on technique/software used, but generally more than 120 to 130 mL is considered abnormal.

4-2c. What does myocardial uptake of the PET imaging agents ^{13}N-ammonia (^{13}NH$_3$) and rubidium-82 (^{82}Rb) indicate? The presence of myocardial perfusion.

CASE 4-3

4-3a. What is the diagnosis? Cracked crystal.

4-3b. How was this image obtained? Either with a radioactive cobalt or technetium point source or a sheet source.

4-3c. How often is this type of image obtained? Uniformity scans are done daily.

CASE 4-4

4-4a. What is the diagnosis in this patient who was in an auto accident 5 years earlier? Splenosis.

4-4b. What radiopharmaceutical besides technetium-99m sulfur colloid can be used to make this diagnosis? ^{99m}Tc heat-damaged red blood cells.

4-4c. What other entities can cause non-visualization of the spleen on a ^{99m}Tc sulfur colloid scan? Congenital asplenia, sickle cell disease, and functional asplenia.

CASE 4-5

4-5a. What is the diagnosis? High probability for pulmonary embolism.

4-5b. What is the approximate number and size of ^{99m}Tc-MAA particles administered? About 400,000.

4-5c. If this patient has pulmonary hypertension, what is the likelihood that pulmonary emboli are the cause, and why is this information important? With pulmonary hypertension and a high probability scan, there is a 95% chance that the hypertension is due to PE and may be surgically treatable (which is not the case for other etiologies).

CASE 4-6

4-6a. What is the diagnosis? Polyostotic Paget disease.

4-6b. What are the pertinent associated findings on the pelvis radiograph? Expansion of the left iliac wing and ischial sclerosis.

4-6c. Do the lytic lesions associated with Paget disease show increased radionuclide uptake on a bone scan? Yes.

CASE 4-7

4-7a. What is the diagnosis? Acute tubular necrosis (ATN).

4-7b. Could dehydration produce the same pattern? Yes.

4-7c. Would chronic renal disease produce the same pattern? No. With chronic renal disease, there is slow clearance of activity from the soft tissues and slow uptake in the renal parenchyma.

CASE 4-8

4-8a. What type of scan is this? Iodine-131 MIBG. There are clearly focal skeletal abnormalities. The poor statistical quality and resolution suggests a high energy radionuclide. A sodium iodide-131 scan would not have liver and spleen activity.

4-8b. What is the diagnosis? Pheochromocytoma with osseous metastases.

4-8c. What other pathological entities show increased activity with this radiopharmaceutical? Carcinoid, neuroblastoma, medullary thyroid carcinoma, and paraganglioma.

CASE 4-9

4-9a. What is the likely diagnosis? Lymphoma.

4-9b. What is the significance of the splenic activity? The stage is at least III$_S$.

4-9c. What is the size threshold for detection of a lesion on FDG PET? About 6 mm.

CASE 4-10

4-10a. What is the most likely diagnosis? Most cold thyroid nodules are due to colloid cysts, but about 10% to 20% may be thyroid cancer.

4-10b. What is the differential diagnosis? A solitary cold nodule is a nonspecific finding. The common differential includes thyroid adenoma, colloid cyst, or thyroid cancer.

4-10c. What is the next step in management? If not a simple cyst on ultrasound, fine-needle aspiration.

CASE 4-11

4-11a. Can a pregnant technologist or physician be actively involved with nuclear medicine patients? Yes, as long as dose limits are not exceeded.

4-11b. Under the ALARA principle, what procedures would you consider restricting the technologist from performing? Generally, radiopharmacy duties and radioiodine therapies are likely to involve the most risk.

4-11c. What are the dose limits for the embryo/fetus? The fetus is subject to a dose limit of greater than 500 mrem (greater than 5 mSv) *after* pregnancy is declared. The employee is not required to declare the pregnancy.

CASE 5-1

5-1a. What is the likely diagnosis? Normal pressure hydrocephalus (NPH).

5-1b. What characteristics differentiate this from a normal study? Prominent ventricular entry with persistence and lack of "ascent" of activity over the cerebral convexities at 24 hours.

5-1c. Identify the anatomy on these images. In this case, the heart-shaped central activity is abnormal entry into the bodies and anterior horns of the lateral ventricles. The bilateral adjacent foci are the temporal horns of the ventricles. Activity immediately below this is in the basal cisterns. In normal patients, activity is seen on the anterior view as a trident with activity in the interhemispheric (central) and sylvian (bilateral) cisterns with no ventricular activity.

CASE 5-2

5-2a. What is the major finding? Hydronephrosis and markedly dilated bladder.

5-2b. What is the likely cause? Transitional cell carcinoma, as evidenced by the

irregular mass near the uterovesicular junction.

5-2c. What is the value of ^{18}F-FDG PET in this entity? FDG PET is of limited value because a large percentage of renal and bladder cancers do not accumulate FDG to an appreciable amount, and urinary excretion of ^{18}F-FDG hinders visualization. FDG PET/CT is more valuable for the detection of regional and distant metastases than in the evaluation of the primary tumor.

CASE 5-3

5-3a. What is the finding? Gastrointestinal hemorrhage at the hepatic flexure of the colon. (Activity in the heart, aorta, and iliac vessels identifies this as a ^{99m}Tc RBC scan.)

5-3b. What bleeding rate is necessary to reliably detect the bleeding with angiography and scintigraphy? 1.0 mL/minute with angiography and 0.2 mL/minute on scintigraphy.

5-3c. If the study had been negative, what would be the next step in management? Imaging can be continued or, if the patient appears to be bleeding again within 24 hours after ^{99m}Tc RBC administration, he or she can be returned for reimaging without reinjection to assess for intermittent bleeding.

CASE 5-4

5-4a. What is the diagnosis? Infected long-stem right hip prosthesis. The study is abnormal on all three phases of the bone scan, as evidenced by markedly increased activity along the entire shaft length.

5-4b. What other nuclear medicine techniques are more appropriate in this setting? ^{111}In-leukocyte scan combined with ^{99m}Tc-sulfur colloid marrow imaging is the procedure of choice for suspected prosthetic joint infections, especially in the case of an equivocal bone scan.

5-4c. What pattern is typically seen on MDP scans with hip prosthesis loosening? Increased activity primarily at the tip of the shaft and near the lesser trochanter. These are the sites with most stress and motion as a result of loosening.

CASE 5-5

5-5a. What type of examination is this? ^{99m}Tc-sestamibi parathyroid scan.

5-5b. What is the most likely diagnosis? Ectopic mediastinal parathyroid adenoma.

5-5c. What other entities might this represent? Many other primary tumors or metastases can have increased activity on sestamibi scans, including thyroid and breast cancer, thymoma, and even fibroadenomas.

CASE 5-6

5-6a. What is the diagnosis in this patient with a rising CEA? Colon cancer metastatic to the liver and para-aortic lymph nodes, as seen on an ^{18}F-FDG PET/CT scan.

5-6b. What is the best test for suspected liver metastases from colon cancer? Contrast-enhanced MRI is the most sensitive, especially for small metastases.

5-6c. What is the role of FDG PET/CT in staging colorectal cancer? Endoscopic ultrasound and endoscopy are best for assessing the primary tumor. PET/CT is valuable for assessing nodal and extranodal metastases, with PET being more sensitive than CT.

CASE 5-7

5-7a. What is the diagnosis? This patient had a cavitary squamous cell lung cancer with rib involvement, as seen on a ^{18}F-FDG PET/CT scan. A large lung abscess could appear in this manner.

5-7b. What is the hot spot in the right supraclavicular region? This was an attenuation correction artifact caused by the cardiac pacing device seen on the chest radiograph.

5-7c. Which set of images is not attenuation-corrected? The lower row of images is not attenuation corrected, the evidence being that the skin activity is prominent and the artifact, as a result of the pacemaker, is not seen.

CASE 5-8

5-8a. What is included in the differential diagnosis? In this case, markedly reduced trapping of the radiopharmaceutical is a result of subacute thyroiditis as seen on this ^{99m}Tc-pertechnetate scan (note the prominent salivary, blood pool, and background activity). This may also be seen in patients receiving thyroid hormone replacement, ectopic endogenous thyroid hormone production (such as "struma ovarii"), or primary or secondary hypothyroidism.

5-8b. Would this pattern likely be due to prior stable iodine ingestion? No. While that would reduce uptake on a radioiodine scan, it has very little effect on trapping of ^{99m}Tc-pertechnetate scan.

5-8c. What scan patterns might be seen with chronic forms of thyroiditis? The scintigraphic presentation of chronic thyroiditis is very variable and can have diffusely uniform increased activity (mimicking Graves disease), coarsely patchy distribution (mimicking a multinodular gland), generally decreased activity, or even appear normal. Thyromegaly is usually the presenting clinical finding.

CASE 5-9

5-9a. What is the diagnosis? LV anteroseptal myocardial ischemia.

5-9b. What would be the implications if the left ventricle dilated on the stress images? In the presence of CAD, transient ischemic dilatation (TID) correlates with high-risk disease (left main or multivessel involvement) and a worse prognosis.

5-9c. What is the mechanism of transient ischemic dilatation? Underlying mechanisms for transient ischemic dilatation include transient stress-induced diffuse subendocardial hypoperfusion, producing an apparent cavity dilatation, ischemic systolic dysfunction, and perhaps in some instances, physical cavity dilatation.

CASE 5-10

5-10a. Assuming a normal chest radiograph, what is the diagnosis? The normal ventilation with diffuse bilateral, multiple small perfusion defects is somewhat nonspecific. In this case, the diagnosis is diffuse vasculitis.

5-10b. What modified PIOPED II probability category would this represent? Very low.

5-10c. What is the differential diagnosis in this case? Fat or tumor emboli could have a similar appearance.

CASE 5-11

5-11a. What methods are used for disposal of radioactive syringes? Either return to the commercial radiopharmacy that supplied the material or decay in storage.

5-11b. Is the method shown here appropriate? No, there is no radioactive label visible on the container.

5-11c. How long is storage required? Can only be done for byproduct material with half-lives of less than 120 days. These materials should be stored for 10 half-lives, when the measured dose rate is indistinguishable from background. Radioactive labels are then removed before disposal with ordinary waste. Decay and disposal records must be maintained.

CASE 6-1

6-1a. What type of scan is this? Hepatobiliary scan, as evidenced by the sequential images, initial cardiac blood pool activity that gets cleared by the liver and with no visualization of the spleen.

6-1b. What is the diagnosis? "Liver scan" sign as a result of intrahepatic cholestasis (hepatitis) or acute/subacute common bile duct obstruction (usually a stone).

6-1c. Is this radiopharmaceutical conjugated by the liver? No, in contrast to bile, iminodiacetic acid agents are not conjugated before excretion.

CASE 6-2

6-2a. What is the diagnosis in this post-traumatic patient? Cerebrospinal fluid rhinorrhea as diagnosed by activity in the nasopharynx.

6-2b. How is the patient prepared for this procedure? Pledgets are placed in the ear or nose, wherever the leak is suspected.

6-2c. With normal images, can a "normal" diagnosis be made for this procedure? No. A CSF leak must be substantial to be visualized. Counting the pledgets in a well counter is necessary to exclude or diagnose a leak.

CASE 6-3

6-3a. What is the diagnosis? Infected axillary-femoral graft. Incidental note of right nephrectomy.

6-3b. What criteria should be used in making the diagnosis? ^{18}F-FDG scanning should not be used within the first 2 to 4 months of surgical placement in cases of suspected graft infection. Inhomogeneous, mild, or moderate uptake should be considered as nondiagnostic. FDG has good sensitivity (about 90%) but poor specificity (about 60%) for the diagnosis of graft infection.

6-3c. What is the value of ^{99m}Tc-WBC compared with FDG PET/CT in this setting? FDG PET/CT is a good initial test, although ^{99m}Tc-WBC should be used in questionable cases because it is more specific for infection.

CASE 6-4

6-4a. What is the diagnosis? Fibrous dysplasia, as seen on a radionuclide bone scan and rib radiograph.

6-4b. Are multiple enchondromas typically "hot" on a bone scan? Yes.

6-4c. What are physiologic factors that cause increased activity on bone scans? Increased osteoid formation, increased blood flow, increased mineralization of osteoid, and interrupted sympathetic nerve supply.

CASE 6-5

6-5a. What is the most likely diagnosis? Parathyroid adenoma, as seen on a ^{99m}Tc-sestamibi scan.

6-5b. Could this lesion be a thyroid adenoma? Very unlikely, because on the SPECT/CT it is separate from the thyroid gland.

6-5c. What method could be used to help locate the lesion at surgery, and how would the patient be prepared? Often a small gamma probe is used during surgery, but the patient needs to receive ^{99m}Tc-sestamibi 2 to 4 hours before surgery.

CASE 6-6

6-6a. What is the diagnosis? Aspergillosis, although lung cancer should be considered in the differential diagnosis on this ^{18}F-FDG PET/CT scan.

6-6b. Is metastatic disease present? There are multiple hypermetabolic ipsilateral hilar and mediastinal lymph nodes. In this case, these were a result of infected or reactive lymph nodes, not metastasis.

6-6c. What is the role of ^{18}FDG PET/CT in infection? FDG is very sensitive for the detection of both infection and inflammation; however, it is very nonspecific. Hyperplastic and neoplastic lymph nodes may also be hypermetabolic. ^{18}F-FDG is useful for the evaluation of FUO, sarcoidosis, and vascular graft infection. It is generally better than gallium-67 citrate in these settings.

CASE 6-7

6-7a. What is the diagnosis? Reversible ischemia of the septum, anterior wall, apex, and distal inferior wall with septal dyskinesia, as seen on a gated ^{99m}Tc-sestamibi scan using exercise stress.

6-7b. What parameters are used to determine if physical exercise stress was adequate in this patient? The determination of peak stress varies with the institution, but it is generally considered to be maximal when chest pain or significant ECG changes appear, when the patient's heart rate reaches 85% of the predicted maximum heart rate (frequently defined as 220 beats/minute minus the patient's age in years), or when the heart rate–blood pressure product (maximum heart rate achieved multiplied by the maximum systolic blood pressure) exceeds a value of 25,000. If none of these conditions is met, the stress is generally deemed submaximal.

6-7c. What degree of coronary artery stenosis is important? When the narrowing of a coronary artery diameter is less than 50% of the diameter of the vessel, the effect on blood flow generally is clinically insignificant. As diameter narrowing approaches 70%, the lesions become much more hemodynamically significant, particularly during exercise. To be significant at rest, 90% or greater narrowing is usually required.

CASE 6-8

6-8a. What is the diagnosis? Lytic sternal metastasis, as seen on a ^{99m}Tc bone scan.

6-8b. What cancer types often produce predominantly lytic bone metastases? Kidney, lung, thyroid.

6-8c. What tumor type most often causes single sternal metastases? Breast cancer.

CASE 6-9

6-9a. What is the most likely diagnosis? Toxic thyroid adenoma, as visualized on a ^{99m}Tc-pertechnetate thyroid scan.

6-9b. Could this lesion be malignant? Yes. Although rare (less than 1%), nodules that are hot on ^{99m}Tc-pertechnetate scans can be thyroid cancer. A thyroid cancer would not be hotter than the normal thyroid tissue on an iodine-123 scan.

6-9c. Does the remainder of the gland appear normal? No. The activity in the rest of the gland is decreased because of the autonomous nodule producing too much hormone and inhibiting pituitary production of circulating TSH.

CASE 6-10

6-10a. What is the diagnosis? Pneumonia.

6-10b. What is meant by the term "triple match"? The term *triple match* is often used to refer to matched ventilation/perfusion abnormalities accompanied by a corresponding chest radiographic abnormality of the same size, usually, but not always, an airspace opacity.

6-10c. What probability of PE is associated with a triple match? Matching ventilation/perfusion defects corresponding to chest radiographic opacities isolated to the upper and middle lung zones imply a very low (less than 10%) probability of pulmonary embolus, whereas similar findings in the lower lung zones represent an intermediate or moderate (20% to 80%) probability of pulmonary embolus.

CASE 6-11

6-11a. What specific paperwork is required to administer this radiopharmaceutical? A "written directive," which is essentially a special prescription required for diagnostic procedures exceeding 30 μCi (1.1 MBq) of sodium iodide-131 and all other radioisotopic therapy procedures.

6-11b. Who must supervise the administration? The medical directive and supervision must be performed by an authorized user (AU) who has had specific training and prior experience with such procedures.

6-11c. Under what conditions can a patient be released after therapeutic administration of I-131? Release of nuclear medicine patients is allowed under NRC regulations, based on a certain amount of administered activity or dose rate (e.g., 33 mCi [1.2 GBq] or less of iodine-131 or 7 mrem [70 μSv]/hr or less at 1 meter for iodine-131). Patients also can be released with much higher activities, based on patient-specific calculations and if the effective dose to family or caregiver is not likely to exceed 0.5 rem (5 mSv).

CASE 7-1

7-1a. What is the diagnosis? Right-to-left shunt on a ^{99m}Tc-MAA lung perfusion scan.

7-1b. If you suspected such a shunt was present, should you have done this procedure at all or modified the procedure? It is common practice to limit the number of particles in the presence of a right-to-left shunt from about 400,000 to about 100,000.

7-1c. What causes "hot spots" in the lung on a ^{99m}Tc-MAA perfusion scan and are they clinically significant? Withdrawal of blood into the syringe containing ^{99m}Tc-MAA before injection may result in labeling of small clots or clumping of the MAA. Once injected, they lodge in the pulmonary capillary bed, causing "hot spots" that are not clinically significant.

CASE 7-2

7-2a. Is this likely to represent chronic cholecystits? No, the linear activity that accumulates in the pericholecystic liver parenchyma of the right lobe is the "rim sign," indicative of acute cholecystitis.

7-2b. Is there a need to alert the clinician, and if so, why? Yes. About 40% of patients with the rim sign have a perforated or gangrenous gallbladder.

7-2c. Is there an advantage to slow infusion of CCK over more than 10 minutes in performing a gallbladder ejection fraction study? Yes, the patient is likely to have less abdominal discomfort than with rapid injection. Be aware that normal gallbladder ejection fraction values vary, depending on the infusion duration.

CASE 7-3

7-3a. What is the diagnosis? Hyperparathyroidism with ^{99m}Tc-MDP activity in the lungs, thyroid, kidneys, and stomach as a result of so-called *metastatic calcification*.

7-3b. What are the two common bone scan presentations of this entity? (1) Increased activity in the skull, extremities, and around the large joints; and (2) soft-tissue activity in the lungs, kidneys, and/or stomach.

7-3c. What are common clinical symptoms and findings associated with this entity? Nephrolithiasis, weakness, fatigue, and bone and joint pain (sometimes referred to as "stones, bones, and groans").

CASE 7-4

7-4a. What is the diagnosis? Inferior wall myocardial wall infarction with severe inferior wall hypokinesis.

7-4b. What is hibernating myocardium? Hibernating myocardium is the result of chronic hypoperfusion and ischemia. This leads to reduced cellular metabolism that is sufficient to sustain viability but inadequate to permit contractile function. Areas of hibernating myocardium usually present as segments of decreased perfusion and absent or diminished contractility.

7-4c. What is stunned myocardium? Stunning is the result of ischemic and reperfusion injury secondary to an acute coronary artery occlusion that has reopened before significant myocardial infarction can occur. Areas of stunned myocardium usually present with normal or near-normal perfusion but with absent or diminished contractility.

CASE 7-5

7-5a. What is the diagnosis? Chondroblastoma, as evidenced by a single trochanteric lesion in a relatively young person (no degenerative changes).

7-5b. What would a septic hip look like on a bone scan? There would be increased activity on both sides of the hip joint.

7-5c. What are other diagnostic considerations? Fibrous dysplasia, infection (tuberculosis), and much less likely giant cell tumor, bone cyst, osteosarcoma, eosinophilic granuloma, or aneurysmal bone cyst. The latter are unlikely a result of either the location of this lesion or its intense uptake.

CASE 7-6

7-6a. What is the diagnosis? Bilateral renal artery stenosis.

7-6b. What is the mechanism by which captopril works? In renal artery stenosis, the efferent blood vessels constrict to maintain filtration pressure in the glomeruli. After administration of an ACE inhibitor, the efferent renal blood vessels become dilated, reducing glomerular filtration pressure with the affected kidney(s) retaining activity in the tubules because of diminished washout of the tubular activity. Thus, when ^{99m}Tc-MAG3 is used, the affected kidney(s) presents as a persistent "nephrogram" after captopril is administered.

7-6c. Is known severe renal artery stenosis a relative contraindication to this procedure? Yes, the drop in intrarenal blood pressure from captopril can induce acute renal failure.

CASE 7-7

7-7a. What are the findings? Decreased metabolic activity in the left temporal lobe at the site of the seizure focus.

7-7b. What is the differential? This is a case of interictal (between seizures) temporal lobe epilepsy, but similar findings can be seen with a low-grade temporal tumor, stroke, or radiation necrosis.

7-7c. What pattern of metabolism is seen with imaging during a seizure (ictal imaging)? Increased activity at the site of seizure focus.

CASE 7-8

7-8a. What is the diagnosis? Lingual thyroid, as seen on a ^{99m}Tc-pertechnetate thyroid scan.

7-8b. What is the usual thyroid function status in these patients? About 70% of these patients are hypothyroid, and 10% have cretinism.

7-8c. What is the pathogenesis of this entity? Embryologically, thyroid tissue originates near the base of the tongue and migrates caudally. But when the migration is arrested, ectopic positioning results, commonly at the base of the tongue, producing a lingual thyroid gland.

CASE 7-9

7-9a. Is this a GI bleeding study? No. It is a Meckel diverticulum study using ^{99m}Tc-pertechnetate, as evidenced by the prompt gastric wall activity and minimal blood pool activity.

7-9b. Does a negative result mean that there is no Meckel diverticulum present? No. A Meckel diverticulum can still be present. However, it does mean that ectopic gastric mucosa is not likely to be present, which is generally the cause of bleeding.

7-9c. What premedication(s) can increase the sensitivity of this procedure? H_2 blockers (cimetidine) reduce the release of pertechnetate from gastric mucosa, pentagastrin can enhance mucosal uptake, and glucagon decreases bowel movement during imaging.

CASE 7-10

7-10a. What is the diagnosis? Multivessel coronary artery disease. Large anteroapical infarct with akinesis, small inferior wall infarct, reduced left ventricle (LV) ejection fraction, and dilated LV.

7-10b. What are the adverse reactions associated with dipyridamole pharmacologic stress and how are they treated? Dipyridamole may cause chest discomfort, headaches, dizziness, flushing, and nausea. These side effects may be rapidly reduced by the intravenous administration of aminophylline (100 to 200 mg). This antidote should be readily available during the procedure.

7-10c. What are the side effects and method of treatment for adverse reactions to adenosine stress? Side effects with adenosine are more common than those with dipyridamole and occur in 75% of patients. The three most common side effects are flushing, shortness of breath, and chest pain. These are usually transient and require no action or treatment. An uncommon, but more serious, side effect is atrioventricular block, which usually occurs in the first few minutes of infusion and is also transient. First-degree and second-degree block are more common. Because the biologic half-life of adenosine is extremely short (less than 10 seconds), its effects may be reversed by simply stopping infusion and beginning any specific treatments, if necessary.

CASE 7-11

7-11a. The beaker contained 370 MBq (10 mCi) of iodine-131. What category spill is this? This is classified as a major spill (greater than 1 mCi [37 MBq] of iodine-131). See Appendix I and Table I-1.

7-11b. What are the actions that need to be taken? For a major spill, the RSO must be notified and involved. Nonaffected persons should vacate the area, the spill should be covered (do not attempt to clean up), and the area secured. Contaminated persons should remove affected clothing and wash with soap and warm water.

7-11c. Are additional actions potentially needed due to the nature of this radiopharmaceutical? With radioiodine, the authorized user (AU) and RSO may consider giving potassium-iodide as a thyroid blocking agent and later doing either urine or thyroid counts to assess possible internal contamination for affected persons.

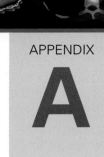

Characteristics of Radionuclides for Imaging and Therapy

NUCLIDE	SYMBOL	HALF-LIFE	DECAY MODE	MAJOR EMISSIONS (MeV)*
Carbon-11	$^{11}_{6}C$	20.3 min	β+	γ 0.511 (200%)
Cesium-137	$^{137}_{55}Cs$	30 yr	β–	γ 0.660 (85%)
Chromium-51	$^{51}_{24}Cr$	27.8 day	E.C.	γ 0.320 (10%)
Cobalt-57	$^{57}_{27}Co$	270 day	E.C.	γ 0.122 (86%) γ 0.136 (11%)
Cobalt-58	$^{58}_{27}Co$	71.3 day	E.C. and β+	γ 0.811 (99%) γ 0.511 (31%)
Cobalt-60	$^{60}_{27}Co$	5.26 yr	β–	γ 1.173 (100%) γ 1.332 (100%)
Fluorine-18	$^{18}_{9}F$	109 min	E.C. and β+	γ 0.511 (194%)
Gadolinium-153	$^{153}_{64}Gd$	240 day	E.C.	γ 0.100 (55%) γ 0.040 γ 0.048†
Gallium-67	$^{67}_{31}Ga$	78.1 hr	E.C.	γ 0.093 (38%) γ 0.184 (24%) γ 0.296 (16%) γ 0.388 (4%)
Gallium-68	$^{68}_{31}Ga$	68.3 min	E.C. and β+	γ 0.511 (178%) γ 1.077 (3%)
Indium-111	$^{111}_{49}In$	67 hr	E.C.	γ 0.172 (90%) γ 0.247 (94%)
Iodine-123	$^{123}_{53}I$	13 hr	E.C.	γ 0.159 (83%)
Iodine-125	$^{125}_{53}I$	60 day	E.C.	γ 0.027 (76%)
Iodine-131	$^{131}_{53}I$	8.06 day	β–	γ 0.284 (6%) γ 0.364 (82%) γ 0.637 (7%) β 0.192 (90%)
Krypton-81m	$^{81m}_{36}Kr$	13 sec	I.T.	γ 0.191 (66%)
Molybdenum-99	$^{99}_{42}Mo$	66.7 hr	β–	γ 0.181 (8%) γ 0.740 (14%) γ 0.778 (5%)
Nitrogen-13	$^{13}_{7}N$	10 min	β+	γ 0.511 (200%)

Continued

NUCLIDE	SYMBOL	HALF-LIFE	DECAY MODE	MAJOR EMISSIONS (MeV)*
Oxygen-15	$^{15}_{8}$O	124 sec	β+	γ 0.511 (200%)
Phosphorus-32	$^{32}_{15}$P	14.3 day	β–	β 0.695 (100%)
Rhenium-186	$^{186}_{75}$Re	90 hr	E.C.	γ 0.137 (9%) β 1.07 max. (93%)
Rubidium-82	$^{82}_{37}$Rb	1.3 min	E.C. and β+	γ 0.511 (189%) γ 0.777 (13%)
Samarium-153	$^{153}_{62}$Sm	46.3 hr		γ 0.103 (30%) β 0.640 (30%) β 0.710 (50%) β 0.810 (20%)
Strontium-87m	$^{87m}_{38}$Sr	2.8 hr	I.T. and E.C.	γ 0.388 (83%)
Strontium-89	$^{89}_{38}$Sr	50.5 day	β–	β 1.463 max. (100%)
Technetium-99m	$^{99m}_{43}$Tc	6.03 hr	I.T.	γ 0.140 (88%)
Thallium-201	$^{201}_{81}$Tl	73 hr	E.C.	γ 0.135 (2%) γ 0.167 (8%) (Hg daughter x-rays 0.069–0.081)
Xenon-127	$^{127}_{54}$Xe	36.4 day	E.C.	γ 0.145 (4%) γ 0.172 (25%) γ 0.203 (68%) γ 0.375 (18%)
Xenon-133	$^{133}_{54}$Xe	5.3 day	β–	γ 0.081 (36%)

Adapted from Dillman LT, Von der Lage FC. Radionuclide Decay Schemes and Nuclear Parameters for Use in Radiation Dose Estimation. New York: Society of Nuclear Medicine; 1975.

  β+, Positron (beta plus) decay; *β–*, beta decay; *E.C.*, electron capture; *I.T.*, isomeric transition.

  *Mean energy. Information in parentheses refers to the percentage of emissions of that type that occurs from disintegration. For example, carbon-11 gives off a gamma ray of 0.511 MeV 200% of the time; i.e., two gamma rays are emitted per disintegration.

  †From Europium 153.

Radioactivity Conversion Table for International System (SI) Units (Becquerels to Curies)

0.05 MBq = 1.4 μCi	90.0 MBq = 2.43 mCi	875.0 MBq = 23.7 mCi
0.1 MBq = 2.7 μCi	100.0 MBq = 2.70 mCi	900.0 MBq = 24.3 mCi
0.2 MBq = 5.4 μCi	125.0 MBq = 3.38 mCi	925.0 MBq = 25.0 mCi
0.3 MBq = 8.1 μCi	150.0 MBq = 4.05 mCi	950.0 MBq = 25.7 mCi
0.4 MBq = 10.8 μCi	175.0 MBq = 4.73 mCi	975.0 MBq = 26.4 mCi
0.5 MBq = 13.5 μCi	200.0 MBq = 5.41 mCi	1.0 GBq = 27.0 mCi
0.6 MBq = 16.2 μCi	225.0 MBq = 6.08 mCi	1.1 GBq = 29.7 mCi
0.7 MBq = 18.9 μCi	250.0 MBq = 6.76 mCi	1.2 GBq = 32.4 mCi
0.8 MBq = 21.6 μCi	275.0 MBq = 7.43 mCi	1.3 GBq = 35.1 mCi
0.9 MBq = 24.3 μCi	300.0 MBq = 8.11 mCi	1.4 GBq = 37.8 mCi
1.0 MBq = 27.0 μCi	325.0 MBq = 8.78 mCi	1.5 GBq = 40.5 mCi
2.0 MBq = 54.1 μCi	350.0 MBq = 9.46 mCi	1.6 GBq = 43.2 mCi
3.0 MBq = 81.1 μCi	375.0 MBq = 10.1 mCi	1.7 GBq = 46.0 mCi
4.0 MBq = 108 μCi	400.0 MBq = 10.8 mCi	1.8 GBq = 48.7 mCi
5.0 MBq = 135 μCi	425.0 MBq = 11.5 mCi	1.9 GBq = 51.3 mCi
6.0 MBq = 162 μCi	450.0 MBq = 12.2 mCi	2.0 GBq = 54.1 mCi
7.0 MBq = 189 μCi	475.0 MBq = 12.8 mCi	2.2 GBq = 59.5 mCi
8.0 MBq = 216 μCi	500.0 MBq = 13.5 mCi	2.4 GBq = 64.9 mCi
9.0 MBq = 243 μCi	525.0 MBq = 14.2 mCi	2.6 GBq = 70.3 mCi
10.0 MBq = 270 μCi	550.0 MBq = 14.9 mCi	2.8 GBq = 75.7 mCi
15.0 MBq = 405 μCi	575.0 MBq = 15.5 mCi	3.0 GBq = 81.1 mCi
20.0 MBq = 541 μCi	600.0 MBq = 16.2 mCi	3.2 GBq = 86.5 mCi
25.0 MBq = 676 μCi	625.0 MBq = 16.9 mCi	3.4 GBq = 91.9 mCi
30.0 MBq = 811 μCi	650.0 MBq = 17.6 mCi	3.6 GBq = 97.3 mCi
35.0 MBq = 946 μCi	675.0 MBq = 18.2 mCi	3.8 GBq = 103 mCi
40.0 MBq = 1.08 mCi	700.0 MBq = 18.9 mCi	4.0 GBq = 108 mCi
45.0 MBq = 1.22 mCi	725.0 MBq = 19.6 mCi	5.0 GBq = 135 mCi
50.0 MBq = 1.35 mCi	750.0 MBq = 20.3 mCi	6.0 GBq = 162 mCi
55.0 MBq = 1.49 mCi	775.0 MBq = 20.9 mCi	7.0 GBq = 189 mCi
60.0 MBq = 1.62 mCi	800.0 MBq = 21.6 mCi	8.0 GBq = 216 mCi
70.0 MBq = 1.89 mCi	825.0 MBq = 22.3 mCi	9.0 GBq = 243 mCi
80.0 MBq = 2.16 mCi	850.0 MBq = 23.0 mCi	10.0 GBq = 270 mCi

Note for conversion: MBq/37 = mCi

B-2

Radioactivity Conversion Table for International System (SI) Units (Curies to Becquerels)

1.0 µCi = 0.037 MBq	450.0 µCi = 16.7 MBq	17.0 mCi = 629 MBq
2.0 µCi = 0.074 MBq	500.0 µCi = 18.5 MBq	18.0 mCi = 666 MBq
3.0 µCi = 0.111 MBq	600.0 µCi = 22.2 MBq	19.0 mCi = 703 MBq
4.0 µCi = 0.148 MBq	700.0 µCi = 25.9 MBq	20.0 mCi = 740 MBq
5.0 µCi = 0.185 MBq	800.0 µCi = 29.6 MBq	21.0 mCi = 777 MBq
6.0 µCi = 0.222 MBq	900.0 µCi = 33.3 MBq	22.0 mCi = 814 MBq
7.0 µCi = 0.259 MBq	1.0 mCi = 37.0 MBq	23.0 mCi = 851 MBq
8.0 µCi = 0.296 MBq	1.5 mCi = 55.5 MBq	24.0 mCi = 888 MBq
9.0 µCi = 0.333 MBq	2.0 mCi = 74.0 MBq	25.0 mCi = 925 MBq
10.0 µCi = 0.370 MBq	2.5 mCi = 92.5 MBq	30.0 mCi = 1.11 GBq
15.0 µCi = 0.555 MBq	3.0 mCi = 111 MBq	35.0 mCi = 1.30 GBq
20.0 µCi = 0.740 MBq	3.5 mCi = 130 MBq	40.0 mCi = 1.48 GBq
25.0 µCi = 0.925 MBq	4.0 mCi = 148 MBq	45.0 mCi = 1.67 GBq
30.0 µCi = 1.11 MBq	4.5 mCi = 167 MBq	50.0 mCi = 1.85 GBq
35.0 µCi = 1.30 MBq	5.0 mCi = 185 MBq	60.0 mCi = 2.22 GBq
40.0 µCi = 1.48 MBq	5.5 mCi = 204 MBq	65.0 mCi = 2.41 GBq
45.0 µCi = 1.67 MBq	6.0 mCi = 222 MBq	70.0 mCi = 2.59 GBq
50.0 µCi = 1.85 MBq	6.5 mCi = 241 MBq	80.0 mCi = 2.96 GBq
60.0 µCi = 2.22 MBq	7.0 mCi = 259 MBq	90.0 mCi = 3.33 GBq
70.0 µCi = 2.59 MBq	7.5 mCi = 278 MBq	95.0 mCi = 3.52 GBq
80.0 µCi = 2.96 MBq	8.0 mCi = 296 MBq	100.0 mCi = 3.70 GBq
90.0 µCi = 3.33 MBq	8.5 mCi = 315 MBq	110.0 mCi = 4.07 GBq
100.0 µCi = 3.70 MBq	9.0 mCi = 333 MBq	120.0 mCi = 4.44 GBq
125.0 µCi = 4.63 MBq	9.5 mCi = 366 MBq	130.0 mCi = 4.81 GBq
150.0 µCi = 5.55 MBq	10.0 mCi = 370 MBq	140.0 mCi = 5.18 GBq
175.0 µCi = 6.48 MBq	11.0 mCi = 407 MBq	150.0 mCi = 5.55 GBq
200.0 µCi = 7.40 MBq	12.0 mCi = 444 MBq	175.0 mCi = 6.48 GBq
250.0 µCi = 9.25 MBq	13.0 mCi = 481 MBq	200.0 mCi = 7.40 GBq
300.0 µCi = 11.1 MBq	14.0 mCi = 518 MBq	250.0 mCi = 9.25 GBq
350.0 µCi = 13.0 MBq	15.0 mCi = 555 MBq	300.0 mCi = 11.1 GBq
400.0 µCi = 14.8 MBq	16.0 mCi = 592 MBq	400.0 mCi = 14.8 GBq

Note for conversion: mCi × 37 = MBq

C-1

Technetium-99m Decay and Generation Tables

The table that follows may be used to determine the amount of technetium-99m (^{99m}Tc) remaining in a sample after a given period of time using the following formula: original activity (mCi or Bq) at time T multiplied by the fraction remaining. Time is given in hours and minutes.

The table on the next page may be used to determine the yield of technetium-99m from a Mo-99/Tc-99m generator when eluted at a particular time interval after the previous elution.

^{99m}Tc Decay Chart

TIME	FRACTION REMAINING	TIME	FRACTION REMAINING
0:00	1.000	3:00	0.707
0:10	0.981	3:10	0.694
0:20	0.962	3:20	0.680
0:30	0.944	3:30	0.667
0:40	0.926	3:40	0.655
0:50	0.908	3:50	0.642
1:00	0.891	4:00	0.630
1:10	0.874	4:10	0.618
1:20	0.857	4:20	0.606
1:30	0.841	4:30	0.595
1:40	0.825	4:40	0.583
1:50	0.809	4:50	0.572
2:00	0.794	5:00	0.561
2:10	0.779	5:10	0.551
2:20	0.764	5:20	0.540
2:30	0.749	5:30	0.530
2:40	0.735	5:40	0.520
2:50	0.721	5:50	0.510

Molybdenum-99/99mTc Generator Yield

HOURS SINCE PREVIOUS ELUTION	99MTC YIELD (PERCENTAGE OF PREVIOUS ELUTION)
1	9
2	18
3	26
4	33
5	39
6	45
7	50
8	54
10	62
12	69
18	80
24	87

99mTc activity reaches maximum in 22.9 hr (transient equilibrium).

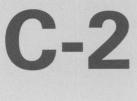

C-2 Other Radionuclide* Decay Tables

Flourine-18

TIME (HOURS)	FRACTION REMAINING
0.25	0.910
0.50	0.827
0.75	0.753
1.00	0.685
1.25	0.623
1.50	0.567
1.75	0.515
2.00	0.469
2.50	0.387
3.00	0.321
4.00	0.219
5.00	0.150
6.00	0.103
12.00	0.011

Gallium-67

TIME (HOURS)	FRACTION REMAINING
0	1.00
6	0.95
12	0.90
18	0.85
24	0.81
36	0.73
48	0.65
60	0.59
72	0.53
90	0.45
120	0.35
168	0.23

Indium-111

TIME (DAY)	FRACTION REMAINING
0	1.000
1	0.781
2	0.610
3	0.476
4	0.372
5	0.290

Iodine-123

TIME (HOURS)	FRACTION REMAINING
0	1.00
3	0.854
6	0.730
12	0.535
15	0.455
18	0.389
21	0.332
24	0.284
30	0.207

*A decay calculator for many radionuclides is available on the Web at http://ordose.ornl.gov/decay.cfm Accessed July 4, 2011.

Iodine-131

TIME (DAY)	DECAY FACTOR
0	1.000
1	0.918
2	0.841
3	0.771
4	0.707
5	0.648
6	0.595
7	0.545
8	0.500
9	0.458
10	0.421
11	0.386
12	0.354
13	0.324
14	0.297
15	0.273
16	0.250
17	0.229
18	0.210
19	0.193
20	0.177

Strontium-89

TIME (DAY)	DECAY FACTOR
0	1.00
6	0.92
8	0.90
10	0.87
12	0.85
14	0.83
16	0.80
18	0.78
20	0.76
22	0.74
24	0.72
26	0.70
28	0.68

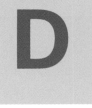

Injection Techniques and Pediatric Dosages

INJECTION TECHNIQUES

Each of the two commonly used rapid bolus injection techniques, when properly executed, provides a high-quality bolus of radiopharmaceutical, assuming patent venous pathways and adequate cardiac function.

Oldendorf Tourniquet Method

In the Oldendorf method, first the blood pressure is taken to determine diastolic and systolic pressures in the arm to be used for injection. The blood pressure cuff is then inflated to a level above diastolic pressure but less than systolic pressure. The pressure in the cuff is left at this level for 1 to 2 minutes to allow engorgement of the venous system in the lower arm, thereby building up a considerable back pressure that will constitute the forward momentum of the injected bolus. The cuff is then inflated above systolic pressure to prevent further entry of blood into the veins. At this point, a venipuncture of an antecubital vein (preferably a basilic vein) is performed, if not already done. Next, the radiopharmaceutical, in a volume of less than 1 mL, is injected, and the cuff is removed from the arm with a single swift motion. It is important to leave the needle in place until the dynamic images are complete so that no pressure on the venipuncture site is instituted.

Intravenous Push Method

The intravenous push technique is simpler than the Oldendorf method and is, in general, more commonly used. The technique requires a special tubing setup with an additional intravenous entry site for the introduction of the radiopharmaceutical. Antecubital venipuncture is performed in the usual way, preferably by using a large-bore needle. The end of the intravenous push tubing is connected to a syringe containing 25 to 30 mL of normal saline. Once the needle is in place, the radiopharmaceutical is injected into the distal tubing through the rubber entry portal, immediately followed by rapid injection of the saline, which propels the bolus to the right heart.

PEDIATRIC DOSAGES

Pediatric doses of radiopharmaceuticals ideally should be kept as low as possible. A balance must be achieved between the smaller doses needed in a small patient and the minimum dose needed to get a statistically valid examination in a reasonable time period. Simple reduction of an adult dose per unit weight necessitates an extremely long imaging time, and the image may be compromised by patient motion.

Surveys have indicated that doses administered to children and adolescents of the same age and size vary widely, often by a factor of 3 and sometimes more. Recently, North American consensus guidelines have been developed in an attempt to limit radiation exposure while maintaining diagnostic quality. The suggested administered activities for 11 radiopharmaceuticals are seen in Table D-1. Additional guidelines from the European Association of Nuclear Medicine with more radiopharmaceuticals are shown in Tables D-2 and D-3.

The European pediatric dosage system uses a baseline activity value (Table D-2), based on classes (A, B, and C) of radionuclide, multiplied by a factor (Table D-3), based on the patient's weight. If the resulting activity is less than the minimum recommended activity, the minimum activity is administered.

TABLE D-1	Recommended Pediatric Administered Activity for Various Examinations *North American Consensus Guidelines*				
EXAMINATION	**RADIOPHAR-MACEUTICAL**	**ACTIVITY BASED ON WEIGHT**	**MINIMUM ACTIVITY**	**MAXIMUM ACTIVITY**	**COMMENTS**
		MBq/kg (mCi/kg)	MBq (mCi)	MBq (mCi)	
Adrenal	^{123}I-MIBG	5.2 (0.14)	37 (1.0)	370 (10)	See Table D-2 for patients over 10 kg
Gastroesophageal liquid emptying	^{99m}Tc-sulfur colloid	NA	9.25 (0.25)	37 (1.0)	
Gastric emptying (solid)	^{99m}Tc-sulfur colloid	NA	9.25 (0.25)	18.5 (0.5)	
Meckel diverticulum scan	^{99m}TcO$_4^-$	1.85 (0.05)	9.25 (0.25)		
Bone scan	^{9m}Tc-MDP	9.3 (0.25)	37 (1.0)		See also Table D-2
Lung scan	^{99m}Tc-MAA (with Tc-DTPA V)	2.59 (0.07)			
	^{99m}Tc-MAA (without Tc-DTPA V)	1.11 (0.03)	14.8 (0.4)		
Renal scan	^{99m}Tc-MAG3 (without flow)	3.7 (0.1)	37 (1.0)	148 (4.0)	
	^{99m}Tc-MAG3 (with flow)	5.5 (0.15)	18.5 (0.5)		
	^{99m}Tc DMSA	1.85 (0.05)	18.5 (0.5)		
Cystography	^{99m}Tc	NA	NA	≤37 (1.0) for each bladder filling cycle	
Hepatobiliary scan	^{99m}Tc-IDA	1.85 (0.05)	18.5 (0.5)		May be considered for neonatal jaundice
Tumor (PET/CT)	^{18}F-FDG	3.7-5.2 (0.10-0.14)	37 (1.0)		The lower end should be considered in smaller patients
Brain (PET/CT)	^{18}F-FDG	3.7 (0.10)	37 (1.0)		
Bone (PET/CT)	^{18}F- Na-fluoride	2.22 (18.5)	18.5 (0.5)		

DMSA, dimercaptosuccinic acid; *DTPA,* diethylenetriamine pentaacetic acid; *FDG,* fluorodeoxyglucose; ^{123}*I,* iodine-123; *IDA,* iminodiacetic acid; *MAA,* macroaggregated albumin; *MAG3,* mertiatide; *MDP,* methylene diphosphonate; *NA,* not applicable; *PET/CT,* positron emission tomography/computed tomography; ^{99m}*Tc,* Technetium-99m; ^{99m}*TcO$_4^-$,* pertechnetate.

TABLE D-2	Class, Baseline Activity Multiplier, and Minimum Activity for Pediatric and Adolescent Examinations

RADIOPHARMACEUTICAL	CLASS	BASELINE ACTIVITY FOR CALCULATIONAL PURPOSES ONLY (MBq)*	MINIMUM RECOMMENDED ACTIVITY (MBq)
^{123}I (thyroid)	C	0.6	3
^{123}I-hippuran (abnormal renal function)	B	5.3	10
^{123}I-hippuran (normal renal function)	A	12.8	10
^{123}I MIBG	B	28.0	80
^{131}I MIBG	B	5.6	35
^{18}F-FDG (2D)	B	25.9	26
^{18}F-FDG (3D) recommended in children	B	14.0	14
^{18}F-fluorine (2D)	B	25.9	26
^{18}F-fluorine (3D) recommended in children	B	14.0	14
^{67}Ga-citrate	B	5.6	10
^{99m}Tc-colloid (gastric reflux)	B	2.8	10
^{99m}Tc-colloid (liver/spleen)	B	5.6	15
^{99m}Tc-colloid (marrow)	B	21.0	20
^{99m}Tc-DMSA (renal cortex)	A	17.0	15
^{99m}Tc-DTPA (abnormal renal function)	B	14.0	20
^{99m}Tc-DTPA (normal renal function)	A	34.0	20
^{99m}Tc-ECD (brain perfusion)	B	32.0	110
^{99m}Tc-HMPAO (brain)	B	51.8	100
^{99m}Tc-HMPAO (white blood cells)	B	35.0	40
^{99m}Tc-IDA (biliary)	B	10.5	20
^{99m}Tc-MAA (lung perfusion)	B	5.6	10
^{99m}Tc-MAG3 (renal function)	A	11.9	15
^{99m}Tc-MDP	B	35.0	40
^{99m}Tc-pertechnetate (cystography)	B	1.4	20
^{99m}Tc-pertechnetate (Meckel scan)	B	10.5	20
^{99m}Tc-Pertechnetate (cardiac first pass)	B	35.0	80
^{99m}Tc-pertechnetate (thyroid)	B	5.6	10
^{99m}Tc-RBC (blood pool)	B	56.0	80
^{99m}Tc-sestamibi or tetrofosmin (cardiac) Rest 2-day protocol	B	42.0-63.0	80
^{99m}Tc-sestamibi or tetrofosmin (cardiac) Stress 2-day protocol	B	42.0-63.0	80
^{99m}Tc-sestamibi or tetrofosmin (cardiac) Rest 1-day protocol	B	28.0	80
^{99m}Tc-sestamibi or tetrofosmin (cardiac) Stress 1-day protocol	B	84.0	80
^{99m}Tc-RBC denatured (spleen)	B	2.8	20

Tables D-2 and D-3 adapted from the European Association of Nuclear Medicine. Lassman M, Biassoni L, Monsieurs M, et al. The new EANM pediatric dosage card. Eur J Nucl Med Mol Imaging 2007; 34(5):796-98 and Lassman M, Biassoni L, Monsieurs M, et al. The new EANM pediatric dosage card: additional notes with respect to F-18. Eur J Nucl Med Mol Imaging 2008; 35(11):2141.

2D, 2-dimensional acquisition; *3D*, 3-dimensional acquisition; *DMSA*, dimercaptosuccinic acid; *DTPA*, diethylenetriamine pentaacetic acid; *ECD*, bicisate; *FDG*, fluorodeoxyglucose; *HMPAO*, exametazine; *IDA*, iminodiacetic acid; *MAA*, macroaggregated albumin; *MAG3*, mercaptoacetyltriglycine; *MDP*, methylene diphosphonate; *MIBG*, metaiodobenzylguanidine; *RBC*, red blood cell.

*Note for conversion: MBq/37 = mCi.

| TABLE D-3 | Multiple of Baseline Activity | | | | | | |

WEIGHT (KG)	CLASS A	CLASS B	CLASS C	WEIGHT (KG)	CLASS A	CLASS B	CLASS C
3	1	1	1	32	3.77	7.29	14.00
4	1.12	1.14	1.33	34	3.88	7.72	15.00
6	1.47	1.71	2.00	36	4.00	8.00	16.00
8	1.71	2.14	3.00	38	4.18	8.43	17.00
10	1.94	2.71	3.67	40	4.29	8.86	18.00
12	2.18	3.14	4.67	42	4.41	9.14	19.00
14	2.35	3.57	5.67	44	4.53	9.57	20.00
16	2.53	4.00	6.33	46	4.65	10.00	21.00
18	2.71	4.43	7.33	48	4.77	10.29	22.00
20	2.88	4.86	8.33	50	4.88	10.71	23.00
22	3.06	5.29	9.33	52-54	5.00	11.29	24.67
24	3.18	5.71	10.00	56-58	5.24	12.00	26.67
26	3.35	6.14	11.00	60-62	5.47	12.71	28.67
28	3.47	6.43	12.00	64-66	5.65	13.43	31.00
30	3.65	6.86	13.00	68	5.77	14.00	32.33

An example of the use of Tables D-2 and D-3 is as follows: We wish to perform a ^{99m}Tc-DMSA scan on a 16-kg child and want to know how much activity to inject. Table D-2 indicates the Class is A, the baseline activity for calculation is 17.0 MBq, and the minimum activity should be at least 15 MBq. Table D-3 indicates the multiplication factor to use for a 16-kg child and a Class A radiopharmaceutical is 2.53. Multiplying 17.0 MBq by 2.53 = 43 MBq (1.16 mCi).

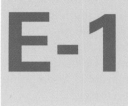

This appendix is provided as a guide to the technical aspects of various imaging procedures. Some of the less common procedures have not been included, and the procedures described herein may need to be adjusted, depending on the equipment available. The protocols for PET examinations are at the end of this appendix. Each nuclear medicine laboratory should have a standardized procedures manual; this appendix may be used as a beginning point for the development of such a manual. The reader is also referred to manufacturers' recommendations and the procedure guidelines in the practice management section of the Society of Nuclear Medicine website (http://www.snm.org). Suggested administered activities for pediatric and adolescent examinations are given in Appendix D.

BRAIN DEATH OR CEREBRAL BLOOD FLOW SCAN

Procedure imaging time
    20 to 30 minutes
Radiopharmaceutical
    Technetium-99m (^{99m}Tc), diethylenetriamine pentaacetic acid (DTPA), or glucoheptonate. Brain-specific agents such as ^{99m}Tc hexamethylpropyleneamine oxime (HMPAO), single-photon emission computed tomography (SPECT) scan, and ^{99m}Tc ethyl cysteinate dimer (ECD), also called Tc-Bicisate, can be used, but there is no clear evidence that they are more accurate. They do obviate the need for a very good bolus injection.
Method of administration
    Bolus IV injection
Normal adult administered activity
    15 to 30 mCi (555 MBq to 1.11 GBq)
Injection-to-imaging time
    Immediate
Conflicting examinations and medications
    None

Patient preparation
    None necessary, although some institutions put a rubber band or tourniquet around the head just above ears to help diminish scalp blood flow. This should not be done in patients with a history of head trauma. Patient should be normally ventilated.
Technique
    Collimator
        High-resolution or ultra-high-resolution; field of view (FOV) should include from the level of the common carotids to the skull vertex.
    Dynamic flow imaging time
        Blood flow images: 1 to 3 seconds/frame for at least 60 seconds. Flow images should start before the arrival of the bolus in the neck.
    Routine views
        Immediate blood pool anterior and anterior image at 5 minutes each. Many institutions also obtain posterior and both lateral views. Note: If brain-specific images are obtained, initial images as described previously are obtained as well as planar and SPECT images obtained after 20 minutes.
    Patient positioning
        Sitting or supine
    Photopeak selection
        140-keV (15% to 20% window)
Dosimetry: rads/mCi (mGy/MBq) of administered activity
    DTPA
        Effective dose   0.02 (0.005)
        Bladder wall   0.19 (0.05)
    HMPAO (also called *Ceretec* or *exametazime*)
        Effective dose   0.034 (0.009)
        Kidneys   0.126 (0.034)
    ECD (Bicisate or Neurolite)
        Effective dose   0.030 (0.008)
        Kidneys   0.033 (0.009)
        Bladder wall   0.185 (0.05)

SPECT BRAIN IMAGING

Procedure imaging time
　30 to 60 minutes
Instrumentation
　SPECT camera
Radiopharmaceutical
　^{99m}Tc-HMPAO (Exametazime unstabilized or stabilized), ^{99m}Tc-ECD
　For unstabilized ^{99m}Tc-HMPAO, inject no sooner than 10 minutes after preparation and not more than 30 minutes after preparation. For seizure disorders, inject within 1 minute after reconstitution. For stabilized ^{99m}Tc-HMPAO, inject no sooner than 10 minutes after preparation and no more than 4 hours after preparation. For ^{99m}Tc-ECD, inject no sooner than 10 minutes after preparation and no more than 4 hours after preparation.
Method of administration
　Place patient in a quiet, dimly lit room and instruct him or her to keep eyes and ears open. The patient should be seated or reclining comfortably. IV access should be placed at least 10 minutes before injection. The patient should not speak or read, and there should be little or no interaction before, during, or up to 5 minutes after injection.
Normal administered activity
　15 to 30 mCi (555 MBq to 1.11 GBq), children 0.2 to 0.3 mCi/kg (7.4 to 11.1 MBq/kg). Minimum dose, 3 to 5 mCi (111 to 185 MBq).
Injection-to-imaging time
　90 minutes or later for stabilized or unstabilized ^{99m}Tc-HMPAO, although images obtained after 40 minutes will be interpretable; 45-minute delay for ^{99m}Tc-ECD, although images obtained after 20 minutes will be interpretable. If possible, all imaging should be obtained within 4 hours of injection.
Conflicting examinations and medications
　None
Patient preparation
　Patient should be instructed, if possible, to avoid caffeine, alcohol, or other drugs known to affect cerebral blood flow. If sedation is required, it should be given after the injection. Patient should void before study for maximum comfort.
Technique
　Collimator
　　Low-energy, high-resolution or ultrahigh-resolution, or fan beam; all-purpose

Acquisition
　128 × 128 or greater acquisition matrix; 3-degree or better angular sampling. Acquisition pixel size should be one third to one half of the expected resolution. Low-pass Butterworth filters should be used for processing in all three dimensions. Attenuation correction should be performed.
Routine views
　360-degree arc of rotation single head camera; however, multiple head detectors may produce better images.
Patient positioning
　Supine
Photopeak selection
　140-keV ^{99m}Tc (20% window)
Dosimetry: rads/mCi (mGy/MBq) administered
　HMPAO (also called *Ceretec* or *exametazime*)

	rads/mCi	(mGy/MBq)
Effective dose	0.034	(0.009)
Kidneys	0.126	(0.034)

　ECD (Bicisate or Neurolite)

	rads/mCi	(mGy/MBq)
Effective dose	0.030	(0.008)
Kidneys	0.033	(0.009)
Bladder wall	0.185	(0.05)

Comments
　Vasodilatory challenge with acetazolamide (Diamox) may be ordered for evaluation of cerebrovascular reserve in transient ischemic attack, completed stroke, or vascular anomalies. Known sulfa allergy is a contraindication, and the procedure is usually avoided within 3 days of an acute stroke. The challenge study is usually done first, and, if normal, the baseline study may be omitted. The dosage is 1000 mg in 10 mL sterile water by slow IV push (over 2 minutes) and 14 mg/kg for children. Wait 10 to 20 minutes before injecting tracer. The patient should void immediately before acquisition.

CISTERNOGRAM

Procedure imaging time
　30 minutes for each set
Instrumentation
　Planar gamma camera
Radiopharmaceutical
　Indium-111 (^{111}In)-DTPA
Method of administration
　Spinal subarachnoid space injection
Normal adult administered activity
　0.5 mCi (18.5 MBq)

Injection-to-imaging time
2 hours, 6 hours, 24 hours, 48 hours, and 72 hours (as needed)

Conflicting examination and medications
Acetazolamide (Diamox) can cause false-positive results

Patient preparation
If the clinical diagnosis is cerebrospinal fluid (CSF) rhinorrhea or otorrhea, the patient's nose and ears should be packed with pledgets before injection for later counting.

Technique
Collimator
Low-energy, all-purpose, parallel-hole
Counts
1. 50- to 100-k counts for ^{111}In
2. Cobalt (^{57}Co) for 50-k counts transmission scan (if useful for anatomic definition)

Routine views
1. Anterior transmission scan: position patient's head between ^{57}Co sheet source and collimator surface. Peak in ^{57}Co by after photopeak determination. Set intensity, but collect only 50-k counts. Do not advance film or image. Remove sheet source from behind patient. Peak detector for ^{111}In. Collect 100-k counts.
2. Lateral transmission scan
3. Anterior head
4. Lateral head (same lateral as transmission scan)

Patient positioning
Supine. If a large CSF leak is suspected in a specific area, the patient may be positioned with that portion dependent.

Photopeak selection
^{57}Co (for transmission images); ^{111}In-DTPA 173-keV (20% window)

Dosimetry: rads/mCi (mGy/MBq) of administered activity

Effective dose	0.6 (0.162)
Spinal cord	12.0 to 20.0 (3.2 to 5.4)

Comments
For CSF rhinorrhea or otorrhea, count all pledget samples in well counter after removal from nose and ears. Note: Remove the pledgets and place each in a separate counting vial at time of removal, labeling each vial with its location.

THYROID SCAN (⁹⁹ᵐTᴄ-PERTECHNETATE)

Procedure imaging time
15 minutes

Radiopharmaceutical
^{99m}Tc-sodium pertechnetate

Method of administration
IV injection

Normal administered activity
2 to 10 mCi (75 to 370 MBq). For 5-year-old child, 15 to 70 µCi/kg (1 to 5 MBq/kg)

Injection-to-imaging time
15 to 30 minutes

Conflicting examinations and medications
None

Patient preparation
None

Technique
Collimator
Low-energy parallel and pinhole
Counts
100- to 250-k counts per image or 5 minutes

Patient positioning
1. Supine
2. Extend neck forward by placing a positioning sponge under back of neck

Routine views
1. Anterior view of the thyroid to include salivary glands, using parallel collimator
2. Pinhole views of thyroid only, in anterior and both anterior oblique positions (positioned so that the thyroid gland fills two thirds of the FOV)

Photopeak selection
140-keV (20% window)

Dosimetry: rads/mCi (mGy/MBq) of administered activity

Effective dose	0.05 (0.01)
Gonads	0.01 to 0.04 (0.003 to 0.011)
Thyroid	0.12 to 0.20 (0.04 to 0.06)
Stomach and colon	0.10 to 0.30 (0.03 to 0.08)

Comments
Remind the patient not to swallow while the camera is imaging. Drinking water is sometimes useful to eliminate confusing esophageal activity.

THYROID SCAN AND UPTAKE (IODINE-123)

Procedure imaging time
1 hour

Radiopharmaceutical
Iodine-123 (^{123}I) sodium iodide

Method of administration
Oral

Normal administered activity
  200 to 600 μCi (7.4 to 25 MBq). For 5-year-old child, 3 to 10 μCi/kg (0.1 to 0.3 MBq/kg)
Administration-to-imaging time
  3 to 24 hours
Conflicting examinations and medications
  1. Radiographic procedures using IV iodine contrast media (e.g., IV pyelogram, computed tomography [CT] scan with contrast)
  2. Other radiographic procedures using iodine contrast media (e.g., myelogram, oral cholecystogram)
  3. Exogenous T_3 or T_4 (liothyronine, levo-thyroxine)
  4. Thyroid-blocking agents such as propyl-thiouracil, perchlorate, and methimazole
  5. Oral iodides in medications containing iodine (e.g., kelp preparations, vitamins, Lugol's solution)
  6. If necessary, do a pertechnetate ($^{99m}TcO_4^-$) scan.
Patient preparation
  Scanning dose to be administered 3 to 24 hours before scanning. Patient should be NPO overnight before examination. If patient is pregnant or lactating, consider using $^{99m}TcO_4^-$
Technique
  Collimator
    Pinhole
  Counts
    50- to 100-k counts per image or 10 minutes/image
  Routine views
    Anterior, right, and left anterior oblique
  Patient positioning
    Supine, neck extended
  Photopeak selection
    159-keV (20% window)
Dosimetry: rads/mCi (mGy/MBq) of administered activity
  Effective dose 0.81 (0.22)
                  0.40 (0.11) uptake 0%
  Gonads   0.01 to 0.03 (0.003 to 0.008)
  Thyroid   16.6 (4.5) assuming 35% uptake
  Stomach   0.22 (0.06)
Comments
  1. Iodine uptake is normally measured at 24 hours, although rarely it is also measured at 6 hours. It is measured with a sodium iodide probe.
  2. Patient's thyroid should be palpated by the physician.

THYROID CANCER SCAN

Procedure imaging time
  1 to 2 hours
Radiopharmaceutical
  ^{131}I-sodium iodide or ^{123}I-sodium iodide
Method of administration
  Oral
Normal adult administered activity
  1 to 5 mCi (37 to 185 MBq) ^{131}I-sodium iodide
  1 to 2 mCi (37 to 74 MBq) ^{123}I-sodium iodide
  10 to 20 mCi (370 to 740 MBq) ^{99m}Tc-sestamibi
Injection-to-imaging time
  72 hours (96 hours, if needed) ^{131}I sodium iodide
  24 hours for ^{123}I sodium iodide
  15 minutes for ^{99m}Tc-sestamibi
Conflicting examinations and medications
  Iodine-containing medications and contrast agents
Patient preparation
  For radioiodine 2 weeks off T_3 replacement or 4 to 6 weeks off T_4 replacement. In some patients, the use of rTSH (thyrogen) may be useful to supplement thyroid hormone withdrawal. Some institutions use a low iodine diet 3 to 10 days before administration of tracer.
Technique
  Whole-body scan or spot views of head, neck, chest, and other clinically suspect areas
  Collimator
    Medium- or high-energy-^{131}I-sodium iodide or low-energy for ^{123}I-sodium iodide or ^{99m}Tc
  Counts
    200-k counts or 10-minute spot views
  Routine views
    Anterior and posterior whole-body views
  Patient positioning
    Supine
  Photopeak selection
    364-keV (20% window) for ^{131}I-sodium iodide or 159-keV (20% window) ^{123}I-sodium iodide
    Absorbed dose with thyroid removed or ablated.
Dosimetry: rads/mCi (mGy/MBq) of administered activity
  ^{123}I   Effective dose 0.50 (0.135)
                    Bladder wall   0.33 (0.09)
  ^{131}I   Whole body 0.27 (0.073)
                    Bladder wall   2.3 (0.62)
  ^{99m}Tc sestamibi (Cardiolite)
    Effective dose 0.03 (0.008)
    Gallbladder   0.14 (0.038)

Comments

1. This scan for metastatic disease is done only after ablation of normal thyroid tissue.
2. Serum thyroid-stimulating hormone (TSH) levels should be above 40 mU/mL before start.
3. Scanning can also be done 7 to 10 days after a cancer therapy treatment with [131]I.
4. Scanning with ^{123}I may prevent stunning of thyroid remnant or metastases.
5. Occasionally, scans are done by using ^{18}F-FDG, ^{99m}Tc-sestamibi or thallium-201 (^{201}Tl) chloride to locate nonfunctioning metastases.

PARATHYROID SCAN

Procedure imaging time
  2 hours
Radiopharmaceutical
  ^{99m}Tc-sestamibi
Method of administration
  IV administration
Normal adult administered activity
  20 mCi (740 MBq)
Injection-to-imaging time
  5 minutes
Conflicting examinations and medications
  None
Patient preparation
  None
Technique
  Collimator
    Low-energy, high-resolution, or pinhole
  Counts/time
    Acquire image for 10 minutes, and if digital acquisition use a 128 × 128 or larger matrix.
  Routine views
    Anterior images of the neck at 5, 20, and 120 minutes after injection. A single anterior large-FOV image should also be obtained that includes the mediastinum.
  Patient positioning
    Supine
  Photopeak selection
    140-keV (20% window)
Dosimetry: rads/mCi (mGy/MBq) of administered activity
  Effective dose   0.03 (0.008)
  Gallbladder   0.14 (0.04)

REST GATED EQUILIBRIUM VENTRICULOGRAPHY*

Procedure imaging time
  30 minutes

Radiopharmaceutical
  ^{99m}Tc-labeled red blood cells (RBCs). See RBC labeling procedures at the end of this appendix. We prefer the modified in vivo method for this examination.
Method of administration
  IV injection
Normal adult administered activity
  15 to 30 mCi (555 MBq to 1110 MBq)
Injection-to-imaging time
  Immediate
Conflicting examinations and medications
  None
Patient preparation
  Fasting for 3 to 4 hours before the study is preferred
Technique
  Collimator
    Low-energy, all-purpose, or high-resolution parallel-hole
  Counts
    3 to 7 million counts with a minimum of 16 and preferably 32 to 64 frames per second
  Patient positioning
  Supine or upright
  Photopeak selection
    140-keV (20% window)
Dosimetry: rads/mCi (mGy/MBq) of administered activity
  Effective dose   0.026 (0.007)
  Heart   0.085 (0.023)
Comments
  In vivo RBC labeling.
    1. Take a vial of cold pyrophosphate and dilute with 1 to 3 mL of *sterile* saline (not bacteriostatic). Shake the mixture, and let it stand for 5 minutes. Without injecting air into the vial, withdraw the contents into a 3-mL syringe, avoiding inclusion of an air bubble.
    2. Inject patient with cold pyrophosphate (0.8 to 1 mg stannous chloride).
    3. After 20 minutes, inject the radiopharmaceutical.
    4. Connect electrocardiogram leads to patient 5 to 10 cm below the axilla bilaterally. Remember to abrade the skin well enough so that the leads have good contact.
    5. Place the patient in the supine position on an imaging table with left side toward the camera.

*Stress study and computer operation vary widely and are not presented here.

SPECT MYOCARDIAL PERFUSION IMAGING

Procedure imaging time
  30 minutes for each set of images
Instrumentation
  SPECT camera
Radiopharmaceutical
  ^{99m}Tc-sestamibi, ^{201}Tl-chloride,
  ^{99m}Tc-teboroxime, or ^{99m}Tc-tetrofosmin
Method of administration
  IV injection
Normal adult administered activity (same day stress-rest)

^{99m}Tc-sestamibi	20 to 30 mCi (750 to 1100 MBq)
^{201}Tl-chloride	3 to 5 mCi (111 to 185 MBq)
^{99m}Tc-teboroxime	30 to 50 mCi (1110 to 1850 MBq)
^{99m}Tc-tetrofosmin	20 to 40 mCi (750 to 1500 MBq)

Injection-to-imaging time
  For post-stress images, immediate for thallium, 30 to 90 minutes for sestamibi.
Conflicting examinations and medications
  Discontinue calcium antagonists, β-blockers, and nitrates, if possible.
  With thallium, increased myocardial uptake has been reported with dipyridamole, furosemide, isoproterenol sodium bicarbonate (IV), and dexamethasone; decreased myocardial uptake with propranolol, digitalis, doxorubicin, phenytoin (Dilantin), lidocaine, and minoxidil.
Patient preparation
  NPO for 4 hours; exercise, if required. In patients with severe coronary disease, it may be advisable to administer nitroglycerin sublingually about 3 minutes before rest injection of the radiopharmaceutical.
Technique
  Collimator
    Low-energy, all-purpose
  Counts and time
    30 to 32 stops for 40 seconds each for ^{201}Tl and 10 seconds for ^{99m}Tc sestamibi
  Routine views
    180- or 360-degree arc of rotation; 180 degrees is preferred from right anterior oblique to left posterior oblique. Either step and shoot acquisition with 32 or 64 stops separated by 3 to 6 degrees or continuous acquisition may be used. The duration for each stop varies but is generally 40 seconds per image for thallium and 25 seconds for technetium radiopharmaceuticals.
Patient positioning
  Supine, left arm overhead
Photopeak technetium
  85-keV (15% window) and possibly 135- to 160-keV for thallium and 140-keV (20% window) for technetium
Dosimetry: rads/mCi (mGy/MBq) of administered activity

^{201}Tl-chloride	
Effective dose	0.52 (0.14)
Kidneys	1.8 (0.48)
Thyroid	0.80 (0.22)
^{99m}Tc-sestamibi	
Effective dose	0.03 (0.008)
Gallbladder	0.14 (0.038)
^{99m}Tc-teboroxime	
Effective dose	0.041 (0.011)
Colon	0.13 (0.035)
^{99m}Tc-tetrofosmin (Myoview)	
Effective dose	0.025 (0.007)
Gallbladder	0.10 (0.027)

Comments
1. Process for short- and long-axis views.
2. Parametric images such as "bull's eye" maps can be used to map perfusion and motion and to quantitate washout.
3. Use 64 × 64 matrix, Butterworth filter, 0.4 cutoff.
4. Attenuation correction significantly reduces artifacts.

EXERCISE PROTOCOL USING A BRUCE MULTISTAGE OR MODIFIED BRUCE TREADMILL EXERCISE PROTOCOL

Patient preparation
  Initial imaging
  Within 10 to 15 minutes after injection, perform SPECT imaging. Time should be long enough to permit clearance of liver activity when using ^{99m}Tc-sestamibi or ^{99m}Tc-tetrofosmin. This is usually 15 to 30 minutes after a stress injection.
  After-exercise instructions
    Only light food intake; minimal physical exertion
  Redistribution imaging
    3 to 4 hours after injection
Contraindications
  Unstable angina with recent (less than 48 hours) angina or congestive heart failure,

documented acute myocardial infarction within 2 to 4 days of testing, uncontrolled systemic (systolic greater than 220 mm Hg, diastolic greater than 120 mm Hg) or pulmonary hypertension, untreated life-threatening arrhythmias, uncompensated congestive failure, advanced atrioventricular block (without a pacemaker), acute myocarditis, acute pericarditis, severe mitral or aortic stenosis, severe obstructive cardiomyopathy, and acute systemic illness. Relative contraindications to exercise stress include conditions that may interfere with exercise such as neuralgic, arthritic, or orthopedic conditions or severe pulmonary or peripheral vascular disease.

DIPYRIDAMOLE PHARMACOLOGIC STRESS PROCEDURE*

Patient preparation
  NPO 4 to 6 hours; withhold caffeine-containing beverages for at least 12 hours and preferably 24 hours.
Drug administered
  IV infusion of dipyridamole in antecubital vein with patient supine; rate, 0.5 mg/kg over 4 minutes in 20 to 40 mL of normal saline.
Radiopharmaceutical administered
  IV administration of any of the radiopharmaceutical listed above 3 minutes after dipyridamole infusion, with patient supine or upright.
Imaging
  Begin 3 to 4 minutes after thallium injection; SPECT imaging; repeat in 3 to 4 hours. For technetium radiopharmaceuticals, postinjection imaging time is not as critical and may be done at 30 to 60 minutes.
Comments
  Side effects may be reversed by IV administration of 100 to 200 mg of aminophylline over 1 minute. No caffeine or theophylline for 12 hours before procedure.
  *Possibly reinject before delayed imaging.

ADENOSINE PHARMACOLOGIC STRESS PROCEDURE

Patient preparation
  Contraindicated in patients with second- or third-degree atrioventricular block, sinus node disease, or asthma. Withhold dipyridamole for 12 to 24 hours before adenosine.
Drug administered
  Adenosine, 140 mcg/kg/minute peripheral IV infusion over 6 minutes (total dose, 0.84 mg/kg)

or 50 mcg/kg/minute increased to 75, 100, and 140 mcg/kg/minute each minute to 7 minutes.
Radiopharmaceutical administered
  Administered at the midpoint (3 minutes) of the infusion
Imaging
  As for dipyridamole
Comments
  Side effects of hypertension, flushing, chest discomfort, dyspnea, headache, dizziness, or gastrointestinal discomfort may occur and usually resolve quickly, although theophylline (50 to 125 mg slow IV injection) may be necessary in rare cases.

PULMONARY VENTILATION SCAN (XENON)

Procedure imaging time
  5 minutes
Instrumentation
  Large-FOV camera, if available
Radiopharmaceutical
  ^{133}Xe
Method of administration
  Gas is inspired through an enclosed ventilation system with appropriate mouthpiece or face mask.
Normal adult administered activity
  4 to 20 mCi (185 to 740 MBq). (If done after perfusion scan, dose may have to be 20 mCi [740 MBq]).
  Dose for children, 0.3 mCi/kg (10 to 12 MBq/kg) with a minimum of 3 mCi (100 to 120 MBq)
Conflicting examination and medications
  None
Patient preparation
  None
Technique
  Collimator
    Low-energy, all-purpose, parallel-hole
  Counts
    All images are taken for 10 to 15 seconds.
  Routine views
    All views are performed in the posterior position unless otherwise specified by the physician.
  1. Begin ^{133}Xe and obtain 10-second inspiration image (1000-k counts).
  2. Record three equilibrium images (300-k counts).
  3. Exhaust ^{133}Xe and record 10- to 40-second images until the bulk of the gas has left the lungs.

Patient positioning
  Sitting, preferably. Supine is also acceptable.
Photopeak selection
  81-keV (25% window)
Dosimetry: rads/mCi (mGy/MBq) of administered activity

Effective dose	0.003 (0.0007)
Lung	0.004 (0.001)

Comments
  An exhaust system or xenon trap should be available for expired xenon. Room must be negative pressure.

PULMONARY VENTILATION SCAN (DTPA AEROSOL)

Procedure imaging time
  15 minutes
Instrumentation
  Large-FOV camera, if available
Radiopharmaceutical
  ^{99m}Tc-diethylenetriamine pentaacetic acid (DTPA) aerosol
Method of administration
  Nebulizer connected to a mouthpiece. The nose should be occluded. Patient performing tidal breathing in the upright position, if possible.
Normal adult administered activity
  25 to 35 mCi (900 to 1300 MBq) in the nebulizer from which the patient receives about 0.5 to 1.0 mCi (20 to 40 MBq).
Conflicting examination and medications
  None
Patient preparation
  None
Technique
  Collimator
    Low-energy, all-purpose, parallel-hole
  Photopeak selection
    140-keV (20% window)
  Counts
    When the camera sees 1000 counts per second, discontinue nebulizer and then do images for 100-k counts per image
  Routine views
  Anterior, posterior, and four obliques
  Patient positioning
    Sitting, preferably. Supine is also acceptable.
Dosimetry: rads/mCi (mGy/MBq) of administered activity

Effective dose	0.026 (0.007)
Bladder	0.17 (0.046)

Comments
  Should usually be performed before the ^{99m}Tc-macroaggregated albumin (MAA) perfusion scan.

PULMONARY PERFUSION SCAN

Procedure imaging time
  30 minutes
Radiopharmaceutical
  ^{99m}Tc-macroaggregated albumin (MAA), about 300,000 particles; however, this can be reduced to 100,000 to 200,000 in persons with known right-to-left shunts, infants, and children.
Method of administration
  Before injection the patient should, if possible, cough and take several deep breaths. Invert syringe immediately before injection to resuspend particles. With the patient supine, or as close to supine as possible, begin slow IV injection in antecubital vein during three to five respiratory cycles.
Normal adult administered activity
  5 mCi (185 MBq); reduce to 3 mCi (111 MBq) if expecting to do xenon study afterward.
Injection-to-imaging time
  Immediate
Conflicting examinations and medications
  None
Patient preparation
  None
Technique
  Collimator
    Low-energy, all-purpose, parallel-hole
  Counts
    500-k counts
  Routine views
  1. Posterior
  2. Left posterior oblique
  3. Left lateral
  4. Left anterior oblique
  5. Anterior
  6. Right anterior oblique
  7. Right lateral
  8. Right posterior oblique
  Patient positioning
    Preferably sitting, although supine is acceptable
  Photopeak selection
    140-keV (20% window)
Dosimetry: rads/mCi (mGy/MBq) of administered activity

Effective dose	0.044 (0.012)
Lung	0.25 (0.068)

Comments

If blood is introduced into the syringe containing the radiopharmaceutical, the injection must be completed immediately or small blood clots entrapping the radiopharmaceutical may cause hot spots in the lung. If the injected particles are too small, they will accumulate in the liver and spleen.

In patients with right-to-left shunts, young children and patients with pulmonary hypertension reduce the number of particles to about 60,000 to 100,000.

A chest radiograph is used for correlation. It should be obtained within an hour or so but be no more than 24 hours.

A well-flushed indwelling line can be used. Do not administer in the distal port of a Swan-Ganz catheter or any indwelling line or port that contains a filter (e.g., chemotherapy line).

LIVER AND SPLEEN SCAN

Procedure imaging time
　30 minutes
Radiopharmaceutical
　^{99m}Tc-sulfur or albumin colloid
Method of administration
　IV injection; bolus injection in antecubital vein for dynamic imaging. Invert syringe before injecting to resuspend particles.
Normal adult administered activity
　4 to 6 mCi (148 to 222 MBq)
Injection-to-imaging time
　20 minutes
Conflicting examinations and medications
　1. Recent upper gastrointestinal series or barium enema with retained barium
　2. Increased bone marrow uptake will occur with nitrosoureas or if the colloid size is too small.
　3. Increased spleen uptake will occur with nitrosoureas, recent halothane, or methylcellulose.
　　Decreased spleen uptake can occur as a result of chemotherapy, epinephrine, and antimalarials.
　4. Lung uptake can be increased as a result of aluminum antacids, iron preparations, virilizing androgens, Mg^2_preparations, niacin, colloid size too large, Al^3_in preparation, and particle clumping.
Patient preparation
　None

Technique
　Collimator
　　Low-energy, all-purpose, parallel-hole
　Counts
　　1. 1000-k counts: anterior supine
　　2. 500-k counts: all other views
　Routine views
　　1. Anterior supine
　　2. Anterior supine with lead marker
　　3. Anterior erect, if possible
　　4. Right anterior oblique
　　5. Right lateral
　　6. Right posterior oblique
　　7. Posterior
　　8. Left lateral
　Optional views
　　In patients who require supine imaging, obtain anterior erect view whenever possible.
　Patient positioning
　　Supine
　Photopeak selection
　　140-keV (20% window)
Dosimetry: rads/mCi (mGy/MBq) of administered activity

Effective dose	0.034 (0.009)
Spleen	0.27 (0.07)

Comments
　1. Breast-shadow artifact is often seen in women. Eliminate artifact by moving right breast away from liver in anterior and right anterior oblique views.
　2. Selective splenic imaging can be performed by using an UltraTag kit for red cells and injecting 1 to 3 mCi (40 to 110 MBq) of heat damaged ^{99m}Tc-labeled RBCs. Cells are typically damaged by heating to 49° C to 50° C in a water bath for 20 minutes.
　3. Blood pool imaging is done for evaluation of cavernous hemangioma after red cell labeling and administration of 20 to 25 mCi (740 to 925 MBq). SPECT imaging is very helpful.

SPECT LIVER AND SPLEEN IMAGING

Procedure imaging time
　30 minutes
Instrumentation
　SPECT camera
Radiopharmaceutical
　^{99m}Tc-sulfur or albumin colloid

Method of administration
IV injection
Normal adult administered activity
6 mCi (222 MBq)
Injection-to-imaging time
20 minutes
Conflicting examinations and medications
Retained barium
Patient preparation
None
Technique
Collimator
Low-energy, high-resolution
Counts and time
60 to 64 stops for 30 seconds each
Routine views
360-degree arc of rotation
Patient positioning
Supine; both arms over head
Photopeak selection
140-keV (20% window)
Dosimetry: rads/mCi (mGy/MBq) of administered activity

Effective dose	0.034 (0.009)
Spleen	0.27 (0.07)

Comments
128 × 128 matrix, if available

HEPATOBILIARY SCAN
Procedure imaging time
1 to 4 hours
Radiopharmaceutical
^{99m}Tc-diisopropyl iminodiacetic acid (DIS-IDA; disofenin) or bromotrimethyl IDA (BrIDA; mebrofenin). Extraction of mebrofenin is significantly better than disofenin in moderate to severe hepatic dysfunction
Method of administration
IV injection; bolus injection in antecubital vein for dynamic imaging
Normal administered activity
3 to 5 mCi (111 to 185 MBq). Higher activities may be needed in patient with hyperbilirubinemia 5 to 10 mCi (185 to 370 MBq). For infants and children, the administered activity is 0.05 to 0.2 mCi/ kg (2 to 7 MBq/kg) with a minimum of 0.4 to 0.5 mCi (15 to 20 MBq)
Injection-to-imaging time
5 minutes
Conflicting examinations and medications
1. Retained barium.
2. Serum bilirubin level above 20 mg/dL may cause a nondiagnostic examination owing to poor hepatocellular function.

3. Delayed biliary-to-bowel transit will occur in patients who have received narcotic analgesics.
4. Liver uptake and excretion will be decreased by chronic high-dose nicotinic acid therapy, and phenobarbital will enhance hepatic excretion.
Patient preparation
NPO for 2 hours and preferably 4 hours before procedure. If the patient has fasted for more than 24 hours or is on total parenteral nutrition, the gallbladder may not fill. In these cases, it may be necessary to pretreat with sincalide (see following).
Technique
Collimator
Low-energy, all-purpose, parallel-hole, or high-resolution
Routine views
Serial images with continuous computer acquisition in anterior position (1 frame per minute for 30 to 60 minutes) reformatted at 4- to 6-minute images for filming or digital display.
If visualization of gallbladder is questionable, obtain right lateral view.
Patient positioning
Supine
Photopeak selection
140-keV (20% window)
Dosimetry: rads/mCi (mGy/MBq) of administered activity

Effective dose	0.06 (0.017)
Gallbladder	0.41 (0.11)

Comments
1. If gallbladder is not seen by 45 minutes, delayed images should be taken at 15-minute intervals until 2 hours after injection, and then hourly until 4 hours. An alternative is to administer morphine (0.04 mg/kg or 2 mg in 10 mL saline IV over 5 to 10 minutes) at 1 hour and continue imaging for 45 minutes or until gallbladder visualizes.
2. If gallbladder is visualized but activity is not seen in the small bowel by 1 hour after injection, or a gallbladder ejection fraction is needed, consider using sincalide (0.02 mcg/kg in 10 mL of normal saline IV over 3 to 10 minutes). This can also be used for evaluation of the gallbladder ejection fraction by administering sincalide when the gallbladder is filled (usually at 1 hour). Slower infusion over 15 to 60 minutes is preferred by some for more complete

gallbladder emptying and less abdominal discomfort. With a 15- or 60-minute infusion, the normal gallbladder EF is equal to or greater than 40% and 38%, respectively.

3. If duodenal activity is confusing, have the patient drink water; wait 10 minutes, and take another view. A left anterior oblique image may also separate duodenal loop activity from the gallbladder.

4. If the patient is being studied for a bile leak, 2- to 4-hour delayed imaging (possibly with decubitus views) may be needed

5. Delayed imaging at 24 hours may be necessary in infants with suspected biliary atresia.

MECKEL DIVERTICULUM SCAN

Procedure imaging time
  ½ to 1 hour
Radiopharmaceutical
  ^{99m}Tc-sodium pertechnetate
Method of administration
  IV injection
Normal administered activity
  8 to 12 mCi (296 to 444 MBq) or 200 to 300 μCi/kg (7.4 to 11.1 MBq/kg) in children and at least 2.0 mCi (74 MBq)
Injection-to-imaging time
  Immediate
Conflicting examinations and medications
  1. Increased gastric will be caused by Pentagastrin and Cimetidine. Decreased gastric mucosa activity will be caused by Al^3_ ion (antacids) and perchlorate.
  2. Recent upper gastrointestinal series can leave attenuating barium in abdomen.
  3. Recent in vivo RBC labeling study with IV administration of stannous ion
Patient preparation
  See following comments.
Technique
  Collimator
    Low-energy, all-purpose, parallel-hole
  Counts
    All static images: 300- to 500-k counts or continuous cine imaging over the lower midabdomen above the bladder
  Routine views
  1. Sequential anterior abdominal images at 30- to 60-second intervals that can be reformatted at 5-minute intervals for 30 to 60 minutes.
  2. Right lateral midabdomen at 45 minutes.
  Patient positioning
    Supine

Photopeak selection
  140-keV (20% window)
Dosimetry: rads/mCi (mGy/MBq) of administered activity
  Effective   0.048 (0.013) in an adult,
    dose   0.15 (0.04) in a 5-year-old child
  Colon   0.23 (0.06) in an adult, 0.78
                (0.21) in a 5-year-old child
Comments
  Premedication may increase the sensitivity of the study but is not necessary for a high-quality study. Cimetidine (20 mg/kg in children or 10 to 20 mg/kg in neonates) given orally for 2 days before the study is the most common method. In adults, cimetidine should be administered at a rate of 300 mg in 100 mL of dextrose 5% in water (D5W) over 20 minutes, with imaging starting 1 hour later. It may also be given 300 mg orally four times a day before the study. Ranitidine may be substituted for cimetidine. Ranitidine dosage is 1 mg/kg IV for infants children and adults infused over 20 minutes, with imaging starting 1 hour later, or 2 mg/kg/dose PO for children and 150 mg/dose for adults. Famotidine can also be used.
  Pentagastrin (6 mcg/kg given subcutaneously 5 to 15 minutes before the study) can be used, but, because it increases peristalsis, glucagon (30 mcg/kg for an adult [maximum 0.5 mg] and 5 mcg/kg for a child, IV 10 minutes before the study) is also necessary.

GASTROINTESTINAL BLEEDING SCAN

Procedure imaging time
  1 to 2 hours
Radiopharmaceutical
  ^{99m}Tc-labeled RBCs
Method of administration
  IV injection (see RBC labeling procedures at end of this appendix). We prefer the UltraTag method for this study.
Normal adult administered activity
  20 mCi (740 MBq) IV
Injection-to-imaging time
  Immediate
Conflicting examinations and medications
  1. Recent upper gastrointestinal series
  2. Recent barium enema
Patient preparation
  None
Technique
  Collimator
    Low-level, all-purpose, parallel-hole

Counts
  Collect 500-k counts per image with camera.
Routine views
  Sequential anterior abdominal images taken at 5- to 10-minute intervals for 1 hour or continuous dynamic acquisition for 1 to 2 hours. Computer acquisition 128 × 128 matrix, 10 to 60 seconds per frame and cine replay at 1-minute frames × 60 is often helpful.
Optional views
  Oblique images may be helpful in locating an abnormality.
Patient positioning
  Supine
Photopeak selection
  140-keV (20%) window)
Dosimetry: rads/mCi (mGy/MBq) of administered activity
  Effective dose   0.026 (0.007)
  Heart   0.085 (0.023)
Comments
  Delayed images over 24 hours may be needed to document an intermittent bleed.

ESOPHAGEAL TRANSIT

Procedure imaging time
  20 minutes
Radiopharmaceutical
  ^{99m}Tc-sulfur colloid in 15 mL of water
Method of administration
  Oral
Normal adult administered activity
  0.1 to 1.0 mCi (3.7 to 37 MBq)
Ingestion-to-imaging time
  Immediate
Conflicting examinations and medications
  None
Patient preparation
  NPO for 4 hours
Technique
  Collimator
    Low-energy
  Counts
    Computer acquisition, initial bolus recorded at 0.25 to 1 second frames × 240, 64 × 64 matrix. Additional data acquisition for 10 minutes when the patient may be asked to dry swallow may be helpful.
  Routine views
    Posterior, swallow radiopharmaceutical as a bolus, dry swallow at 30 seconds three or four times

Patient positioning
  Sitting
Photopeak selection
  140-keV (20% window)
Dosimetry: rads/mCi (mGy/MBq) of administered activity
  Effective dose   0.089 (0.024)
  Colon   0.48 (0.13)
Comments
  1. A computer is required.
  2. In a normal person, the esophageal bolus transit time is less than 5 seconds.

GASTROESOPHAGEAL REFLUX

Procedure imaging time
  1 to 2 hours
Radiopharmaceutical
  ^{99m}Tc-sulfur or albumin colloid in 150 mL of orange juice and 150 mL of 0.1 N HCl
Method of administration
  Oral
Normal adult administered activity
  300 μCi (11.1 MBq)
Administration-to-imaging time
  Immediate
Conflicting examinations and medications
  None
Patient preparation
  NPO for 4 hours
Technique
  Collimator
    Low-energy
  Counts
    30-second images; computer acquisition mandatory, 5 to 10 seconds per frame for 60 minutes
  Routine views
    Anterior; image with Valsalva maneuver and then with abdominal binder at 0, 20, 40, 60, 80, and 100 mm Hg. Do not use a binder on infants or children.
  Patient positioning
    Upright, supine, or both as needed.
  Photopeak selection
    140-keV (20% window)
Dosimetry: rads/mCi (mGy/MBq) of administered activity
  Effective dose   0.089 (0.024)
  Colon   0.48 (0.13)
Comments
  1. More than 4% reflux is abnormal.
  2. A nasogastric tube may be used in young children for insertion of sulfur colloid.

3. To look for pulmonary aspiration in infants, use 5 µCi/mL (0.19 MBq) in milk or formula (for a total of 500 µCi or 18.5 MBq). Image over lungs at 4, 6, and 12 hours as needed.

GASTRIC EMPTYING

Procedure imaging time
    4 hours
Radiopharmaceutical
    Liquid phase, ^{111}In-DTPA (diethylenetriamine pentaacetic acid), or ^{99m}Tc-DTPA in 300 mL water, orange juice, or milk
    Solid phase, ^{99m}Tc-sulfur colloid in scrambled egg whites (e.g., Egg-beaters) placed in between two slices of white bread and with 30 g of jam or jelly. Eaten with 120 mL of water
Method of administration
    Oral; the meal should optimally be ingested within 10 minutes.
Normal adult administered activity
    Liquid phase, 0.1 to 0.2 mCi (3.7 to 7.4 MBq) of ^{111}In-DTPA in 300 mL
    Solid phase, 0.5 to 1.0 mCi (18.5 to 37 MBq) of ^{99m}Tc-sulfur colloid
Administration-to-imaging time
    Immediate
Conflicting examinations, conditions, and medications
    Drugs affecting gastric motility. Two-day cessation of aluminum hydroxide, atropine, narcotics, nifedipine, progesterone, octreotide, theophylline, benzodiazepine, phentolamine, and propantheline. Gastric emptying enhanced by Reglan. Prokinetic drugs such as metoclopramide, tegaserod, domperidone, and erythromycin stopped 2 days before exam unless the purpose is to test their efficacy.
    Optimally premenopausal women should be studied on days 1 through 10 of their menstrual cycle to avoid effects of hormonal variation on gastrointestinal motility.
Patient preparation
    NPO for 8 hours. Diabetics need to be instructed to bring insulin with them. The dose of insulin is to be adjusted when the meal is given. Blood sugar ideally less than 200 mg/dL.
Technique
    Collimator
        Low-energy for ^{99m}Tc; medium-energy for ^{111}In

Images
    Anterior and posterior. For solid phase, 1-minute images at 1, 30, 60, 120, 180, and 240 minutes, or continuous dynamic acquisition for 90 minutes with liquid-phase imaging
Routine views
    Left anterior oblique only or anterior and posterior sequentially for geometric mean method
Patient positioning
    Sitting between images, standing for imaging
Photopeak selection
    172 and 246-keV (20% windows) for ^{111}In
    140-keV (20% window) for ^{99m}Tc
Dosimetry: rads/mCi (mGy/MBq) of administered activity
    ^{99m}Tc nonabsorbable solid or liquid
        Effective dose   0.089 (0.024)
        Colon   0.41 (0.11)
    ^{111}In nonabsorbable solid or liquid
        Effective dose   1.1 (0.3)
        Colon   7.4 to 7.8 (2.0 to 2.1)
Comments
    1. For solid meal, rapid gastric emptying is less than 70% remaining in the stomach at 30 minutes or less than 30% at 60 minutes. Delayed gastric emptying criteria is more than 90% at 60 minutes, more than 60% at 120 minutes, more than 30% at 180 minutes, or more than 10% at 240 minutes. The 4-hour value is the best discriminator of a normal or abnormal result.
    2. Computer acquisition is essential. Half-time for liquid emptying is done by drawing a region of interest around the stomach and determination of the time it takes to reach half the peak counts or a least-squares fit method to derive a half-emptying time to reach 50% of the peak counts. For solid phase, a geometric mean of anterior and posterior images is obtained to quantify emptying and obtain a time activity curve.

PERITONEAL (LEVEEN) SHUNT PATENCY

Procedure imaging time
    1 to 2 hours
Radiopharmaceutical
    ^{99m}Tc-macroaggregated albumin (MAA) or ^{99m}Tc-sulfur colloid

Method of administration
Intraperitoneal using aseptic technique
Normal adult administered activity
5 to 5 mCi (18.5 to 185 MBq)
Injection-to-imaging time
Immediate
Conflicting examinations and medications
None
Patient preparation
Void before examination; local anesthesia at injection site
Technique
Collimator
Low-energy
Counts
Serial images. If flow is slow, use 2-minute static images. Image as soon as lower portion of tube is seen. At 1 hour, image lungs if MAA was used or the liver if sulfur colloid was used
Routine views
Anterior abdomen and chest
Patient positioning
Supine
Photopeak selection
140-keV (20% window)
Comments
1. Flush needle with 3 to 5 mL of saline. On occasion, normal saline (50 to 200 mL) can be used to facilitate distribution.
2. Abdominal ballottement may facilitate mixing with ascitic fluid.
3. If tube does not appear, delaying views up to 5 hours may be necessary.

SALIVARY GLAND IMAGING
Procedure imaging time
30 minutes
Radiopharmaceutical
^{99m}Tc-pertechnetate
Method of administration
Intravenous
Normal adult administered activity
8 to 12 mCi (296 to 444 MBq)
Injection-to-imaging time
Immediate
Conflicting examinations and medications
None
Patient preparation
None
Technique
Collimator
Low-energy

Counts
Serial images over 30 minutes
Routine views
Anterior; lateral or oblique static images may also be helpful
Patient positioning
Supine
Photopeak selection
140-keV (20% window)
Comments
Lemon juice may be used to stimulate salivary emptying

BONE SCAN (^{99m}-TECHNETIUM)
Procedure imaging time
30 to 60 minutes
Radiopharmaceutical
^{99m}Tc-labeled phosphates and phosphonates
Method of administration
IV injection
Normal administered activity
Adults 20 to 30 mCi (740 MBq to 1.11 GBq)
Markedly obese adults, 300 to 350 μCi/kg (11 to 13 MBq/kg)
Children, 0.25 mCi/kg (9.3 MBq/kg) with a minimum of 1.0 mCi (37 MBq)
Injection-to-imaging time
Immediate to 3 hours (see Comments)
Conflicting examinations and medications
1. Renal uptake can be increased by amphotericin B, aluminum antacids, iron preparations, Al^3_ions in preparation, radiation therapy, recent radiographic contrast sodium diatrizoate, dextrose, gentamycin, and chemotherapy agents, particularly vincristine, doxorubicin, and cyclophosphamide.
2. Breast uptake can be increased by gynecomastia-producing drugs, digitalis, estrogens, cimetidine, spironolactone, and diethylstilbestrol.
3. Stomach uptake can be caused by isotretinoin.
4. Liver uptake can be caused by aluminum antacids, iron preparations, Al^3_ions in preparation, excess Sn^2 ions in preparation, recent radiographic contrast, sodium diatrizoate, and alkaline pH.
5. Spleen uptake can be increased by phenytoin and aluminum preparations.
6. Excessive blood pool activity can be the result of aluminum preparations, iron dextran, or too few Sn^2 ions in preparation.

7. Focal soft tissue or muscle uptake can result from ion dextran injections, calcium gluconate injections, heparin injections, or meperidine injections.

Patient preparation
1. If not contraindicated, the patient should be hydrated, IV or PO (two or more 8-ounce glasses of water).
2. Patient should void before imaging.

Technique
Collimator
Low-energy, high-resolution, or ultrahigh-resolution parallel-hole
Counts
1. 500-k to 1 million counts over the chest with other axial skeletal images for the same time
2. 150- to 250-k counts in extremities
3. Minimum of 1000-k counts per view for whole-body imaging systems
4. Whole-body images usually obtained with a 256 × 256 × 16 or greater matrix and spot images with a 128 × 128 × 16 or 256 × 256 × 16 matrix. The scanning speed should be adjusted so that routine anterior or posterior whole-body delayed images contain more than 1.5 million counts.
Routine views
Anterior and posterior skeleton, lateral skull
Patient positioning
Supine, prone, or sitting
Photopeak selection
140-keV (20% window)

Dosimetry: rads/mCi (mGy/MBq) of administered activity

Effective dose	0.02 (0.006)
Bone surface	0.23 (0.06)

Comments
1. Differential diagnosis of cellulitis from osteomyelitis requires flow study of 30 frames (64 × 64 × 16 or greater matrix at 1 to 3 seconds per frame) and a 3- to 5-minute blood pool image (128 × 128 × 16 or greater matrix and 200- to 300-k counts/image) within 10 minutes of injection over the region of interest. Delayed images at 3 to 4 hours are also necessary.
2. Prevent cold spot artifacts by having patient remove metal objects (e.g., money, lighter, jewelry).
3. Identify region of interest to be imaged before selecting injection site to prevent injection in area of interest.

4. Urine contamination is the most common hot spot artifact. Decontaminate patient, and image again.

SPECT BONE IMAGING

Procedure imaging time
30 minutes
Instrumentation
SPECT camera
Radiopharmaceutical
^{99m}Tc-phosphates or diphosphonates
Method of administration
IV injection
Normal administered activity
Same as for standard bone scan
Injection-to-imaging time
3 hours
Conflicting examinations and medications
Retained barium
Patient preparation
None
Technique
Collimator
High-resolution
Counts and time
60 to 120 stops, 64 × 64 × 16 or greater matrix and 10 to 40 seconds per stop
Routine views
360-degree arc of rotation
Patient positioning
Supine
Photopeak selection
140-keV (20% window)

Dosimetry: rads/mCi (mGy/MBq) of administered activity

Effective dose	0.02 (0.005)
Bone surface	0.23 (0.06)

BONE MARROW SCAN

Procedure imaging time
1 hour
Radiopharmaceutical
^{99m}Tc-sulfur colloid
Method of administration
IV injection
Normal adult administered activity
8 to 10 mCi (296 to 370 MBq)
Injection-to-imaging time
20 minutes
Conflicting examinations and medications
None
Patient preparation
None

Technique
  Collimator
    Low-energy, all-purpose, parallel-hole
  Counts
    All images: 250-k count in bone marrow
  Routine views
  1. Anterior: shoulders, sternum, ribs, pelvis, thighs
  2. Posterior: thorax, lumbar spine, pelvis
  Patient positioning
    Supine or prone or sitting
  Photopeak selection
    140-keV (20% window)
Dosimetry: rads/mCi (mGy/MBq) of administered activity

Effective dose	0.035	(0.009)
Spleen	0.27	(0.07)

Comments
  1. Overlap spot images of regions of interest to prevent loss of information.
  2. Liver and spleen require lead shielding if within region of interest.

RENAL BLOOD FLOW SCAN

Procedure imaging time
  5 minutes
Radiopharmaceutical
  ^{99m}Tc-diethylenetriamine pentaacetic acid (DTPA), glucoheptonate, or mercaptoacetyltriglycine (MAG3)
Method of administration
  IV injection; bolus injection in antecubital vein
Normal adult administered activity
  10 mCi (370 MBq)
Injection-to-imaging time
  Immediate
Conflicting examinations and medications
  None
Patient preparation
  None
Technique
  Collimator
    Low-energy, all-purpose, parallel-hole
  Counts
    500-k count for static image
  Routine views
  1. Dynamic (anterior: transplant; posterior: retroperitoneal): 2 to 3 seconds per frame for 30 seconds
  2. Static (immediate) image
  Patient positioning
    Sitting or supine

Photopeak selection
  140-keV (20% window)
Dosimetry: rads/mCi (mGy/MBq) of administered activity

DTPA		
Effective dose	0.02	(0.005)
Bladder	0.19	(0.05)
MAG3		
Effective dose	0.026	(0.007)
Bladder	0.41	(0.11)
Glucoheptonate		
Effective dose	0.089	(0.024)
Bladder	0.56	(0.15)

RENAL SCAN (A) CORTICAL IMAGING

Procedure imaging time
  20 minutes
Radiopharmaceutical
  ^{99m}Tc-DMSA (cortical agent); if not available ^{99m}Tc-glucoheptonate
Method of administration
  IV administration: bolus injection in antecubital vein in less than 0.5 mL volume using a 22-gauge needle
Normal administered activity
  5 mCi (185 MBq) ^{99m}Tc-DMSA for adults and a minimum of 0.3 mCi (≈11 MBq) in children with a maximum of 3.0 mCi (≈110 MBq)
  10 to 20 mCi (370 to 740 MBq) ^{99m}Tc-glucoheptonate for adults and a 0.05 mCi/kg (1.85 MBq/kg) with a minimum of 0.5 mCi (18 MBq) for children
Injection-to-imaging time
  Immediate and at 2 to 4 hours for DMSA
  Immediate for glucoheptonate
Conflicting examinations and medications
  None
Patient preparation
  None
Technique
  Collimator
    Low-energy, high-resolution, or ultrahigh-resolution
  Counts
    500-k counts for static image on 128 × 128 or 256 × 256 matrix
  Routine views
  1. Dynamic (anterior: transplant; posterior: retroperitoneal), 2 to 3 seconds per frame for 30 seconds
  2. Static imaging immediately after flow study

3. Static imaging 2 hours after flow study
Patient positioning
Supine (or prone for pinhole)
Photopeak selection
140-keV (20% window)
Dosimetry for children: rads/mCi (mGy/MBq) of administered activity

DMSA
Effective dose	0.03	(0.008)
Kidneys	0.66	(0.18)

Glucoheptonate
Effective dose	0.020	(0.005)
Bladder	0.56	(0.15)

Comments
SPECT imaging is very helpful with either 180 or 360-degree sampling on a 128 × 128 matrix.

RENAL SCAN (B) GLOMERULAR FILTRATION

Procedure imaging time
45 minutes
Radiopharmaceutical
^{99m}Tc–diethylenetriamine pentaacetic acid (DTPA) or glucoheptonate
Method of administration
IV injection: bolus injection in antecubital vein
Normal adult administered activity
10 mCi (370 MBq)
Injection-to-imaging time
Immediate
Conflicting examination and medications
None
Patient preparation
None
Technique
Collimator
Low-energy, all-purpose, parallel-hole
Counts
1. First dynamic study: 2 seconds per frame
2. Second dynamic study: 120 seconds per frame
3. Static image for 500-k counts
Routine views
1. A flow study at 2 seconds per image in the anterior position for a transplanted kidney and the posterior position for a retroperitoneal kidney (perfusion study).
2. On completion of the initial flow study, a second phase of dynamic study is performed at 3 minutes per frame with the patient in the same position. The second phase is carried out for 20 minutes after injection (excretion study).

3. A delayed image may be taken in the same position as the previous studies. An upright postvoid image may be useful to assess collecting system drainage.
Patient positioning
Supine or sitting
Photopeak selection
140-keV (20% window)
Dosimetry: rads/mCi (mGy/MBq) of administered activity

DTPA
Effective dose	0.02	(0.005)
Bladder	0.19	(0.05)

RENAL SCAN (C) TUBULAR FUNCTION

Procedure imaging time
30 minutes
Radiopharmaceutical
^{99m}Tc-mercaptoacetyltriglycine (MAG3)
Method of administration
IV injection
Normal adult administered activity
8 mCi (296 MBq)
Injection-to-imaging time
Immediate
Conflicting examinations and medications
None
Patient preparation
None
Technique
Collimator
Low-energy, all-purpose, or high-resolution
Counts
15 dynamic images of 2 minutes each are obtained.
Views
Anterior for transplant evaluation; posterior for native kidneys
Patient positioning
Supine
Photopeak selection
140-keV (20% window)
Dosimetry: rads/mCi (mGy/MBq) of administered activity

MAG3
Effective dose	0.026	(0.007)
Bladder	0.41	(0.11)

Comments
Erect posterior images may be obtained after the patient has ambulated if ureteral obstruction is suspected.

DIURETIC (LASIX) RENOGRAM

Procedure imaging time
  30 to 60 minutes
Radiopharmaceutical
  ^{99m}Tc-DTPA (glomerular agent) or MAG3 (tubular secretion)
Method of administration
  Bolus IV injection in antecubital vein
Normal administered activity
  10 mCi (370 MBq) for adults. For children, 1.9 MBq (50 μCi) per kg of body weight of MAG3 and 3.7 MBq (100 μCi) for DTPA. The minimum administered activity should be 1.0 mCi (37 MBq).
Injection-to-imaging time
  Immediate
Conflicting examinations and medications
  IV iodine contrast media should not be used on the same day that this examination is performed.
Patient preparation
  1. See requisition because some patients may require an indwelling bladder catheter placed before this procedure (particularly in patients with suspected bladder pathology).
  2. Patient should be hydrated unless contraindicated.
  3. Patient must void before imaging.
Technique
  Collimator
    Low-energy, all-purpose, parallel-hole
  Counts and time
    15 to 60 seconds per frame computer acquisition 64 × 64 or 128 × 128 matrix and filmed as 2-minute images for at least 30 minutes
  Routine views
    Posterior
  Patient positioning
    Sitting, if possible
  Photopeak selection
    140-keV (20% window)
Dosimetry: rads/mCi (mGy/MBq) of administered activity

DTPA		
Effective dose		0.020 (0.005)
Bladder		0.19 (0.05)
MAG3		
Effective dose		0.026 (0.007)
Bladder		0.41 (0.11)

Comments
  1. Furosemide (for adults 0.3 mg/kg body weight IV or 20 to 40 mg) is given about 10 to 15 minutes into the study if there appears to be a delay in excretion. Note frame number of administration. For children, 1.0 mg/kg with a usual maximum of 40 mg IV over 1 to 2 minutes.
  2. A region of interest can be drawn around the dilated collecting system and a t½ calculated after administration of furosemide. A half time less than 10 minutes usually means the absence of obstruction, and a half time of more than 20 minutes identifies obstruction. Half time value of 10 to 20 minutes is equivocal.

CAPTOPRIL RENOGRAM FOR DIAGNOSIS OF RENOVASCULAR HYPERTENSION

Procedure imaging time
  1 hour
Radiopharmaceutical
  ^{99m}Tc-DTPA or ^{99m}Tc-MAG3
Method of administration
  Radionuclide administered 1 hour IV after 25 to 50 mg captopril given as single oral dose.
Normal adult dose
  1 to 10 mCi (37 to 370 MBq), ^{99m}Tc-DTPA or ^{99m}Tc-MAG3
Injection-to-imaging time
  Immediate; however, injection of radiopharmaceutical should be done 60 minutes after administration of captopril or 15 minutes after enalaprilat administration.
Conflicting examinations and medications
  Short-acting angiotensin-converting enzyme (ACE) inhibitors, such as captopril, should be withheld 3 days before the study, and longer-acting ACE inhibitors should be withheld for 5 to 7 days before the study. If this is not done, the study still can be performed but with some reduction in sensitivity. The study should not be initiated if systolic blood pressure is below 140 mm Hg.
Patient preparation
  Patient should be hydrated orally. Patients on an oral ACE inhibitor should drink only water and should not eat a solid meal within 4 hours of the study. The recommended dose of captopril is 25 to 50 mg PO. Enalaprilat can also be used at 40 mcg/kg administered intravenously over 3 to 5 minutes with a maximum dose of 2.5 mg.

Technique
  Collimator
    Low-energy or general all-purpose
  Counts and time
    Flow study at 1 or 2 seconds obtained for 1 minute, followed by sequential imaging every 2 to 3 minutes on film or every 30 seconds on computer for 20 minutes. A postvoid image is obtained.
  Routine views
    Posterior blood flow and sequential imaging. In some protocols, patients may receive furosemide (40 mg) 3 minutes after administration of the MAG3.
  Patient positioning
    Supine
  Photopeak selection
    140-keV (20% window)
Dosimetry: rads/mCi (mGy/MBq) of administered activity
  DTPA
    Effective dose   0.020 (0.005)
    Bladder   0.19 (0.05)
  MAG3
    Effective dose   0.026 (0.007)
    Bladder   0.41 (0.11)
Comments
  Patients may become seriously hypotensive with this procedure. It is advisable to establish IV infusion of normal saline before administration of captopril; blood pressure should be recorded every 15 minutes. Many patients who become hypotensive respond to IV fluids without the need for vasopressive drugs.

RADIONUCLIDE CYSTOGRAM IN CHILDREN

Procedure imaging time
  20 minutes
Radiopharmaceutical
  ^{99m}Tc-pertechnetate (preferred); ^{99m}Tc-sulfur colloid or ^{99m}Tc-DTPA are nonabsorbable and can also be used.
Method of administration
  Sterile urethral catheterization. Radiopharmaceutical mixed in 250 to 500 mL of saline or irrigating solution, with shielded bag hung 100 cm above the table or introduced directly into the catheter. Filling usually ends when the patient voids spontaneously, the estimated bladder volume of the bladder is reached, or the flow from the hung solution stops because of back pressure.

Normal administered activity
  0.5 to 1.0 mCi (18.5 to 37 MBq) No more than 1.0 mCi (37 MBq) for each bladder filling cycle.
Infusion-to-imaging time
  Immediate
Conflicting examinations and medications
  None
Patient preparation
  Sterile urethral catheterization
Technique
  Collimator
    Low-energy, high-resolution, or general-purpose
  Routine views
    30-second anterior prevoid and postvoid image
    5-second images during filling and voiding on 128 × 128 matrix with camera positioned under the table
  Patient positioning
    Supine
  Photopeak selection
    140-keV (20% window)
Dosimetry for children: rads/mCi (mGy/MBq) of administered activity
  ^{99m}Tc-pertechnetate, ^{99m}Tc-sulfur colloid, or ^{99m}Tc-DTPA
    Effective dose   0.009 (0.0024)
    Bladder   0.10 (0.027)
Comments
  1. Bladder volume in an individual patient can be approximated in milliliters by the formula (age in years + 2) × 30 mL = bladder volume.
  2. Residual postvoid volume can be quantitated with regions of interest drawn over the bladder on prevoid and postvoid images and requires recording voided volume as follows:
    RV (mL) = [Voided volume (mL) × postvoid bladder counts (ROI)]/[Initial bladder counts (ROI) − postvoid bladder counts (ROI)]
  3. Another method requires an empty bladder and uses the following formula:
    RV (mL) = [Postvoid bladder counts (ROI) × volume infused]/[Initial bladder counts (ROI)]

GALLIUM SCAN FOR TUMOR OR INFECTION

Procedure imaging time
  30 minutes

Radiopharmaceutical
^{67}Ga-citrate

Method of administration
IV injection

Normal administered activity
In adults, 4 to 6 mCi (150 to 220 MBq) for infection; 5 to 10 mCi (185 to 370 MBq) for neoplasm
In children, 0.04 to 0.07 mCi/kg (1.5 to 2.6 MBq/kg) with a minimum dose of 0.25 to 0.5 mCi (9 to 18 MBq)

Injection-to-imaging time
6 and 24 hours for abscess; 48 and 72 hours for tumor imaging

Conflicting examinations and medications
1. Retained barium can cause attenuation.
2. Excessive bone uptake can result from iron preparations, chemotherapy, hemodialysis.
3. Excessive liver uptake can result from iron dextran or phenobarbital.
4. Excessive renal uptake can occur from chemotherapy, furosemide, phenytoin, allopurinol, ampicillin, erythromycin, cephalosporin, ibuprofen, sulfonamides, rifampin, pentamidine, phenylbutazone, and phenobarbital.
5. Stomach uptake also can be increased by chemotherapy and breast uptake increased by reserpine, phenothiazine, metoclopramide, estrogens, and oral contraceptives.
6. Colon uptake will be increased in antibiotic-induced pseudomembranous colitis, especially from clindamycin, cephalosporins, and ampicillin.
7. Prolonged whole-body clearance can occur as a result of vincristine, steroid treatment, or mechlorethamine.
8. Mediastinal and hilar lymph node uptake has been reported in patients taking phenytoin (Dilantin).
9. Lung uptake can be increased as a result of cyclophosphamide, amiodarone, bleomycin, busulfan, and *Bacillus* Calmette-Guerin (BCG).
10. Thymus activity can be increased as a result of radiation therapy, chemotherapy, or antibiotics.

Patient preparation
Bowel preparation after initial images may occasionally be helpful

Technique
Collimator
Medium-energy, parallel-hole, large FOV

Counts
Usually about 10 to 20 minutes per view for planar images. At least 500-k counts per image and 1.5 million to 2 million counts for images of the chest, abdomen, and pelvis. For whole-body images, a scanning speed to achieve an information density of 450 counts/cm^2 or greater than 1.5 million counts for each view.

Patient positioning
Supine

Photopeak selection
93, 184-keV (20% windows). Other photopeaks (296 and 388-keV) can be used.

Routine views
1. Anterior and posterior whole-body images with scanning gamma camera
2. Spot views (optional)

Dosimetry: rads/mCi (mGy/MBq) of administered activity

Effective dose	0.44 (0.12)
Bone surface	2.2 (0.6)

Comments
1. Subtraction views with ^{99m}Tc-sulfur colloid may be considered.
2. SPECT scanning may be useful.

SOMATOSTATIN RECEPTOR SCAN WITH INDIUM-111 PENTETREOTIDE

Procedure imaging time
1 hour

Radiopharmaceutical
^{111}In-pentetreotide (Octreoscan). Should be used within 6 hours of preparation.

Method of administration
IV administration

Normal administered activity
6 mCi (222 MBq) for adults; 0.14 mCi/kg (5 MBq/kg) for children.

Injection-to-imaging time
4 and 24 hours; 48 hours may be needed when there is significant bowel activity at 24 hours.

Conflicting examinations and medications
Consideration should be given to discontinuing octreotide therapy 24 hours before administration of the radiopharmaceutical.
Radiotracer should not be injected into IV lines for, or together with, solutions for total parenteral nutrition.

Patient preparation
Void before imaging

Technique
  Collimator
    Medium-energy, large FOV
  Routine views
    Anterior and posterior views of head, chest, abdomen, pelvis
  Counts
    10 to 15 minutes per image using 512 × 512 or 256 × 256 word matrix. For dual-headed cameras, anterior and posterior whole-body images from head to upper femurs in a 1024 × 512 or 1024 × 256 word matrix for a minimum of 30 minutes (speed 3 cm/min)
  Patient positioning
    Supine
  Photopeak selection
    173 and 247-keV (symmetric 20% window)
Dosimetry: rads/mCi (mGy/MBq) of administered activity

Effective dose	0.19 (0.05)
Spleen	2.11 (0.57)

Comments
  1. In patients suspected of having insulinoma, an IV infusion of glucose should be available because of the potential for inducing severe hypoglycemia.
  2. SPECT imaging may be very helpful, and images are usually obtained at 24 hours with 3-degree angular sampling. 128 × 128 matrix, 360-degree rotation, and 20 to 30 seconds per stop

LYMPHOSCINTIGRAPHY (SENTINEL NODE LOCALIZATION)

Procedure imaging time
  30 minutes
Radiopharmaceutical
  Filtered (0.22 micron millipore filter) ^{99m}Tc-sulfur colloid in 0.1 mL
Method of administration
  Intradermal or peritumoral, 4 to 8 injections within 1 cm that surround the biopsy or tumor site. Finger massage at each site may promote drainage. High pressure of intradermal injection can cause leakage upon needle removal, and site should be covered with bandage or cotton ball.
Normal administered activity
  100 µCi (3.7 MBq)
Injection-to-imaging time
  Immediate
Conflicting examination and medications
  None

Patient preparation
  None
Technique
  Collimator
    Low-energy, all-purpose, parallel-hole
  Counts/time
    Sequential or continuous imaging after injections for 30 to 60 minutes. Continuous images of 30 seconds per frame or sequential images every 5 minutes.
  Routine views
    Over area of injection and with FOV to include expected drainage direction. Injection site may need to be covered with a piece of lead to discern lymphatic drainage. Transmission and oblique views are often helpful for localization.
  Patient positioning
    Usually supine or prone. Breast cancer patients should be positioned with the arm in as close to the same position as the surgery will be done because there is a marked effect of arm position on the perceived location of the sentinel node.
  Photopeak selection
    140-keV (20% window)
Dosimetry: rads/mCi (mGy/MBq) of administered activity (local radiation dose has been ignored and effective dose is calculated assuming 20% of administered activity is absorbed)

Effective dose	0.0071 (0.002)
Spleen	0.057 (0.015)

Comments
  1. Skin is usually marked over the sentinel node.
  2. For trunk lesions, axillary as well as inguinal view should be included; for lesions of the head and neck anterior, posterior and oblique images should be obtained; and for extremity lesion, in-transit nodes around the knee or elbow should also be imaged. For breast cancer patients, oblique axillary and triangulation views are usually obtained.
  3. Mild (not vigorous or prolonged) massaging of the breast following injection may improve distribution of radiotracer. The larger the breast, the slower is the migration of activity.
  4. Use of a gamma probe in the operating room can be done 0.5 to 3 hours after injection to help localize the node, and a sentinel node typically has 10 times the

background counts taken at a location remote from the injection site.

BREAST IMAGING WITH BREAST-SPECIFIC GAMMA CAMERA

Procedure imaging time
  1 hour
Radiopharmaceutical
  99mTc-sestamibi
Method of administration
  Intravenous followed by 10 mL saline flush. Preferable to inject on side opposite the suspected abnormality
Normal administered activity
  25 mCi (925 MBq)
Injection-to-imaging time
  5 minutes
Conflicting examination and medications
  None
Patient preparation
  None
Technique
  Equipment
  High-resolution small field-of-view gamma camera
  Routine views
    Planar imaging begins at 5 minutes; acquired for 10 minutes each or 175-k counts
    Right and left craniocaudal; right and left mediolateral oblique
  Patient positioning
Seated
  Photopeak selection
  140-keV (20% window)
Dosimetry: rads/mCi (mGy/MBq) of administered activity (local radiation dose has been ignored and effective dose is calculated assuming 20% of administered activity is absorbed)
  Effective dose   0.033 (0.009)
  Gallbladder   0.14 (0.039)
Comments
  1. Additional views such as axillary tail, cleavage, implant displacement, 90-degree lateral, and exaggerated craniocaudal views may also be helpful.
  2. Homogeneous, patchy, or diffusely increased uptake is often normal, especially if it is correlated with mammographic findings
  3. Anatomy (BIRADS 1-4). Intensity of focal uptake in malignant lesions is highly variable. Moderate to intense focal uptake with well-delineated contours is strongly suggestive of malignancy (BIRADS 5).

LEUKOCYTE (WHITE BLOOD CELL) SCAN

Procedure imaging time
  1 hour
Radiopharmaceutical
  111In autologous oxine-labeled or 99mTc-HMPAO (Ceretec, Amersham) leukocytes
  Only the unstabilized form of HMPAO should be utilized.
Method of administration
  IV administration
Normal administered activity
  In adults, 500 μCi (18.5 MBq) of 111In; in children, 7.5 to 15 μCi/kg (0.25 to 0.5 MBq/kg), with a minimum administered activity of 50 to 75 μCi (1.85 to 2.3 MBq)
  In adults, 10 to 20 mCi (370 to 740 MBq) for 99mTc-HMPAO; in children, 0.1 to 0.2 mCi/kg (3.7 to 7.4 MBq/kg) for HMPAO, with a minimum of 0.5 to 1.0 mCi (18 to 37 MBq).
Injection-to-imaging time
  1 to 4 hours and 16 to 24 hours for 111In oxine leukocytes
  0.5 to 4 hours for 99mTc-HMPAO (exametazime). With HMPAO, early imaging of the abdomen and pelvis is essential because of hepatobiliary excretion and bowel transit, and 15-minute images at 8 hours after injection may be needed for pulmonary infection or osteomyelitis.
Conflicting examinations and medications
  Patients on antibiotics or with altered chemotaxis may have false-negative examination results.
Patient preparation
  None
Technique
  Collimator
    Medium-energy for 111In and low-energy all-purpose for 99mTc; 500-k counts per view
  Routine views
    Anterior and posterior views of head, chest, abdomen, pelvis
  Counts
    10 to 20 minutes per image for 111In oxine leukocytes
    800-k or 5 to 10 minutes per view for 99mTc-HMPAO
  Patient positioning
    Supine
  Photopeak selection
    Dual: 173- and 247-keV (20% window) for 111In
    140-keV (20% window) for 99mTc

Dosimetry: rads/mCi (mGy/MBq) of administered activity

^{111}In leukocytes

Effective dose	1.3 (0.36)
Spleen	20.0 (5.4)

^{99m}Tc-exametazime (HMPAO)

Effective dose	0.041 (0.011)
Spleen	0.56 (0.15)

Comments

1. Leukocytes are obtained from 20 to 80 mL of venous blood in adults. The minimum volume of blood needed for a child is about 10 to 15 mL.
2. It is difficult to obtain enough cells to label in leukopenic (less than 4000 cells/μL) patients.
3. Labeled cells should be reinjected as soon as possible and no later than 3 to 4 hours after obtaining the sample.
4. Gallium scintigraphy is usually preferred for patients with neutropenia, fever of unknown origin, or nonsuppurative, granulomatous, or lymphocyte-mediated infections.

PET/CT TUMOR IMAGING WITH FLUORINE-18 FLUORO-2-DEOXYGLUCOSE

Procedure imaging time
  30 to 60 minutes
Radiopharmaceutical
  Fluorine-18 fluoro-2-deoxyglucose (^{18}F-FDG)
Method of administration
  IV administration. For brain imaging, for several minutes before FDG administration and for 30 minutes after, the patient should be in a quiet and darkened room.
Normal adult administered activity
  10 to 20 mCi (370 to 740 MBq)
Injection-to-imaging time
  30 to 60 minutes. Void before imaging.
Conflicting examination and medications
  High serum glucose level will reduce tumor uptake.
Patient preparation
  Patients should fast at least 4 hours; this will reduce serum insulin levels to near basal levels and diminish uptake by some organs such as the heart.
  Some institutions will check the blood glucose level, but many do not.
Technique
  Collimator
    None in 3D acquisition; present in 2D acquisition
  Counts/time

Routine views
  Whole body. Usually from just below the brain to the knees. This may require up to 10 bed positions with overlap fields by one or more of the acquisition slices.
Patient positioning
  Supine. For neoplasms of the head or neck, the arms should be down, and for lesions of the chest, the arms should be up. For lesions of the neck that may have mediastinal or pulmonary involvement, it may be necessary to do imaging twice with the arms in both positions
Photopeak selection
  300- or 350- to 650-keV for BGO, 435- to 590- or 665-keV for NaI.
Dosimetry: rads/mCi (mGy/MBq) of administered activity

Effective dose	0.07 (0.019)
Bladder	0.60 (0.16)

Comments
  Attenuation correction can be performed with cesium, germanium, or CT.
  IV and oral contrast can be used with positron emission tomography (PET)/CT; however, the barium should be oral glucose-free 1.3% to 2.1% barium sulfate 500 to 750 mL 60 to 90 minutes before FDG injection. High-density barium should be avoided. Another 100 to 200 mL of oral barium is given 30 minutes after the FDG injection. The patient then sits or lies quietly, and the CT scan is performed just before the PET scan and uses IV contrast (300 mg I/mL) 80 mL at 3 mL/sec to achieve arterial contrast, followed by another 60 mL at 2 mL/sec for venous and parenchymal enhancement.

POSITRON EMISSION TOMOGRAPHY CARDIAC IMAGING WITH FLUORINE-18 FLUORO-2 DEOXYGLUCOSE

Procedure imaging time
  30 to 60 minutes
Radiopharmaceutical
  ^{18}F-FDG
Method of administration
  IV administration. Normal adult administered activity
  10 to 20 mCi (370 to 740 MBq)
Injection-to-imaging time
  30 to 60 minutes; void before imaging
Conflicting examination and medications
  Caffeine will increase cardiac uptake.

Patient preparation

Patient should eat a light, nonfat, high-carbohydrate breakfast or lunch or have a glucose solution (1 to 3 hours before FDG injection) to change the heart from fatty acid to glucose metabolism.

Some institutions will check the blood glucose level, but many do not.

Technique

Collimator

None in 3D acquisition; present in 2D acquisition

Counts/time

20-minute static acquisition

Routine views

Chest

Patient positioning

Supine with arms raised

Photopeak selection

300- or 350- to 650-keV for BGO, 435- to 590- or 665-keV for NaI.

Dosimetry: rads/mCi (mGy/MBq) of administered activity

Effective dose	0.07 (0.019)
Bladder	0.60 (0.16)

Comments

Attenuation correction can be performed with cesium, germanium, or CT.

Compare to myocardial perfusion images.

POSITRON EMISSION TOMOGRAPHY BRAIN IMAGING WITH FLUORINE-18 FLUORO-2-DEOXYGLUCOSE

Procedure imaging time

30 to 60 minutes

Radiopharmaceutical

^{18}F-FDG

Method of administration

IV administration. For brain imaging, for several minutes before FDG administration and for 30 minutes after, the patient should be in a quiet and darkened room.

Normal adult administered activity

10 to 20 mCi (370 to 740 MBq)

Injection-to-imaging time

60 minutes; void before imaging

Conflicting examination and medications

High serum glucose level will reduce tumor uptake.

Patient preparation

Patients should fast at least 4 hours; this will reduce serum insulin levels to near basal levels

and diminish uptake by some organs such as the heart.

Some institutions will check the blood glucose level, but many do not.

Technique

Collimator

None in 3D acquisition; present in 2D acquisition

Counts/time

6-minute static acquisition in the 3D mode or 20-minute acquisition in the 2D mode

Routine views

Head

Patient positioning

Supine with arms down

Photopeak selection

300- or 350- to 650-keV for BGO, 435- to 590- or 665-keV for NaI.

Dosimetry: rads/mCi (mGy/MBq) of administered activity

Effective dose	0.07 (0.019)
Bladder	0.60 (0.16)

Comments

Attenuation correction can be performed with cesium, germanium, or CT.

Fusion with CT or MRI images is desirable.

POSITRON EMISSION TOMOGRAPHY CARDIAC REST/STRESS IMAGING WITH RUBIDIUM-82 OR NITROGEN-13 AMMONIA

Procedure imaging time

30 minutes with rubidium-82 (^{82}Rb), 90 minutes with nitrogen-13 (^{13}N)-ammonia

Radiopharmaceutical

^{82}Rb from strontium-82 (^{82}Sr) generator system or ^{13}N-ammonia

Method of administration

IV administration

Normal adult administered activity

With rubidium 50 mCi (1850 MBq) at rest and 50 mCi (1850 MBq) for stress

With ^{13}N-ammonia, 10 to 20 (370 to 740 MBq) at rest and 10 to 20 mCi (370 to 740 MBq) at stress

Injection-to-imaging time

70 seconds with the patient at rest

6-minute rest emission scan performed

Transmission scan for attenuation correction (when using ^{13}N-ammonia, there must be 45 minutes between rest and stress injections to allow for radioactive decay as a result of the longer half-life of ^{13}N)

3 to 4 minutes dipyridamole infusion

Reinject for stress

6-minute stress emission scan performed

Conflicting examination and medications

    None

Patient preparation

Technique

    Collimator

        None in 3D acquisition; present in 2D acquisition

    Counts/time

        20 to 40 million counts for each 6-minute emission scan

    Routine views

        Chest

    Patient positioning

        Supine arms down

    Photopeak selection

        300- or 350- to 650-keV for BGO, 435- to 590- or 665-keV for NaI; CPET.

Dosimetry: rads/mCi (mGy/MBq) of administered activity

    ^{82}Rb

Effective dose	0.013 (0.004)

    ^{13}N-ammonia

Effective dose	0.007 (0.002)

Comments

1. Cost for a ^{82}Rb from ^{82}Sr generator system is about $20,000 or more for a month.
2. ^{13}N-ammonia requires an on-site cyclotron.

BONE SCAN PET/CT (FLUORINE-18)

Procedure imaging time

    30 minutes

Radiopharmaceutical

    ^{18}F-fluoride

Method of administration

    IV injection

Normal administered activity

    Adults 5 to 10 mCi (185 MBq to 370 MBq)

    Children, 0.06 mCi/kg (2.22 MBq/kg), with a range of 0.5 to 5.0 mCi (18.5 to 185 MBq)

Injection-to-imaging time

    30 minutes to 1 hour and 90 to 120 minutes for high-quality images of extremities

Conflicting examinations and medications

    None

Patient preparation

1. If not contraindicated, the patient should be hydrated.
2. Patient should void before imaging.
3. There is no need for fasting unless the CT scan portion is being done with intravenous contrast.

Technique

    Acquisition

        2D or 3D, although 3D is preferred

2 to 5 minutes per bed position

128×128 matrix

Iterative processing; reconstruction protocols used for ^{18}F-FDG PET can be used

Maximum intensity projection display

    Patient positioning

        Supine

    Photopeak selection

        511-keV

Dosimetry: rads/mCi (mGy/MBq) of administered activity (adult)

Effective dose	0.089 (0.024)
Bladder	0.81 (0.22)

Comments

    Radiation doses per unit activity from ^{18}F-fluoride scans are about four times higher than with ^{99m}Tc-MDP. When the CT dose is added, the effective dose to the patient is about seven times higher than for a ^{99m}Tc-MDP scan.

RED BLOOD CELL LABELING TECHNIQUES

1. In vitro commercial kit (UltraTag, Mallinckrodt): Results in 98% labeling. Add 1 to 3 mL of blood (heparin or anticoagulant citrate dextrose solution (ACD) as an anticoagulant) to reagent vial (stannous chloride sodium citrate and dextrose). Allow to react for 5 minutes. Add syringe 1 (sodium hypochlorite) and mix by gently inverting four to five times. Add syringe 2 (citric acid, sodium citrate, and dextrose) and mix. Add 10 to 100 mCi (370 to 700 MBq) of ^{99m}Tc-pertechnetate to vial. Mix and allow to react for 20 minutes.
2. In vivo: Add 3 mL saline to Mallinckrodt stannous pyrophosphate kit. Wait 5 minutes and inject intravenously. Wait 10 to 20 minutes and inject 20 mCi (740 MBq) ^{99m}TcO$_4^-$. Results in 60% to 80% labeling, with remaining activity in kidneys, bladder, stomach, thyroid, and salivary glands.
3. Modified in vivo: Results in about 85% to 90% labeling. Add 3 mL of normal sterile

saline to Mallinckrodt stannous pyrophosphate kit. Wait 5 minutes and then inject 1 mL intravenously. Wait 20 minutes. Using a 20-gauge needle, draw 10 mL of patient's blood into a syringe containing 20 mCi (740 MBq) of $^{99m}TcO_4^-$ and 0.5 mL of heparin. Allow this mixture to incubate for 10 minutes at room temperature before reinjecting into the patient. Patients with low hematocrit counts may need more than 10 minutes of incubation.

Reduced RBC labeling efficiency in patients on heparin, methyldopa, hydralazine, quinidine, digoxin, prazosin, propranolol, doxorubicin, and recent iodinated contrast media.

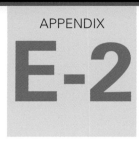

Abnormal Radiopharmaceutical Distribution as a Result of Medications and Other Extrinsic Factors

FINDINGS	CAUSE
Bone Imaging ^{99m}Tc Diphosphonates	
Renal uptake	Amphotericin B
	Aluminum antacids
	Iron preparations
	Al^{3+} ions in preparation
	Radiation therapy
	Radiographic contrast—sodium diatrizoate
	Chemotherapy agents
	Vincristine
	Doxorubicin
	Cyclophosphamide
	Gentamicin
	Dextrose
Breast uptake	Gynecomastia-producing drugs
	Digitalis
	Estrogens
	Cimetidine
	Spironolactone
	Diethylstilbestrol
Stomach uptake	Isotretinoin
Liver uptake	Aluminum antacids
	Iron preparations
	Al^{3+} ions in preparation
	Excess Sn^{2+} ions in preparation
	Radiographic contrast—sodium diatrizoate
	Alkaline pH
Spleen uptake	Phenytoin
	Aluminum preparations
Excessive blood pool activity	Iron dextran
	Aluminum preparations
	Too few Sn^{2+} ions in preparation
Myocardial activity	Doxorubicin
	Recent electrocardioversion
Excessive soft tissue uptake	Iron dextran injections (focal)
	Iodinated antiseptics
	Calcium gluconate injections
	Heparin injections (focal)
	Meperidine injections (focal)

Continued

FINDINGS	CAUSE
Muscle activity	ε-Aminocaproic acid Intramuscular injections
Decreased skeletal uptake	Corticosteroids Etidronate therapy Iron compounds Phospho-Soda Recent cold diphosphonate (hours) Vitamin D$_3$
Increased calvarial activity ("sickle sign")	Cytotoxic chemotherapy Calcium carbonate antacids

Regionally increased skeletal uptake	Regional chemoperfusion
	    Melphalan
	    Actinomycin

Labeled Leukocyte Imaging—^{111}In	
Reduced or absent abscess uptake, (false-negative results)	Antibiotics Lidocaine Procainamide Corticosteroids Hyperalimentation
Lung activity	Cell clumping as a result of excessive agitation
Colon activity	Antibiotic-induced pseudomembranous colitis
Liver and Spleen Imaging—^{99m}Tc Sulfur Colloid	
Increased bone marrow uptake	Nitrosoureas Colloid size too small
Increased spleen uptake	Nitrosoureas Halothane Methylcellulose
Decreased spleen uptake	Chemotherapy Epinephrine Antimalarials Thorium dioxide (Thorotrast)
Lung uptake	Aluminum antacids Iron preparation Virilizing androgens Mg^{2+} preparation Niacin Colloid size too large Al^{3+} in preparation Particle clumping
Focal areas of decreased liver activity	Estrogens
Hepatobiliary Imaging—^{99m}Tc IDA Derivatives	

Delayed biliary-to-bowel transit	Narcotic analgesics
	    Morphine
	    Demerol
	Phenobarbital

Decreased liver uptake and excretion	Chronic high-dose nicotinic acid therapy
Enhanced hepatobiliary excretion	Phenobarbital
Nonvisualization of the gallbladder (false-positive results)	Hepatic artery chemotherapy infusion
Prolonged gallbladder activity and decreased contractile response to stimulation	Atropine
^{18}F-FDG PET Imaging	
Decreased tumor uptake	Elevated glucose levels Elevated insulin levels

Continued

FINDINGS	CAUSE
Increased muscle uptake (generalized)	Elevated insulin levels Elevated glucose levels
Increased cardiac uptake	Elevated insulin levels Elevated glucose levels Caffeine and possibly nicotine
Decreased cardiac uptake	Fasting
Focally increased brain uptake	External stimulation (light and noise during or shortly after injection)

^{67}Ga Citrate Imaging

FINDINGS	CAUSE

Excessive bone uptake	Iron preparation
	Gadopentetate
	Chemotherapy
	    Methotrexate
	    Cisplatin
	    Vincristine
	    Mechlorethamine
	Hemodialysis

Excessive liver uptake	Iron dextran Phenobarbital
Excessive renal uptake	Doxorubicin Bleomycin Cisplatin Vinblastine Furosemide Phenytoin Allopurinol Cephalosporin Ampicillin Ibuprofen Sulfonamides Methicillin Erythromycin Rifampin Pentamidine Phenylbutazone Phenobarbital Phenazone

Stomach uptake	Chemotherapy
	    Doxorubicin
	    Bleomycin
	    Cisplatin
	    Vinblastine

Breast uptake	Estrogens
	    Diethylstilbestrol
	    Oral contraceptives
	Reserpine
	Phenothiazine
	Metoclopramide

Colon uptake pseudomembranous colitis, especially:	Antibiotic-induced Clindamycin Cephalosporins Ampicillin
Decreased abscess uptake	Prior treatment with iron dextran, deferoxamine
Prolonged whole-body clearance	Vincristine Steroid treatment Mechlorethamine
Mediastinal and hilar lymph node uptake	Phenytoin (Dilantin)

Continued

FINDINGS	CAUSE
Lung uptake	Cyclophosphamide
	Amiodarone
	Bleomycin
	Busulfan
	BCG
Thymus activity	Chemotherapy/radiation therapy
	Antibiotics

Blood Pool Imaging—^{99m}Tc-Labeled Red Blood Cells

Reduced red blood cell labeling efficiency	Heparin
	Methyldopa
	Hydralazine
	Quinidine
	Digoxin
	Prazosin
	Propranolol
	Doxorubicin
	Iodinated contrast media

Myocardial Perfusion Imaging—^{201}Tl Chloride

Increased myocardial uptake	Dipyridamole
	Furosemide
	Isoproterenol
	Sodium bicarbonate (IV)
	Dexamethasone
Decreased myocardial uptake	Propranolol
	Digitalis
	Doxorubicin
	Phenytoin (Dilantin)
	Lidocaine
	Minoxidil

Meckel Diverticulum Imaging—^{99m}Tc Pertechnetate

Increased gastric mucosa activity	Pentagastrin
	Cimetidine
Decreased gastric mucosa activity	Al^{3+} ion (antacids)
	Perchlorate

Lung Perfusion Imaging—^{99m}Tc-Labeled MAA

Focal hot spots or patchy distribution in lungs	Mg^{2+} sulfate therapy/clot formation
Increased liver uptake	Particles too small

Thyroid Uptake and Imaging Radionuclides (^{131}I, ^{123}I)

See Chapter 4, Table 4-1 and Box 4-1.

Gastric Emptying Studies—any Radiopharmaceutical

Delayed gastric emptying	Aluminum hydroxide
	Narcotics
	Propantheline
Shortened gastric emptying	Reglan

Cerebral Cisternography—^{111}In DTPA

Ventricular entry and stasis (false-positive results)	Acetazolamide (Diamox)

Nonradioactive Pharmaceuticals in Nuclear Medicine*

PHARMACEUTICAL	INDICATION	ADULT DOSE
Acetazolamide (Diamox)	Brain perfusion	1 g in 10 mL sterile water, IV over 2 min for adults (14 mg/kg for children) 10-20 min before injecting tracer
Adenosine (Adenocard)	Cardiac stress	140 mcg/kg/min for 6 min, or 50 mcg/kg/min increased to 75, 100, and 140 mcg/kg/min each min to 7 min
Bethanechol (Urecholine)	Gastric emptying	2.5-5 mg subcutaneously
Captopril (Capoten)	Renovascular hypertension evaluation	25-50 mg orally before study
Cholecystokinin (Sincalide or Kinevac)	Hepatobiliary imaging	0.02 mcg/kg in 10 mL saline IV over 3-60 min
Cimetidine (Tagamet)	Meckel diverticulum imaging	Adult 300 mg/four times daily, pediatric 20 mg/kg in 20 mL saline IV over 20 min
Dipyridamole (Persantine)	Cardiac stress	0.57 mg/kg IV over 4 min in 20-40 mL of normal saline
Dobutamine (Dobutrex)	Cardiac stress	Incremental dose rate of 15 mcg/kg/min up to 40 mcg/kg/min every 3 min
Enalaprilat (Vasotec IV)	Renovascular hypertension evaluation	0.04 mg/kg in 10 mL saline IV over 3-5 min maximum dose 2.5 mg
Furosemide (Lasix)	Renal imaging	Adult 20-40 mg, pediatric 1.0 mg/kg given IV over 1-2 min
Glucagon	Meckel diverticulum imaging	Adult 0.5 mg, pediatric 5 mcg/kg given IV or IM
Morphine (Astramorph, Duramorph)	Hepatobiliary imaging	0.04 mg/kg diluted in 10 mL saline, IV over 3-5 min (range, 2.0-4.5 mg)
Pentagastrin (Peptavlon)	Meckel diverticulum imaging	6 mcg/kg 5-15 min before study
Phenobarbital (Luminal)	Hepatobiliary imaging	5 mg/kg/day for 5 days

Adapted from Park HM, Duncan K. Nonradioactive pharmaceuticals in nuclear medicine. J Nucl Med Technol 1994; 22:240-49.

*Many of these drugs can cause hypotension, dizziness, nausea, vomiting, respiratory depression, and headache, and the patients often require careful monitoring after administration.

SUGGESTED READINGS

Saremi F, Jadvar H, Siegel ME. Pharmacologic interventions in nuclear radiology: indications, imaging protocols, and clinical results. RadioGraphics 2002;22:477.

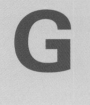

APPENDIX

G Pregnancy and Breastfeeding

PREGNANCY

Many clinicians are concerned about ordering radionuclide scans for a pregnant patient. The question most frequently arises in connection with lung and hepatobiliary scans. In general, if the scan is medically indicated and would be performed on a nonpregnant female, it is indicated during pregnancy. There are some facts to be kept in mind when considering this issue:

1. Radiation-induced fetal abnormalities have not been reported at fetal absorbed dose levels below 10 rads (0.1 Gy). The risk of spontaneous congenital abnormalities is between 3% and 6%.

2. The risk of radiation carcinogenesis may be higher for the embryo/fetus and children than for adults, but the risk is not likely to exceed 1 in 1000 per rad (10 mGy). The spontaneous cancer risk in the United States is about 1 in 3 (33%).

3. Iodine will cross the placenta. The fetal thyroid does not concentrate iodine before about 12 weeks gestational age. After this, the fetal thyroid will avidly accumulate iodine, which can be blocked by administering stable iodine (potassium iodide, 130 mg) to the mother.

4. It is unlikely that the fetal absorbed dose from xenon-133 (^{133}Xe) or a technetium-99m (^{99m}Tc) radiopharmaceutical would exceed 0.5 rad (5 mGy). See Table G-1.

5. A large portion of the fetal absorbed dose from most radiopharmaceuticals comes from the maternal bladder, so hydration and frequent voiding should be encouraged.

6. In many instances, the administered activity can be reduced by half and imaging time increased without significant degradation of the information obtained.

TABLE G-1	Estimated Absorbed Dose to Embryo/Fetus for Selected Radiopharmaceuticals	
RADIOPHARMACEUTICAL	**ABSORBED DOSE IN rad/mCi (mGy/MBq)**
^{18}F-FDG	0.600 (0.162)
^{18}F-fluoride	0.025-0.063 (0.0068-0.017)
^{67}Ga-citrate	0.250 (0.067)
^{99m}Tc-human serum albumin	0.020 (0.005)
^{99m}Tc-macroaggregated albumin	0.035 (0.009)
^{99m}Tc-diphosphonate	0.040 (0.011)
^{99m}Tc-sodium pertechnetate	0.040 (0.011)
^{99m}Tc-glucoheptonate	0.040 (0.011)
^{99m}Tc-DTPA (intravenous or aerosol)	0.035 (0.009)
^{99m}Tc-sestamibi (rest)	0.020-0.055 (0.0054-0.015)
^{99m}Tc-sulfur colloid	0.035 (0.009)

Continued

TABLE G-1	Estimated Absorbed Dose to Embryo/Fetus for Selected Radiopharmaceuticals—cont'd	
RADIOPHARMACEUTICAL	**ABSORBED DOSE IN rad/mCi (mGy/MBq)**	
^{99m}Tc-DISIDA	0.030 (0.008)	
^{99m}Tc-red blood cells*	0.060 (0.016)	
^{99m}Tc-tetrofosmin	0.013-0.036 (0.0036-0.0096)	
^{111}In leukocytes*	0.400 (0.110)	
^{123}I sodium iodide (15% uptake)	0.035 (0.009)	
^{131}I sodium iodide (15% uptake)	0.100 (0.027)	
^{201}Tl chloride*	0.300 (0.080)	
^{133}Xe†	0.001 (0.0003)	

Data adapted from Protection in Nuclear Medicine and Ultrasound Diagnostic Procedures in Children, report no. 73. Washington, DC, National Council on Radiation Protection and Measurements, 1983; Smith EM, Warner GG. Estimates of radiation dose to the embryo from nuclear medicine procedures. J Nucl Med 1976; 17:836; and Russell JR, Stabin MG, Sparks RB, et al. Health Phys 1997; 73(5):756-69.

*In instances in which no data on embryonic or fetal absorbed dose were available, either the maternal whole-body dose or the gonadal dose was used. To be conservative, the largest of these two quantities was chosen.

†Value of 0.10 before 10 weeks gestational age.

BREASTFEEDING

Federal regulations (10 CFR 35.75) require that if the dose to a breastfeeding infant or child could exceed 100 mrem (1 mSv), assuming there was no interruption of breastfeeding, the licensee must give (1) guidance on the interruption or cessation of breastfeeding, and (2) information on the consequences of failure to follow guidance. In general, diagnostic procedures involving radionuclides other than radioiodine would have no measurable consequences, and instructions would be directed at keeping doses as low as reasonably achievable. Specific requirements are shown in Table G-2. Recommendations on breastfeeding cessation differ between the U.S. Nuclear Regulatory Commission (NRC) and the International Commission for Radiological Protection (ICRP) for some radiopharmaceuticals. It should be noted that the cessation times are guidance and not regulatory requirements.

TABLE G-2	Activities of Radiopharmaceuticals That Require Instructions and Records When Administered to Patients Who Are Breastfeeding an Infant or Child		
RADIOPHARMACEUTICAL	**COLUMN 1 ACTIVITY ABOVE WHICH INSTRUCTIONS ARE REQUIRED MBq (mCi)**	**COLUMN 2 ACTIVITY ABOVE WHICH A RECORD IS REQUIRED MBq (mCi)**	**COLUMN 3 EXAMPLES OF RECOMMENDED DURATION OF INTERRUPTION OF BREASTFEEDING**
^{11}C-labeled agents			Not necessary*
^{13}N-labeled agents			Not necessary*
^{15}O-labeled agents			Not necessary*
^{18}F-FDG			Not necessary*
^{67}Ga-citrate	1 (0.04)	7 (0.2)	1 month for 150 MBq (4 mCi) 2 weeks for 50 MBq (1.3 mCi) 1 week for 7 MBq (0.2 mCi) >3 weeks*
^{51}Cr-EDTA	60 (1.6)	300 (8)	Not necessary*
^{81}Kr-gas			Not necessary*

| TABLE G-2 | Activities of Radiopharmaceuticals That Require Instructions and Records When Administered to Patients Who Are Breastfeeding an Infant or Child—cont'd |

RADIOPHARMACEUTICAL	COLUMN 1 ACTIVITY ABOVE WHICH INSTRUCTIONS ARE REQUIRED MBq (mCi)	COLUMN 2 ACTIVITY ABOVE WHICH A RECORD IS REQUIRED MBq (mCi)	COLUMN 3 EXAMPLES OF RECOMMENDED DURATION OF INTERRUPTION OF BREASTFEEDING
^{99m}Tc-DTPA	1000 (30)	6000 (150)	Not necessary*
^{99m}Tc-MAA	50 (1.3)	200 (6.5)	12 hr for 150 MBq (4 mCi)
^{99m}Tc-pertechnetate	100 (3)	600 (15)	24 hr for 1100 MBq (30 mCi) 12 hr for 440 MBq (12 mCi)
^{99m}Tc-DISIDA	1000 (30)	6000 (150)	Not necessary
^{99m}Tc-glucoheptonate	1000 (30)	6000 (170)	Not necessary
^{99m}Tc-HMPAO			Not necessary*
^{99m}Tc-MIBI	1000 (30)	6000 (150)	Not necessary
^{99m}Tc-MDP	1000 (30)	6000 (150)	Not necessary
^{99m}Tc-red blood cell in vivo labeling	400 (10)	2000 (50)	6 hr for 740 MBq (20 mCi) 12 hr*
^{99m}Tc-red blood cell in vitro labeling	1000 (30)	6000 (150)	Not necessary
^{99m}Tc-sulfur colloid	300 (7)	1000 (35)	6 hr for 440 MBq (12 mCi) Not necessary*
^{99m}Tc-DTPA aerosol	1000 (30)	6000 (150)	Not necessary*
^{99m}Tc-MAG3	1000 (30)	6000 (150)	Not necessary*
^{99m}Tc-white blood cells	100 (4)	600 (15)	24 hr for 1100 MBq (5 mCi) 12 hr for 440 MBq (2 mCi)
^{111}In-white blood cells	10 (0.2)	40 (1)	1 week for 20 MBq (0.5 mCi) Not necessary*
^{111}In-octreotide			Not necessary*
^{131}I-NaI	0.01 (0.0004)	0.07 (0.002)	Complete cessation (for this infant or child)
^{123}I-NaI	20 (0.5)	100 (3)	Not necessary 3 weeks* (as a result of possible ^{131}I contamination)
^{123}I-MIBG	70 (2)	400 (10)	24 hr for 370 MBq (10 mCi) 12 hr for 150 MBq (4 mCi) >3 weeks* (as a result of possible ^{131}I contamination)
^{133}Xe-gas			Not necessary*
^{201}Tl-chloride	40 (1)	200 (5)	2 weeks for 110 MBq (3 mCi) 48 hr*

The duration of interruption of breastfeeding is selected to reduce the maximum dose to a newborn infant to less than 1 mSv (0.1 rem), although the regulatory limit is 5 mSv (0.5 rem). The actual doses that would be received by most infants would be far below 1 mSv (0.1 rem). Of course, the physician may use discretion in the recommendation, increasing or decreasing the duration of interruption.

Notes: Activities are rounded to one significant figure, except when it was considered appropriate to use two significant figures. Details of the calculations are shown in NUREG-1492, Regulatory Analysis on Criteria for the Release of Patients Administered Radioactive Material.

If there is not necessary recommendation in Column 3 of this table, the maximum activity normally administered is below the activities that require instructions on interruption or discontinuation of breastfeeding.

Agreement state regulations may vary. Agreement state licensees should check with their state regulations prior to using these values.

*International Commission on Radiological Protection, Radiation Dose to Patients from Radiopharmaceuticals. Annex D. Recommendations on breastfeeding interruptions. ICRP Publication 106, Annals of the ICRP 38(1-2):163-165, 2008.

H-1

General Considerations for Hospitalized Patients Receiving Radionuclide Therapy

1. It is important for the patient to understand the nature of the radionuclide treatment. Patient cooperation is important in minimizing unnecessary incidents and exposure.

2. Before administration of the radionuclide, the procedures and special precautions should be reviewed with the nursing staff. The nursing staff must have specific written instructions for each procedure and should review them before the patient arrives in the room.

3. Immediately after the return of the treated patient to the hospital room from the nuclear medicine department, a radiation safety officer (RSO) should survey the patient and surrounding areas to determine distance and time restrictions for hospital personnel and visitors in the patient's room. These distances and times are recorded on a form in the patient's chart and listed on the caution sign on the patient's door. These signs and labels should remain posted until removal is ordered by the RSO.

4. Hospital personnel and allowed visitors should position themselves as far from the patient as is reasonable except for necessary bedside care. A distance of 2 m is normally acceptable. In some cases, the RSO may determine that mobile lead shields are needed to reduce exposure to others in adjacent areas. Specific restrictions are noted by the RSO on the room door and in the hospital chart.

5. It is not advisable for pregnant women or children younger than 18 years to enter the hospital room.

6. Dosimeters are required for all hospital personnel who are likely to receive in excess of 25% of the dose-equivalent limit for radiation workers. The RSO identifies hospital personnel within this category and issues the appropriate dosimeters to them.

7. Pregnant personnel should not routinely be assigned to the care of patients under treatment with radioactive materials.

8. Patients receiving radionuclide therapy should be assigned a private room and restricted to the room unless an exception is authorized by the RSO.

9. Limits for release of radionuclide therapy patients from hospitals are given in the U.S. Nuclear Regulatory Commission regulatory guide 8-39, published in April 1997. Patient release criteria have been outlined in Chapter 13. Patients may be released on the basis of administered activity or dose rate. The specifics for common radionuclides are shown in Table H-1A. There are patients who may be released but who have a level of activity that requires them to be supplied with written instructions on how to maintain doses to other individuals as low as reasonably achievable. These activities and dose rates are shown in Table H-1B. Patients may also be released if the calculated maximum likely effective dose to another individual (family and caregivers) is no greater than 0.5 rem (5 mSv). This method requires use of a formula. The recordkeeping requirements are shown in Table H-1C.

TABLE H–1A	Activities and Dose Rates for Authorizing Patient Release*	
	COLUMN 1	**COLUMN 2**
RADIONUCLIDE	**ACTIVITY AT OR BELOW WHICH PATIENTS MAY BE RELEASED GBq (mCi)**	**DOSE RATE AT 1 M AT OR BELOW WHICH PATIENTS MAY BE RELEASED mSv/hr (mrem/hr)†**
^{198}Au	3.5 (93)	0.21 (21)
^{51}Cr	4.8 (130)	0.02 (2)
^{67}Ga	8.7 (240)	0.18 (18)
^{123}I	6.0 (160)	0.26 (26)
^{125}I	0.25 (7)	0.01 (1)
^{131}I	1.2 (33)	0.07 (7)
^{111}In	2.4 (64)	0.2 (20)
^{32}P	—‡	—‡
^{186}Re	28 (770)	0.15 (15)
^{188}Re	29 (790)	0.20 (20)
^{47}Sc	11 (310)	0.17 (17)
^{153}Sm	26 (700)	0.3 (30)
^{117m}Sn	1.1 (29)	0.04 (4)
^{89}Sr	—‡	—‡
^{99m}Tc	28 (760)	0.58 (58)
^{201}Tl	16 (430)	0.19 (19)
^{90}Y	—‡	—‡
^{169}Yb	0.37 (10)	0.02 (2)

The gigabecquerel values were calculated based on the millicurie values and the conversion factor from millicuries to gigabecquerels. The dose rate values were calculated based on the millicurie values and the exposure rate constants.

In general, the values are rounded to two significant figures. However, values less than 0.35 GBq (10 mCi) or 0.1 mSv (10 mrem) per hour are rounded to one significant figure. Details of the calculations are provided in NUREG-1492.

Agreement state regulations may vary. Agreement state licensees should check with their state regulations prior to using these values.

*The activity values were computed based on 5 mSv (0.5 rem) total effective dose equivalent.

†If the release is based on the dose rate at 1 m in Column 2, the licensee must maintain a record as required by 10 CFR 35.75(c) because the measurement includes shielding by tissue. See Regulatory Position 3.1, Records of Release, for information on records.

‡Activity and dose rate limits are not applicable in this case because of the minimal exposures to members of the public resulting from activities normally administered for diagnostic or therapeutic purposes.

TABLE H–1B	Activities and Dose Rates Above Which Instructions Should Be Given When Authorizing Patient Release*	

	COLUMN 1	COLUMN 2
RADIONUCLIDE	**ACTIVITY ABOVE WHICH INSTRUCTIONS ARE REQUIRED GBq (mCi)**	**DOSE RATE AT 1 M ABOVE WHICH INSTRUCTIONS ARE REQUIRED mSv/hr (mrem/hr)**
^{198}Au	0.69 (19)	0.04 (4)
^{51}Cr	0.96 (26)	0.004 (0.4)
^{67}Ga	1.7 (47)	0.04 (4)
^{123}I	1.2 (33)	0.05 (5)
^{125}I	0.05 (1)	0.002 (0.2)
^{131}I	0.24 (7)	0.02 (2)
^{111}In	0.47 (13)	0.04 (4)
^{32}P	—†	—†
^{186}Re	5.7 (150)	0.03 (3)
^{188}Re	5.8 (160)	0.04 (4)
^{47}Sc	2.3 (62)	0.03 (3)
^{153}Sm	5.2 (140)	0.06 (6)
^{117m}Sn	0.21 (6)	0.009 (0.9)
^{89}Sr	—†	—†
^{99m}Tc	5.6 (150)	0.12 (12)
^{201}Tl	3.1 (85)	0.04 (4)
^{90}Y	—†	—†
^{169}Yb	0.073 (2)	0.004 0.4

The gigabecquerel values were calculated based on the millicurie values and the conversion factor from millicuries to gigabecquerels. The dose rate values were calculated based on the millicurie values and the exposure rate constants.

In general, the values are rounded to two significant figures. However, values less than 0.37 GBq (10 mCi) or 0.1 mSv (10 mrem) per hour are rounded to one significant figure. Details of the calculations are provided in NUREG-1492.

Agreement state regulations may vary. Agreement state licensees should check with their state regulations prior to using these values. Abbreviations are the same as in Table H-1A.

*The activity values were computed based on 1 mSv (0.1 rem) total effective dose equivalent.

†Activity and dose rate limits are not applicable in this case because of the minimal exposures to members of the public resulting from activities normally administered for diagnostic or therapeutic purposes.

TABLE H-1C Summary of Release Criteria, Required Instructions to Patients, and Records To Be Maintained

PATIENT GROUP	BASIS FOR RELEASE	CRITERIA FOR RELEASE	INSTRUCTIONS NEEDED	RELEASE RECORD REQUIRED
All patients, including patients who are breastfeeding an infant or child	Administered activity	Administered activity ≤ Column 1 of Table H-1A	Yes—if administered activity > Column 1 of Table H-1B	No
	Retained activity	Retained activity ≤ Column 1 of Table H-1A	Yes—if retained activity > Column 1 of Table H-1B	Yes
	Measured dose rate	Measured dose rate ≤ Column 2 of Table H-1A	Yes—if dose > Column 2 of Table H-1B	Yes
	Patient-specific calculations	Calculated effective dose to other individuals ≤5 mSv (0.5 rem)	Yes—if calculated effective dose to other individuals >1 mSv (0.1 rem)	Yes
Patients who are breastfeeding an infant or child	All of the above bases for release		Additional instructions required if administered activity > Column 1 of Table G-2, or licensee calculated dose from breastfeeding >1 mSv (0.1 rem) to the infant or child	Records that instructions were provided are required if administered activity > Column 2 of Table G-2, or licensee calculated dose from breastfeeding >5 mSv (0.5 rem) to the infant or child

APPENDIX

H-2

Special Considerations and Requirements for Iodine-131 Therapy

The following are useful for hospitalized patients, and they can be adapted for home use if patients with more than 33 mCi (1.2 GBq) of iodine-131 (^{131}I) are released. See also information in chapters 4 and 13.

1. All patients in this category shall be in a private room with a toilet.

2. The door must be posted with a radioactive materials sign, and a note must be posted on the door or in the patient's chart explaining where and how long visitors may stay in the patient's room.

3. Visits by people younger than 18 years of age should be authorized only on a patient-by-patient basis with approval of the authorized user and after consultation with the radiation safety officer (RSO).

4. A survey of the patient's room and surrounding areas should be conducted as soon as practicable after administration of treatment dose. The results of daily surveys can be used to recalculate permitted staying times of various visitors. Film or thermoluminescent dosimeter badges should be worn by the nurses attending the patient.

5. Patients containing ^{131}I shall be confined to their rooms except for special medical or nursing purposes approved by the nuclear medicine or radiation therapy departments and the RSO. The patient should remain in bed during visits.

6. If possible, there should be no pregnant visitors or nurses attending the patient.

7. Staff should wear disposable gloves, discard them in a designated waste container located just inside the room, and wash their hands after leaving the room.

8. Disposable plates and cups and other disposable items should be used, and after use they should be discarded in a specifically designated container.

9. All items such as clothing, bed linens, and surgical dressings may be either surveyed before removal from the room or placed in a designated container and held for decay.

10. Urine, feces, and vomitus from ^{131}I therapy patients may be disposed of by way of the sewer or stored for decay in the radioactive waste storage area. The method of disposal should be determined by the RSO.

11. If the urine from ^{131}I patients is to be collected (not a Nuclear Regulatory Commission requirement), special containers should be provided by the RSO. The patient should be encouraged to collect his or her urine in the container. If the patient is bedridden, the urinal or bedpan should be flushed several times with hot soapy water after each use.

12. The same toilet should be used by the patient at all times and should be flushed several times after each use.

13. Precautions should be taken to ensure that no urine or vomitus is spilled on the floor or bed. If any part of the patient's room is suspected of being contaminated, the RSO should be notified.

14. If a therapy patient needs emergency surgery or dies, the RSO and the nuclear medicine or radiation therapy departments should be notified immediately.

15. After the patient is released from the room, the room should be surveyed and may not be reassigned until removable contamination is less than 2000 disintegrations/minute/100 cm^2. Final survey of the room should include areas likely to have been contaminated, such as the toilet area and items likely to have been touched by the patient, such as the telephone and doorknobs.

16. The thyroid burden of each person who helped prepare or administer a liquid dosage of ^{131}I should be measured within 3 days after administration of the doses. The records should include each thyroid burden measurement, the date of measurement, the name of the person measured, and the initials of the person who made the measurements. These records must be maintained indefinitely.
17. If the patient is released and not hospitalized, staying in a hotel (rather than home) should be strongly discouraged.

NURSING INSTRUCTIONS

1. Only the amount of time required for ordinary nursing care should be spent near the patient.
2. Visitors should be limited to those 18 years of age or older, unless specified.
3. The patient should remain in bed. All visitors should remain at least 2 meters from the patient.
4. The patient should be confined to the room, except by special approval of the RSO.
5. No pregnant nurse, visitor, or attendant should be permitted in the room, if possible. Attending personnel should wear disposable gloves.
6. If a spill of urine or radioactive material is encountered, the RSO should be notified.

Emergency Procedures for Spills of Radioactive Materials

Accidental spillage of radioactive material is rare; however, spills may occur in the laboratory, in public areas such as the hall, in the freight elevator, or in any hospital room or ward through contamination by a patient's body fluids. Spill procedures should be posted in the restricted areas where radioactive materials are used or stored and should specifically state the names and telephone numbers of persons to be notified (e.g., radiation safety officer [RSO]). They should also include instructions about area evacuation, spill containment, decontamination, and reentry.

Major radiation accidents or serious spills of radioactive contamination have rarely involved medical or allied health personnel. Usually spills in hospitals involve only small amounts of radioactivity (Table I-1), in which the main concern is the spread of the contamination (e.g., from shoes or contaminated clothing into public areas). The following is a general outline of the procedure to be followed in the event of a radioactive spill. The reader is also referred to NRC NUREG 1556 Volume 9 Appendix N.

MINOR SPILLS*

1. Notify persons in the area that a spill has occurred.
2. Prevent the spread of contamination by covering the spill with absorbent paper.
3. Wear gloves and protective clothing such as a lab coat and booties, and clean up the spill using absorbent paper. Carefully fold the absorbent paper with clean side out and place in a "caution radioactive material" labeled plastic bag for transfer to a radioactive waste container. Also put contaminated gloves and any other contaminated disposable material in the bag.

4. Survey the area with a low-range radiation detection survey instrument sufficiently sensitive to detect the radionuclide. Check for removable contamination to ensure contamination levels are below trigger levels. Check the area around the spill as well as hands, clothing, and shoes for contamination.
5. Report the incident to the RSO.

MAJOR SPILLS

1. Clear the area. Notify all persons not involved in the spill to vacate the room.
2. Prevent the spread of contamination by covering the spill with "caution radioactive material" -labeled absorbent paper, but do not attempt to clean it up. To prevent the spread of contamination, clearly indicate the boundaries of the spill, and limit the movement of all personnel who may be contaminated.
3. Shield the source, if possible. Do this only if it can be done without further contamination or a significant increase in radiation exposure.
4. Close the room and lock the door, or secure the area to prevent entry.
5. Notify the RSO immediately.
6. Decontaminate the personnel by removing contaminated clothing and flushing contaminated skin with lukewarm water, then washing it with mild soap. If contamination remains, the RSO may consider inducing perspiration. Then wash the affected area again to remove any contamination that was released.

For short-lived radionuclides, decay may be used rather than decontamination. A report to the NRC may be required.

---

*The differentiation of major and minor and which procedure to implement is incident-specific and dependent on a number of variables (e.g., number of individuals involved or other hazards present).

TABLE I–1	General Guidance on the Amount of Radioactivity that Differentiates Minor from Major Spills		
RADIONUCLIDE	**MILLICURIES (MBq)**	**RADIONUCLIDE**	**MILLICURIES (MBq)**
Phosphorus-32	1 (37)	Technetium-99m	100 (3700)
Chromium-51	100 (3700)	Indium-111	10 (370)
Cobalt-57	10 (370)	Iodine-123	10 (370)
Cobalt-58	10 (370)	Iodine-125	1 (37)
Iron-59	1 (37)	Iodine-131	1 (37)
Cobalt-60	1 (37)	Samarium-153	10 (370)
Gallium-67	10 (370)	Ytterbium-169	10 (370)
Selenium-75	1 (37)	Mercury-197	10 (370)
Strontium-85	10 (370)	Gold-198	10 (370)
Strontium-89	1 (37)	Thallium-201	100 (3700)

SURFACE CONTAMINATION LIMITS

Recommended limits for surface contamination in restricted areas are 2000 dpm/100 cm^2 for iodine and indium and 20,000 dpm/100 cm^2 for gallium-67, technetium-99m, and thallium-201. Limits for unrestricted areas are an average of 1000 dpm (16.7 Bq)/100 cm^2 for iodine and 5000 dpm (83.3 Bq)/100 cm^2 for gallium-67, technetium-99m, and thallium-201. With regard to removable contamination in unrestricted areas, the limits are 100 dpm (1.67 Bq) and 200 dpm (3.3 Bq)/100 cm^2, respectively.

EMERGENCY SURGERY OF PATIENTS WHO HAVE RECEIVED THERAPEUTIC AMOUNTS OF RADIONUCLIDES

The following procedure may be used:
1. If surgery is performed within the first 24 hours following the administration of iodine-131, fluids (e.g., blood, urine) will be carefully removed and contained in a closed system.
2. Protective eyewear will be worn.
3. The radiation safety staff will direct personnel in methods to keep doses as low as reasonably achievable in a practical fashion.

4. If an injury (such as a cut) or a tear in a glove occurs, the individual will be monitored to see whether contamination occurred and whether any action is necessary.

EMERGENCY AUTOPSY OF PATIENTS WHO HAVE RECEIVED THERAPEUTIC AMOUNTS OF RADIONUCLIDES

The following procedure may be used:
1. Immediately notify the authorized user in charge of the patient and the RSO upon death of a therapy patient.
2. An autopsy will be performed only after consultation and permission from the RSO.
3. Protective eyewear will be worn. Consider the need for protection against exposure from high-energy beta rays in cases involving therapy with phosphorus-32 and yttrium-90.
4. Remove tissues containing large activities early to help reduce exposure. Shield and dispose of tissues in accordance with license conditions.
5. If an injury (such as a cut) or a tear in a glove occurs, the individual will be monitored to see whether contamination occurred and whether any action is necessary.

Index